Laparoscopic and Robot-Assisted Surgery in Urology

Jens-Uwe Stolzenburg · Ingolf A. Türk
Evangelos N. Liatsikos *(Editors)*

Laparoscopic and Robot-Assisted Surgery in Urology

Atlas of Standard Procedures

Springer

Prof. Dr. Jens-Uwe Stolzenburg
Prof. Dr., FRCS (Ed), FRCS (Eng)
Professor and Chairman
Department of Urology
Head of International Training Centre
of Urologic Laparoscopy
University of Leipzig
Liebigstraße 20, 04103 Leipzig, Germany

Prof. Evangelos N. Liatsikos
Ass. Professor of Urology
Department of Urology
University of Patras, School of Medicine
26500 RIO, Patras, Greece

Prof. Ingolf A. Türk
Professor and Chairman
Department of Urology
Director Robot Assisted Surgery Program
St. Elizabeth's Medical Center
Professor of Urology
Tufts University, School of Medicine
11 Nevins Street, Suite 501
Boston, MA 02135, USA

ISBN 978-3-642-00890-0 e-ISBN 978-3-642-00891-7
DOI 10.1007/978-3-642-00891-7
Springer Heidelberg Dordrecht London New York

Library of Congress Control Number: 2011927116

Cover design: eStudioCalamar, Figueres/Berlin
Projektmanagement, typesetting and reproduction of the figures:
Fotosatz-Service Köhler GmbH – Reinhold Schöberl, Würzburg

Printed on acid-free paper

Springer is part of Springer Science+Business Media (www.springer.com)

Preface

Laparoscopic urologic surgery has been well established in the management of urologic patients for more than two decades. The majority of oncological and reconstructive urologic surgery can be performed by a laparoscopic approach providing significant advantages for the patient. Technical issues and the requirement of a high level of laparoscopic skill have limited the wide acceptance of the laparoscopic approach. Thus, several laparoscopic procedures are performed only by specialised surgeons in laparoscopy centres. Since these institutions have accumulated vast experience in the field of laparoscopic surgery in the course of time, the task of training the next generation of laparoscopic urologic surgeons as well as the wide distribution of the laparoscopic surgical craft is their responsibility. Single-port surgery has also evolved significantly in recent years and generated great enthusiasm among experienced laparoscopists.

In addition, the robot-assisted approach for laparoscopic surgery has been introduced during the last decade, a further step in the evolution of laparoscopic surgery. Robot-assisted surgery has been rapidly adopted by several institutions. The high cost of the system has been balanced by the superior intraoperative conditions for the surgeon and its promising operative outcome.

The lack of an atlas describing both pure laparoscopic and robot-assisted urological surgery led us to introduce this atlas of laparoscopic and robotic urology, describing step by step all the urologic procedures performed using these methods. Several hundred figures obtained during the surgical experience of experts in the field of laparoscopic and robotic surgery have been included in an attempt to demonstrate the anatomical and technical issues of each procedure.

Every procedure is described in a concise manner, allowing surgeons in training to gain perspective on laparoscopic and robotic surgery step by step. Basic issues such as patient position and trocar placement for each procedure are presented in detail, including 3D drawings, in an attempt to help the laparoscopic surgeons in their initial experience in the aforementioned fields. Moreover, experienced laparoscopic/robotic surgeons could enrich their technical armamentarium with the numerous tips and tricks outlined by the contributing surgeons. The aim of the editors was to provide an atlas that could accompany a surgeon for many years to come. We hope that this publication achieves this purpose. Enjoy reading the book!

We would like to thank Jens Mondry (Director, Moonsoft, Germany) for his outstanding contribution of computer imaging and design creations. Furthermore, the authors gratefully acknowledge the assistance of Phuc Ho Thi in preparing the endoscopic figures in all chapters. Finally, we would like to express our gratitude to all contributing authors for their significant scientific input.

Leipzig, January 2011

Jens-Uwe Stolzenburg
Ingolf Türk
Evangelos Liatsikos

Contents

Contributors

Abulsorour, Sherif, Dr. Department of Urology, Klinikum Dortmund GmbH, Münsterstr. 240, D-44145 Dortmund

Anderson, Christopher, MBChB, FCS(SA), FRCS (Urol) Department Urology, St George's hospital, Blackshaw Rd, Tooting, London SW170QT, United Kingdom, cja@blueyonder.co.uk

Astigueta, JuanCarlos, MD Instituto Medico la Floresta, Centro de Cirugia Robotica y de invasion minima, Caracas, Venezuela

Bachmann, Alexander, Prof., Dr. Department of Urology, University Hospital Basel, Spitalstrasse 21, 4031 Basel, Switzerland, bachmanna@uhbs.ch

Backhaus, Miguel, Dr. Servicio de Urología., Fundación IVO., C/Beltrán Báguena, 8 46009, Valencia, Spain

Beerlage, Harry P., MD, Dr. Urologist, Jeroen Bosch Hospital, Department of Urology, PO Box 90153, 5200 ME's-Hertogenbosch, The Netherlands, hpbeerlage@hotmail.com

Brandina, Ricardo, MD Department of Urology, Keck school of Medicine, University of Southern California, 1441 Eastlake Ave, Suite 7416; Los Angeles, CA 90033, USA

Breda, Alberto, MD Department of Urology, Autonoma University, Fundació Puigvert, Barcelona, Spain, albbred@hotmail.com

Buendia, Camilo Mejia, MD Instituto Medico la Floresta, Centro de Cirugia Robotica y de invasion minima, Caracas, Venezuela

Casey, Rowan, MD FRCSI (Urol), Department of Urology, University of Leipzig, Liebigstraße 20, 04103 Leipzig, Germany, rowcasey@rcsi.ie

Cortés, Roberto Garza, MD Instituto Medico la Floresta, Centro de Cirugia Robotica y de invasion minima, Caracas, Venezuela

Dalpiaz, Orietta, Dr. Department of Urology, Klinikum Dortmund, Münsterstr. 240, 44145 Dortmund, Germany

Deger, Serdar, Prof., Dr. Paracelsus Krankenhaus Ruit, Hedelfingerstraße 166, 73760 Ostfildern, Germany, s.deger@kk-es.de

Denaeyer, Geert, MD Department of Urology O.L.Vrouw Clinic, Moorselbaan 164, 9300 Aalst, Belgium

Desai, Mihir, Prof., MD Department of Urology, Keck school of Medicine, University of Southern California, 1441 Eastlake Ave, Suite 7416; Los Angeles, CA 90033, USA, adityadesai2003@gmail.com

Dietel, Anja, Dr.med. Department of Urology, University of Leipzig, Liebigstraße 20, 04103 Leipzig, Germany, Anja.Dietel@medizin.uni-leipzig.de

Do, Hoang Minh, Dr. Dept. of Urology, University of Leipzig, Liebigstraße 20, 04103 Leipzig, Germany, HoangDo.Minh@medizin.uni-leipzig.de

Dunn, Ian, MBChB, FRCS (Urol) Departement of Urology, Monklands Hospital, NHS Lanarkshire, Scotland

Ficarra, Vincenzo, MD Department of Urology O.L.Vrouw Clinic, Moorselbaan 164, 9300 Aalst, Belgium

Ganzer, Roman, Dr. Department of Urology, University of Regensburg, Krankenhaus St. Josef, 93053 Regensburg, Germany, roman.ganzer@gmx.de

Giedelman, Camilo, MD Instituto Medico la Floresta, Centro de Cirugia Robotica y de invasion minima, Caracas, Venezuela

Gill, Inderbir S. Department of Urology, Keck school of Medicine, University of Southern California, 1441 Eastlake Ave, Suite 7416, Los Angeles, CA 90033, USA

Gonsior, Andreas, Dr. Department of Urology, Head of International Training Centre of Urologic Laparoscopy, University of Leipzig, Liebigstraße 20, 04103 Leipzig

Gözen/Gozen, Ali Serdar, Dr. Department of Urology, SLK Kliniken Heilbronn, Am Gesundbrunnen 20, 74078 Heilbronn, Germany

Guballa, Christoph, Dr. Department of Urology, Klinikum Dortmund, Münsterstr. 240, 44145 Dortmund, Germany

Guillonneau, Bertrand, Prof., MD Memorial Sloan Kettering Cancer Center, New York, NY, USA, guillonb@mskcc.org

Gürkan, Leven, Dr. Department of Urology, SLK Kliniken Heilbronn, Am Gesundbrunnen 20, 74078 Heilbronn, Germany

Häfner, Tim, Dr. Department of Urology, Head of International Training Centre of Urologic Laparoscopy, University of Leipzig, Liebigstraße 20, 04103 Leipzig

Ho Thi, Phuc, Dr. Department of Urology, Head of International Training Centre of Urologic Laparoscopy, University of Leipzig, Liebigstraße 20, 04103 Leipzig

Hosseini, Abolfazl, MD Dept of Urology, Karolinska University Hospital, 17176 Stockholm, Sweden

Hruza, Marcel, Dr. Department of Urology, SLK Kliniken Heilbronn, Am Gesundbrunnen 20, 74078 Heilbronn, Germany

Janetschek, Günter, Prof., Dr. Medical University Salzburg, Dept. of Urology, Müllner Hauptstr. 48,5020 Salzburg, Austria, g.janetschek@salk.at

Jonsson, Martin N, MD Dept of Urology, Karolinska University Hospital, 17176 Stockholm, Sweden

Kallidonis, Panagiotis, Dr. Department of Urology, University of Patras, School of Medicine, 26500 RIO, Patras, Greece

Kamradt, Jörn, Dr. University Clinics of Saarland, Department of Urology, Kirrbergerstr., 66421 Homburg/Saar, Germany

Klein, Jan Thorsten, Dr. Department of Urology, SLK Kliniken Heilbronn, Am Gesundbrunnen 20, 74078 Heilbronn, Germany

Kreutzer, Niklas, Dr. Department of Urology, Klinikum Dortmund GmbH, Münsterstr. 240, 44145 Dortmund, Germany, niklas.kreutzer@klinikumdo.de

Liatsikos, Evangelos N., Ass. Prof., MD, PhD Department of Urology, University of Patras, School of Medicine, 26500 RIO, Patras, Greece, Liatsikos@yahoo.com

Mc Neill, Alan, MBChB, FRCS (Urol) Western General Hospital, Crewe Road Edinburgh, EH4 2XU, Scotland, Alan.McNeill@luht.scot.nhs.uk

Mills, Robert, FRCS (Urol) The Norfolk and Norwich University Hospital, Colney Lane, Norwich, NR4 7UY, United Kingdom

Mondry, Jens Director Moonsoft, Otto-Schott-Str. 2, 07745 Jena, Germany

Morillo, Eudo Herrera, MD Instituto Medico la Floresta, Centro de Cirugia Robotica y de invasion minima, Caracas, Venezuela

Mottrie, Alexandre, Dr., MD Department of Urology O.L.Vrouw Clinic, Moorselbaan 164, 9300 Aalst, Belgium, a.mottrie@telenet.be

Neuhaus, Jochen, Dr. rer. nat. Department of Urology, Head of International Training Centre of Urologic Laparoscopy, University of Leipzig, Liebigstraße 20, 04103 Leipzig, Germany

Orth, Stefan, Dr. Department of Urology, Klinikum Dortmund, Münsterstr. 240, 44145 Dortmund, Germany, stefan.orth@klinikumdo.de

Pini, Giovannalberto, Dr. Department of Urology, SLK Kliniken Heilbronn, Am Gesundbrunnen 20, 74078 Heilbronn, Germany

Rassweiler, Jens, Prof., Dr. Department of Urology, SLK Kliniken Heilbronn, Am Gesundbrunnen 20, 74078 Heilbronn, Germany, jens.rassweiler@slk-kliniken.de

Rayala, Heidi, MD Memorial Sloan Kettering Cancer Center, New York, USA

Rehman, Jamil, MD Department of Urology O.L.Vrouw Clinic, Moorselbaan 164, 9300 Aalst, Belgium

Riddek/Riddick, Tony, MBChB, FRCS (Urol) Western General Hospital, Crewe Road Edinburgh, EH4 2XU, Scotland

Sangalli, Mattia, MD Department of Urology O.L.Vrouw Clinic, Moorselbaan 164, 9300 Aalst, Belgium

Schulze, Michael, Dr. Department of Urology, SLK Kliniken Heilbronn, Am Gesundbrunnen 20, 74078 Heilbronn, Germany

Schumacher, Martin C., MD Dept of Urology, Karolinska University Hospital, 17176 Stockholm, Sweden

Schwalenberg, Thilo, Dr. University of Leipzig, Dept. of Urology Liebigstraße 20, 04103 Leipzig, Germany, Thilo.Schwalenberg@medizin.uni-leipzig.de

Siemer, Stefan, Prof., Dr. University Clinics of Saarland, Department of Urology, Kirrbergerstr., 66421 Homburg/Saar, Germany, stefan.siemer@uniklinikum-saarland.de

Sotelo, René, Dr., MD Instituto Medico la Floresta, Centro de Cirugia Robotica y de invasion minima, Caracas, Venezuela, renesotelo@cantv.net

Stöckle, Michael, Prof. Dr. Chairman Department of Urology, University Clinics of Saarland, Kirrbergerstr., D-66421 Homburg/Saar, Germany

Stolzenburg, Jens-Uwe, Prof. Dr., FRCS (Ed), FRCS (Eng) Professor and Chairman, Department of Urology, Head of International Training Centre of Urologic Laparoscopy, University of Leipzig, Liebigstraße 20, 04103 Leipzig, Germany, Jens-Uwe.Stolzenburg@medizin.uni-leipzig.de

Suardi, Nazareno, MD Department of Urology O.L.Vrouw Clinic, Moorselbaan 164, 9300 Aalst, Belgium

Subotic, Svetozar, Dr. Department of Urology, University Hospital Basel, Spitalstrasse 21, 4031 Basel, Switzerland

Teber, Dogu, Dr. Department of Urology, SLK Kliniken Heilbronn, Am Gesundbrunnen 20, 74078 Heilbronn, Germany

Tenke, Peter, Prof. Dr. The Hopsital adress, Jahn ferenc South-Pest Teaching Hospital, 1204 Budapest Köves. s. 1, Hungaria, tenke.peter@jahndelpest.hu

Thomas, Ben G., MBChB, FRCS (Urol) Western General Hospital, Crewe Road Edinburgh, EH4 2XU, Scotland

Till, Holger, Prof., Dr. Professor and Chairman, Department of Paediatric Surgery, University of Leipzig, Liebigstraße 22, 04103 Leipzig, Holger.Till@medizin.uni-leipzig.de

Truß, Michael C., Prof. Dr. Chairman Department of Urology, Klinikum Dortmund, Münsterstr. 240, 44145 Dortmund, Germany

Türk, Ingolf A., Prof., MD Professor and chairman of department of Urology, Director Robot Assisted Surgery Program, St. Elizabeth's Medical Center, Professor of Urology, Tufts University, School of Medicine, 11 Nevins Street, Suite 501, Boston, MA 02135

Turner, Kevin, MA DM FRCS (Urol) Department of Urology, Royal Bournemouth Hospital, BH7 7DW, Bournemouth, United Kingdom, Kevin.Turner@rbch.nhs.uk

Waldschmidt, Ulrike, Dr. Department of Paediatric Surgery, University of Leipzig, Liebigstraße 22, 04103 Leipzig, Germany

Wiklund, N. Peter, Prof., MD Dept of Urology, Karolinska University Hospital, SE-171 76 Stockholm, Sweden, Peter.Wiklund@karolinska.se

Winkler, Mathias, MD, FRCS (Urol) Imperial College NHS Trust, Charing Cross Hospital, Fulham Palace Road, London W6 8RF, United Kingdom

Wissing, Florian, Dr. Department of Urology, Klinikum Dortmund, Münsterstr. 240, 44145 Dortmund, Germany

Wyler, Stephen, Dr. Department of Urology, University Hospital Basel, Spitalstrasse 21, 4031 Basel, Switzerland

Zehnder, Pascal, MD Department of Urology, Keck school of Medicine, University of Southern California, 1441 Eastlake Ave, Suite 7416; Los Angeles, CA 90033, USA

Zimmermann, R., Dr. Medical University Salzburg, Dept. of Urology, Müllner Hauptstr. 48 5020 Salzburg, Austria

Chapter 1

Upper Urinary Tract (Kidney, Ureter and Adrenal Gland)

CONTENTS

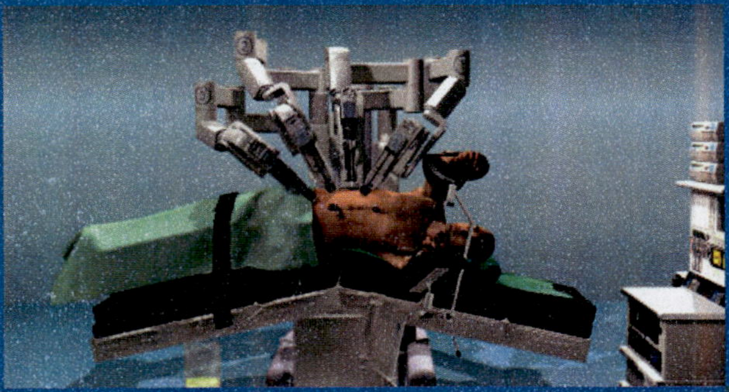

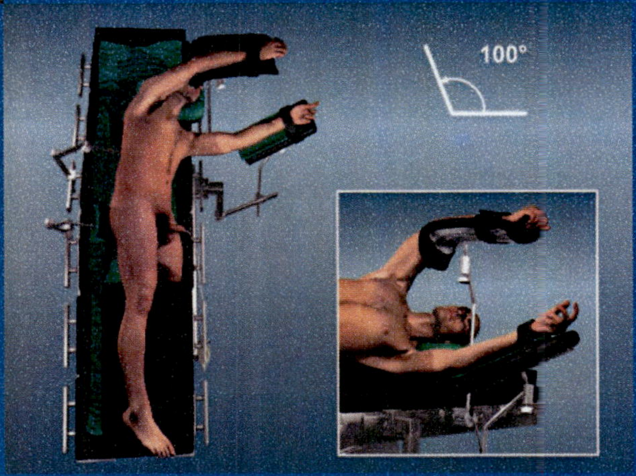

J.-U. Stolzenburg, I. Türk, E. Liatsikos: *Laparoscopic and Robot-Assisted Surgery in Urology*
DOI: 10.1007/978-3-642-00891-7_1, © Springer-Verlag Berlin Heidelberg 2011

1.1 Patient Position for Kidney Surgery

Jens-Uwe Stolzenburg, Rowan Casey, Jens Mondry, Minh Do, Anja Dietel,
Tim Haefner, Thilo Schwalenberg, Evangelos Liatsikos

Step 1: Lateral position

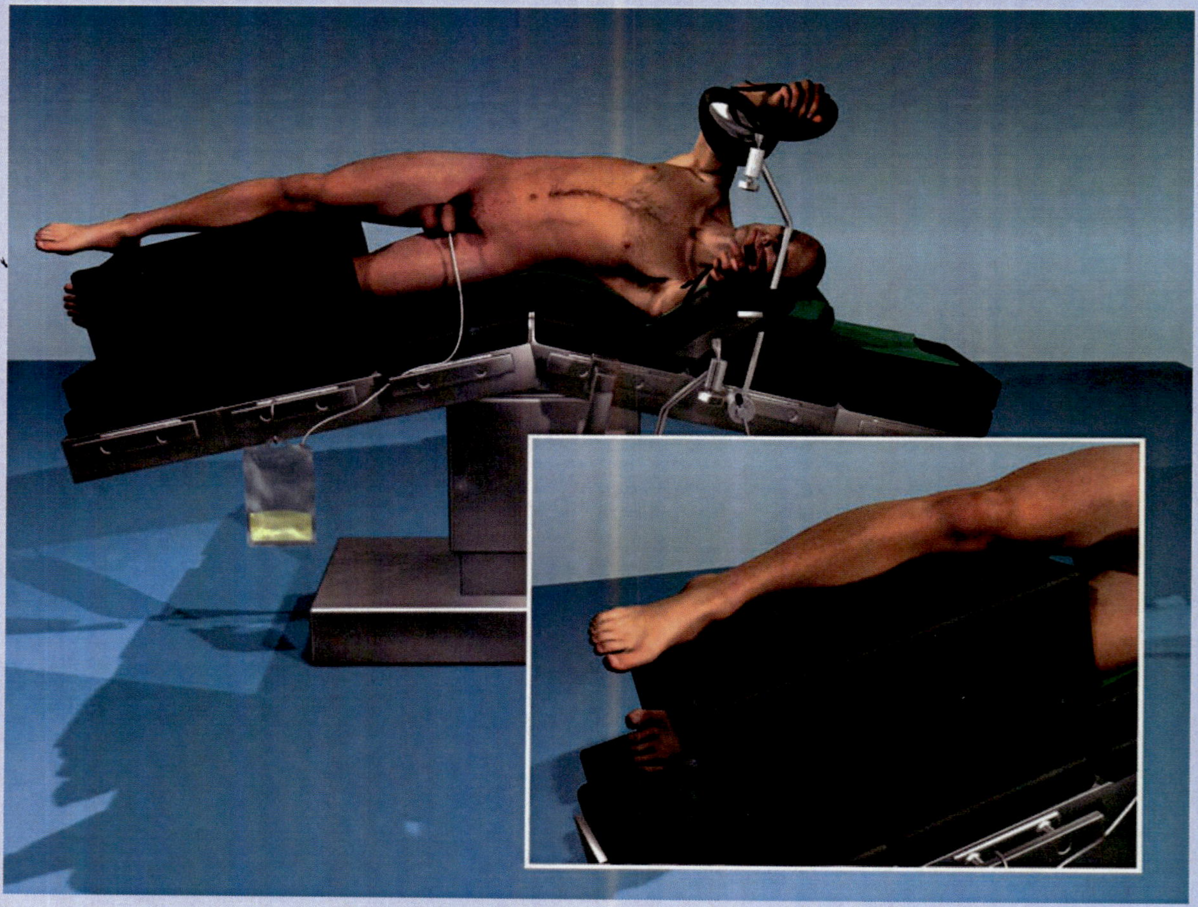

Whilst the patient is supine, following induction of anaesthesia, a urinary catheter is inserted. The patient is now rotated to the lateral position and the urinary bag is placed either at the top or bottom end of the bed for access by the anaesthetist. The legs are separated and protected with either pillows or a specially designed foam or rubber device between them as seen in the inset, in order to relieve any weight on pressure points, while the legs are slightly flexed at the knees. All other bony points, including shoulders and hips, are protected by the rubber or foam mat that is positioned on the operating table. The head and neck are supported with either pillows or a rubber head ring in order to maintain them in a neutral position. Depending on the softness of the table mattress, an axillary rubber roll may be required (not illustrated in these images) to prevent brachial plexus injury.

Step 2: Flexion of the table

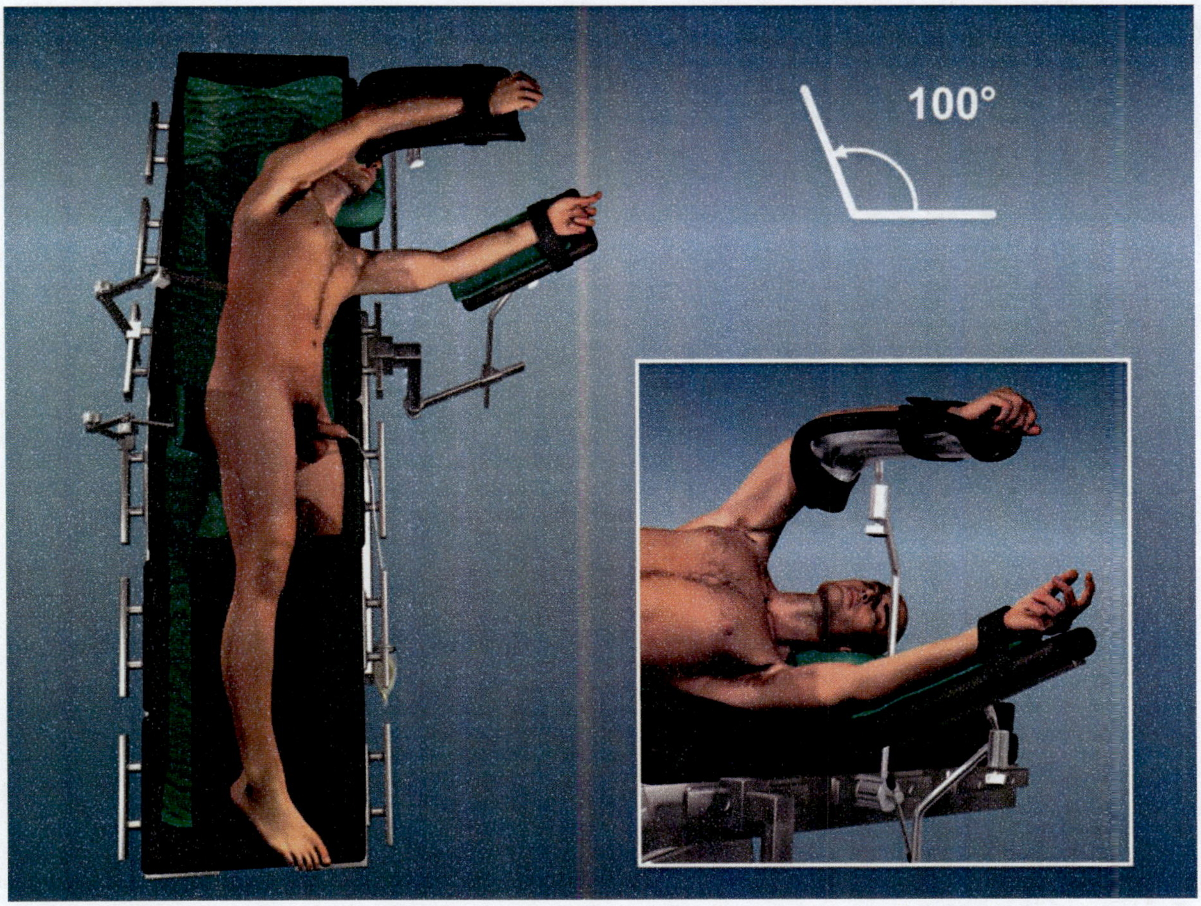

A patient with right-sided renal pathology is positioned in the left lateral position at an angle of 110° to the horizontal. The table is broken at the level of the umbilicus by approximately 10–15°. The patient is positioned on the table towards the edge of the table facing the surgeons. This prevents interference of the instruments with the table during the procedure and facilitates surgeon ergonomics. As can be seen in Step 2 inset, the patient's arms are slightly flexed at the elbow and the arm boards are positioned approximately 100–110° towards the head. They are both supported appropriately with armrests and all bony and nerve pressure points are well padded. The arms are secured in the rests with Velcro strapping, leaving both forearms and antecubital fossae available to the anaesthetist at all stages. Both the anaesthetist and the surgeon should finally check the position of the arms together to make sure that there is no interference with laparoscopic instrument movements during the procedure.

Step 3: Fixation of the patient

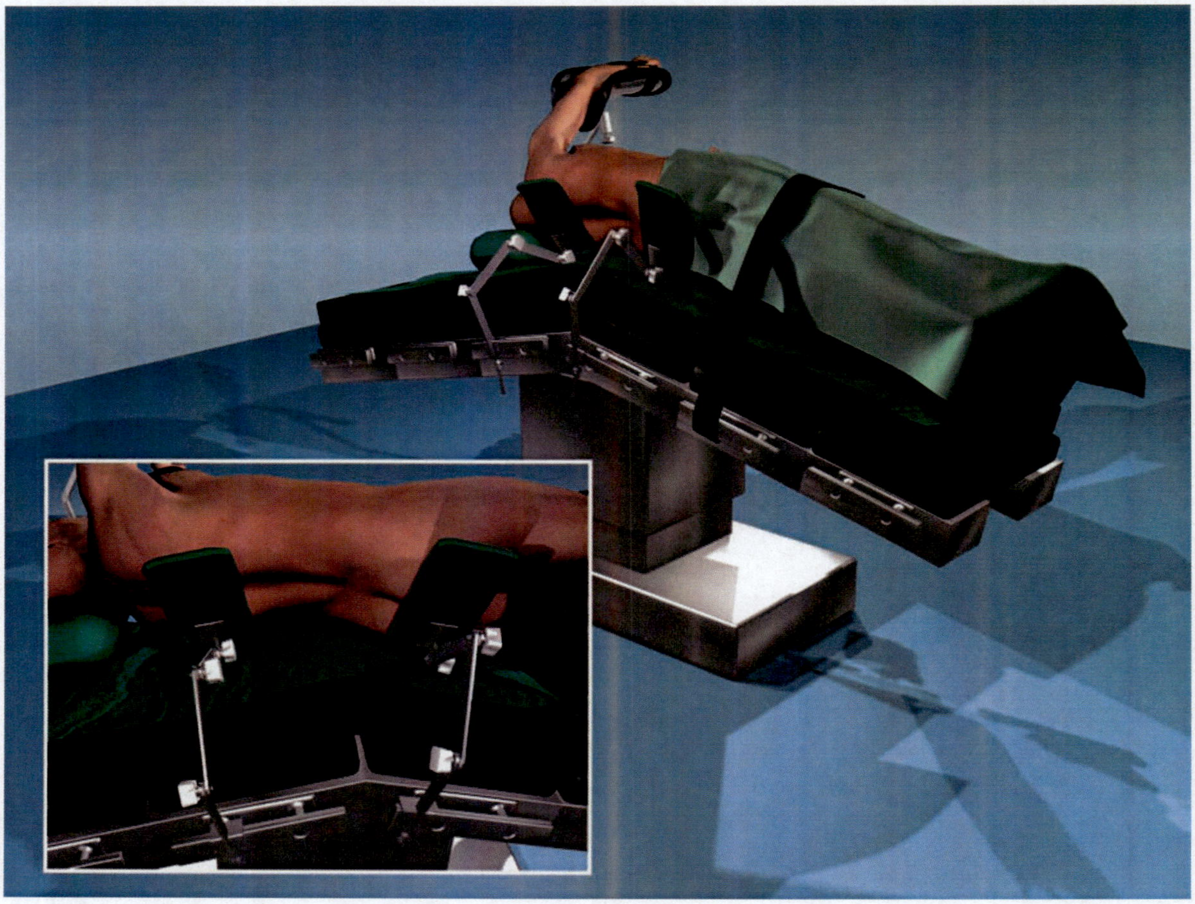

The patient's thoracic and lumbar areas are supported in the lateral position with table attachments which are well padded and which must be securely fixed to the table because the patient is rotated posteriorly (see previous step). The patient is firmly supported with Velcro tapes across both forearms and secured with a wide-diameter belt at the level of the pelvis. Following this the patient can easily and safely be rotated to another position such as a modified lateral decubitus. This may be necessary in order to allow gravity to facilitate a change in position of the bowel or kidney. It also allows optimum positioning at the beginning of the procedure to place the umbilical trocar. A Bair Hugger or blanket is is used to cover the patient to assist maintenance of body temperature. It must also be noted that sequential compressing stockings should be fitted to all patients prior to surgery.

Step 4: Entire operative setup

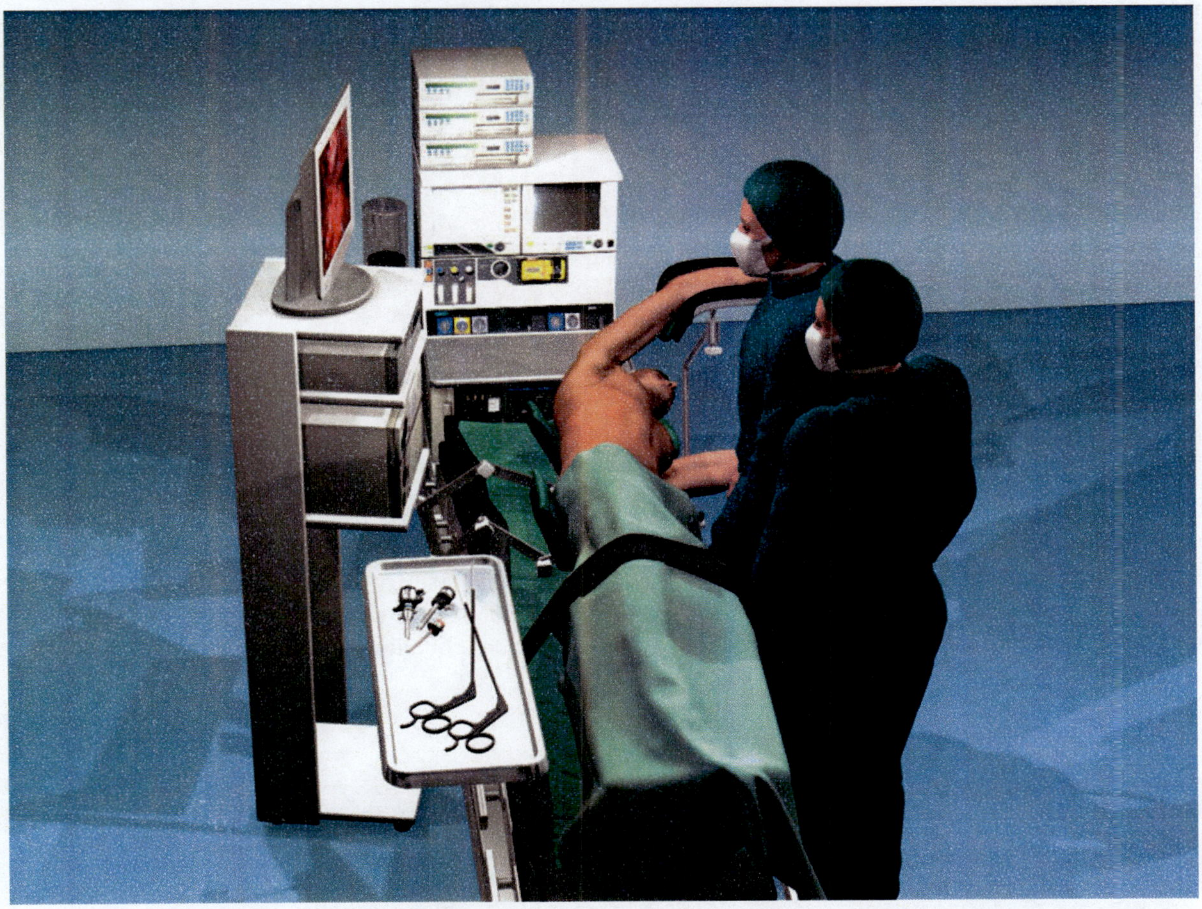

Step 4 gives an overview of the entire theatre set up. The operator and the assistant are positioned on the same side. The monitor is at eye level facing the surgeon at the opposite side of the patient. The screen should be positioned so that the surgeon can maintain a natural head position considering that the procedure can take longer then 2 h. The scrub nurse and the instrument table can be placed at the bottom of the table, either opposite or on the same side as the surgeon but should not interfere with the surgeons' view or laparoscopic range of movement.

Step 5: Anatomical landmarks I

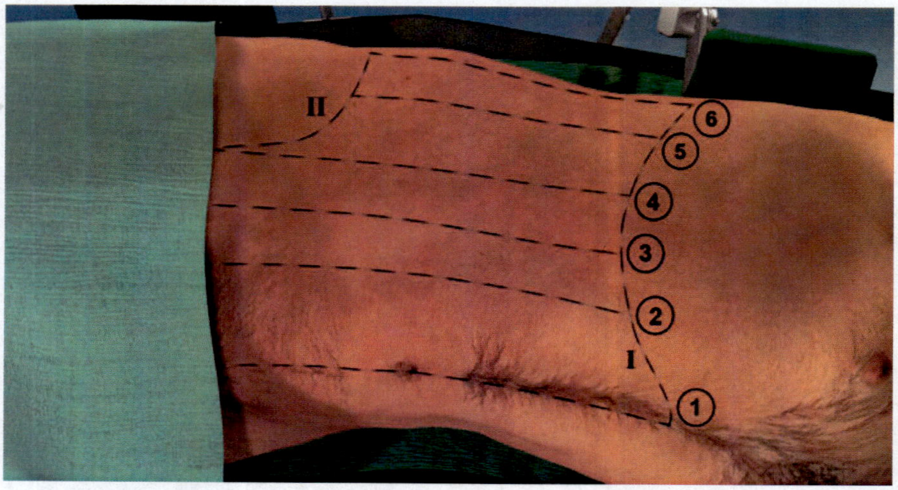

Trocar access is demonstrated in all the chapters. We represent trocar placement along a number of imaginary lines guided by anatomical landmarks on the patient. For transperitoneal access, the most important lines are demonstrated in the following two figures.

1 = midline, 2 = para-rectal line, 3 = mid-clavicular line, 4 = anterior axillary line, 5 = midaxillary line, and 6 = posterior axillary line. These anatomical landmarks are bounded by the subcostal margin superiorly (I) and the iliac crest inferiorly (II).

Step 6: Anatomical landmarks II

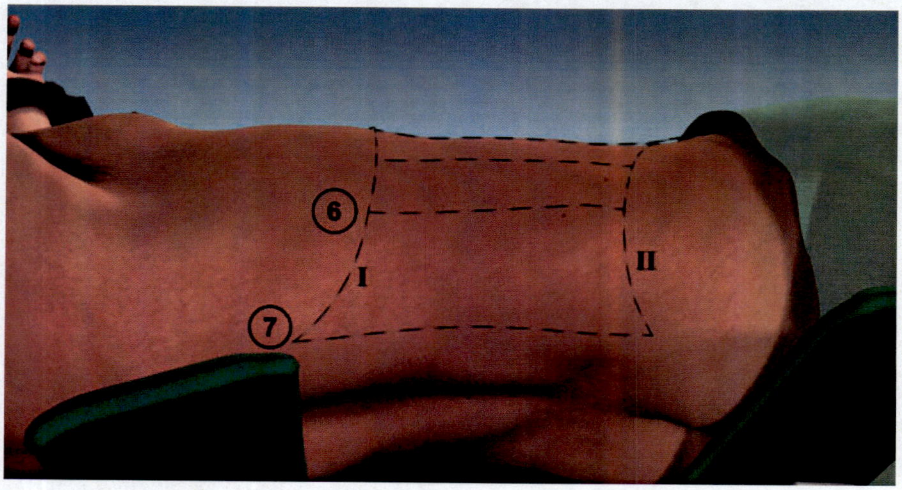

Similarly, for access to the retroperitoneal space with trocars the imaginary lines demonstrated in Step 5 include: 5 = midaxillary line, 6 = posterior axillary line, 7 = paralumbar line, I = subcostal margin and II = iliac crest. The majority of cases use the posterior axillary line for initial trocar access to develop the retroperitoneal space with a balloon trocar and allow direct visual control for insertion of the other trocars. Depending on the procedure and surgeon, these trocar placements can vary slightly.

1.2 Trocar Placement – Transperitoneal Access

1.2.1 Minilaparotomy

Rowan Casey, Minh Do, Ho Thi Phuc, Tim Haefner, Andreas Gonsior, Evangelos Liatsikos, Jens-Uwe Stolzenburg

Introduction

A number of methods can be used to enter the peritoneal cavity. These include Veress needle access, VersaStep port insertion (a variation on the Veress needle), the open mini-laparotomy technique and the optical cutting trocar device (Visiport). The camera port can also be placed through a number of anatomical positions (sub-, supra-, and transumbilical, paramedian, pararectal, etc.). Each has a slightly different anatomical arrangement of subcutaneous structures that must be considered. It is vital to remember that the most frequent accident in laparoscopy occurs during the insertion of the Veress needle or the first port. Therefore, a very careful step-by-step approach is required for the correct insertion of all trocars. Poor insertion, apart from leading to vascular or visceral injury, can make the laparoscopic procedure very difficult to accomplish because of poor view or mobility of the trocar.

Step 1: Skin incision

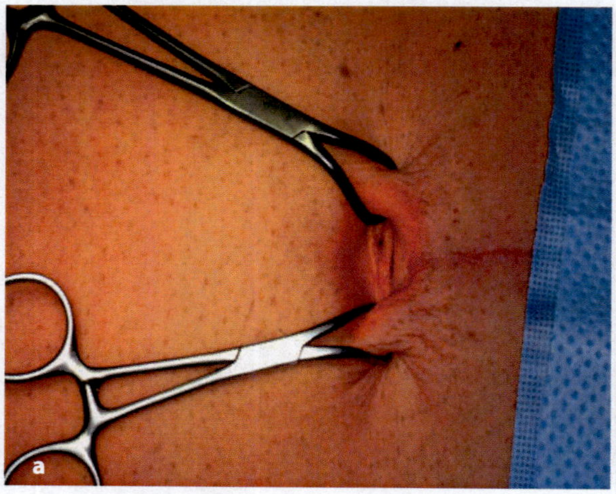

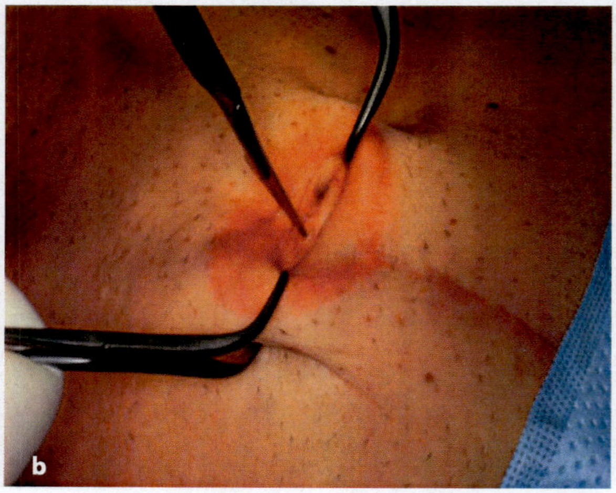

All surgeons are familiar with laparotomy. For this reason this technique is probably the most reliable. In case of previous surgery or major intra-abdominal infection, an open procedure should always be performed. The skin is grasped on either side of the incision with Backhaus clamps and elevated. The skin is then incised with a scalpel to 1.5–2 cm as dictated by the diameter of the port to be inserted. We use a transumbilical incision to directly access the fascia (all the fascial layers join at the umbilicus to form a single layer). It is also possible to perform a semi-circumferential incision at the lower end of the umbilicus.

Step 2: Fascial incision

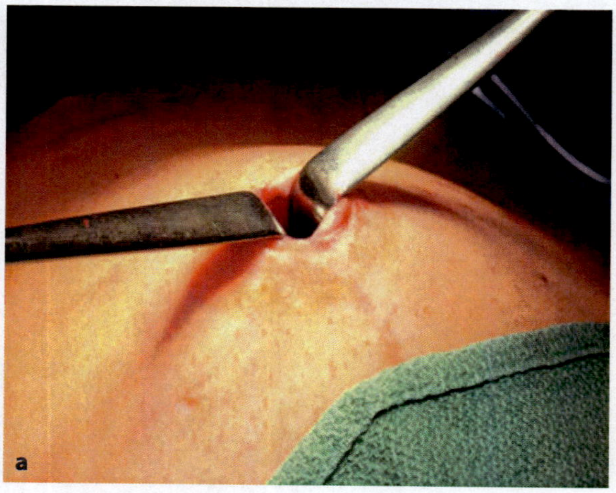

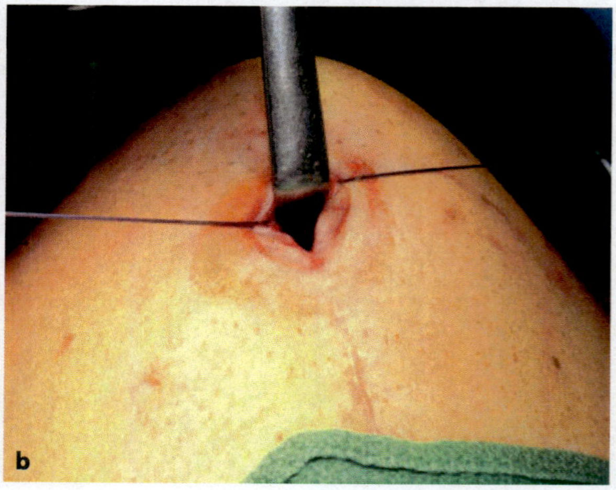

Langenback retractors are used to retract the umbilicus. A small incision is now made in the fascial layer in order to obtain direct access to the peritoneum. With the free edges of the fascia visible, two stay sutures are placed across both sides. This allows better visualisation of the peritoneum, secures it to the trocar and allows closure of the fascia later. The peritoneum is grasped with a forceps or two artery clips and lifted upwards. It can then be incised sharply with scissors to enter the peritoneal cavity.

Step 3: Optical trocar insertion

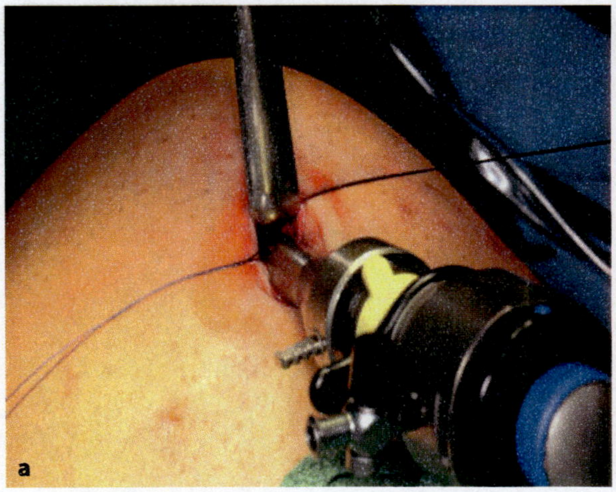
a

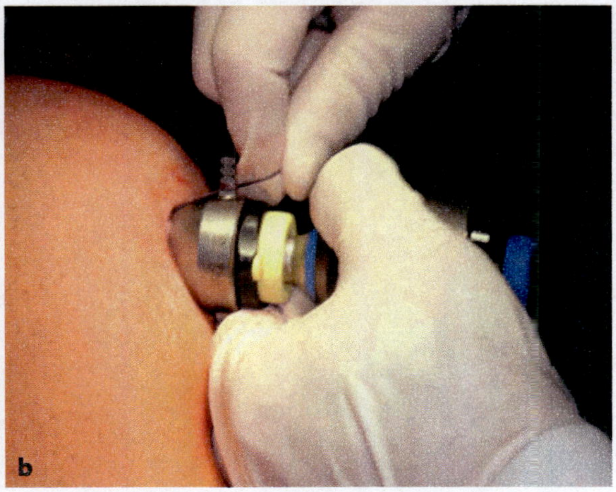
b

When the peritoneum is opened, the retractor is placed in the abdominal cavity and elevated (Step 3a) to guide insertion of the trocar. Now the optical trocar is placed along the retractor into the cavity. We prefer a 10-mm Hassan trocar because it allows adjustment of the length of the port within the abdominal cavity as the port can be moved within the Hassan tip of this trocar. The Hassan trocar is then secured to the fascial sutures as tightly as possible to prevent gas escaping and to secure the port.

Step 4: Gas insufflation

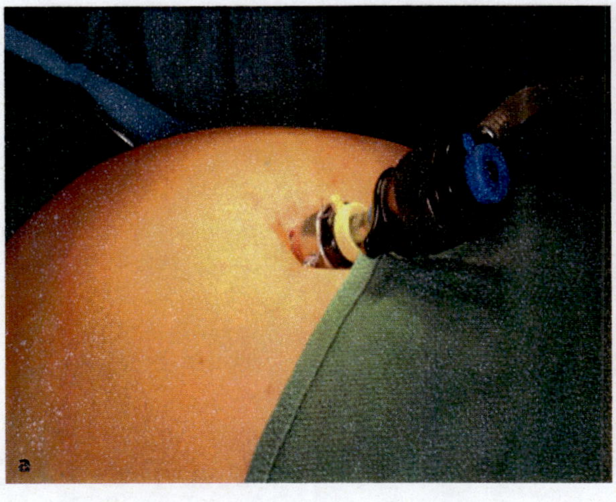
a

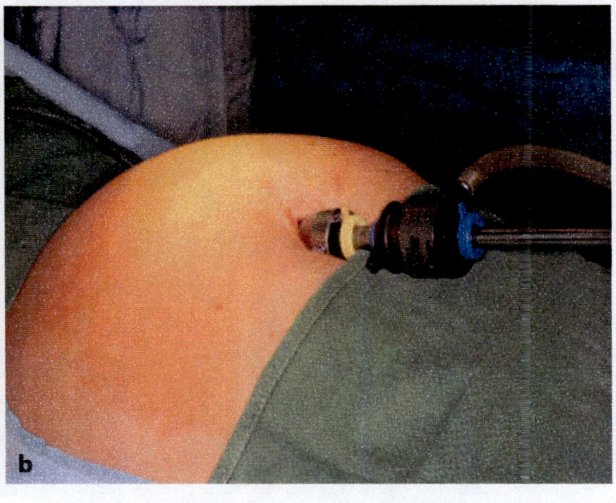
b

The laparoscope is inserted. Gas insufflation is commenced via the trocar valve at high flow. Then the abdominal cavity is inspected for adhesions and any incidental abnormalities. All other port insertions are carried out under direct vision through this port. Before inserting each trocar, the light from the optical trocar can be projected through the abdominal wall to demonstrate underlying blood vessels which should be avoided during further port insertion. The gas tubing can then be changed to another 10-mm port, which helps prevent optic lens cooling and condensation.

1.2.2 Veress Needle Technique

Rowan Casey, Minh Do, Ho Thi Phuc, Andreas Gonsior, Evangelos Liatsikos, Jens-Uwe Stolzenburg

Step 1: Skin incision

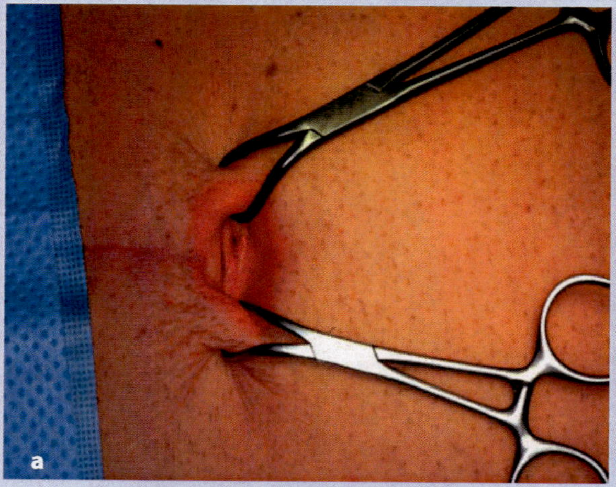

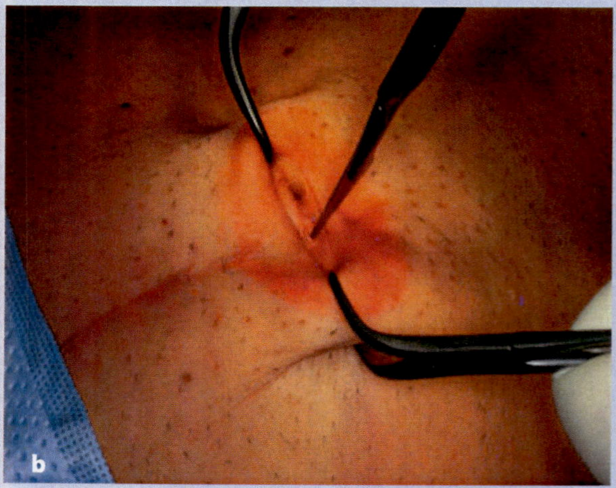

A nasogastric tube must be placed before Veress needle insertion, especially if the puncture is made above the umbilicus to avoid gastric injury. Similarly, the bladder should be emptied for access below the umbilicus. Usually the easiest site to place the Veress needle is via the umbilicus as all fascial layers converge to a single fascia. The paraumbilical skin is elevated on both sides with Backhaus clamps and a 1.5-cm horizontal skin incision is made with a scalpel. Before insertion, the needle must be tested. At the tip, there is a spring-loaded blunt stylet inside the needle which extends beyond the tip of the needle. The stylet retracts as the needle is pushed against tissue and automatically advances as the cavity is penetrated.

Step 2: Veress needle insertion and position check

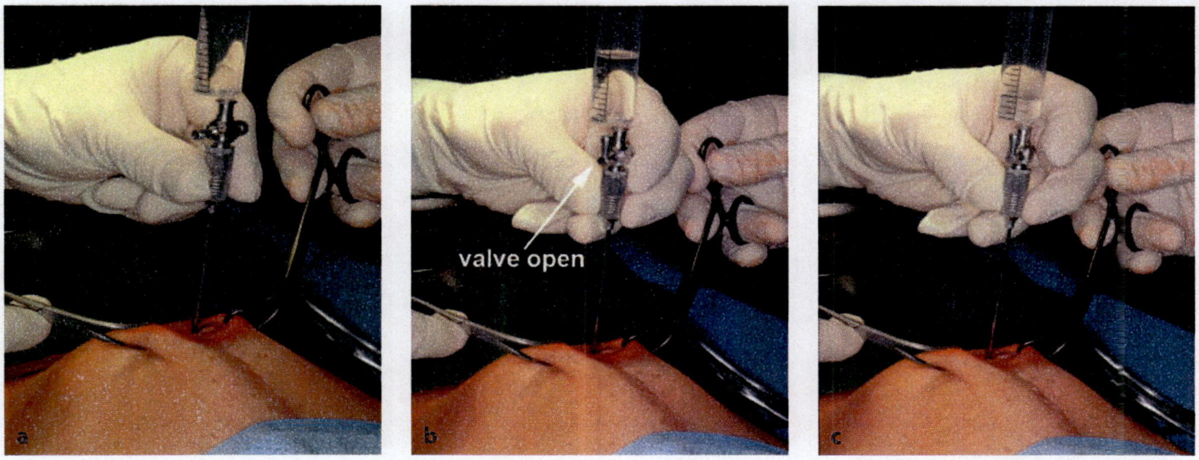

The abdominal wall is lifted up with the Backhaus clamps. A 10-cc syringe without a plunger is filled with water and attached to the Veress needle with the valve closed. The needle is placed against the fascial layer and the valve is opened. Between the thumb and index finger, the needle is advanced into the peritoneal cavity at a 90° angle to the fascia. The needle passes with a click through the fascia and peritoneum. If the needle is correctly in the abdominal cavity the water level in the syringe starts to drop (Step 2c). If water or air can be aspirated back, then the needle may be in the preperitoneal space.

Step 3: Gas insufflation

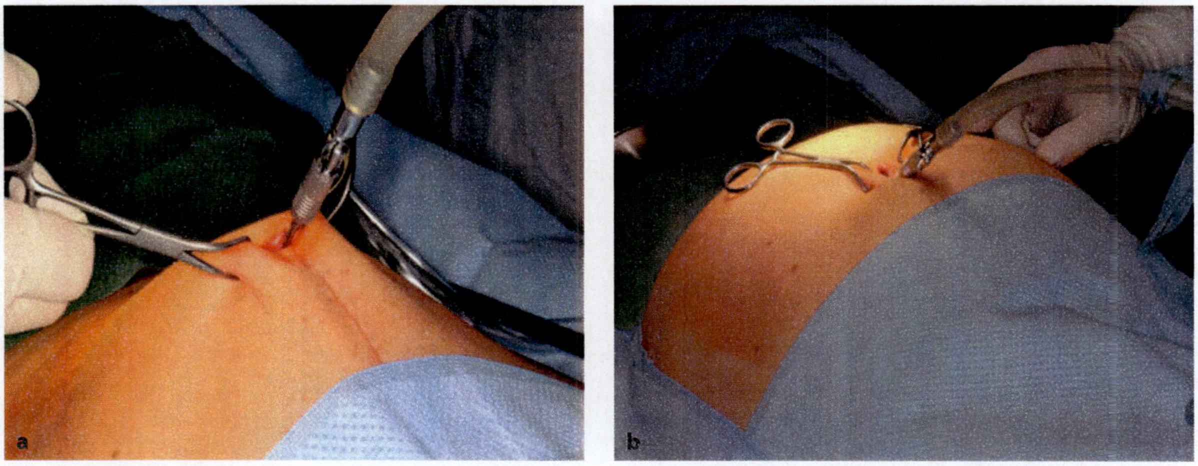

The Veress needle is advanced further into the abdominal cavity gently and the syringe is removed (Step 3a). Gas is insufflated initially at low flow into the peritoneal cavity to a pressure of 12 mmHg, as in Step 3b. Percussion in the area of the liver or spleen can be done to check for resonance (tympanism) before starting high flow. If the pressure alarm on the gas insufflator rings, this implies that either the patient is not relaxed sufficiently or the tip of the Veress needle may be blocked by omentum or bowel. The needle should be slightly withdrawn and repositioned.

Step 4: First port insertion

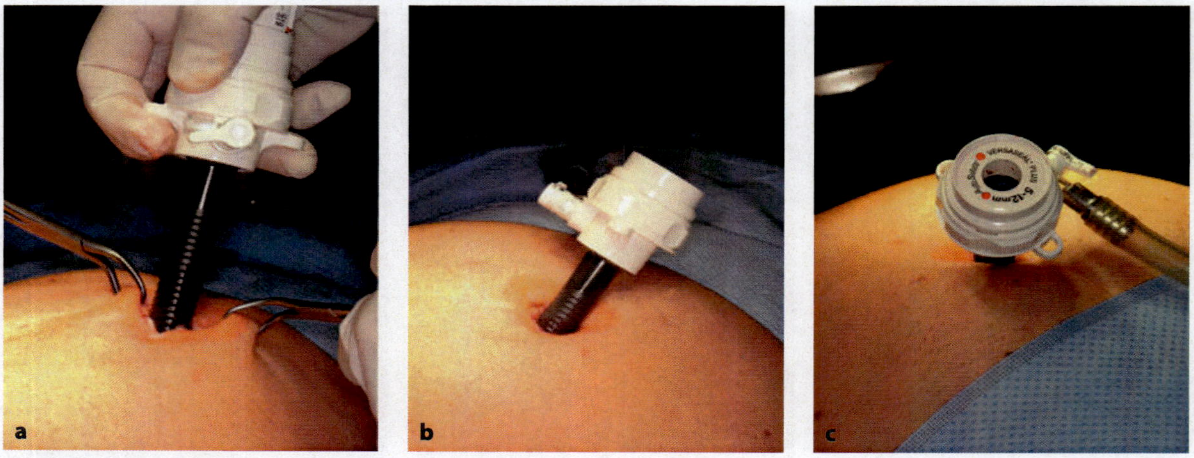

The abdomen is now distended sufficiently to at least 2 l and a pressure of 12 mmHg. This allows sufficient resistance to port insertion. The Veress needle is then withdrawn. A 5- to 12-mm safety port with a retractable blade is inserted into the peritoneal cavity with careful hand control in a slight left to right twisting motion. This is inserted at 90° to the abdominal wall or slightly in the direction of the operating field (Step 4a, Step 4b, Step 4c). Excessively oblique port insertion (especially in obesity) risks abdominal wall injury and reduced port mobility. When the first port is placed, the valve is opened so gas leakage can be heard and confirm the intraperitoneal position. The insufflator is connected and the optic device is inserted. Perform visual inspection to ensure that no injury has occurred during this blind insertion. Place additional ports under direct visual control.

1.2.3 Versaport Technique

Rowan Casey, Minh Do, Ho Thi Phuc, Andreas Gonsior, Evangelos Liatsikos, Jens-Uwe Stolzenburg

Step 1: Skin incision

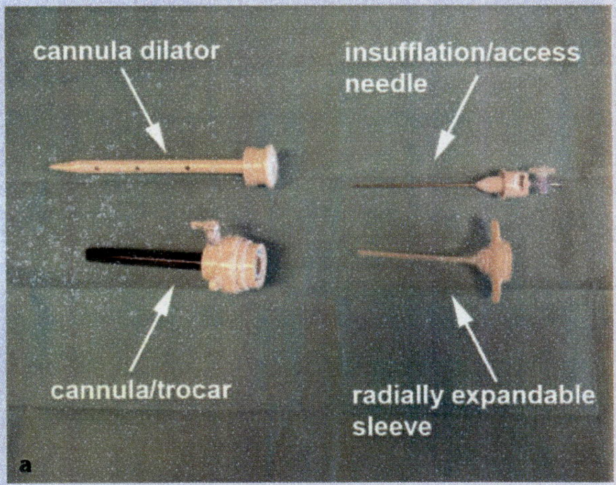

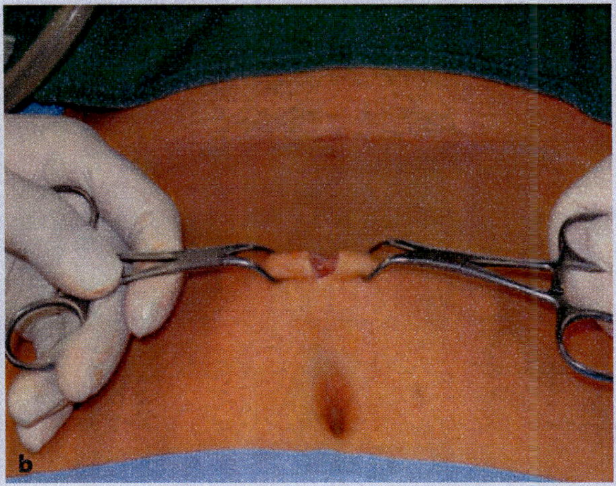

The insufflation/access needle used to establish pneumoperitoneum is a 14-G stainless steel needle surrounded by a radially expandable sleeve (Step 1a). There is a spring-loaded blunt stylet inside the needle extending beyond the tip of the needle. The stylet retracts as the needle is advanced but automatically advances as the peritoneal cavity is entered. This needle is reusable with other expandable sleeves during one patient procedure. The radially expandable sleeve is designed to lock together with the insufflations/access needle (Step 1a). The dilator/cannula comprises a blunt dilator and hollow cannula with a valve to establish pneumoperitoneum. A skin incision matching the diameter of the trocar is made (Step 1b).

Step 2: Peritoneal access

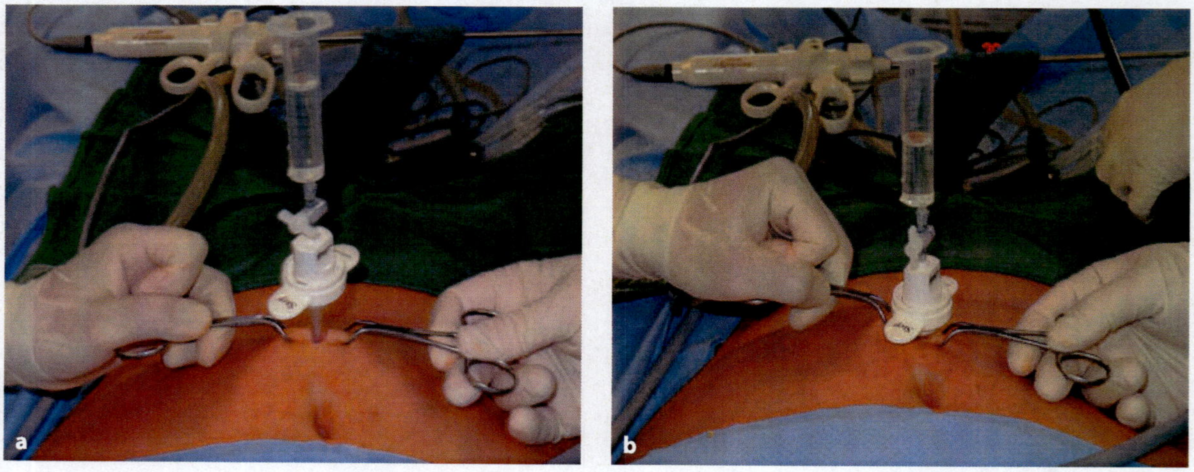

Insert the bare insufflation/access needle into the peritoneal cavity using conventional Veress access techniques. Alternatively, as in this case, both can be inserted initially as a Veress needle technique in order to create the pneumoperitoneum. This can also be the case for secondary port insertion. Using this technique, greater resistance will be felt at the tissue level given its larger diameter. The water drop test is used to confirm correct entry into the peritoneum. The water level in the syringe can be seen to be falling between Steps 2a and 2b.

Step 3: Gas insufflation

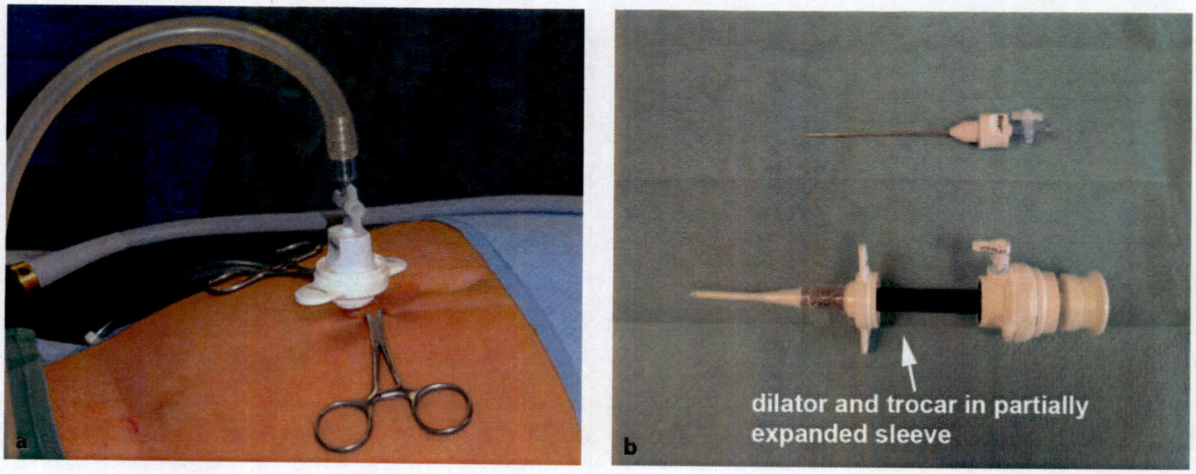

The pneumoperitoneum is now created through the insufflation needle and expandable trocar (Step 3a). Once the pneumoperitoneum is created, remove the insufflation/access needle from the sleeve. The dilator/cannula will be inserted next with a twisting motion through the radial expanding sleeve. Step 3b demonstrates the partially inserted trocar and the sleeve dilation. If it is inserted at an angle there is a danger of the sleeve tearing, which should be replaced, making sure the damaged sleeve is removed intact.

Step 4: Trocar insertion

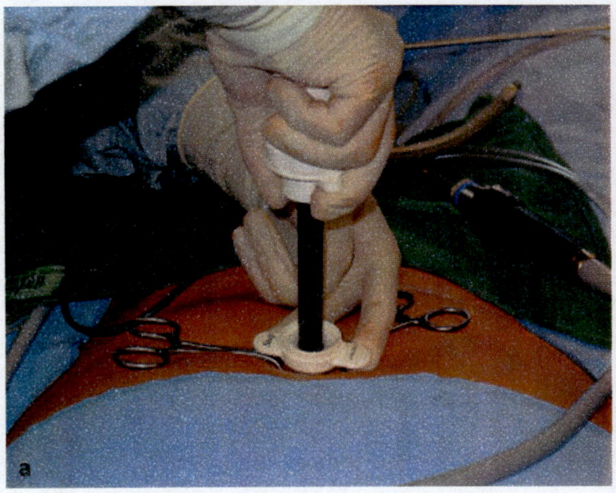

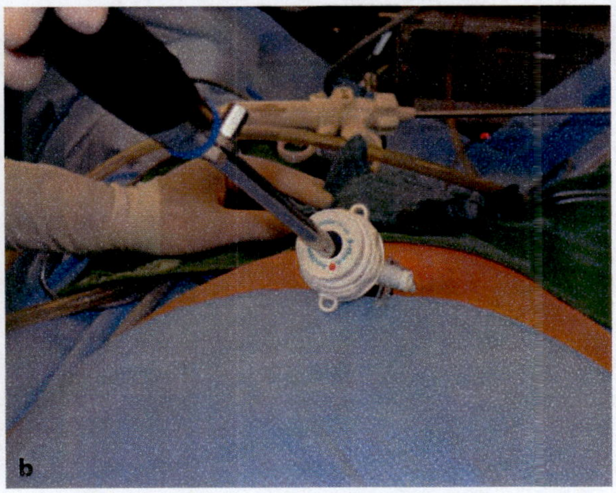

Whilst holding the sleeve handle, insert the dilator and cannula straight through the centre of the sleeve (Step 4a). Then remove the dilator leaving the cannula and radially expanding sleeve in situ. The gas source can be attached at this point. The cannula can be removed from the sleeve and a larger or smaller one can be inserted as a stepping-up or -down technique. When removing the cannula and sleeve from the abdominal cavity, desufflate the abdomen first. Leave the laparoscope in place in the cannula. Remove the cannula and expanding sleeve over the laparoscope, thus preventing viscera from entering the defect and allowing visualisation of the sleeve removal (Step 4b).

1.2.4 Visiport Technique

Rowan Casey, Minh Do, Ho Thi Phuc, Andreas Gonsior, Evangelos Liatsikos, Jens-Uwe Stolzenburg

Step 1: Insertion of the camera into the Visiport

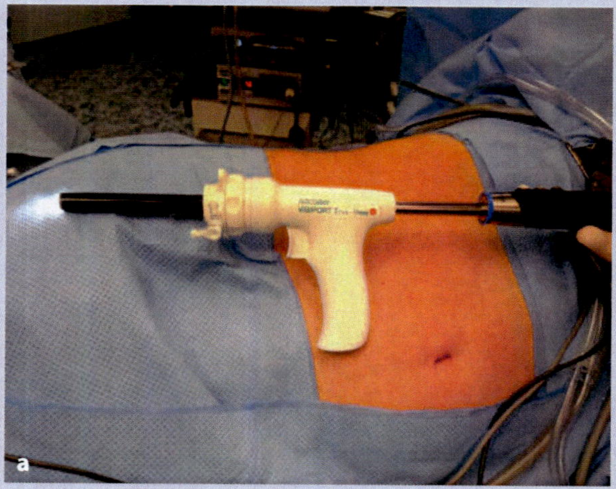

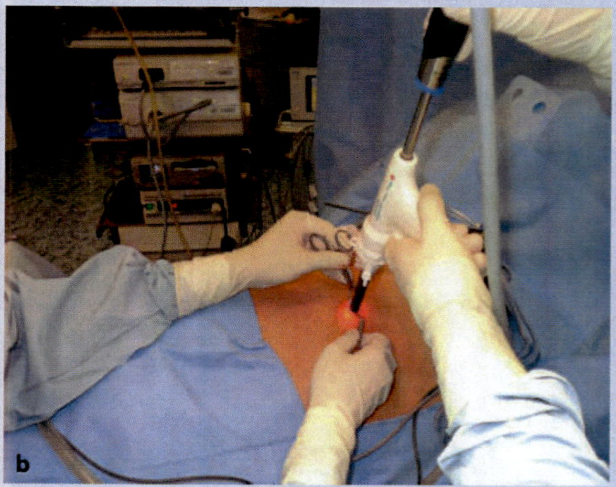

The Visiport pistol handle is inserted into the trocar port and the optic is inserted into the Visiport handle (Step 1a). The optic can be white-balanced within the trocar held against a white gauze. A 1.5- to 2-cm incision is made in the skin at the site of optical trocar placement just large enough to allow the optical trocar to be inserted. Insufflation with a Veress needle first may be used at the discretion of the surgeon but is usually not necessary. We use Backhaus clamps to elevate the skin. Uniform and direct pressure with the trocar against the skin is applied (Step 1b).

Step 2: Construction of the Visiport

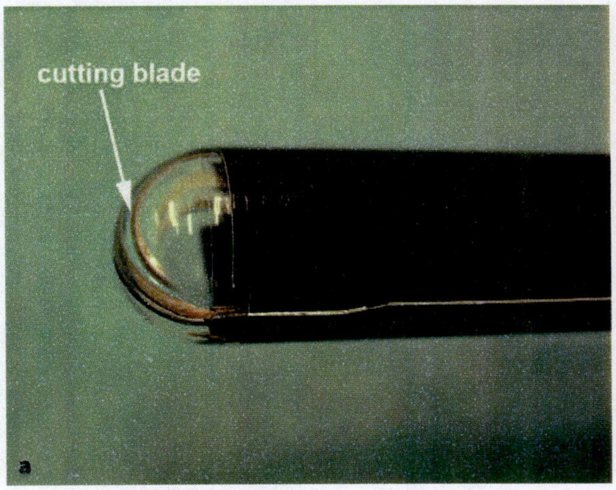

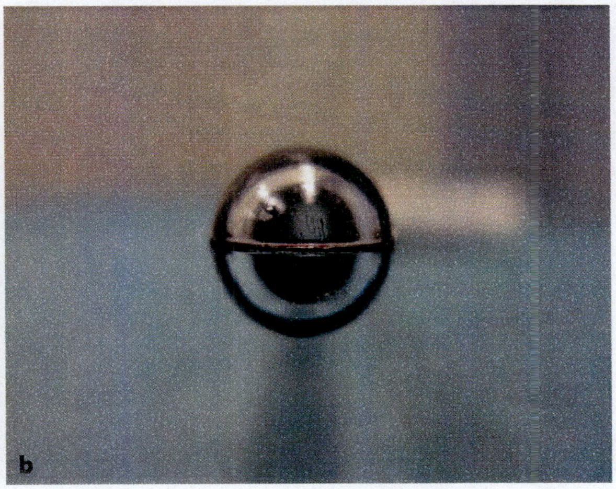

The device can be advanced through the layers of the abdominal wall with a gentle twisting motion and pressure on the trocar whilst intermittently deploying the blade. The blade should only be deployed when the surgeon is sure of the position of the blade within the abdominal wall using the optical trocar and visual landmarks (see Step 5). The blade is deployed 1 mm and immediately retracts after the trigger is pulled. Thus the Visiport allows a combination of blunt and sharp dissection.

Step 3: Port insertion

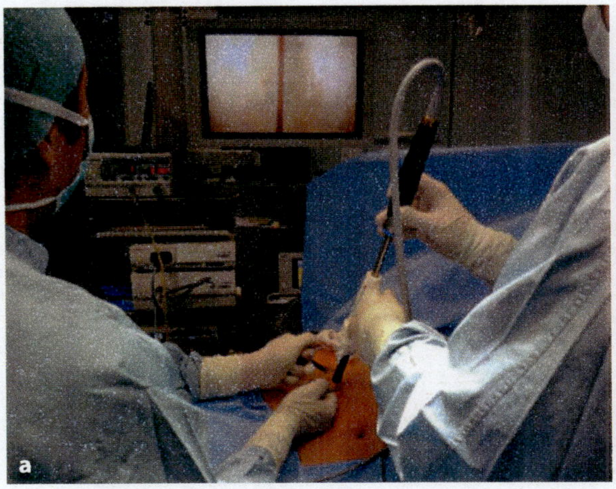

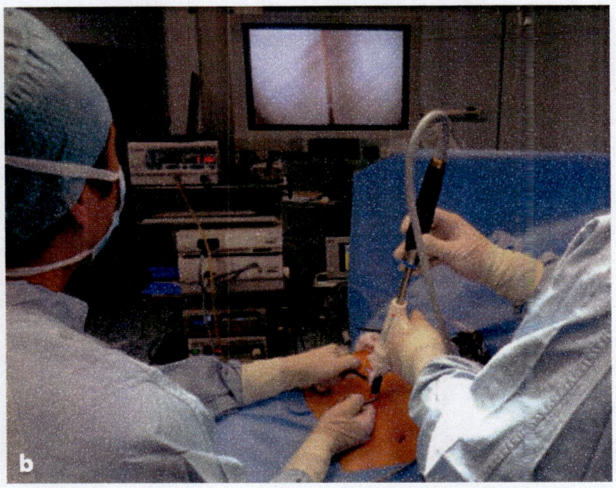

The Visiport can be rotated as it passes through the tissue to allow tissue separation. Direct visualisation of the tissue layers during primary port insertion is vital, especially in obese patients. The first structure to pass through is the subcutaneous fat, as can be seen on the monitor in Step 3a. The fascia is seen next and can be recognised by its parallel fibres (Step 3b). The fascia can be easily separated whilst deploying, rotating and advancing the Visiport with gentle pressure. The rectus muscle will then be encountered and separated. The optic device/trocar must be perpendicular to the abdominal wall and not become obliquely angled.

Step 4: Port insertion

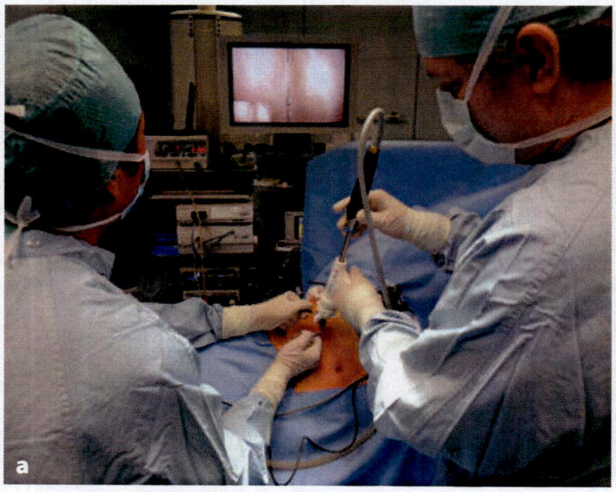

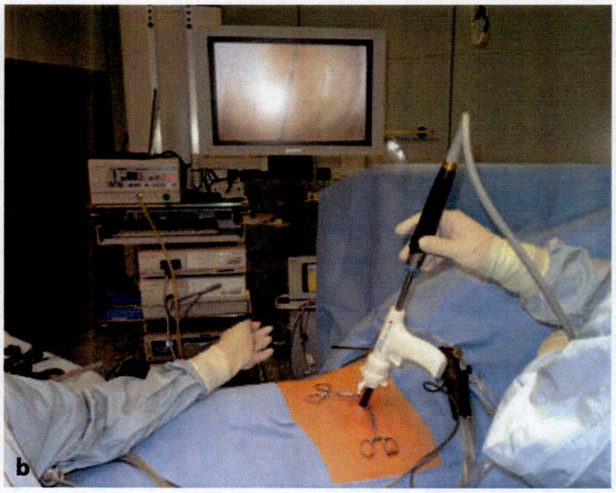

When the muscle comes into view, the same technique is used to advance the port. The muscle fibres can be seen and dissection should be carried out with the cutting blade parallel to these fibres with a gentle twisting motion (Step 4a). Then the posterior fascial layer and preperitoneal fat and space come into view (Step 4b).

The abdominal viscera may be seen through the peritoneal lining. Before penetrating the peritoneal lining, it may be helpful to adjust the angle of the Visiport approach to avoid contact with any intraperitoneal structures upon penetration. The trigger is squeezed and the peritoneum is penetrated with gentle pressure.

Step 5: Layers that should be encountered during port insertion

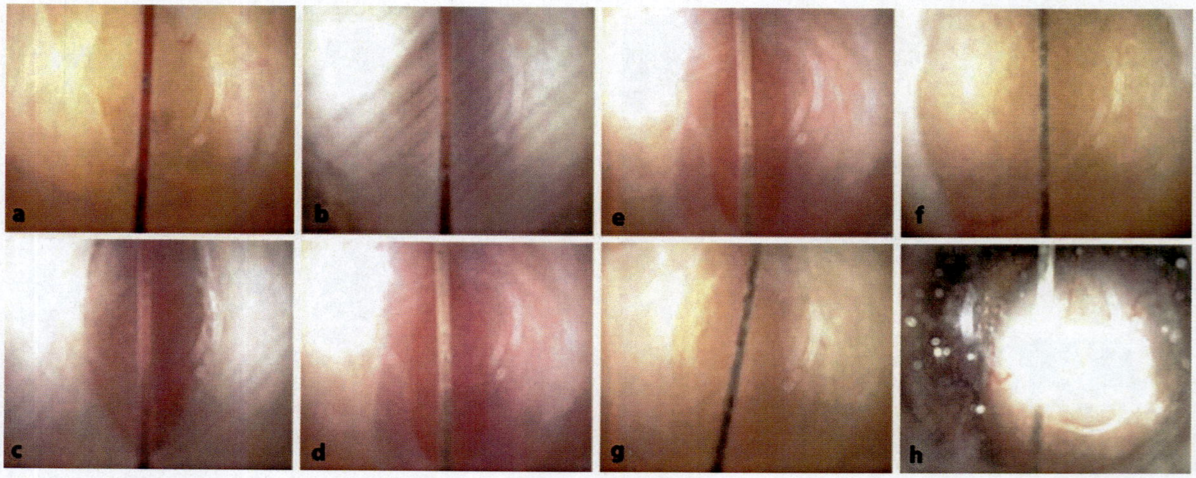

These series of illustrations demonstrate the various layers that should be encountered sequentially as follows: (a) subcutaneous fatty layer; (b) fascial layer; (c) splitting the fascial layer; (d) muscle fibres; (e) posterior fascial layer (if present); (f) preperitoneal fatty layer; (g) peritoneal layer (with contents possibly visible through this layer) and (h) intra-abdominal contents (bowel with blood vessels on serosa).

Step 6: Removal of Visiport pistol handle and final trocar placement

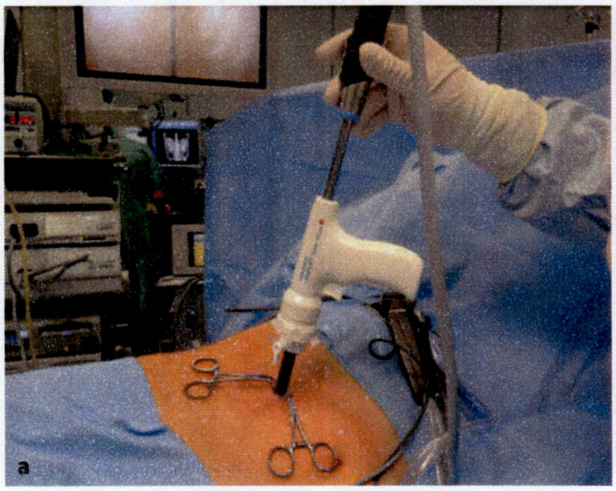

a

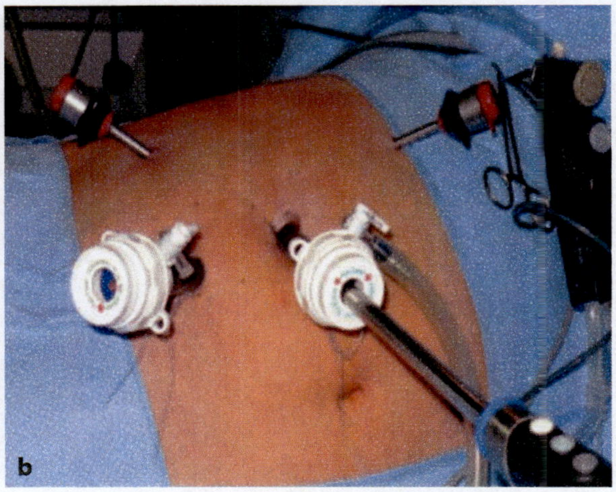

b

The Visiport pistol handle and obturator can now be removed, leaving the trocar sheath in position in the abdominal cavity. The trocar sheath has two eyelets on it that allow suturing to the abdominal wall because there are no threads on the outside of the trocar sheath.

The optic is now re-inserted through the trocar sheath (Step 6b). The other trocars are placed under direct visual control, as shown in this case of transperitoneal nephrectomy.

1.3 Trocar Placement: Retroperitoneal Access

Alexander Bachmann, Svetozar Subotic, Stephen Wyler

Introduction

Wittmoser first explored the retroperitoneal space by performing a lumbar sympathectomy in 1973 [1]. Guar described the use of an inflation balloon in the retroperitoneum to increase space for the laparoscopic approach [2]. The use of the inflation balloon prepared the way for modern retroperitoneoscopic surgery. Even in challenging cases such as dismembered pyeloplasty in children, the retroperitoneoscopic approach is safe and feasible.

The advantage of the retroperitoneal approach is the direct and safe identification of the renal artery. Peritoneal contents are not affected in comparison to the transperitoneal access. To date there are still not significant data to show any superiority between the transperitoneal and retroperitoneal approach. However, the potential risk of injury to abdominal organs is higher with the transperitoneal approach. Finally, the surgeon's preference and experience should determine the access chosen.

Indications

- Adrenalectomy
- Living donor nephrectomy
- Tumour nephrectomy
- Nephroureterectomy
- Nephrolithotomy
- Nephron-sparing surgery
- Ureter reconstruction

Contra-indications

- Obstructive and restrictive lung disorders
- Diseases of the spine
- Previous retroperitoneal surgery

Step 1: Patient position and anatomical landmarks

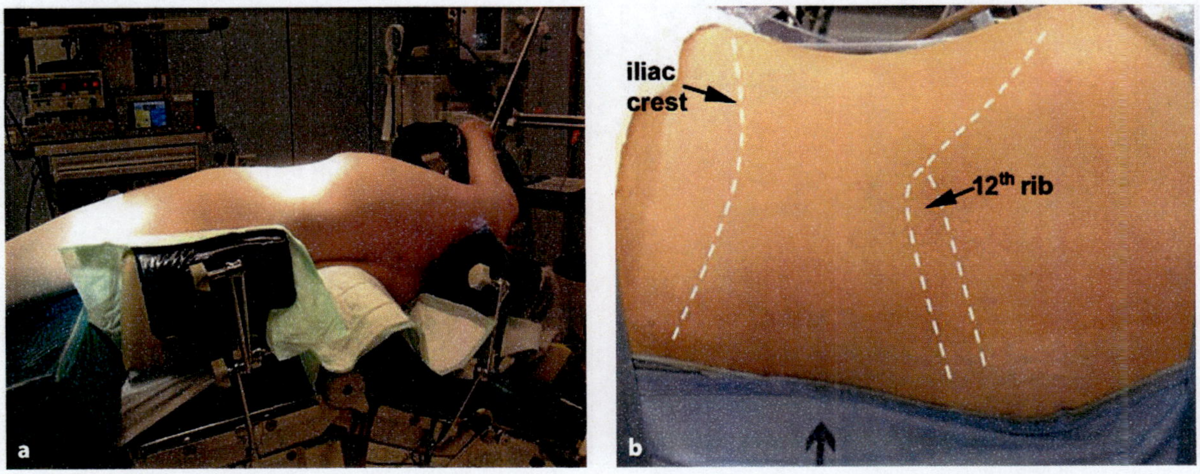

The patient is positioned in a slightly extended flank position. The left arm is placed on an armrest (Step 1a). The first incision is placed at the tip of the 12th rib or 1 cm dorsally (Step 1b). This incision is used for the camera later during the procedure. The retroperitoneal space is accessed in the muscle-free triangle between the external oblique muscle, the latissimus dorsi muscle and the iliac crest. The anatomical landmarks of the tip of the 12th rib, erector spinae muscle and iliac crest are marked and observed prior to the first port placement.

Step 2: Access to the retroperitoneal space

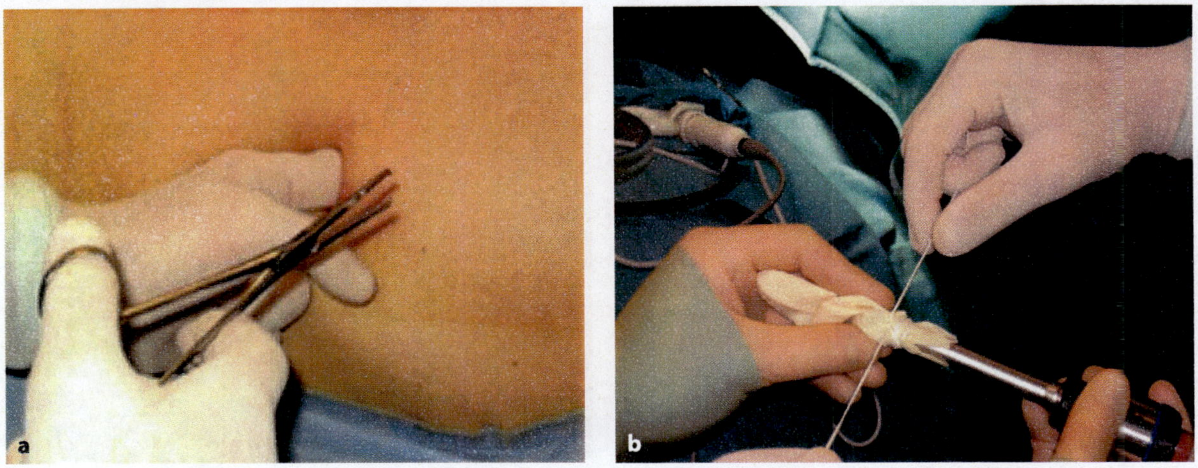

The fascia of the external and internal intercostal muscles are perforated with a blunt forceps (Step 2a). The fascia transversalis is then perforated and the retroperitoneal space is then identified as the 12th rib tip is palpated. The retroperitoneal space is enlarged with digital dissection, allowing the psoas muscle and the lower pole of the kidney to be felt. The retroperitoneal space is dilated with a Herloon balloon device (Aesculap, Tuttlingen, Germany). Alternatively, a self-made dilatation balloon made out of two fingers of a surgical glove can be used (Step 2b).

Step 3: Dissection of the retroperitoneal space

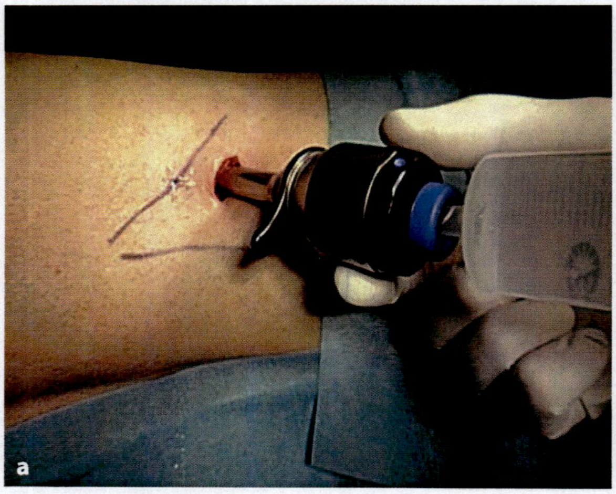
a

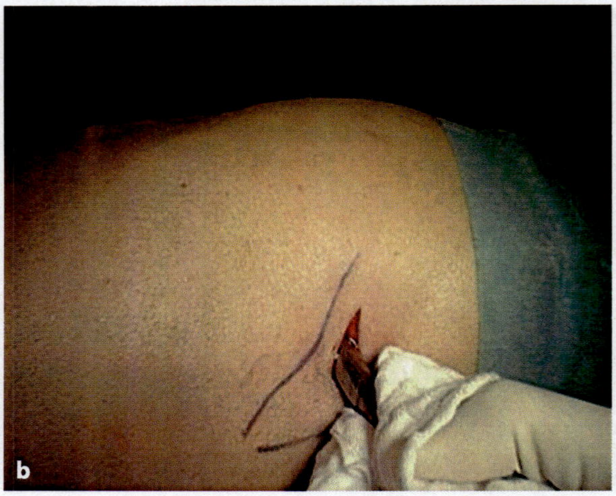
b

This step shows how the self-made dilatation balloon is inserted into the retroperitoneal space after blunt digital dissection. Saline is instilled in the balloon via a 60-ml catheter-tipped syringe through the 10-mm trocar (Step 3a). The retroperitoneal space is enlarged by instilling 800–1,000 ml of saline into the balloon. Balloon filling can be monitored as distension and protrusion on the skin surface (Step 3b). Once the space has been made, gas is insufflated. For beginners, the use of a commercial balloon trocar is recommended.

Step 4: Trocar placement

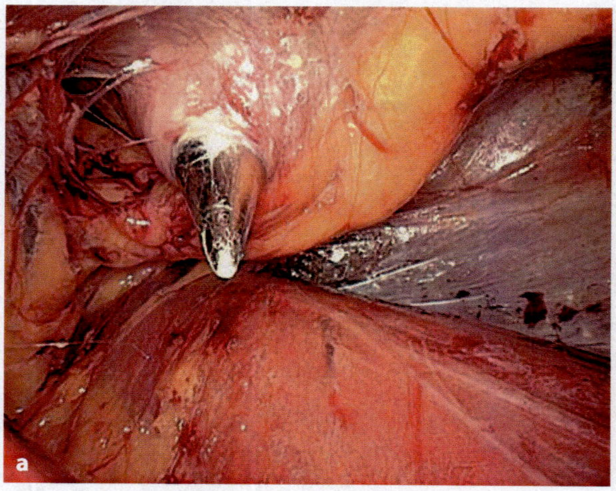
a

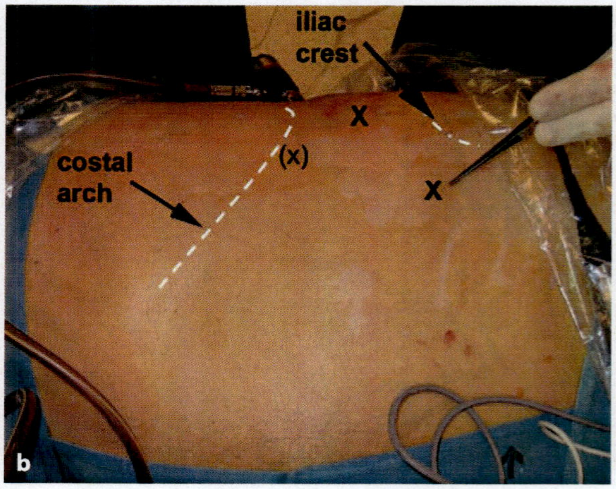

b

After establishing a pneumoretroperitoneum with 14 mmHg of pressure, the additional trocars are inserted depending on which procedure is to be performed. The reference structure that is seen first should be the psoas muscle and must be kept in a horizontal position (Step 4a). The peritoneal reflection is moved ventrally using the camera as a dissector. This enlarges the retroperitoneal space and removes the peritoneum out of the range of the anterior trocar. In Step 4b two 5- to 12-mm trocars and optionally a 5-mm auxiliary trocar are inserted in a typical rhomboid configuration (image shown with ventral view).

Step 5: Retroperitoneoscopy (landmarks)

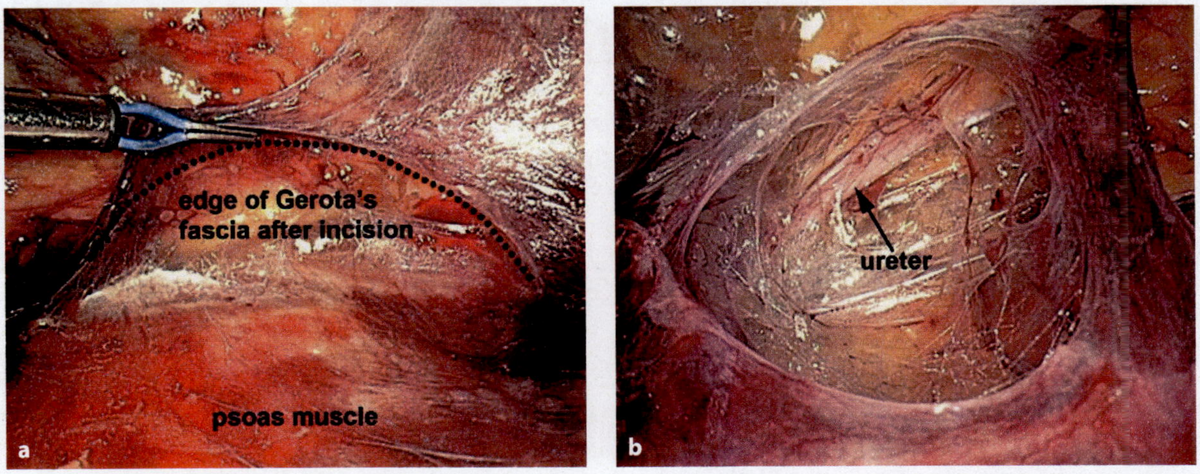

The reference structures now seen in retroperitoneoscopy are the psoas muscle and the edge of the Gerota fascia (Step 5a). After incision of the Gerota fascia, the border of the psoas muscle, the perivascular, perirenal fatty and lymphatic tissue can be identified. It is critical to incise along the border of the psoas muscle in order not to cut any vessels inadvertently. The direct identification of the ureter is often possible (seen in the centre of Step 5b). The ureter guides the surgeon for the further preparation of the kidney. It can be utilised as a reference structure for preparation of the vascular pedicle of the kidney (cranially) or for preparation towards the pelvis.

References

1. Wittmoser R (1973) Die Retroperitoneoskopie als neue Methode der lumbalen Sympathectomie. Fortschr Endosk 4:219–233
2. Gauer D (1992) Laparoscopic operative retroperitoneoscopy: Use of a new device. J Urol 148:1137–1139

1.4 Set up of daVinci Robot for Kidney Surgery

1.4.1 Possible Trocar Positions for Robot-Assisted Kidney Surgery

Evangelos Liatsikos, Panagiotis Kallidonis, Ingolf Tuerk, Christopher Anderson, Harry Beerlage, Jens-Uwe Stolzenburg

Introduction

Robot-assisted surgery of the upper urinary tract includes radical and partial nephrectomy as well as pyeloplasty. Although robot-assisted laparoscopic radical nephrectomy (RALRN) has been reported in very few publications [1], robot-assisted partial nephrectomy (RALPN) and pyeloplasty (RALP) are alternatives to laparoscopic and open surgical approaches [2–5]. All approaches have been introduced in an attempt to provide the advantages of minimally invasive surgery and to overcome the challenges of conventional laparoscopy [1–5]. The performance of the above procedures requires careful preoperative planning and robot setup. All steps of robot setup as well as trocar placement are similar when all of the above procedures are performed by the transperitoneal approach.

Option 1: Lateral trocar placement of four robotic arms for left-sided surgery

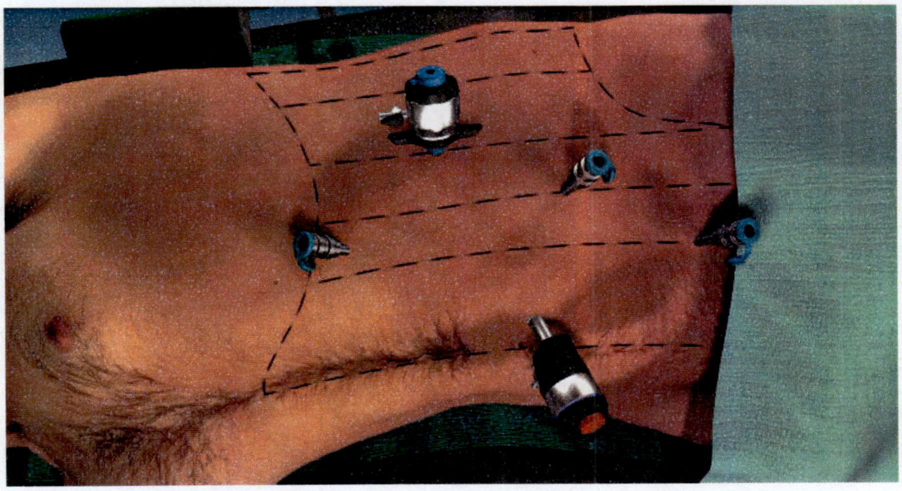

Patient positioning is identical to laparoscopic radical or partial nephrectomy as well as pyeloplasty. The placement of the trocars is similar for both left- and right-sided procedures. The appropriate trocars are inserted with the conventional laparoscopic technique using a Veress needle or the open Hasson technique. The figure presents the site of trocar positioning for the left-sided procedure. The camera is inserted on the anterior axillary line, as shown in the figure. The two robotic working trocars are placed on the midclavicular line. A fourth robotic trocar is positioned on the lateral margin of the rectus muscle near the pubic bone. The assistant conventional trocar is placed on a paraumbilical site.

Option 2: Lateral trocar placement of four robotic arms for right-sided surgery

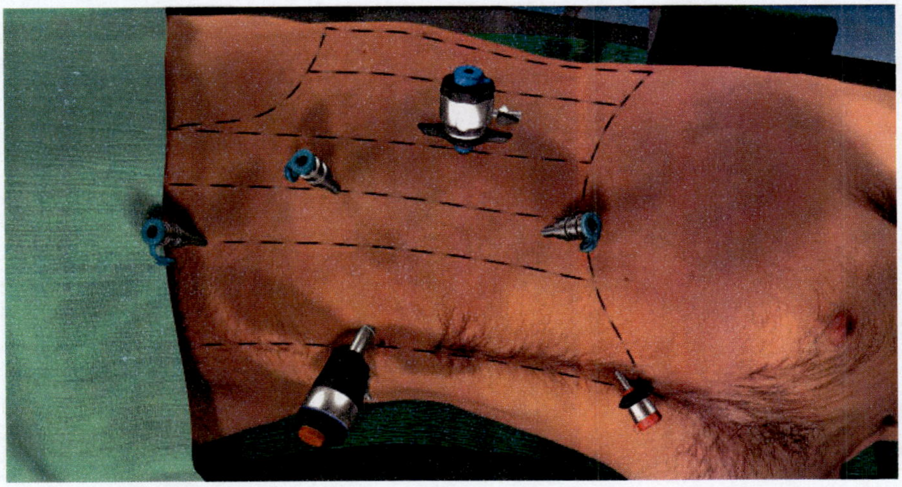

For the right-sided procedure, the robotic and assistant trocar sites remain the same. Nevertheless, an additional conventional laparoscopic trocar is inserted below the xiphoid for liver retraction. This trocar could be either 5 mm or 3 mm. Some surgeons prefer introducing fan retractors or snake-like liver retractors. The robotic working trocars should be carefully inserted to avoid collision between the robotic arms. A distance of approximately 8 cm is usually adequate. Lateral trocar placement facilitates the performance of robotic surgery in obese patients.

Option 3: Lateral trocar placement of three robotic arms for left-sided surgery

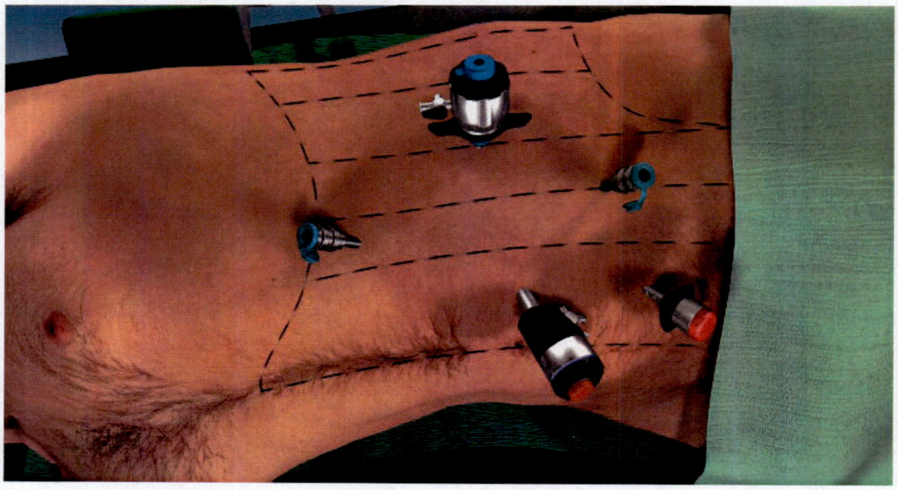

The camera trocar is placed at the anterior-axillary line while the two robotic working ports are positioned on the mid-clavicular line. When inserting the camera as illustrated in the figure, a 0° camera is normally used. A 12-mm conventional laparoscopic assistant trocar is inserted in a paraumbilical site, while a 5-mm port is placed caudally to the 12-mm trocar towards the pubic symphysis. The 5-mm port is usually used for the suction insertion and the 12-mm port for insertion of clips and staplers. The use of three robotic arms is usually sufficient for the performance of the majority of upper urinary tract surgeries.

Option 4: Lateral trocar placement of three robotic arms for right-sided surgery

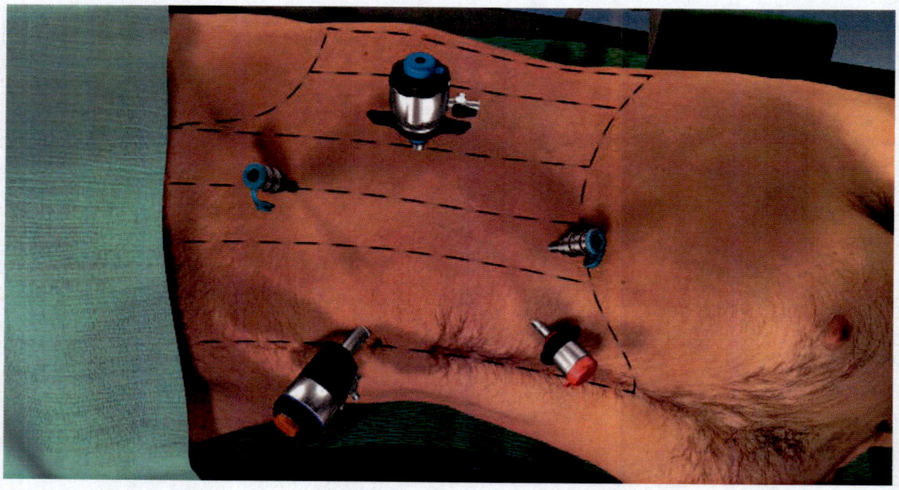

The robotic camera and working ports are inserted in the same site as the afore-mentioned left-sided surgery configuration with utilisation of three robotic arms. The conventional laparoscopic ports used by the assistant are placed paraumbilically (12 mm) and below the xiphoid. Through the latter trocar, a fan retractor or laparoscopic grasper is inserted for liver retraction. The three-arm robotic system is sufficient for kidney surgery. When performing a pyeloplasty, it is very useful to have a fourth robotic arm to facilitate retraction when performing ureteropelvic junction anastomosis. In pyeloplasties, the 5-mm xiphoid instrument could be avoided.

Option 5: Paraumbilical trocar placement of four robotic arms for left-sided surgery

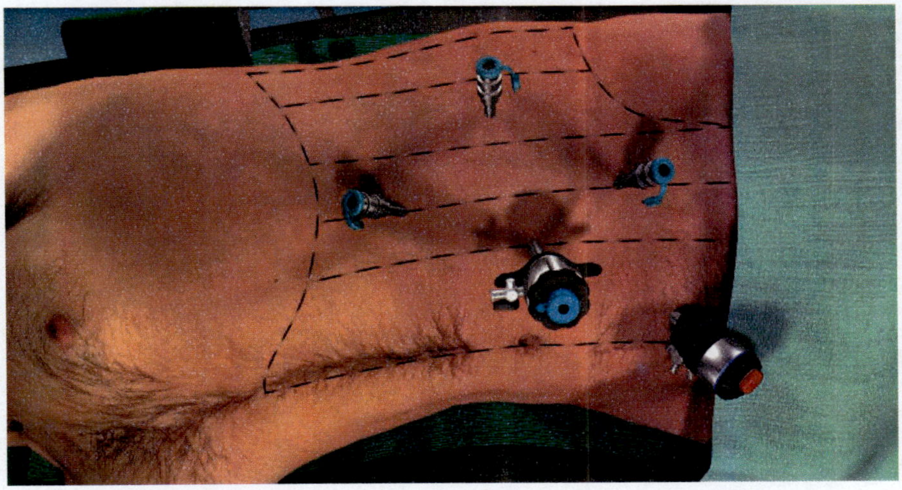

The most commonly used site for camera trocar placement for robotic upper urinary tract surgery is on the lateral margin of the rectus muscle sheath. Most cases of robotic partial, donor and radical nephrectomy have been performed using this trocar placement configuration. The two working trocars are inserted on the midclavicular line, while the trocar for the fourth arm is positioned between the anterior and midaxillary line, as shown in the figure. A 12-mm assistant trocar is placed on the middle or pararectal line near the pubic bone. Care should be taken to minimise collision between the robotic and assistant's instruments.

Option 6: Paraumbilical trocar placement of four robotic arms for right-sided surgery

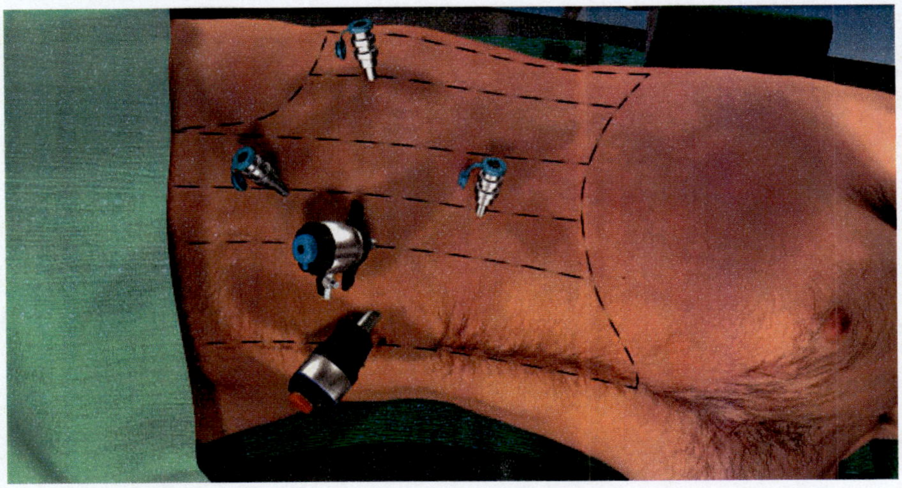

The positioning of the robotic trocars is similar to Option 5. Nevertheless, the 12-mm conventional laparoscopic port controlled by the assistant is positioned either at the level of the umbilicus or more caudally towards the pubic bone. The latter trocar is used for the insertion of large-bore instruments such as staplers, clip applicators and endobags. An additional 5- or 3-mm trocar is often used under the xiphoid for liver retraction. As previously mentioned, this is particularly useful in nephrectomies and partial nephrectomies, facilitating upper pole exposure. When performing pyeloplasties, the latter trocar is rarely needed.

Option 7: Paraumbilical trocar placement of three robotic arms for left-sided surgery

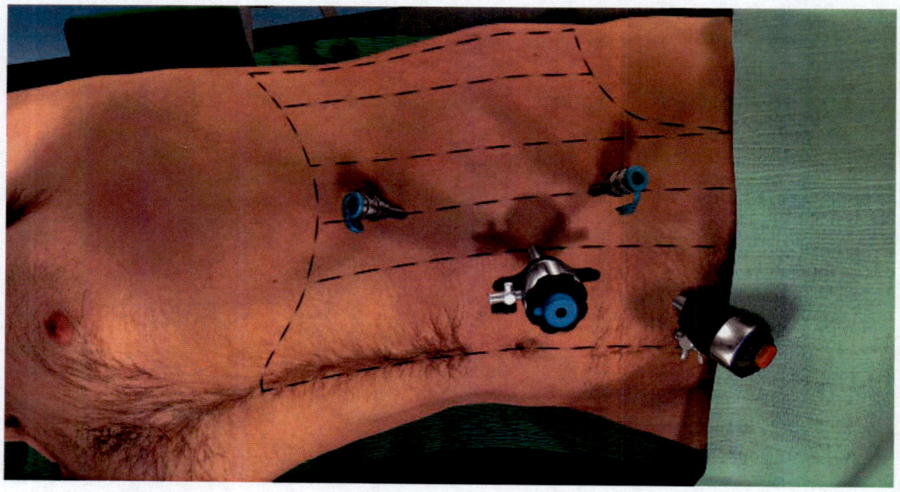

Left-sided surgery using the three-arm robotic system does not require any additional conventional laparoscopic trocars in comparison to a four-arm robotic system. The camera is placed on the lateral margin of the rectus muscle while the two working trocars are positioned on the midclavicular line. The 12-mm laparoscopic trocar is placed on the same imaginary line to the camera caudally near the pubic bone. Although it seems that the three-arm system requires fewer trocars, the use of additional 5-mm laparoscopic trocars may be deemed necessary. The insertion of these ports is based on the surgeon's preference.

Option 8: Paraumbilical trocar placement of three robotic arms for right-sided surgery

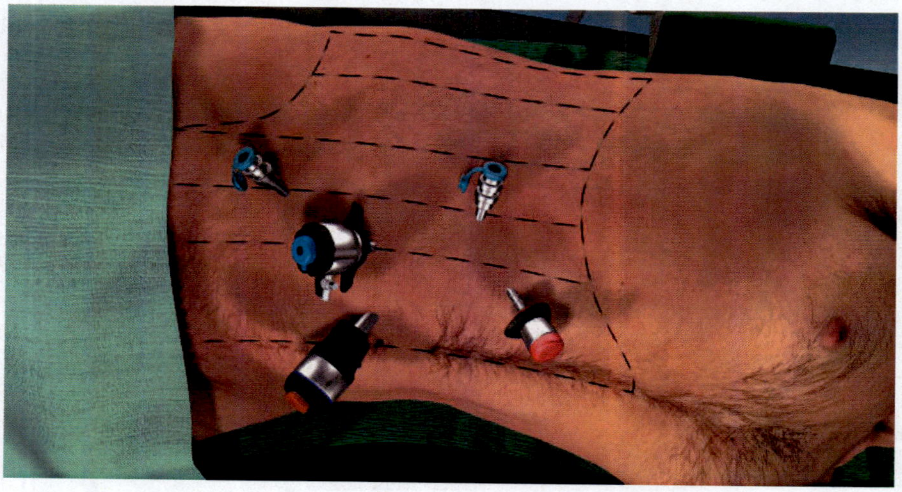

The retraction of the liver is important in right-sided surgery. Thus, the right-sided approach requires the insertion of a 5-mm conventional laparoscopic trocar below the xiphoid. The robotic camera, the working trocar and the assistant 12-mm trocars are on the same sites as the left-sided approach presented in Option 7. The use of all five trocars is the most appropriate for right-sided surgery. When the assistant trocar is positioned paraumbilically, as shown in the figure, there might be collisions with the robotic camera trocar during the operation. If that happens, it is suggested to move the assistant trocar caudally.

Option 9: Umbilical trocar placement of four robotic arms for left-sided surgery

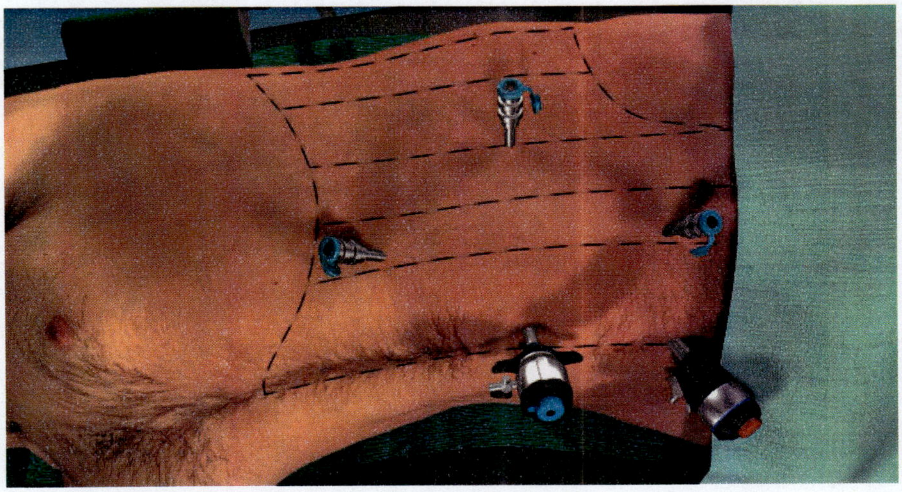

The insertion of the robotic camera trocar at the umbilicus has been described, especially in cases of robot-assisted pyeloplasty. Cameras carrying 30° lenses are used to carry out the procedure. The working trocars are positioned on the midclavicular line; one trocar is placed below the costal margin and the other at the level of the iliac spina. The trocar for the fourth robotic arm is inserted on the anterior axillary line. A 12-mm assistance trocar should be placed on the midline caudally to the camera trocar. Moving the camera trocar at the umbilicus reduces collisions with the remaining robotic trocars.

Option 10: Umbilical trocar placement of four robotic arms for right-sided surgery

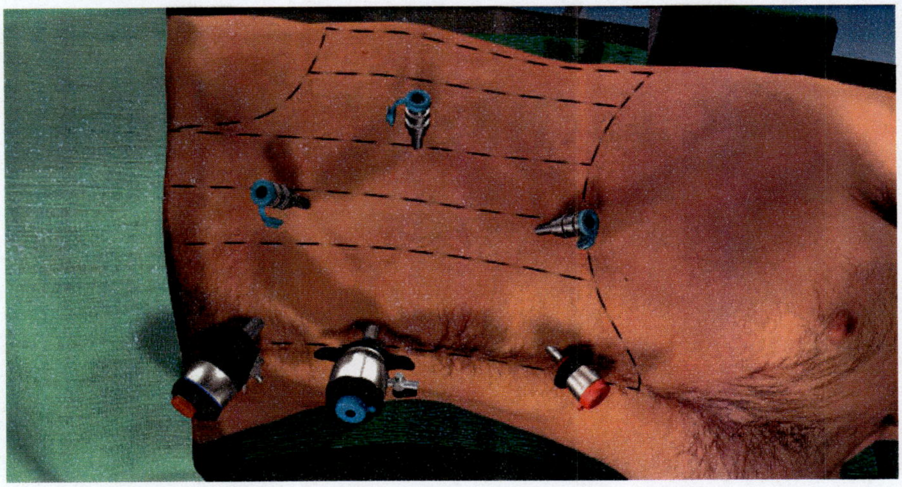

The insertion of the camera and working trocars mirrors the configuration of the umbilical approach for left-sided surgery presented in Option 9. The 12-mm assistant trocar is placed at the same site as in the left-sided surgery. Through an additional 5-mm conventional laparoscopic trocar, an instrument is inserted for liver retraction. The latter trocar is placed below the xiphoid. Use of the four-arm system facilitates the performance of kidney surgery as the fourth arm is used for retraction purposes. Retraction should be performed with great caution because organs such as vessels and the adjacent bowel could be inadvertently injured.

Option 11: Umbilical trocar placement of three robotic arms for left-sided surgery

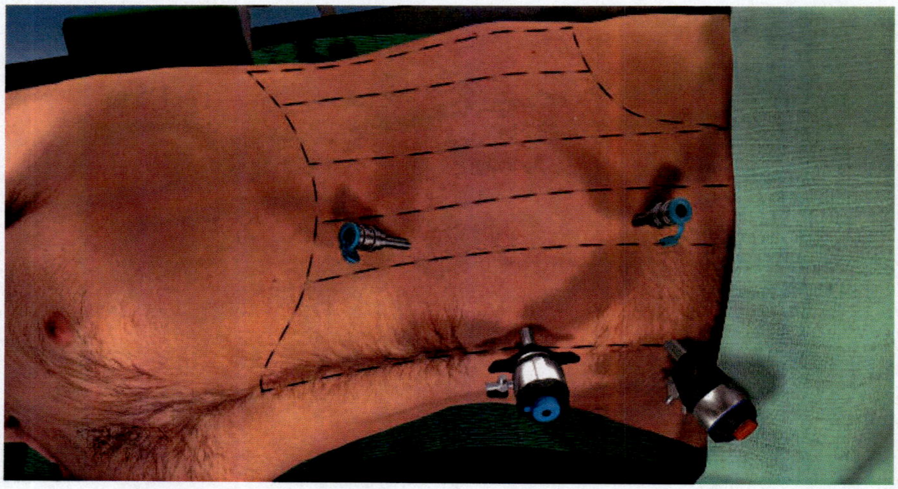

The camera is inserted at the umbilicus. The two robotic trocars are positioned on the midclavicular line while an assistant trocar (12 mm) is inserted on the midline near the pubic bone. Additional trocars and instruments could be inserted if deemed necessary. Performing radical and donor nephrectomy usually does not require the use of more than four trocars unless there is bleeding and continuous use of the suction device is required. Nevertheless, partial nephrectomy and pyeloplasty involve suturing very delicate structures and use of additional trocars should be considered.

Option 12: Umbilical trocar placement of three robotic arms for right-sided surgery

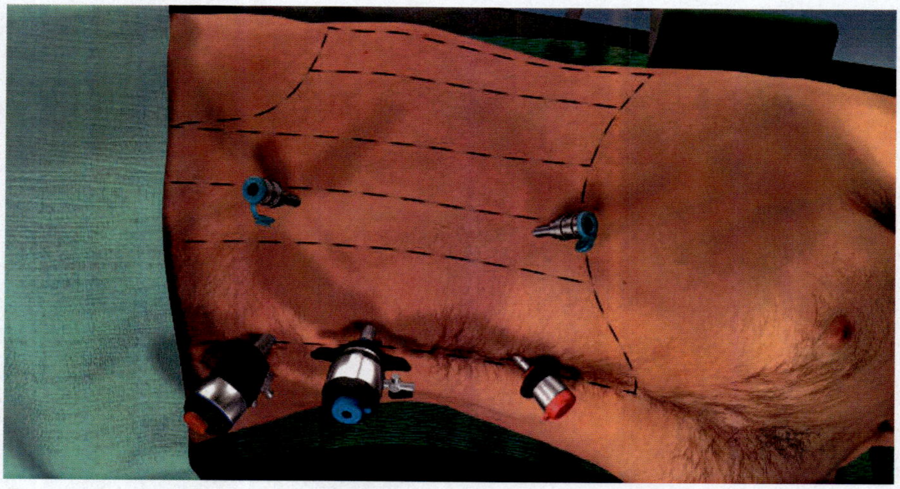

Placement of the ports for the three robotic arms and the insertion site of the 12-mm assistance trocar mirrors the configuration of the left-sided approach (Option 11). The additional 5-mm port for liver retraction is inserted at the usual site below the xiphoid. Often the 12-mm assistant trocar needs to be moved more caudally than shown in the figure to avoid clashing instruments inside the abdominal cavity. If the camera trocar and the 12-mm trocar are in close vicinity, then the Endo-GIA or the clip appliers may collide with the optics. This collision could lead to a cumbersome and/or dangerous approach to the renal hilum.

References

1. Hemal AK, Kumar A (2009) A prospective comparison of laparoscopic and robotic radical nephrectomy for T1-2N0M0 renal cell carcinoma. World J Urol 27:89–94
2. Ljungberg B, Hanbury DC, Kuczyk MA, Merseburger AS et al (2007) Renal cell carcinoma guidelines. Eur Urol 51:1502–1510
3. Aron M, Gill IS (2007) Minimally invasive nephron-sparing surgery (MINSS) for renal tumors. Part I: laparoscopic partial nephrectomy. Eur Urol 51:337–347
4. Singh I (2009) Robot-assisted laparoscopic partial nephrectomy: current review of the technique and literature. J Minim Access Surg 5:87–92
5. Atalla MA, Dovey Z, Kavoussi LR (2010) Laparoscopic versus robotic pyeloplasty: man versus machine. Expert Rev Med Devices 7:27–34

1.4.2 Setup of da Vinci System for Kidney Surgery

Evangelos Liatsikos, Panagiotis Kallidonis, Ingolf Tuerk, Christopher Anderson, Harry Beerlage, Jens-Uwe Stolzenburg

Step 1: Docking of the robotic camera arm

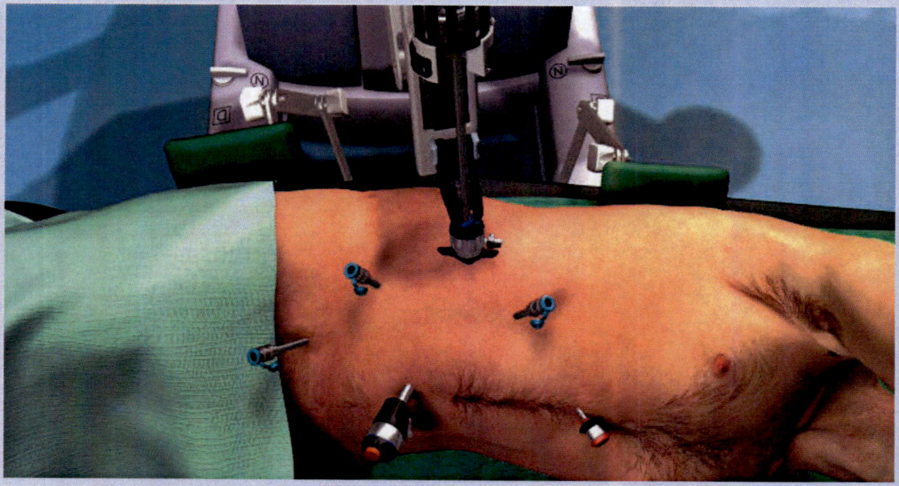

The standard process for the self-diagnostic test, initial calibration and checking the functionality of the system is followed. The draping process is described in the robotic setup for robot-assisted laparoscopic radical prostatectomy and cystectomy. The camera arm is placed first. Zero and 30° optics are used according to the surgeon's preference. When the camera trocar is positioned laterally, as shown in the figure, most surgeons prefer the 0° lens. After docking the camera arm, extra traction can be exerted by the robotic instrument on the abdominal wall, further expanding the available working space.

Step 2: Docking of the second robotic instrument

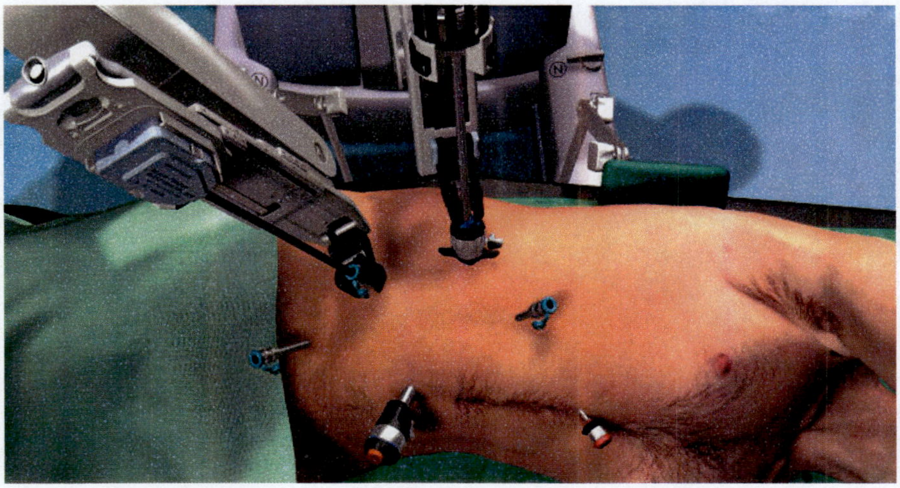

The second robotic instrument is docked according to the surgeon's preference. There is no difference in docking the right or left working instruments. It is important to ensure that the robotic arm is adequately connected to the trocar. The assistant and the nurses need to be alert at all times during docking so that the robotic arms do not exert pressure on any of the patient's body segments. Such compression could become problematic and could generate unexpected injuries. Once the trocar is connected with the robotic arm, the entire unit (arm and trocar) is retracted to its final position.

Step 3: Docking of the third robotic instrument

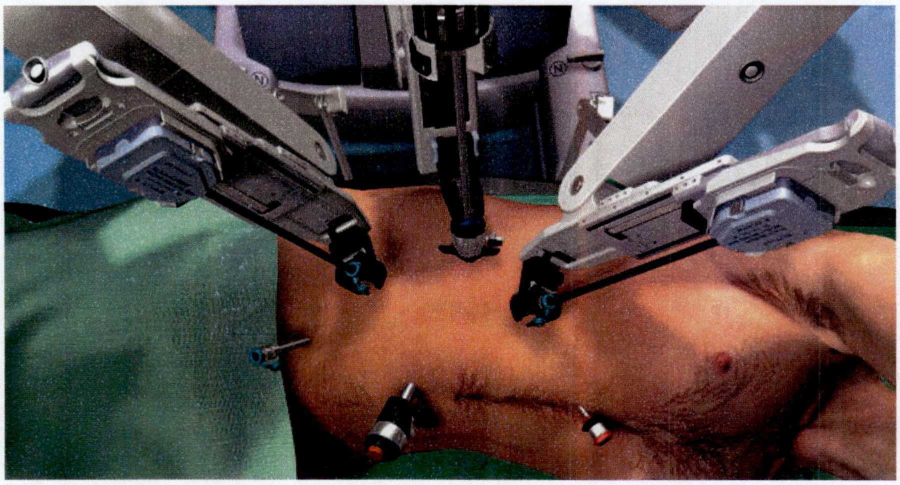

The third robotic arm is docked in a similar fashion as the previous one. In the figure, the third arm is connected to the right subcostal trocar. It is important that this trocar not be inserted in the immediate proximity of the costal margin to void compression trauma to the costal cage itself. It should be emphasised that the surgeon needs to always be alert when inserting the trocars and docking the robotic arms, avoiding injuries to the patient and securing the maximal range of movement for the robotic arms. If the trocar is inserted in an incorrect fashion, one should not hesitate to reposition it before docking the robotic arm.

Step 4: Docking of the fourth robotic instrument

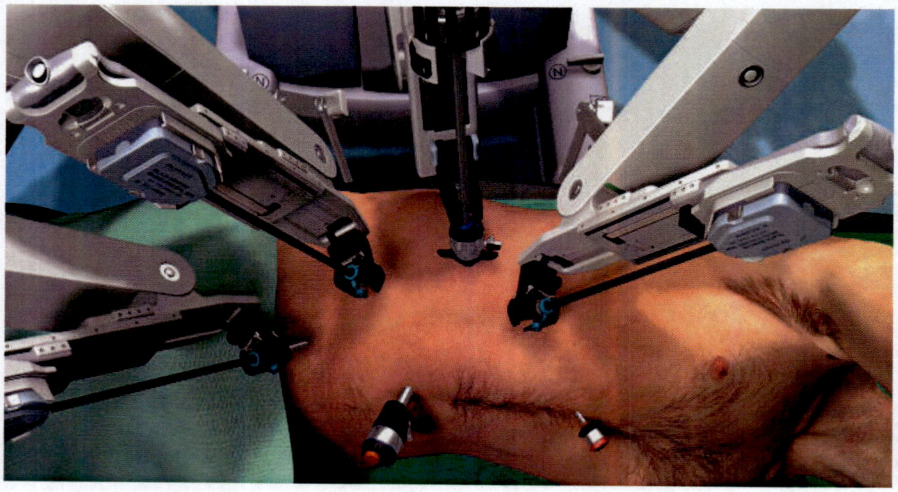

Final disposition of the four robotic arms is now described. The fourth robotic arm should be docked last of all, providing an angle that enables adequate working space for its neighboring arm. It is important to note that the fourth arm is more static than the other arms because it is mainly used for retraction. When docking the fourth arm, one needs to keep in mind that it needs to be away from the main operative field. Finally, the 12-mm trocar inserted in the umbilicus is used by the assistant. An additional 3- or 5-mm trocar is often used for liver retraction when working on the right side.

Step 5: Final robotic setup. Anterior view

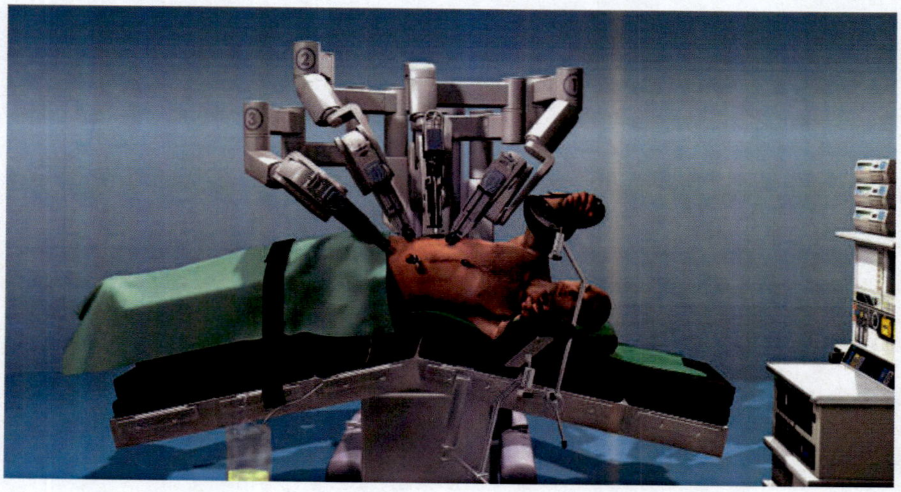

The robotic system is placed for surgical docking on the patient's ventral side. The flexed operating table provides greater space for the robotic arms, thus avoiding their collision. It is extremely important that once the robotic system is docked, the patient's position on the table cannot be changed. In addition, the table cannot be rotated when the robot is docked. If the surgeon needs to change either the patient's position or redirect the operating table, then the robotic system needs to be undocked. When the final patient position is achieved, the system can be redocked and the operation can proceed. The surgeon should ensure that the patient position is the correct one before docking the system to avoid inadvertent delays.

Step 6: Final robotic setup. Operating room overview

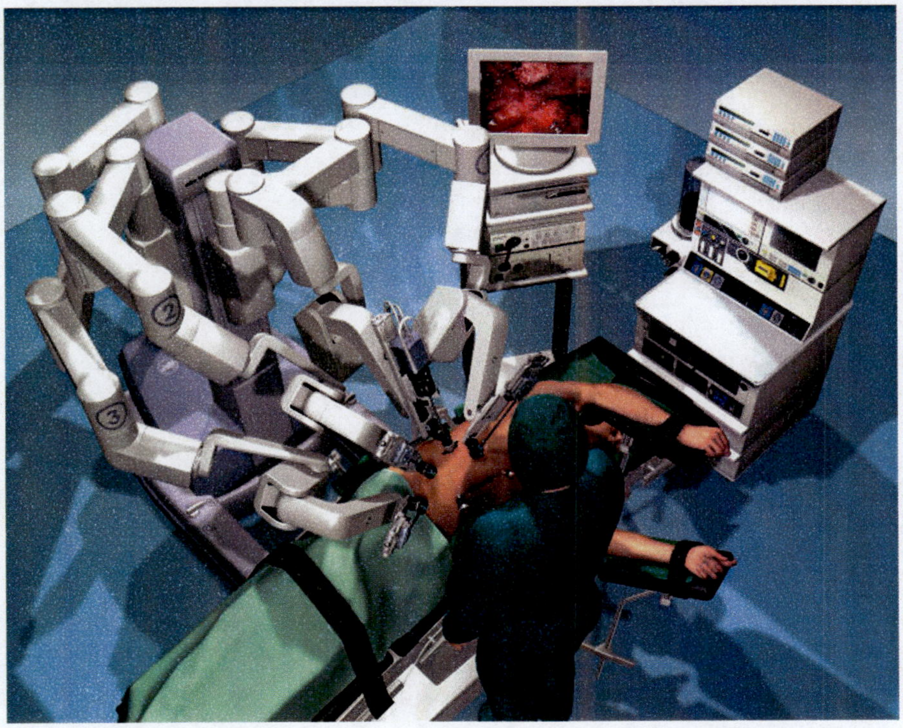

After all arms are activated, the system is ready for performing the procedure. The robotic system is docked over the patient coming over his back side. The figure shows the entire aspect of the operative setup for upper urinary tract surgery. The endoscopic monitor could be positioned on either side of the robotic unit. Most surgeons prefer to position it cephalad to the patient (i.e. in vicinity of the anaesthesia unit), as shown in the figure. When using a fourth robotic arm, it is cumbersome for the assistant to see the monitor if it is positioned caudal to the patient side of the robotic unit.

1.5 Nephropexy

Minh Do, Panagiotis Kallidonis, Rowan Casey, Tony Riddek, Anja Dietel, Holger Till, Phuc Ho Thi, Tim Haefner, Ian Dunn, Evangelos Liatsikos, Jens-Uwe Stolzenburg

Introduction

Nephroptosis is defined as significant displacement of the kidney (>5 cm, or two vertebral bodies), as the patient moves from the supine to erect position [1]. Although common, only the minority of cases are symptomatic. Typical symptoms are loin pain, with haematuria and urinary tract infections seen less commonly. Young thin females are the most common symptomatic patients. Recognition of the condition in the late nineteenth century led to widespread popularisation of nephropexy as a surgical technique. However, the procedure was discredited by the early twentieth century because poor patient selection led to a high rate of unsatisfactory outcomes and complications. More recently, there has been recognition of this disorder as a valid clinical entity [2]. Stricter diagnostic criteria, more robust investigative techniques, and the availability of minimally invasive surgical treatment options have led to a resurgence of nephropexy in carefully selected cases.

We recommend that other than clinical symptoms, the diagnosis of nephroptosis requires the detection of significant renal descent, as described above, and the finding of ureteric obstruction or diminished arterial inflow [3]. This can be achieved using ultrasonography and colour-Doppler imaging, IVU, CT scanning or radionuclide scanning [4]. Whether the procedure is performed open or laparoscopically, the principles remain the same. The kidney must be exposed within the Gerota fascia, it must be immobilised in a more cephalad retroperitoneal position, any associated obstruction should be relieved, and the renal axis must be fixed without tension.

Indications

- All symptomatic cases of nephroptosis with supporting objective radiological evidence

Contra-indications

- No specific contraindications are raised

Preoperative Preparation

- DVT prophylaxis as per local guidelines
- Empty urinary bladder (urinary catherisation if necessary)
- Single-shot broad-spectrum antibiotics

1

Step 1: Patient position and trocar placement

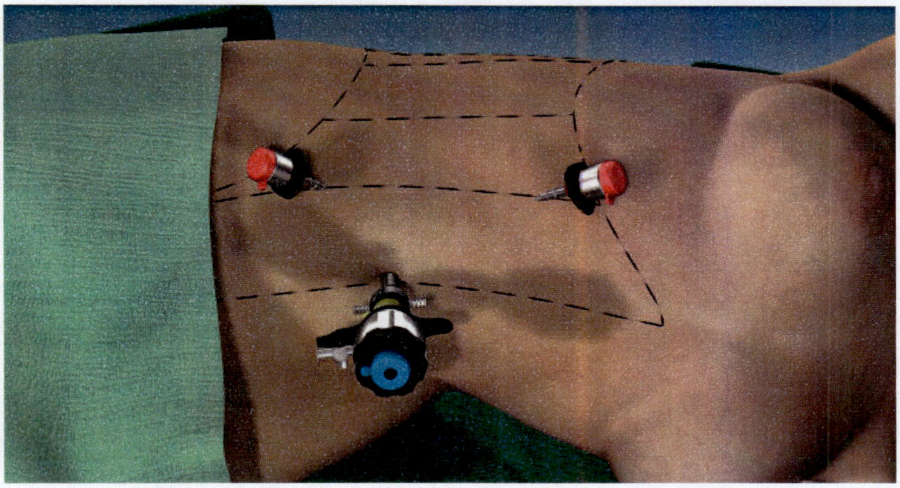

As detailed in Sect. 1.1, the patient is positioned in the lateral position with the operating table flexed. An umbilical 10- to 12-mm trocar is placed for the laparoscope. We prefer using the Hassan type trocar because we perform minilaparotomy to gain access to the abdominal cavity. CO_2 insufflation, to a pressure of 12 mmHg is commenced. Standard trocar placement is to insert two 5-mm ports on the pararectal line above the iliac crest and below the costal margin as shown in Step 1. Nephropexy is also ideally suited to single-port surgery (laparoendoscopic single-site surgery, LESS).

Step 2: Landmarks and mobilisation of the colon

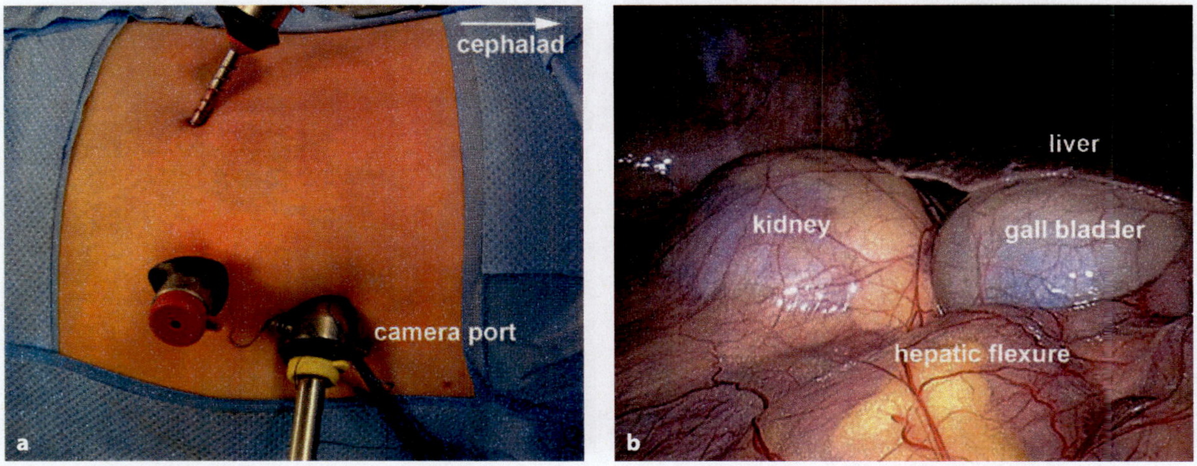

Alternatively, a slightly different port placement can be used as shown in Step 2a. On the right side, this allows additional 5-mm port placement below the costal margin to retract the liver without clashing (surgeon, two working instruments from below; assistant, camera and one forceps to retract the liver). Most nephropexy patients are female and thin, as shown in Step 2b. It should also be noted that there is a paucity of intra-abdominal fat in this typical patient. The anatomical landmarks are easy to identify.

Step 3: Exposure of structures for "pexing"

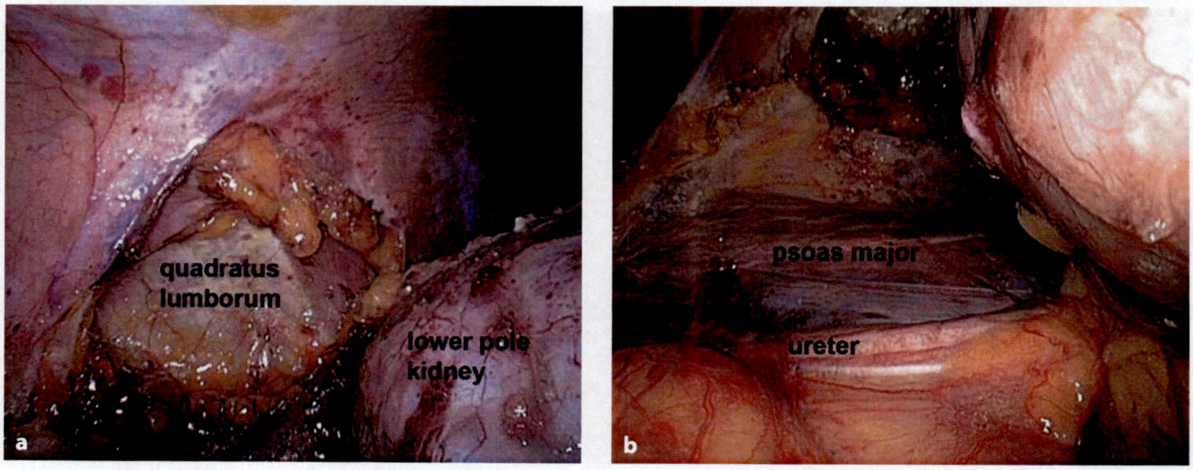

An extra 5-mm port placement to assist was not necessary here. The whole procedure could be performed with two working and one optical trocar. The peritoneum lateral to the kidney is incised to allow exposure of quadratus lumborum, to which the kidney will be "pexed" (Step 3a). The peritoneum over the lower pole of the kidney is also incised, and this incision continued inferiorly to expose the psoas major muscle (Step 3b), with the ureter located here. Exposure of these structures possibly requires extended mobilisation of the colon from the level of iliac vessels to the colonic flexure.

Step 4: First suture placement

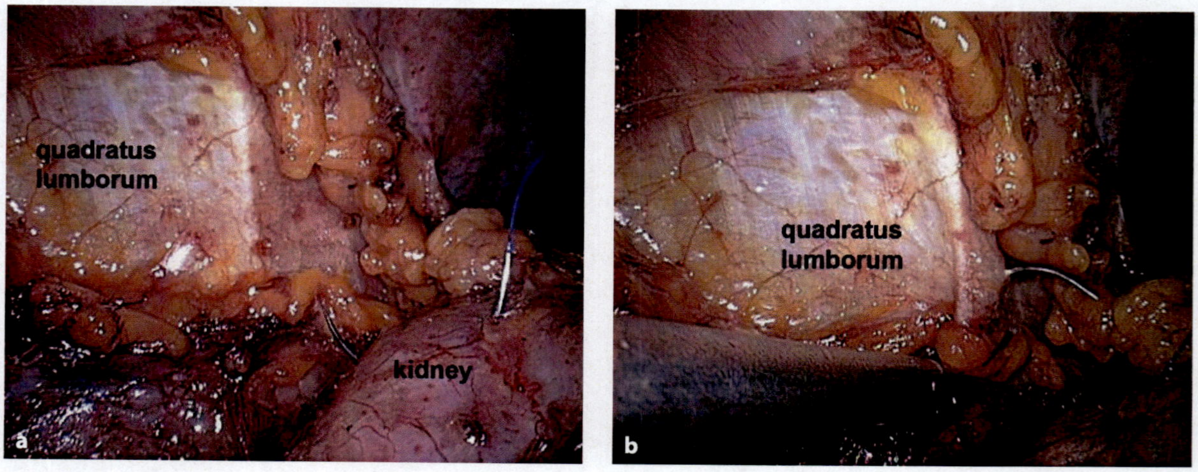

The Gerota fascia must also be opened to allow dissection of perinephric fat from the renal capsule. The perinephric fat is dissected from the anterior and lateral aspects of the kidney, exposing the capsule (Step 4a). To fix the kidney, a minimum of three sutures should be placed and the patient must be placed in a head-down position (about 10–15°). The superolateral aspect of the kidney is sutured to the fascia overlying quadratus lumborum using nonabsorbable 3/0 nylon suture in order to elevate to kidney to a more secure posterolateral position within the retroperitoneum (Step 4b).

Step 5: Second suture placement

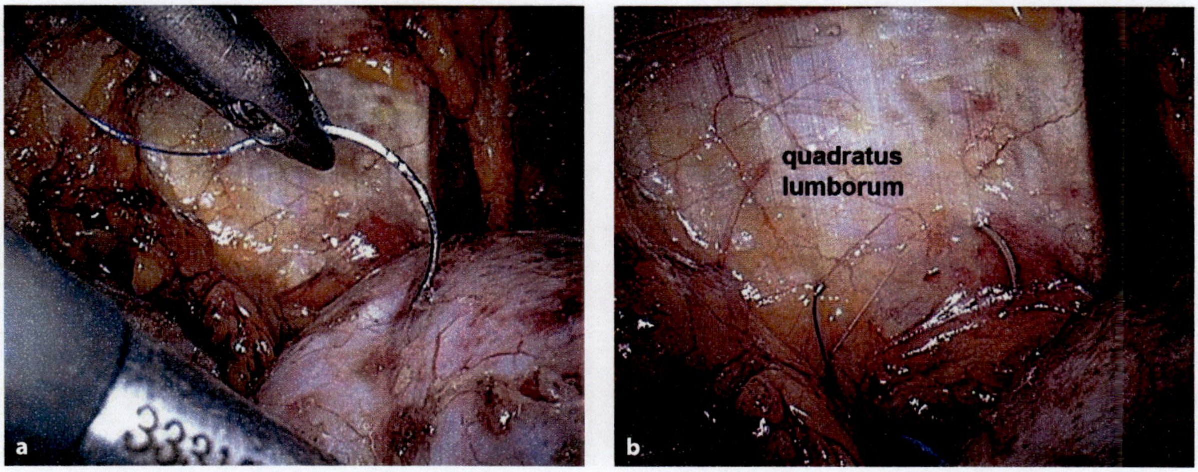

The second lateral suture is placed inferiorly to the first suture. It is placed through sufficient renal capsule laterally and quadratus lumborum fascia in order to provide additional security for the first suture. Both sutures should provide contact between the raw surfaces of both the renal capsule and quadratus lumborum fascia to allow fibrous adhesion tissue to eventually form.

Step 6: Third suture placement

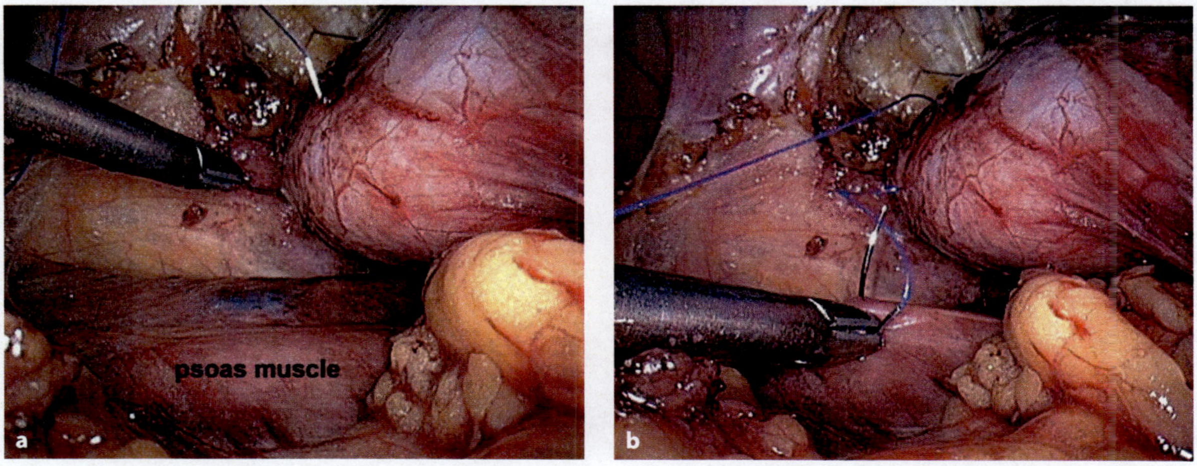

The final suture is placed from the lower pole of the kidney to the body of the psoas major muscle. The suture must be taken sufficiently deep through both structures to prevent the suture from cutting through. This suture which provides additional stability and prevents the lower pole of the kidney from rotating forwards on its vascular pedicle, along with upper sutures provide three-point fixation. It is essential to ensure that the ureter is visualised and protected prior to suturing.

Step 7: Final inspection

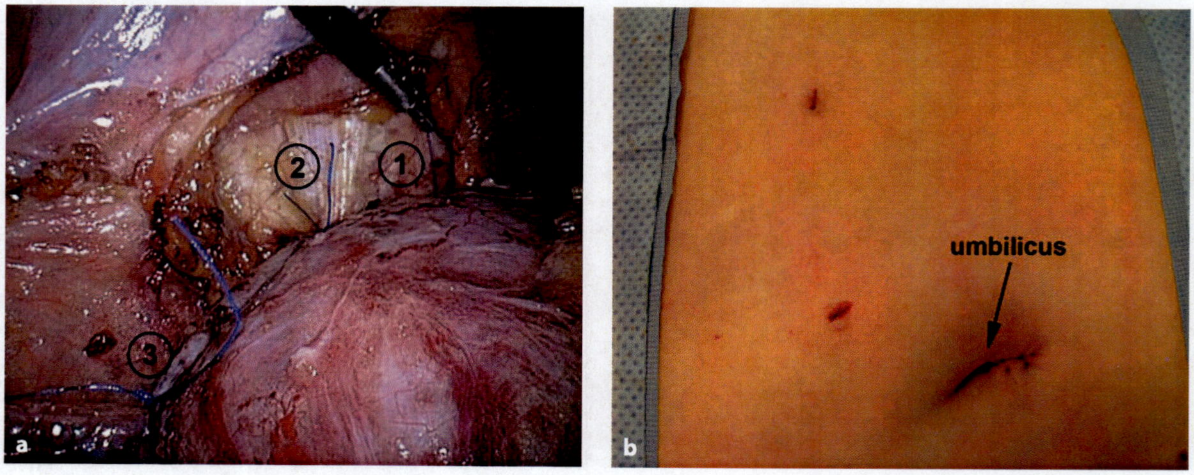

The three sutures placed can be seen "pexing" the kidney superolaterally and inferiorly (Step 7a). The surgical field is inspected for bleeding, which is rarely a problem. There is no need to place a surgical drain following this procedure. The anterior rectus fascia of the optic port site is closed with subcutaneous absorbable sutures, and the skin wounds are closed with subcuticular absorbable sutures (Step 7b).

Postoperative Management

- DVT prophylaxis until mobile
- Bed rest until day 3 to reduce the risk of suture rupture and increase perinephric adhesions
- Oral analgesia is administered as required
- Oral diet and fluids can be re-introduced as tolerated

References

1. Fornara P, Doehn C, Jocham D (1997) Laparoscopic nephropexy: 3-year experience. J Urol 158: 1679–1683
2. Barber NJ, Thompson PM (2004) Nephroptosis and nephropexy-hung up on the past? Eur Urol 46:428–433
3. Bishoff JT, Kavoussi LR (2007) Laparoscopic surgery of the kidney. In Walsh PC, Retik AB, Vaughan ED, Wein AJ (eds) Campbell's Urology, 9th edn., Chapter 51
4. Srirangam, SJ, Pollard AJ, Adeyoju AA, O'Reilly PH (2009) Nephroptosis: seriously misunderstood? BJU International. 103:296–300

1.6 Laparoscopic Endoscopic Single-Site Surgery (LESS): Renal Cyst Deroofing

Minh Do, Rowan Casey, Robert Mills, Anja Dietel, Holger Till, Evangelos Liatsikos, Jens-Uwe Stolzenburg

Introduction

Approximately 36% of the population have simple renal cysts by their eighth decade [1]. These are now detected because of the increased use of abdominal ultrasound and computed tomography in patients undergoing genitourinary assessment or as part of abdominal pain work-up.

A symptomatic large renal cyst dealt with by single session aspiration with or without sclerosant therapy has unacceptably high recurrence rates. Given the major developments in minimally invasive laparoscopic surgery in the last 10 years, laparoscopic cyst deroofing and ablation is now considered a significant advancement on previous decompression techniques [2, 3].

LESS surgery (laparoscopic-endoscopic single-site surgery) is a further development of laparoscopic surgery. It is ideally suited to renal cyst deroofing because of its low level of technical complexity.

Indications

- Symptomatic simple type-1 Bosniak renal or parapelvic cyst (usually larger than 5 cm)

Contra-indications

- Asymptomatic renal cysts
- Renal cysts greater than Bosniak 1 classification
- Severe respiratory or cardiac co-morbidities
- Morbid obesity

Preoperative Preparation

- Full history and examination to exclude other causes of patient symptoms
- Trial of aspiration to determine whether this relieves symptoms
- IVP or ureteral retrograde study to rule out calyceal diverticulum

Step 1: Patient position and trocar placement

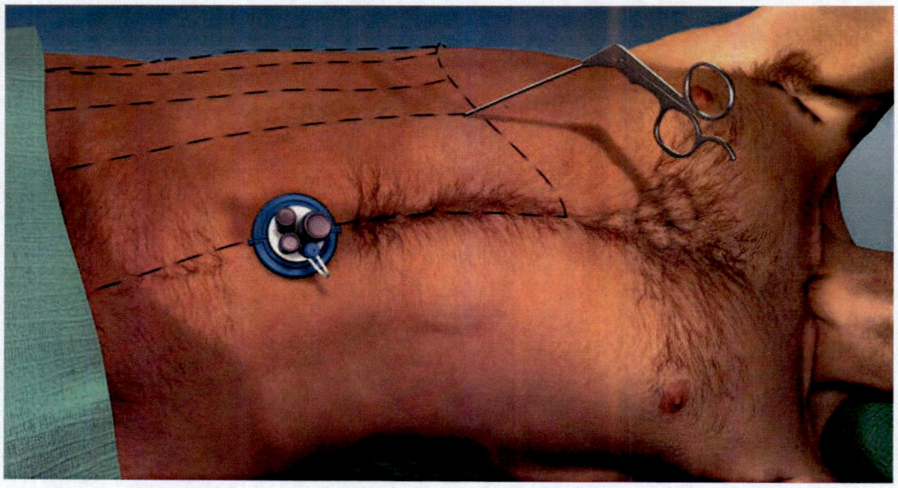

The patient position is fully described in Sect. 1.1. The TriPort (Olympus, USA) is inserted transperitoneally through the umbilicus, as described in Sect. 1.2.1. CO_2 insufflation is commenced to a pressure of 10–12 mmHg.

If necessary, a 3-mm needlescopic grasper is inserted percutaneously, without the need of a trocar, below the costal margin along the pararectal line to allow liver or splenic retraction.

Step 2: Instruments for LESS

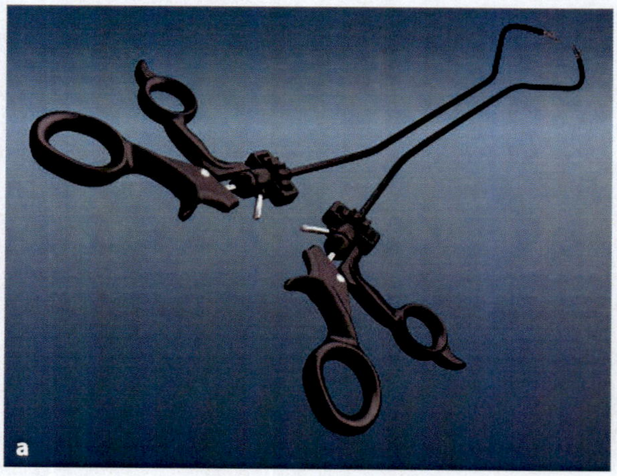

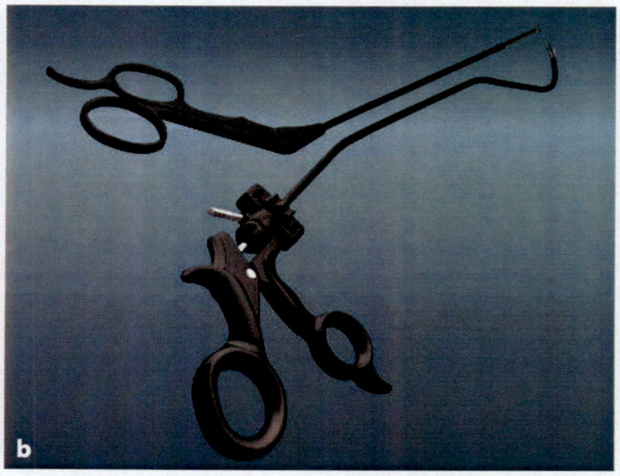

The single-port technique does not provide the potential for triangulation of the instruments used. Innovative instruments have been designed in an attempt to overcome this difficulty. Intraoperative ergonomic issues such as instrument clashing and crossing are significantly minimised by the use of prebent instruments.

Therefore, for LESS we recommend the use of two prebent instruments (Step 2a) or one prebent and one straight instrument (Step 2b).

Step 3: Exposure of the right kidney

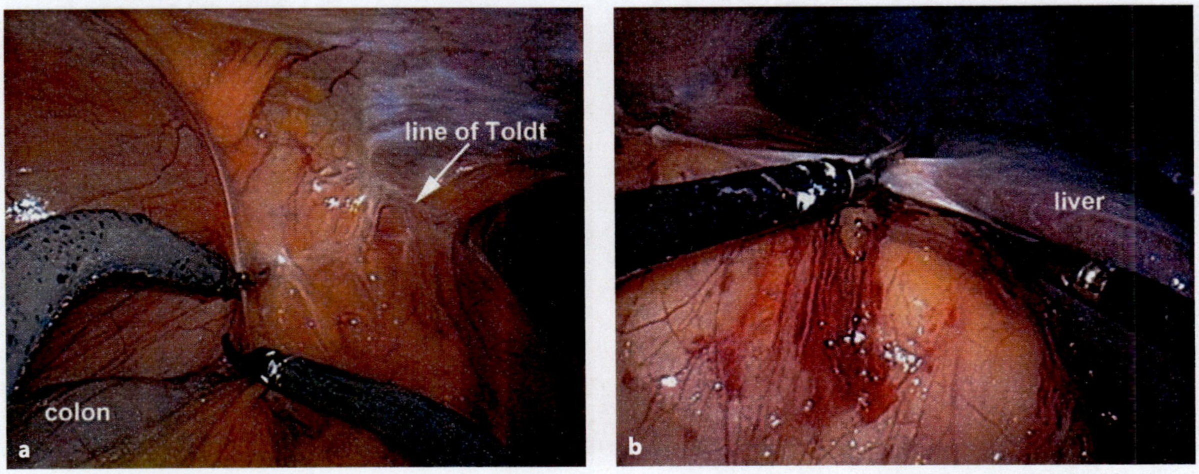

The upper pole of the right kidney containing the cyst is exposed by incising along the white line of Toldt in order to release the hepatic flexure of the colon, which is then reflected (Step 3a). Incising the peritoneal attachments of the right lobe of the liver allows it to be reflected medially (Step 3b). This step of the procedure is performed with the help of two prebended instruments or one prebended instrument and one straigth instrument.

Step 4: Opening of Gerota fascia and exposure of the cyst surface

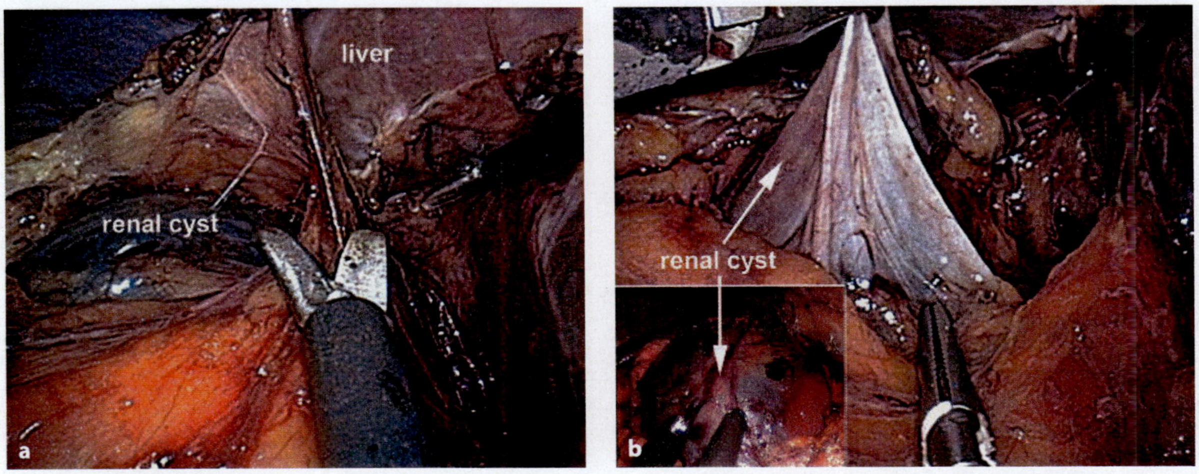

The Gerota fascia is incised and mobilised together with perinephric fat (Step 4a) until the entire surface of the cyst is exposed (inset, Step 4b). If the cyst is not readily apparent intraoperative ultrasound may be required. Depending on the position of the cyst, the kidney may need to be mobilised to see the full extent of the cyst. Once the surface of the cyst has been delineated, it is incised at the junction with the renal parenchyma and the fluid aspirated (Step 4b). This fluid can be sent for cytological analysis if necessary.

Step 5: Cyst deroofing and fulguration

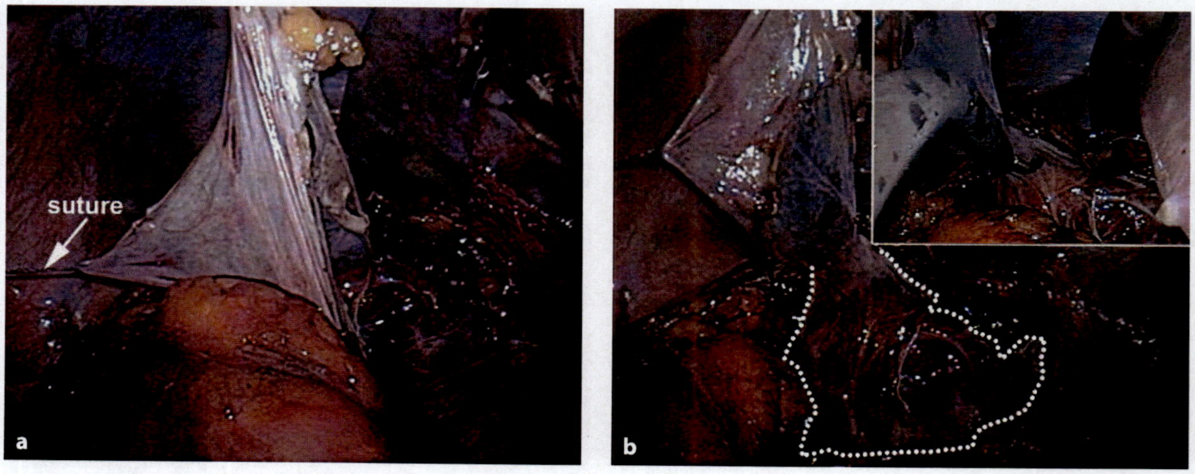

The cyst wall is detached by incising along the junction of the cyst wall with the renal parenchyma. If the cyst wall is very bulky one or two straight needles may be passed through the abdominal wall, through the cyst and back out through the abdominal wall under direct vision. Fixing the suture at the abdominal wall with a clamp aids further dissection by retracting the cyst wall out of the operative field (Step 5b). Step 5b shows the cyst wall just prior to detachment. The final incision is made using prebent scissors (inset, Step 5b).

Step 6: Specimen removal

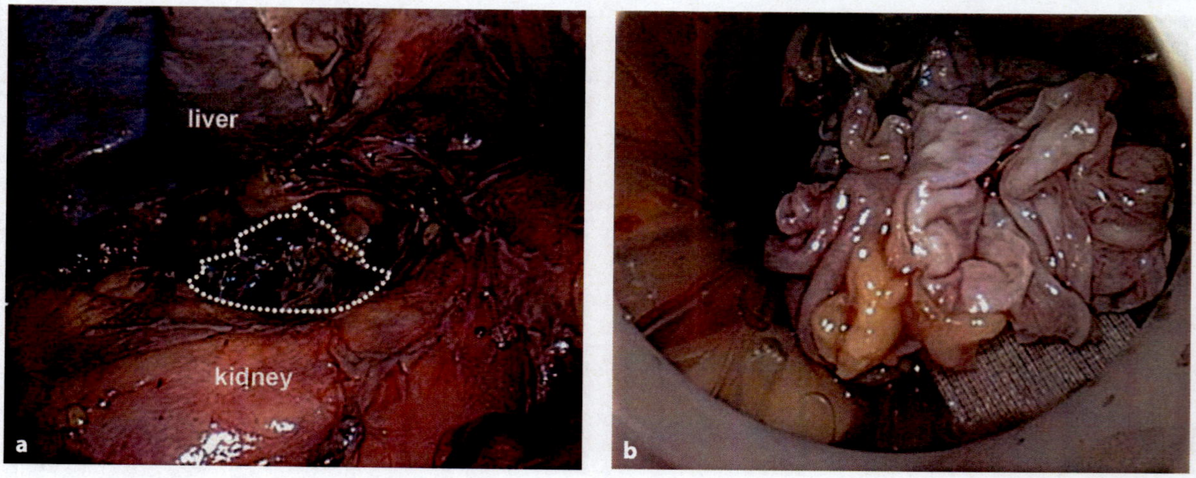

In the final operative view of the kidney, the cavity representing the intrarenal portion of the cyst is marked by the dotted line. The base of the cyst is then fulgurated. We suggest using the bipolar forceps for this step of the procedure. The cyst wall is easily removed via the TriPort and may be sent for histological analysis (Step 6b).

Postoperative Management

- Early mobilisation
- Remove urinary catheter (if inserted) on day 1
- Remove drain (if inserted) on day 1
- Normal activities on day 3

References

1. Terada N, Ichilka K, Matsuta Y, Okubo K, Yoshimura K, Arai Y (2002) The natural history of simple renal cysts. J Urol 167:21–23
2. Arisan S, Dalkilinc A, Caskurlu T, Sonmez N, Guney S, Ergenekon E (2006) Laparoscopic unroofing and aspiration-sclerotherapy in the management of symptomatic simple renal cysts. TSW Urology 6:2296–2301
3. Okeke AA, Mitchelmore AE, Keeley FX Jr, Timoney AG (2003) A comparison of aspiration and sclerotherapy with laparoscopic de-roofing in the management of symptomatic simple renal cysts. BJU Int 92:610–613

1.7 Transperitoneal Laparoscpic Nephrectomy

1.7.1 Simple Laparoscopic Nephrectomy

Minh Do, Rowan Casey, Evangelos Liatsikos, Anja Dietel, Panagiotis Kallidonis, Phuc Ho Thi, Michael Truss, Alan Mc Neill, Holger Till, Jens-Uwe Stolzenburg

Introduction

Simple laparoscopic nephrectomy was first described by Clayman and colleagues [1] in 1991 in a patient with an oncocytoma and since then has developed into the gold standard for minimally invasive surgical treatment of renal disease in properly selected patients.

In the modern era, simple laparoscopic nephrectomy has been demonstrated to be superior to open surgery in terms of analgesic requirements, cosmesis, length of hospital stay, blood loss and return to work [2]. The transperitoneal approach is more favoured by urological surgeons as the intra-abdominal anatomy is more familiar and provides more space than the retroperitoneal approach without any greater perioperative morbidity [3].

Indications

- Hydronephrotic kidneys from chronic PUJ obstruction
- Cystic dysplastic or nonfunctioning kidneys
- Chronically infected kidneys
- Renovascular hypertension

Contra-indications

Absolute Contra-indications

- Extensive intra-abdominal surgery
- Uncorrected coagulopathy
- Uncorrected sepsis
- Marked cardiorespiratory morbidity

Relative Contra-indications

- Perinephric inflammation (e.g. xanthogranulomatous pyelonephritis)
- Morbid obesity

Preoperative Preparation

- CT imaging
- Informed consent (conversion <5%)
- Urinary catheterisation
- Broad-spectrum antibiotic prophylaxis

Step 1: Trocar placement (right kidney)

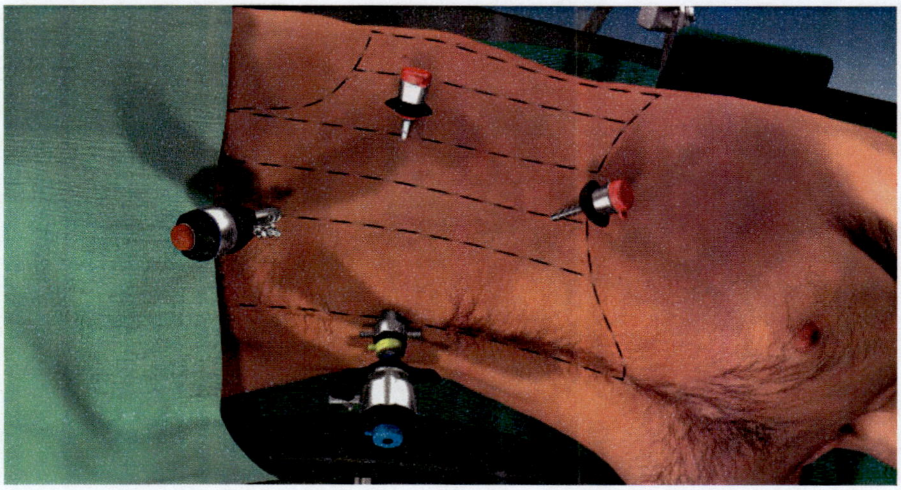

The pneumoperitoneum is created via minilaparotomy with an optical trocar inserted umbilically. CO_2 insufflation at 10–12 mmHg is commenced to allow additional trocars to be inserted under direct vision. As can be seen in Step 1, on the right side a 5-mm trocar is inserted in the midclavicular line just below the costal margin to allow the assistant to retract the liver. A 10- to 12-mm trocar is inserted along the pararectal line at the level of the anterior superior iliac spine and an additional 5-mm trocar is placed at the anterior axillary line above the anterior superior iliac crest.

Step 2: Alternative trocar placement (right kidney)

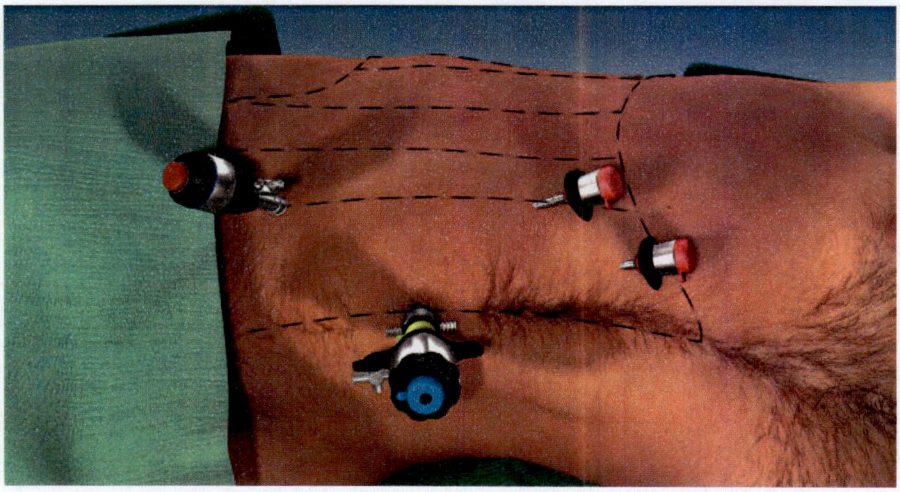

Some surgeons prefer another trocar arrangement to the one shown in this figure. The optical trocar is also placed in the umbilicus. The surgeon works with a 12-mm trocar, which is inserted along the pararectal line at the level of the anterior superior iliac spine, and a 5-mm trocar, which is inserted on the same line subcostally. This arrangement provides perfect triangulation for the surgeon. The assistant uses an additional 5-mm trocar inserted closer to the xiphisternum for retraction (liver) and suction.

Step 3: Trocar placement (left kidney)

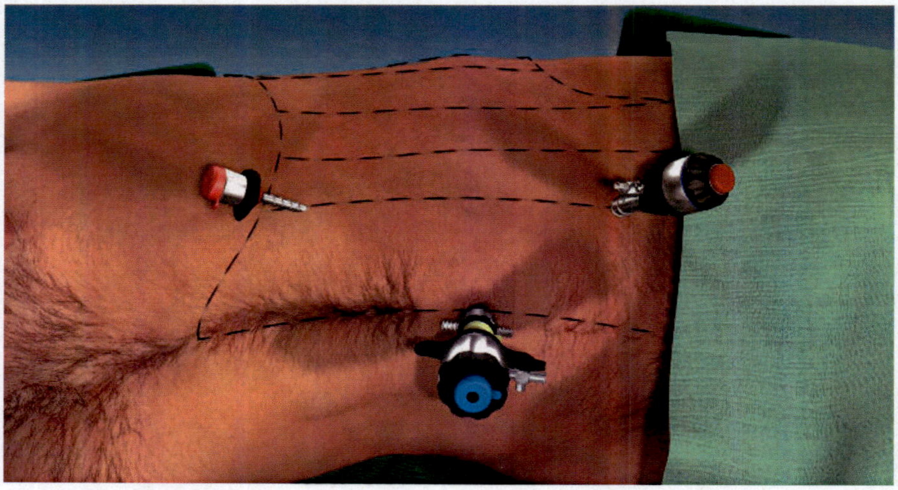

For a left nephrectomy, the same trocar arrangement as on the right side can be used. Using a four-trocar technique as on the right side allows the assistant to assist during the whole procedure with suction or a forceps. This figure demonstrates an alternative trocar placement for left nephrectomy. Especially experienced surgeons prefer to work only with two trocars (1×5 mm, 1×12 mm), which is possible in straightforward cases. In obese patients, the optical trocar is placed on the pararectal line rather than transumbilically and the other trocar positions are adjusted accordingly.

Step 4: Mobilisation of the colon

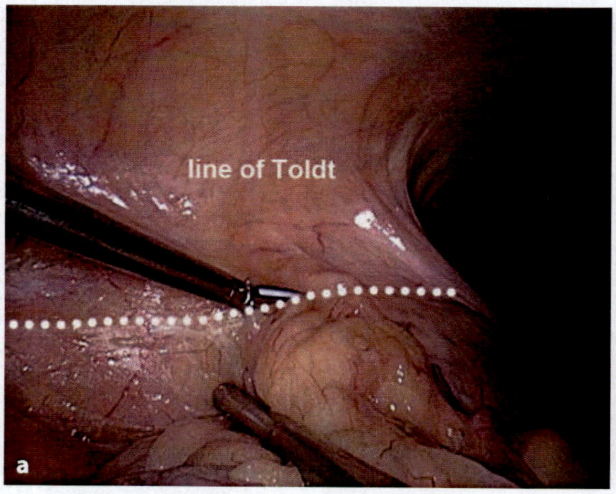

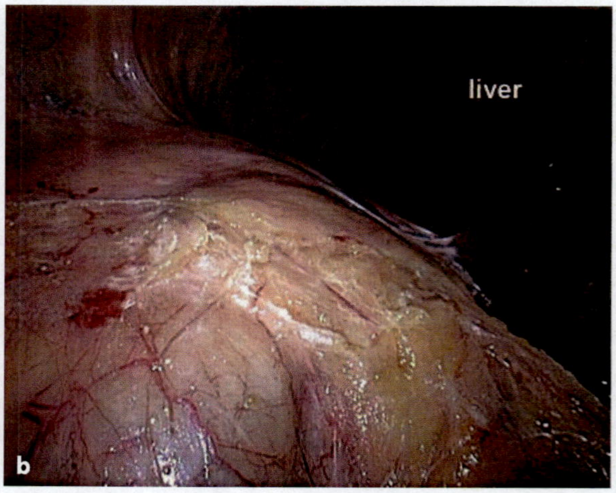

Incise the lateral colonic peritoneal reflection along the line of Toldt to just below the lower pole of the kidney. Leave the peritoneum attached to the lateral and superior pole of the kidney in order to prevent the kidney from falling forward during the procedure (Step 4b). Dissect up to the colonic flexure and either splenocolic or hepatocolic ligaments to allow further colon mobilisation. On the right side, "kocherise" the duodenum to expose the IVC. Injury to the small-bowel mesentery can be avoided by careful medial retraction of the colon and avoidance of too much electrocautery near this area.

Step 5: Ureteric mobilisation

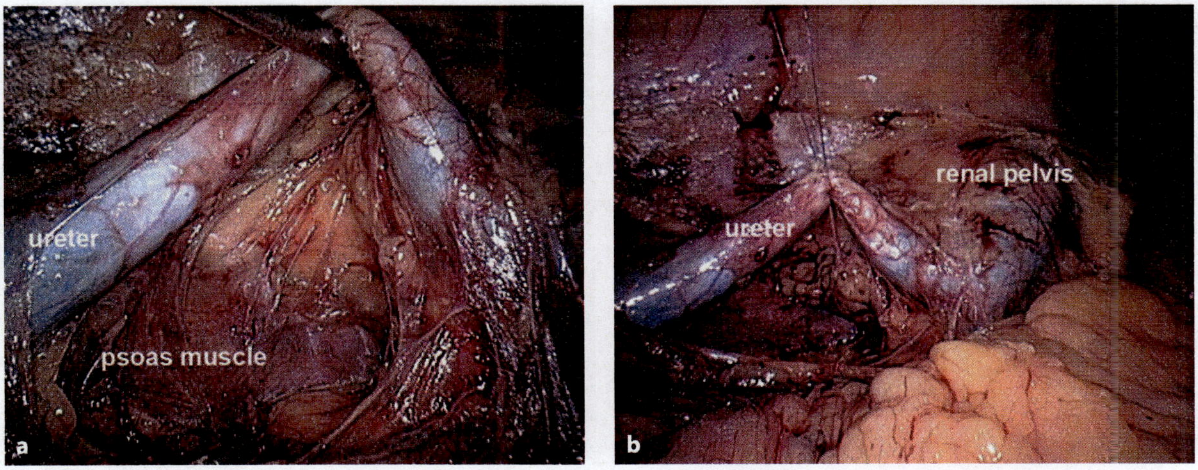

A window is created in the tissue posterior to the ureter (Step 5a). In order to aid proximal dissection of the ureter towards the lower pole, renal pelvis and hilar vessels, the ureter can be looped with a long straight needle passed through the anterior abdominal wall under laparoscopic vision. It is then grasped, passed under the ureter and brought up through the anterior abdominal wall beside its entry point and either sutured or clipped to the other suture end with as much tension as needed to elevate the ureter sufficiently (Step 5b). Once the ureter is elevated it can be dissected up to the lower pole of the kidney along the psoas fascia.

Step 6: Identification of the gonadal and renal vein

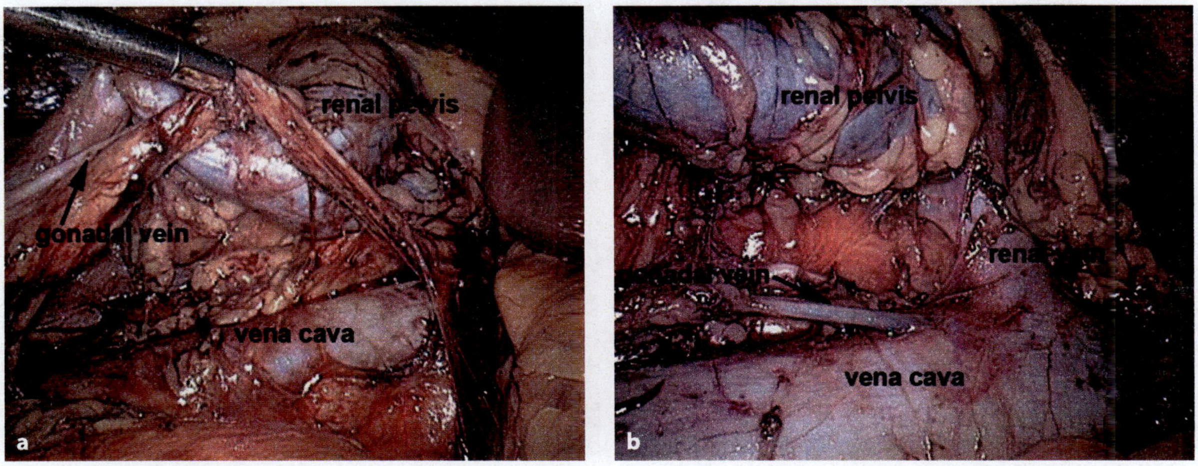

The next step is to identify the gonadal vein, which should lie anterior and lateral to the midureter. The gonadal vein, often surrounded by loose fatty tissue, can be elevated by a laparoscopic grasper and will help locate the ureter but more importantly the inferior vena cava (Step 6a). On the right side, the gonadal vein enters proximally the inferior vena cava directly on its anterior surface (Step 6b). On the left side, it enters the left renal vein directly. The gonadal vein must be mobilised very gently in order to prevent its avulsion.

Step 7: Identification and mobilisation of hilar vessels

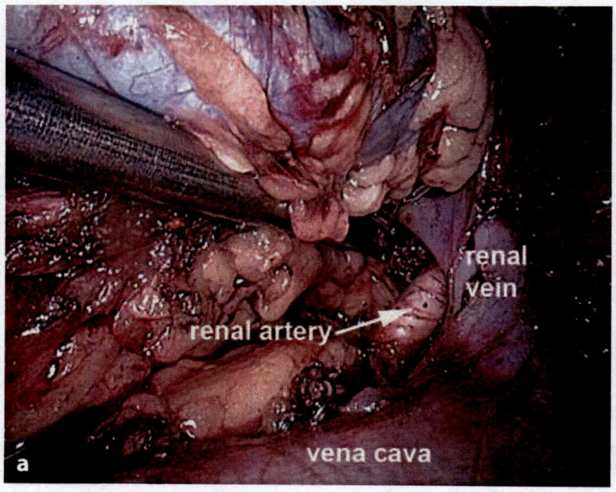

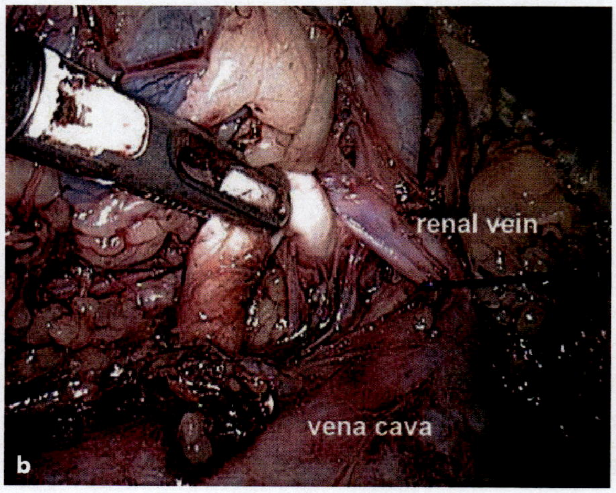

Once the junction between the gonadal vein and IVC (on the right side) or renal vein (on the left side) is determined, then the renal artery requires isolation and dissection. In the majority of cases, it lies directly behind the renal vein (Step 7a). In order to dissect the renal artery, it is necessary to mobilise the renal vein by sharp and blunt dissection. On the right, avoid the adrenal vein, which enters the IVC directly above the renal vein. To aid identification of the renal artery, it is possible to encircle the renal vein with a suture in order to mobilise it with mild tension on a grasper (Step 7b). Identify the renal artery, clean it of adventitia and create a window behind it for Hem-o-lok clips using a right-angled laparoscopic dissector.

Step 8: Clipping of the renal artery and vein

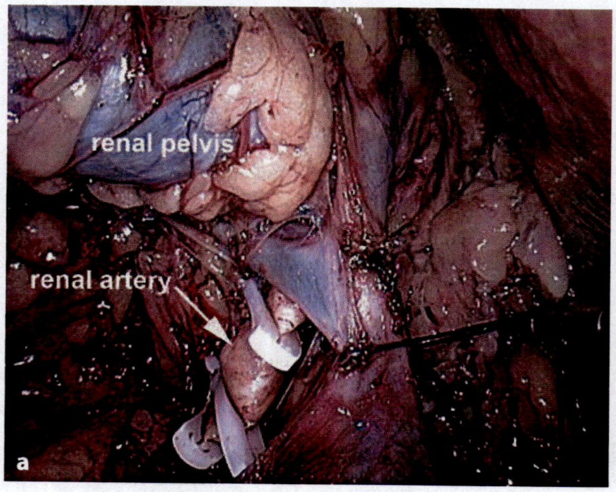

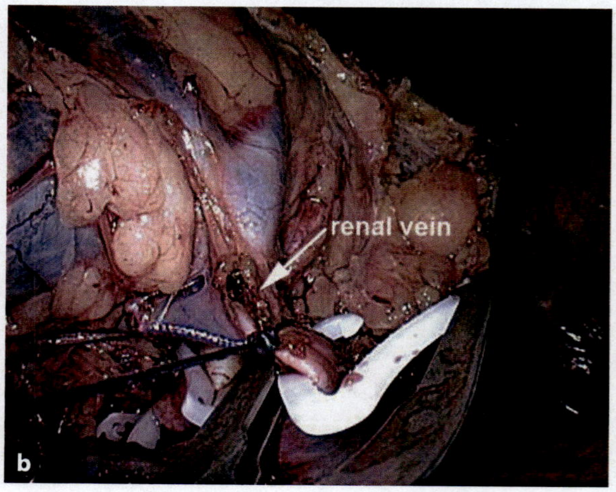

At least two clips are placed on the proximal (aortic) side of the artery and one clip on the distal (kidney) side of the kidney, leaving enough space between them to cut the artery (Step 8a). When dividing the artery, leave a good cuff of arterial tissue on the proximal (aortic) side and make a small cut in the artery initially to ensure it is not actively bleeding. Then the rest of the artery can be transected. The renal vein retraction suture can now be tightened in order to bundle the renal vein so it can be more easily clipped with two Hem-o-lok clips on the proximal (vena cava) side and one distally (kidney side) (Step 8b).

Step 9: Kidney mobilisation

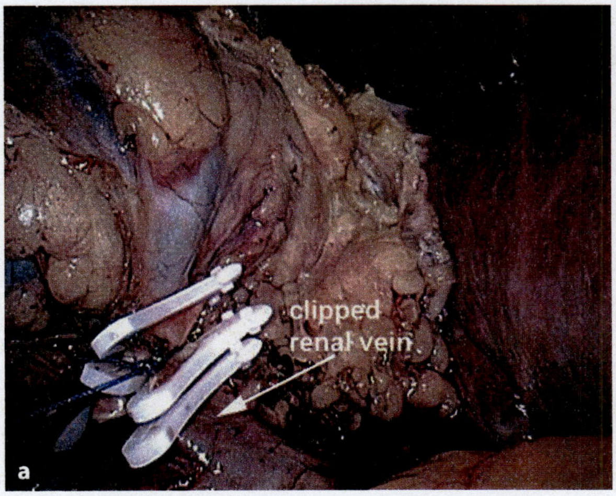

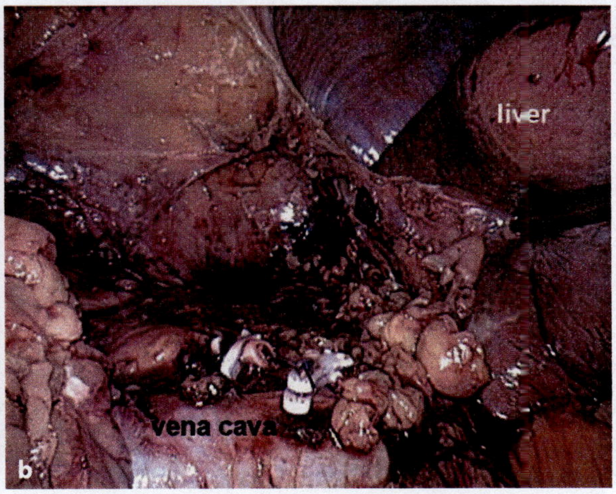

The kidney can now be mobilised medially and supero-medially. Dissect the kidney from the adrenal gland using the ultrasound dissector or bipolar cautery in order to prevent bleeding from the bare surface between them (Step 9b). Avoid damage to the adrenal vein, which enters the IVC posteriorly on the right side, and the renal vein on the left. The kidney can now be mobilised laterally and superiorly from the peritoneal attachments.

Finally, the ureter is divided as low as possible between the two clips. The gas pressure is then reduced to less than 5 mmHg to ensure there is no bleeding. A drain may be placed if necessary. The kidney is placed in a 10-to 12-mm EndoCatch bag and extracted through the 10-to 12-mm port and fascial defects are closed with absorbable suture.

Postoperative Management

- Oral or intramuscular analgesia is sufficient
- Drain removal on day 1 if minimal output (if inserted)
- Normal diet and mobilise on day 1

References

1. Clayman RV, Kavoussi LR, Soper NJ, Dierks SM, Meretyk S, Darcy MD, Roemer FD, Pingleton ED, Thomson PG, Long SR (1991) Laparoscopic nephrectomy: initial case report. J Urol 146:278
2. Dunn MD, Portis AJ, Shelhav AL, Elbashnasy AM, Heidorn C, McDougall EM, Clayman RV (2000) Laparoscopic versus open radical nephrectomy: a 9-year experience. J Urol 164:1153–1159
3. Liao JC, Breda A, Schulam PG (2008) Laparoscopic renal surgery for benign disease. Curr Urol Rep 8:12–18

1.7.2 Radical Nephrectomy

1.7.2.1 Laparoscopic Radical Nephrectomy

Jens-Uwe Stolzenburg, Minh Do, Rowan Casey, Anja Dietel, Alan Mc Neill, Evangelos Liatsikos

Introduction

Since its introduction, laparoscopic nephrectomy has evolved to become an established surgical procedure worldwide. Laparoscopic radical nephrectomy (LRN) is the standard of care for patients with T2 tumours and smaller renal masses not treatable by nephron-sparing surgery. Long-term data indicate that LRN has cancer-free survival rates equivalent to those of open radical nephrectomy. It also appears to have a lower morbidity compared to open surgery based on studies using quality-of-life data. Tumour control rates appear equivalent for T1–T2 tumours. The laparoscopic approach must follow established open surgical oncological principles established by Robson in his seminal paper in 1969 [1]. However, what is currently debated is the role played by adrenalectomy as part of nephrectomy. Some surgeons believe that the adrenal gland should not be removed because of the low probability of ipsilateral adrenal metastases and the associated morbidity. Current 2010 EAU guidelines state that adrenalectomy is not indicated when preoperative staging shows a normal gland, when intraoperative findings do not show a nodule or when there is no obvious direct invasion of the adrenal gland by a large upper-pole tumour.

Indications

- T1–T2 renal carcinoma
- T3 in experienced surgical centres [2, 3]
- Debulking tumour nephrectomy in patients with metastatic RCC with good performance status in combination with immunotherapy

Contra-indications

- Uncorrected bleeding disorders
- Uncorrected paraneoplastic syndromes
- Anaesthetic and cardiorespiratory risks
- Widespread skeletal and solid organ metastases
- Severe hilar adenopathy (relative)
- Renal vein (relative) or caval tumour thrombus
- Cirrhosis/portal hypertension (relative)

Preoperative Preparation

- Full staging with CT (thorax, abdomen, pelvis), MRI (with or without venogram), bone scan as indicated
- Preoperative renal biopsy as per tumour board recommendations

Step 1: Patient position and trocar placement

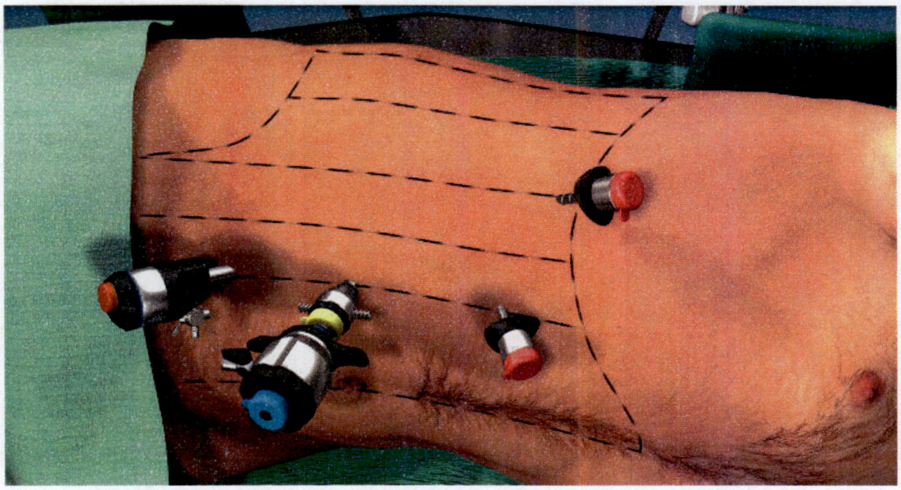

The patient is placed in the standard position as was described in Sect. 1.1. There are different trocar positions possible for nephrectomy, as described in Sect. 1.7.1. Another option is the trocar position shown in the figure. The optical trocar is placed paraumbilically. Either a 0 or 30° optic can be used. The main 10-mm and 5-mm surgeon trocars are placed along the same line. The assistant may require a 5-mm trocar on the anterior axillary line below the costal margin for liver retraction and for suction. This allows good triangulation for the main surgeon but can cause clashing with the assistant's arms outside the ports.

Step 2: Bowel mobilisation

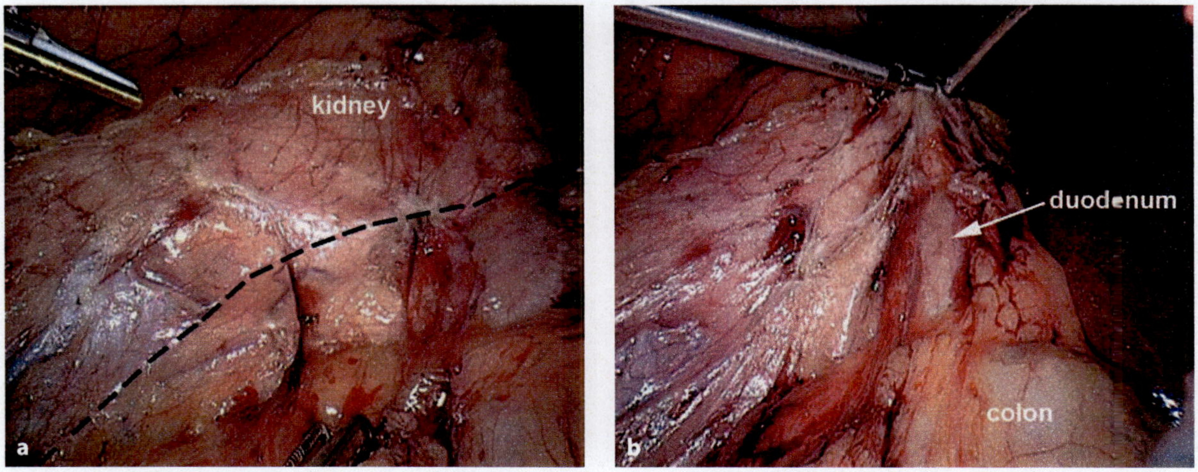

In order to access the retroperitoneal space, the overlying colon must be mobilised medially along the dotted line in Step 2a. We use a combination of SonoSurg and bipolar grasping forceps (operating surgeon) and the sucker as a blunt dissector (assisting surgeon). The colon is mobilised caudally to the iliac vessels. Cranially this mobilisation includes the colon flexure in order to achieve full mobilisation and access the kidney's upper pole and adrenal gland. Step 2b demonstrates the colon and duodenum, both of which need to be mobilised medially. We continue the mobilisation as high as possible over the upper pole at this stage.

Step 3: Ureteric identification and mobilisation

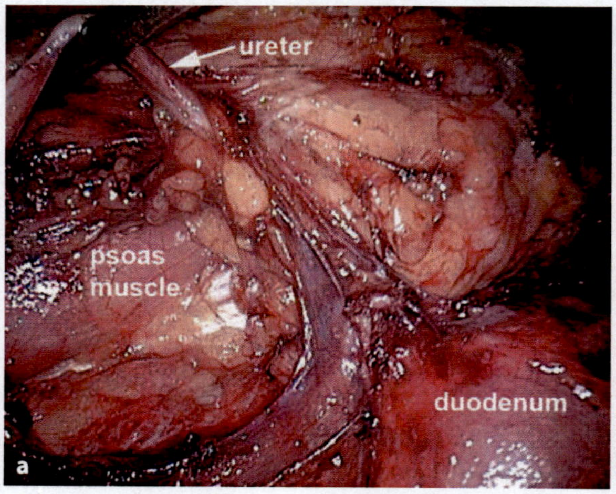

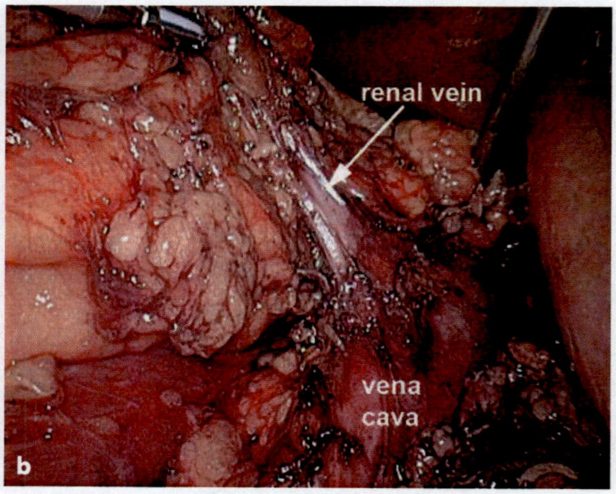

The next structure that should be recognised is the psoas muscle laterally. The ureter is mobilised off the psoas muscle and a window is made behind it (Step 3a) and it is clipped distally. As dissection continues more medially, the gonadal vein or vena cava will be identified next. It is useful to identify the gonadal vein at this stage (not shown) as this provides a direct route to the renal vein on the left and vena cava (just below the renal vein) on the right. A straight needle can be used to encircle the ureter and clamped outside the abdomen to provide traction and this creates a window between the cava and renal hilum that can be developed.

Step 4: Renal hilar mobilisation

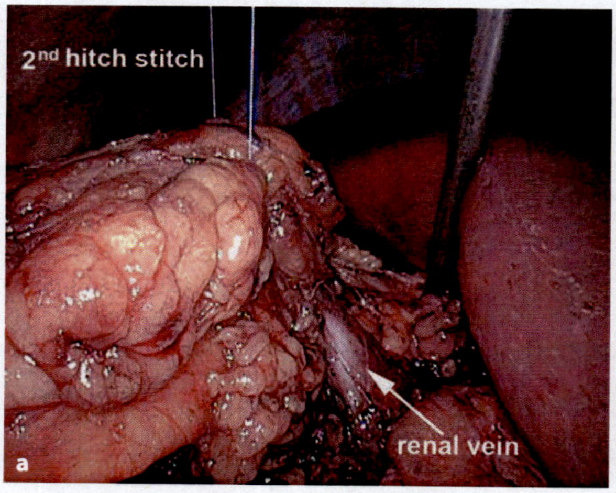

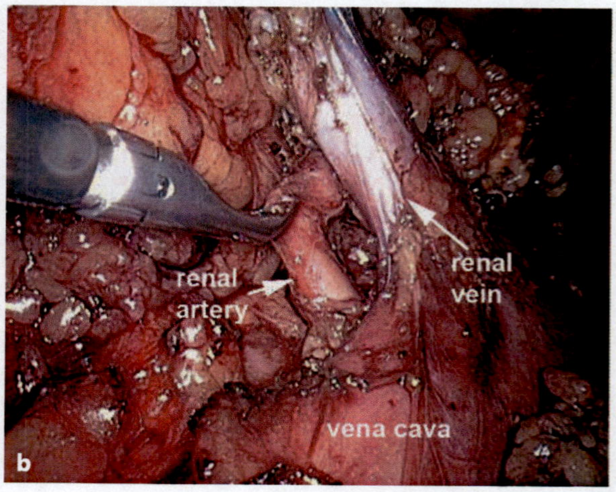

The key to successful mobilisation and identification of structures at the hilum is to have good retraction. This may require insertion of an additional 5-mm port or 3-mm trocarless instrument. In this case, we choose to insert another hitch stitch percutaneously to retract perirenal fat overlying the hilum and provide traction on the renal vein (Step 4a). Dissection of the single renal artery from the vein is aided by a right-angled forceps. The most important aspect of dividing the renal vessels no matter which technique is used is to ensure that the vessels are skeletonised, separated and have a good length available for clipping.

Step 5: Renal hilar division

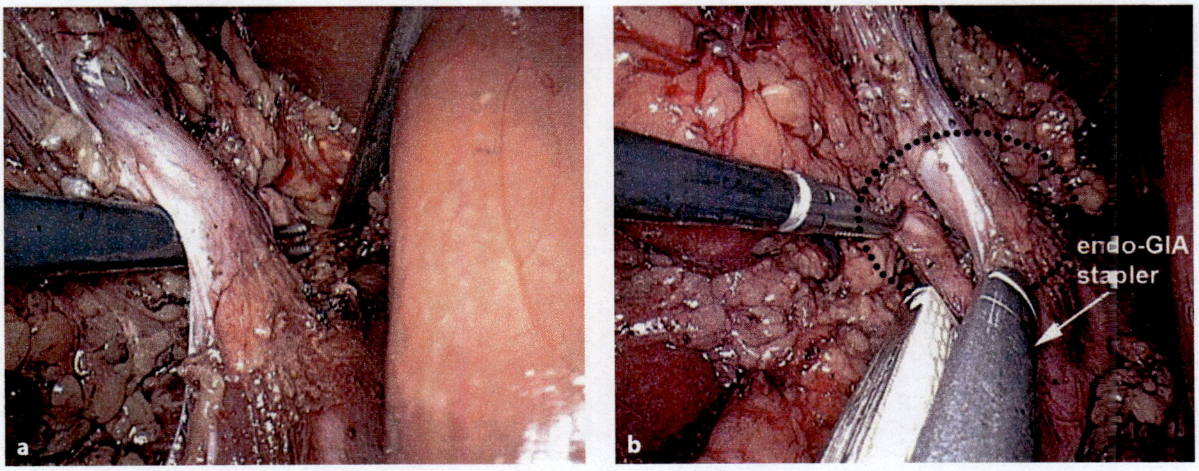

Step 5a shows that it is possible, following dissection above and below the vein, to pass an instrument easily behind it without tissue interposition. One option is to divide both renal artery and vein en-bloc with an endo-GIA stapler (Step 5b). The concerns regarding artery or vein fistula formation appear to be unfounded [4]. However, there have been reports of misfiring in approximately 1–1.7% [5, 6]. When firing the endo-GIA stapler, one must ensure that all tissue is between the markings on the proximal and distal part of the stapler which indicates the staple line.

Step 6: Alternative renal hilar division

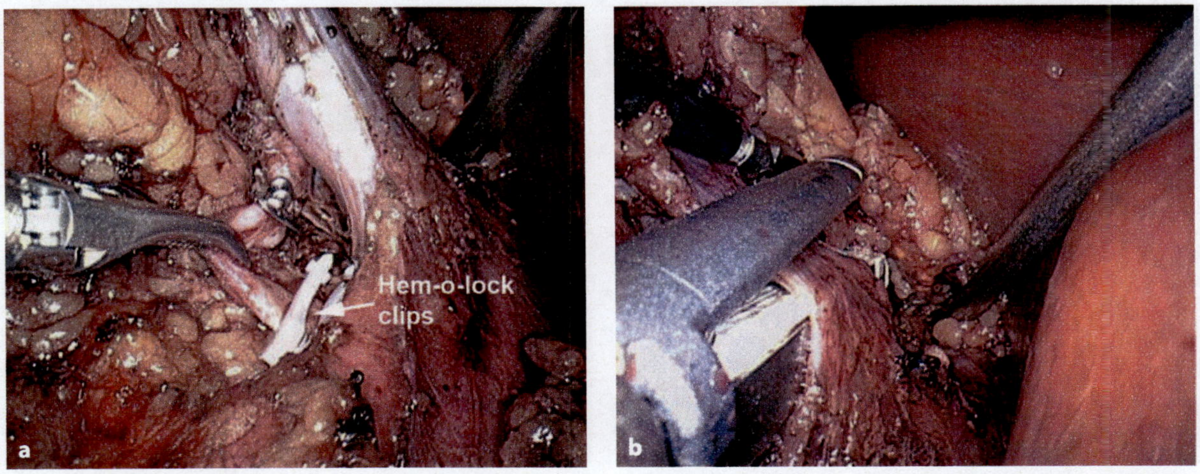

Two Hem-o-lok clips must be placed on the proximal side to divide the renal artery. Distally on the artery, it is possible to use titanium clips, especially if the renal artery mobilised is short (Step 6a). The benefit of the 5-mm assistant trocar is to use suction to provide a window above the vein to retract the perirenal tissue cranially. The renal vein has been completely mobilised and can be easily manipulated to place and endo-GIA stapler across it, especially when the vein is large in diameter (Step 6a). The far end of the stapler must be visible and have no tissue or clip interposition, and the vein must be within its firing marks.

Step 7: Renal vein division and adrenal gland mobilisation

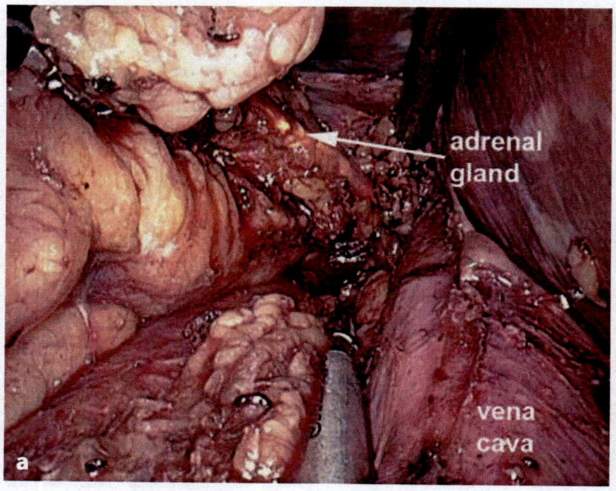

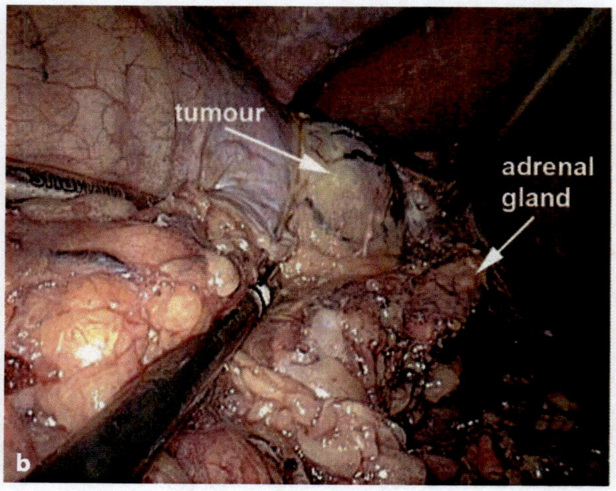

The renal vein has been divided with endo-GIA clips (Step 7a). Progress is now made along the lateral aspect of the vena cava to the adrenal gland, which will be part of the specimen as the tumour is in the upper pole and was suspicious on imaging (Step 7a, b). It was not possible to accurately identify the adrenal artery and vein in this case as they were very small and encased in fat. The SonoSurg device is suitable to coagulate and ligate these vessels if they are small. Otherwise titanium clips or the Ligasure device should be used when the vessels are identified.

Step 8: Kidney mobilisation

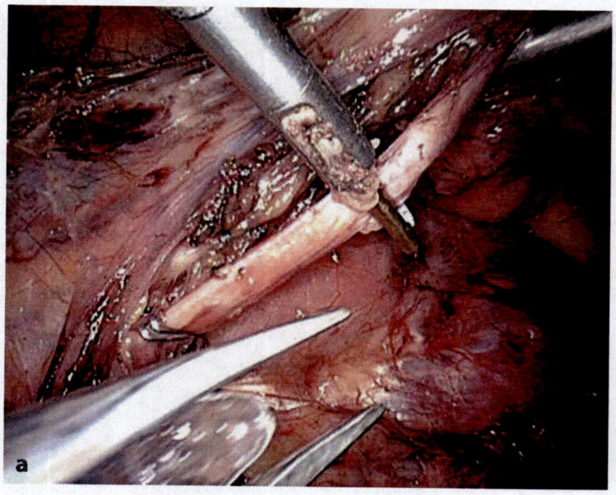

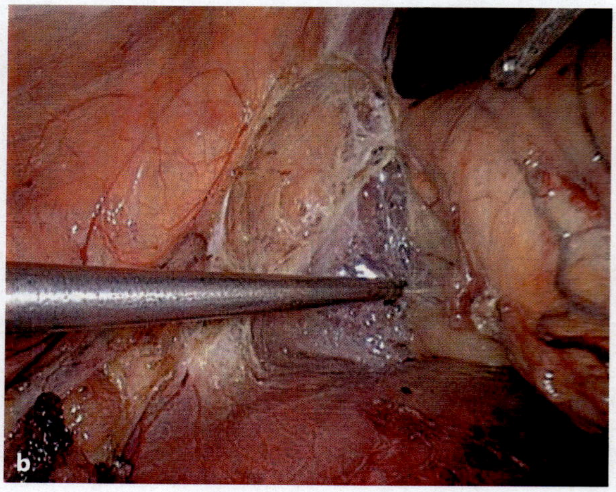

The ureter can now be divided between any clips to allow access and mobilisation of the lower pole of the kidney off the psoas muscle (Step 8a). Now mobilisation of the medial and superior poles of the kidney is carried out. Liver retraction is essential using either suction or a fan retractor. The majority of the kidney can be mobilised bluntly inferiorly and laterally using the instruments to elevate the kidney. Small adhesions and capsular vessels can be divided with the SonoSurg device. Ensure that the adrenal gland is removed completely intact with the specimen.

Step 9: Specimen bagging and final inspection

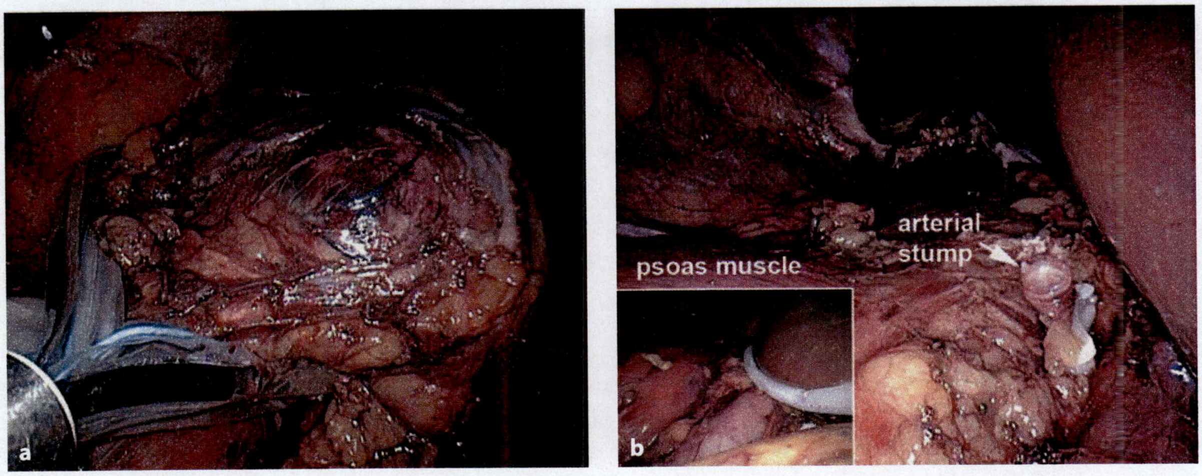

The specimen is placed above the liver or in the renal fossa and is then bagged (Step 9a). Larger specimens may need a large bag, which can only be introduced through a 15-mm port or directly through the skin through the 12-mm port site. If the preoperative imaging suggests a large specimen a 15-mm trocar with a reducer can be inserted during initial trocar placement. As the skin has some compliance, the skin incision should not be as large as the fascial incision when removing the specimen. A final inspection is made for bleeding from the adrenal bed and renal hilar area. A non-suction wide-bore drain is optional (Step 9b, inset).

Postoperative Management

- Light diet first evening
- Drain removal if minimal output on day 1
- Urinary catheter removed when able to ambulate
- Serum creatinine and haemoglobin check day before discharge

References

1. Robson CJ, Churchill BM, Anderson W (1969) The results of radical nephrectomy for renal cell carcinoma. J Urol 101:297–301
2. Bird VG, Shields JM, Azixz M et al (2009) Laparoscopic radical nephrectomy for patients with T2 and T3 renal-cell carcinoma: evaluation of perioperative outcomes. J Endourol 23:1527–1533
3. Bensalah K, Salomon L, Lang H et al (2009) Survival of patients with nonmetastatic pT3 renal tumours: a matched comparison of laparoscopic vs open radical nephrectomy. BJU Int 104:1714–1717
4. Buse S, Gilfrich C, Pfitzenmaier J, Bedke J, Haferkamp A, Hohenfellner M (2008) En bloc stapler ligation of the renal vascular pedicle during laparoscopic nephrectomy. BJU Int 101:878–882
5. Chan D, Bishoff JT, Ratner L, Kavoussi LR, Jarrett TW (2000) Endovascular gastrointestinal stapler device malfunction during laparoscopic nephrectomy: early recognition and management. J Urol 164:319–321
6. Deng DY, Meng MV, Nguyen HT, Bellman GC, Stoller ML (2002) Laparoscopic linear cutting stapler failure. Urology 60:415–419

1.7.2.2 LESS: Radical Nephrectomy

Jens-Uwe Stolzenburg, Anja Dietel, Mathias Winkler, Minh Do, Rowan Casey, Panagiotis Kallidonis, Holger Till, Evangelos Liatsikos

Introduction

The European Association of Urology (EAU) Guidelines (2008) propose laparoscopic radical nephrectomy (LRN) as a first-line treatment approach for renal cell carcinoma. Typically, the laparoscopic approach for the performance of major urologic operations requires three to six ports. In an attempt to minimise port-related morbidity and to avoid multiple scars, a further development of laparoscopy is the concept of laparoendoscopic single-site surgery (LESS). The potential advantages of LESS would appear to be improved cosmetic appearance, reduced wound pain and earlier hospital discharge [1]. However, the technique requires advanced laparoscopic expertise and enhanced spatial awareness [2]. Careful case selection is essential from the beginning [3, 4].

With growing experience, in principle all candidates for conventional laparoscopic tumour nephrectomy are also suitable for LESS procedure. At any stage in the LESS procedure, additional ports can be inserted as needed to ensure the patient's safety, which is the most important criterion. Although many unanswered questions persist and instruments have to be improved, it is also critically important that urologists evaluate these new approaches carefully and scientifically. The LESS procedure itself and the idea of performing complex surgery through a single entry is fascinating and holds enormous potential.

Indications

- Small solid renal tumour proven on cross-sectional imaging and not amenable to partial nephrectomy

Contra-indications

- Uncorrected bleeding diathesis
- Radiological evidence of tumour invasion of the renal vein
- Abdominal aortic aneurysm
- Obesity (relative contraindication)
- Extensive surgical scars in the upper abdomen(relative contraindication)

Preoperative Preparation

- As for laparoscopic or open radical nephrectomy
- Thromboprophylaxis as per local guidelines
- Urinary catheterisation (done in the operative theatre)

Step 1: Operative setup

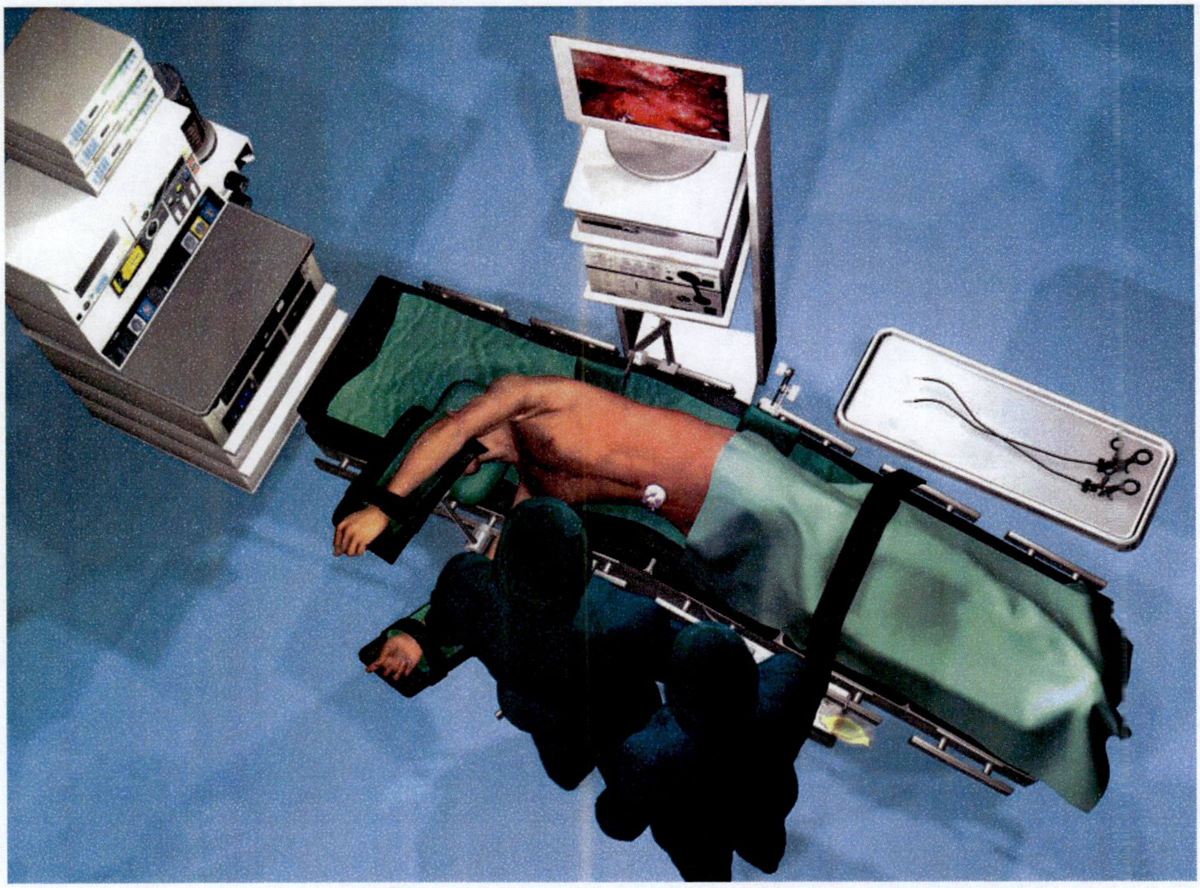

The patient is placed in the lateral decubitus position as described in Sect. 1.1. The surgeon is situated in front of the patient with the assistant positioned cranially to operate the telescope. We find that it is better if the assistant sits down during the procedure in order to allow the surgeon the full range of movement of the instruments without clashing with the assistant. The instrument table can be positioned either on the surgeon's side or on the opposite side. The ideal patient for LESS tumour nephrectomy is slim and has little perinephric fat, although it is may be feasible to expand this to obese patients.

Step 2: Port placement

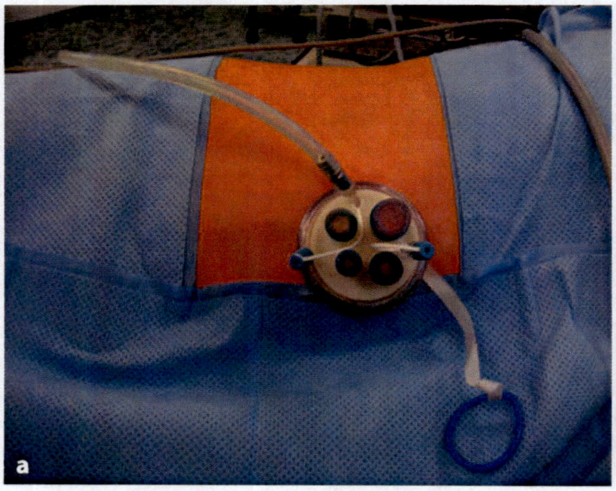

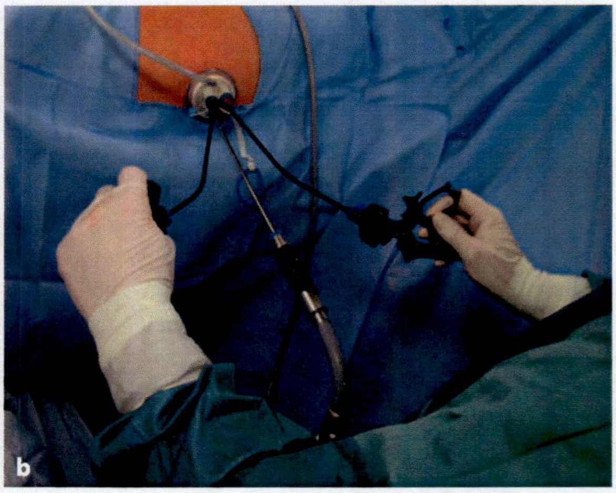

In a slim patient, the QuadPort (Olympus, USA) is placed at the umbilicus after a 2-cm skin incision is made (Step 2a). We recommend the use of specially designed optics for LESS; 30° HD-quality 5-mm extra-long and with a bendable handle (Olympus) or 30° HD-quality 5-mm extra-long (Karl Storz, Tuttlingen, Germany). If they are not available, standard HD 0° or 30° 10-mm optics can be used. The position of the bendable 5-mm 30° telescope to a pair of prebent instruments is shown in Step 2b. This allows for an excellent range of movement without instrument clashing.

Step 3: Port placement in obese patients (right side)

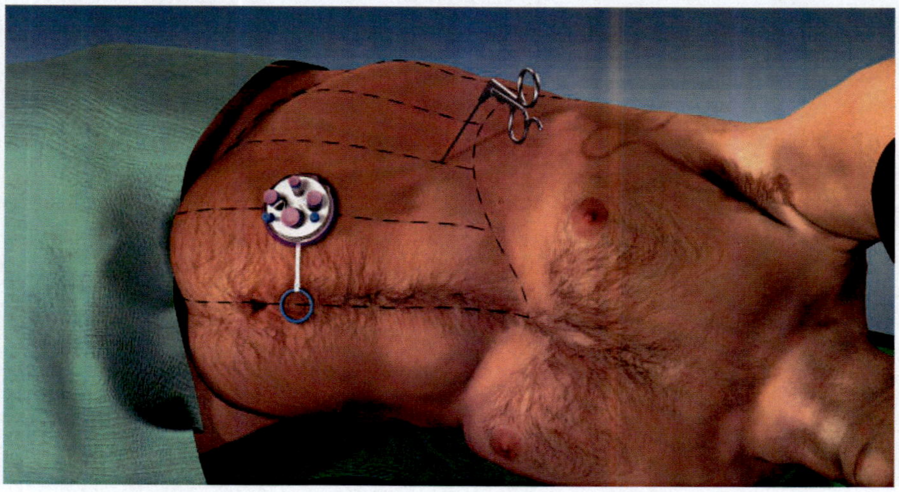

In this obese patient, the QuadPort is placed at the level of the umbilicus on the pararectal line (Step 3a) for more direct access to the kidney without the large bowel interposed. The QuadPort incorporates one 5-mm, two 10-mm and one 15-mm access sheaths for wide instrument choice. On the right side, as shown in the figure, an additional needlescopic instrument is required to retract the liver.

Step 4: Port placement in obese patients and instrument selection

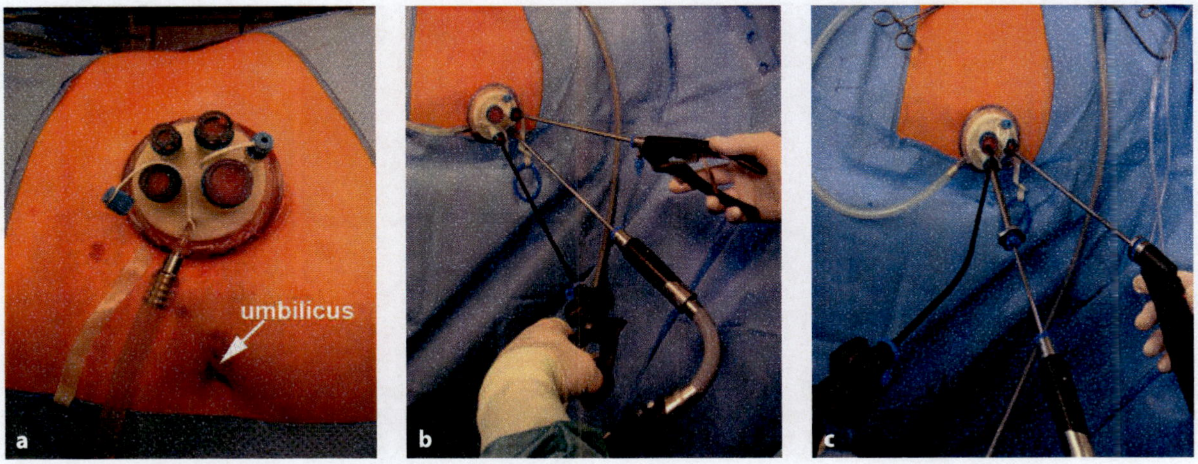

Instead of using two prebent instruments, one straight and one prebent instrument can be used, as shown in Step 4b, c. The combination of one prebent instrument for retraction with a straight dissecting instrument has emerged as the best compromise in our experience for many steps of the procedure. This generation of the Quadport requires permanent lubrication of the port valves. As a result, smudging of the telescope lens is a common problem during telescope insertion. This can be overcome by using a 10-mm reduction sleeve positioned over the telescope prior to insertion (Step 4c).

Step 5: Mobilisation of the descending colon

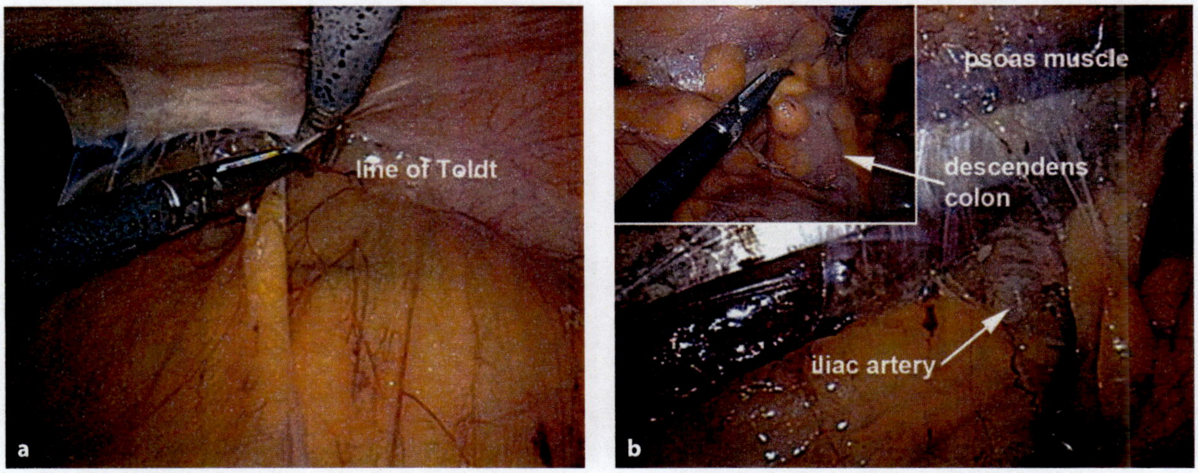

The descending colon and colonic flexure are now mobilised away from the Gerota fascia along the line of Toldt (Step 5a). A left-sided prebent Maryland dissector is used for retraction in combination with prebent scissors in the surgeon's right hand. Alternatively, straight laparoscopic scissors or the SonoSurg device (Olympus) may be appropriate. The psoas muscle and tendon and inferiorly the left common iliac artery are helpful landmarks, which indicate complete colonic mobilsation caudally (Step 5b). Care must be taken to avoid heat injury to the colon if diathermy or a harmonic scalpel is used.

Step 6: Mobilisation of the colonic flexure and spleen

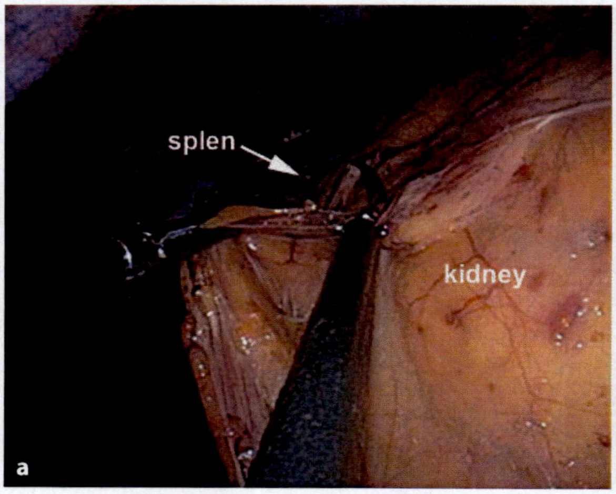

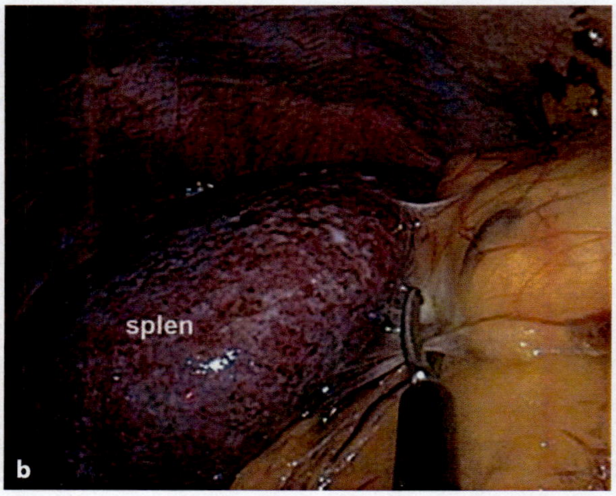

It is well worth spending some time to mobilise the left colonic flexure and spleen completely, which is accomplished with a combination of blunt and sharp dissection (Step 6a). This will avoid iatrogenic splenic tears and facilitate apical renal mobilisation. Once the spleen and colonic flexure is fully mobilised, it should passively fall away from the kidney and make further dissection easier.

Again, in addition to the LESS retracting prebent instrument in the left hand of the surgeon, the ultrasonic scalpel (SonoSurg) or straight scissors are used to dissect. At this stage, the upper pole of the kidney should be mobilised completely from the undersurface of the spleen in order to allow the spleen to be pushed cranially.

Step 7: Mobilisation of the ureter and gonadal vein

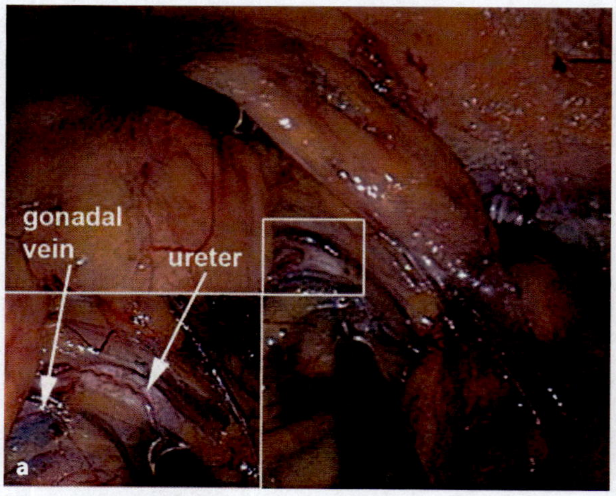

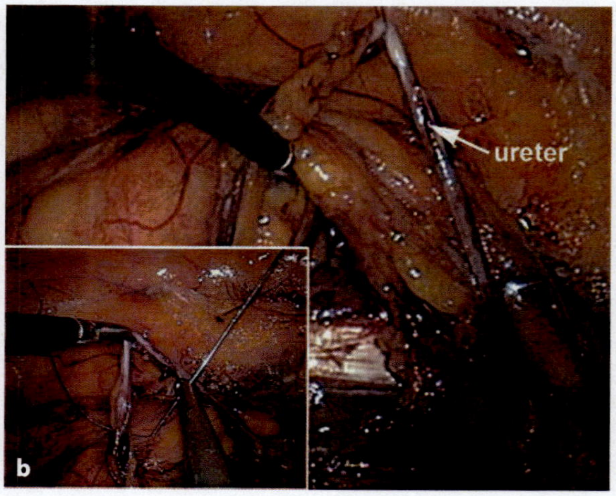

The next step of the procedure is the identification of the ureter to guide further dissection towards the renal pedicle (Step 7a). The ureter is mobilised and retracted laterally. A stay suture provides tension on the ureter to elevate it (Step 7b). This is achieved with a suture on a long straight needle, which is inserted from outside, passed under the ureter, brought back out through the skin and secured with a clip. The tension on this stay suture can be adjusted from outside. If necessary, a second stay suture can be placed in the same manner more proximally.

Step 8: Identification of renal vein and division of testicular vein

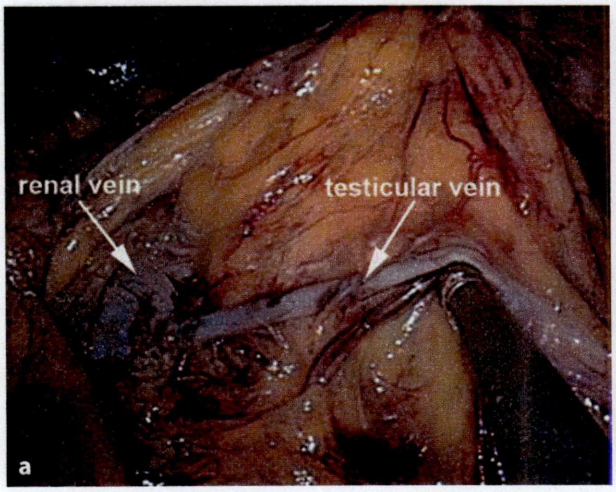

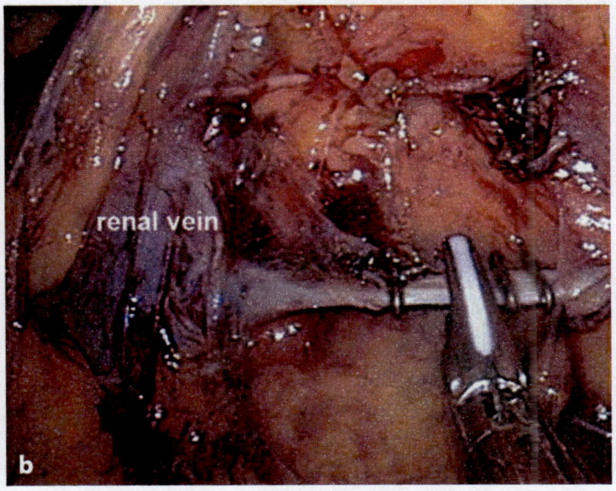

The gonadal (testicular) vein is now dissected off the ureter. Following the gonadal vein guides one to the renal vein, as shown in Step 8a. The distal end of the gonadal vein is double-clipped and in this case the straight ultrasonic scalpel is used to divide the structure (Step 8b). The cranial clip should not be placed too close to the renal vein. This might cause difficulty during application of the Hem-o-lok clips or vascular GIA at the renal vein later in the procedure.

Step 9: Skeletonising of renal pedicle and dissection of renal vein

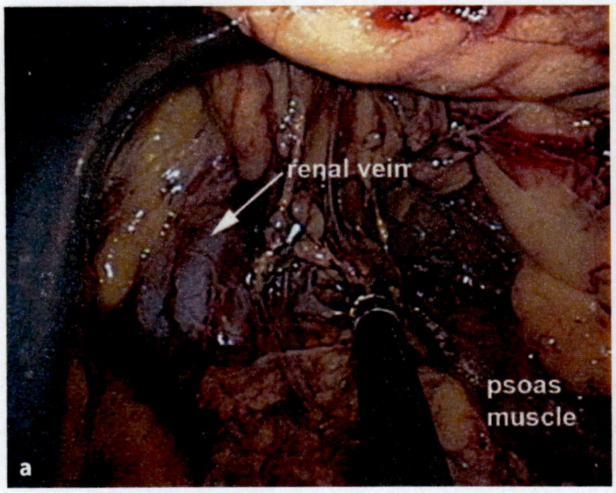

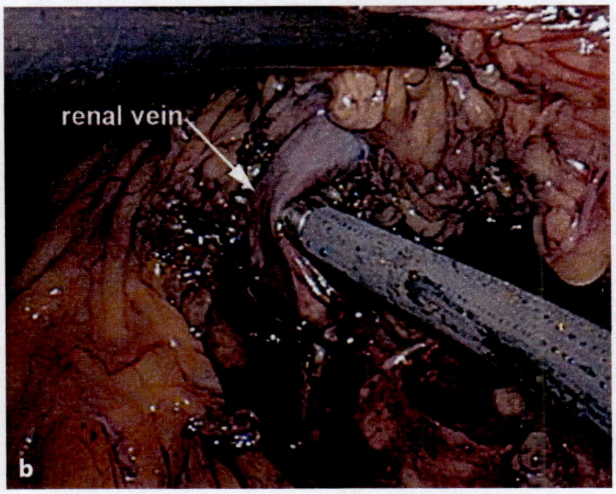

The renal vein is identified and dissected out with a mixture of sharp and blunt instruments. The necessary retraction is achieved with a prebent instrument at all times in the surgeon's left hand. In the right hand, a bipolar forceps (Step 9a) or a prebent dissector (Step 9b) can be used. Be aware of the delicate lumbar veins at the proximal and posterior aspect of the renal vein. These should either be left alone or, if prominent and distal, carefully clipped and divided. The adrenal vein is prone to injury during blunt dissection of the cranial aspect of the renal pedicle. It should be sought out and clipped early.

Step 10: Dissection and clipping of the renal artery

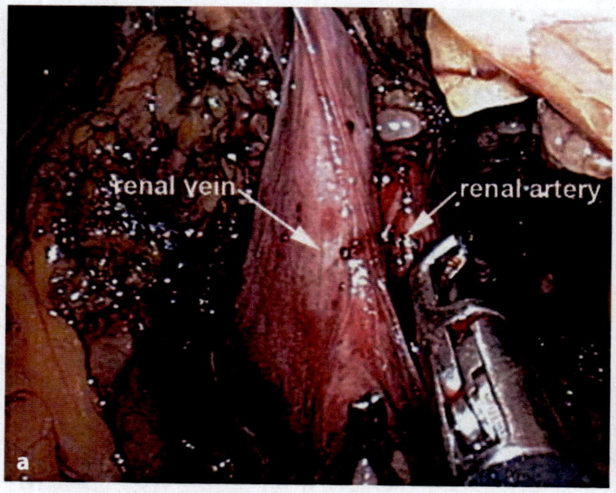

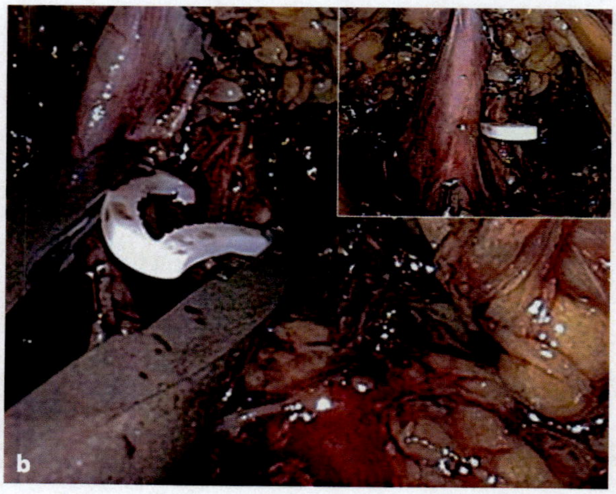

A right-angle dissector from the straight laparoscopic set helps to fully mobilise the posterior aspect of the renal vein from surrounding tissue and to completely mobilise and skeletonise the renal artery (Step 10a). If the renal artery cannot accommodate a minimum of three clips, as in this case, one Hem-o-lok clip is applied to the artery as proximally as possible (Step 10b). Although Hem-o-lok clips are an excellent way of securing a vessel, it is of utmost importance to carefully visualise the hooked tip of the clip behind the vessel before closure of the clip applier. This will ensure the clip is completely around the vessel and avoid accidental injury of the vessel back wall. Then the next step is to clip and divide the vein to obtain safe access to the artery.

Step 11: Division of renal vein and artery

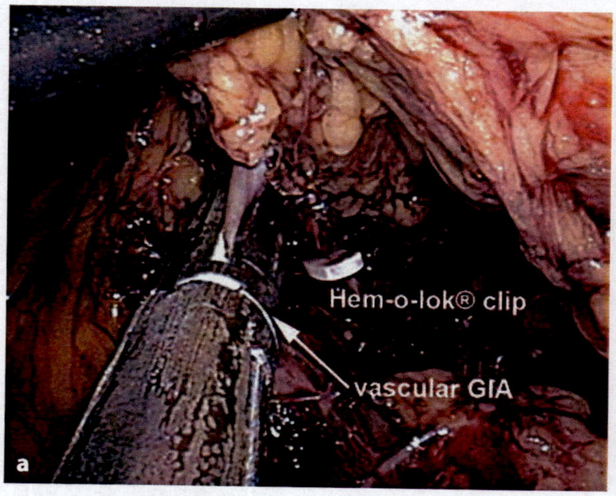

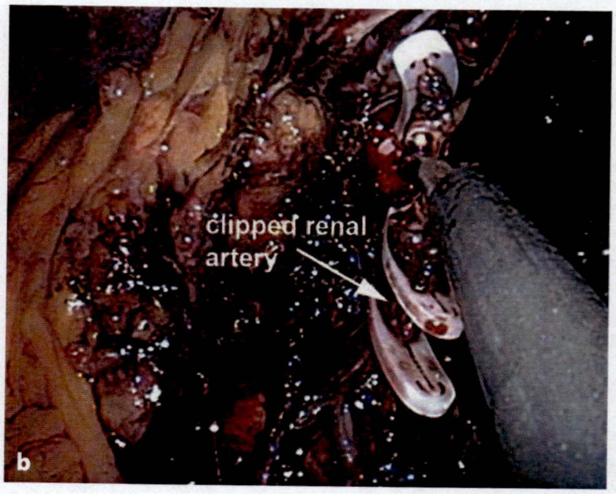

The fully mobilised renal vein is sealed and divided with a vascular endo-GIA stapling device, which is inserted through the 15-mm access sheath of the QuadPort (Step 11a). Division of the renal vein allows further dissection for greater length on the renal artery and facilitates application of two more Hem-o-lok clips to the skeletonised renal artery. The artery is divided with straight scissors, taking care to leave an adequate cuff of tissue at the end of the proximal arterial stump (Step 11b). This should prevent slippage of Hem-o-lok clips and catastrophic haemorrhage. Alternatively, titanium clips may be used, but a minimum of three clips should be applied to the proximal end of the artery. It is also possible to divide the artery and vein en bloc with the vascular GIA.

Step 12: Full mobilisation of the kidney and specimen removal

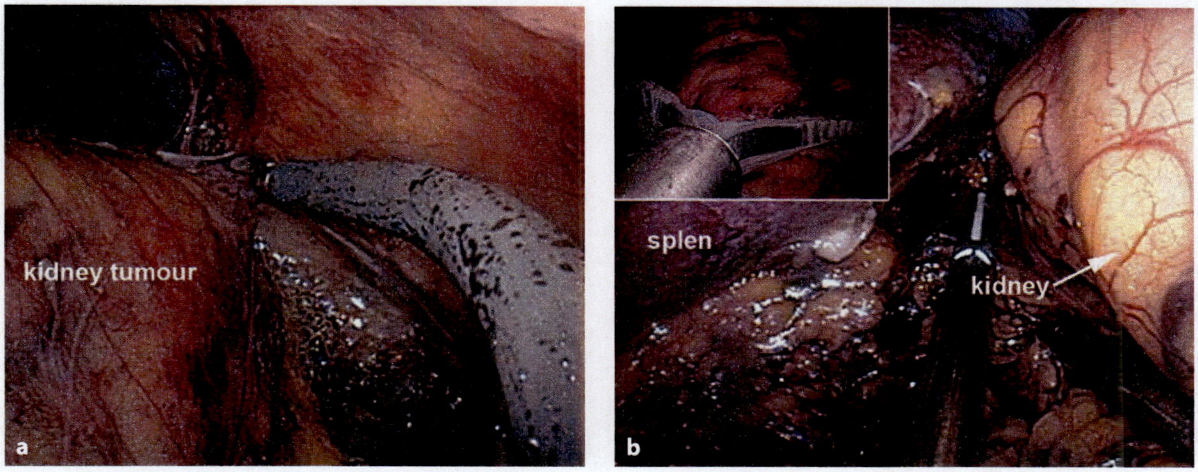

The kidney is now fully mobilised (with or without the adrenal gland depending on the tumour location). The full mobilisation of the spleen at the beginning of the procedure helps to avoid problems during the mobilisation of the superior aspect of the kidney. A large Endo-Catch extractor bag (Covidien, Mansfield, MA, USA) is introduced through the 15-mm access sheath of the QuadPort and used for kidney retrieval (Step 12b). Haemostasis should be checked after bagging the specimen and before removal through the umbilical incision. Reduction of insufflation pressure to 6 mmHg may improve identification of venous bleeding.

Step 13: Extraction wound in a slim patient

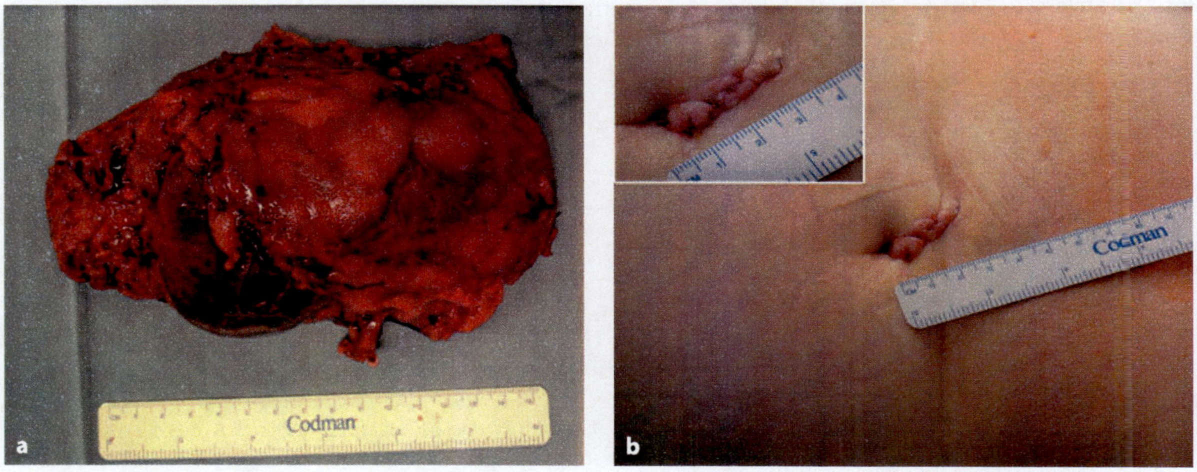

The final operative specimen is shown (Step 13a) and measures 15 cm in length. It is possible to extract specimens of this size through a dilated umbilical LESS incision. The skin can accommodate this given its flexibility. The fascial incision must be larger than the skin incision. The final skin wound is no longer than 3–5 cm. Subcuticular skin closure affords a superior cosmetic appearance (Step 13b). Drain placement is optional. Local anaesthetic infiltration of the wound can be used to reduce analgesic requirements.

Step 14: Extraction wound in an obese patient

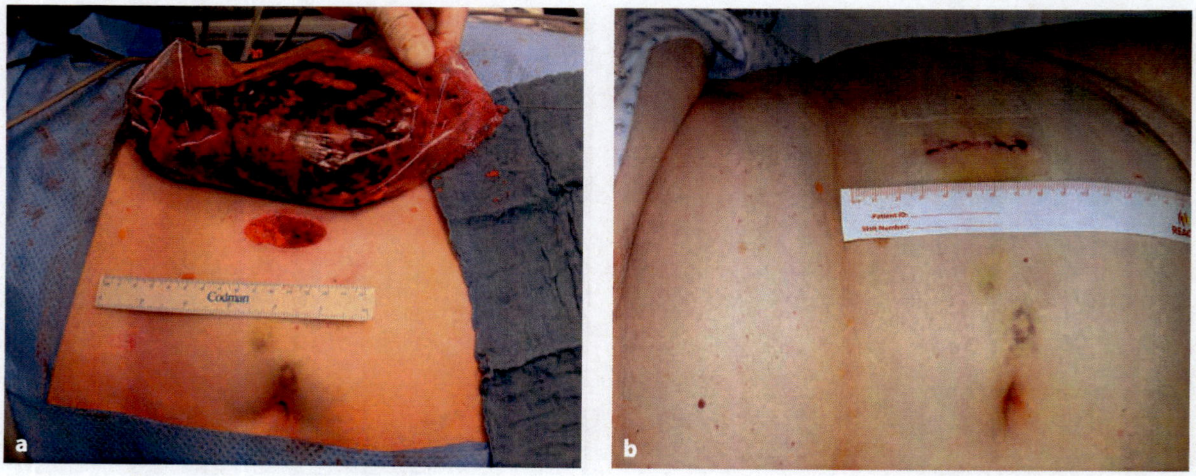

This picture illustrates the extracted specimen and size of the extraction wound if the Quadport is placed paraumbilically. Particular attention should be given to fascial closure to prevent incisional hernias. Although the wound is larger (5–6 cm) than in patients with umbilical port placement, it is still small. It is conceivable that smaller wounds cause less pain, which could ultimately lead to faster mobilisation, especially in obese patients and reduced venous-thromboembolic complications.

Postoperative Management

- Oral or intramuscular analgesia is sufficient
- Drain removal on day 1 if minimal output (if inserted)
- Normal diet and mobilise on day 1

References

1. Park YH, Park JH, Jeong CW, Kim HH (2010) Comparison of laparoscopic single-site radical nephrectomy with conventional laparoscopic radical nephrectomy for localised renal-cell carcinoma. J Endourol 7 24:997–1003
2. Stolzenburg JU, Kallidonis P, Oh MA, Ghulam N, Do M, Haefner T, Dietel A, Sakellaropoulos G, Liatsikos EN (2010) Comparative assessment of laparoscopic single-site surgery instruments to conventional laparoscopic in laboratory setting. J Endourol 24:239–245
3. Desai MM, Berger AK, Brandina R, Aron M, Irwin BH, Canes D, Desai MR, Rao PP, Sotelo R, Stein R, Gill IS (2009) Laparoendoscopic single-site surgery: initial hundred patients. Urology 74:805–812
4. Stolzenburg JU, Kallidonis P, Hellawell G, Do M, Haefner T, Dietel A, Liatsikos EN (2009) Technique of laparoscopic-endoscopic single-site surgery: radical nephrectomy. Eur Urol 56: 644–650

1.8 Retroperitoneal Nephrectomy

Ben G. Thomas, Tony Riddick, Jens-Uwe Stolzenburg, Minh Do, Alan McNeill

Introduction

Laparoscopic nephrectomy, simple or radical, has become the standard approach to nephrectomy as it has been shown to minimise morbidity without compromising the longer-term outcomes [1, 2]. The retroperitoneal approach to laparoscopic nephrectomy offers the advantages of faster access to the hilar vessels and less mobilisation of other structures, shortening overall operating time [3], whilst a transperitoneal approach offers greater working space and more readily identifiable landmarks. The retroperitoneal approach is particularly useful where previous abdominal operations and associated adhesions make a transperitoneal approach more difficult and hazardous. However, a recent randomised trial comparing retroperitoneal and transperitoneal approaches showed no significant differences in ileus or organ injury [3]. The indications for a retroperitoneal approach, given the smaller working space, may be limited by the surgeon's experience, in particular when undertaking tumour nephrectomy for larger renal tumours.

Indications

- Nonfunctioning atrophic kidney
- Radical nephrectomy for T1 and some T2 tumours (depending on the surgeon's experience)
- Laparoscopic donor nephrectomy

Contra-indications

- Cardiorespiratory morbidity
- Morbid obesity
- Uncorrected coagulopathy

Preoperative Preparation

- Thromboprophylaxis
- Usual preoperative work-up

Step 1: Patient position and Visiport placement

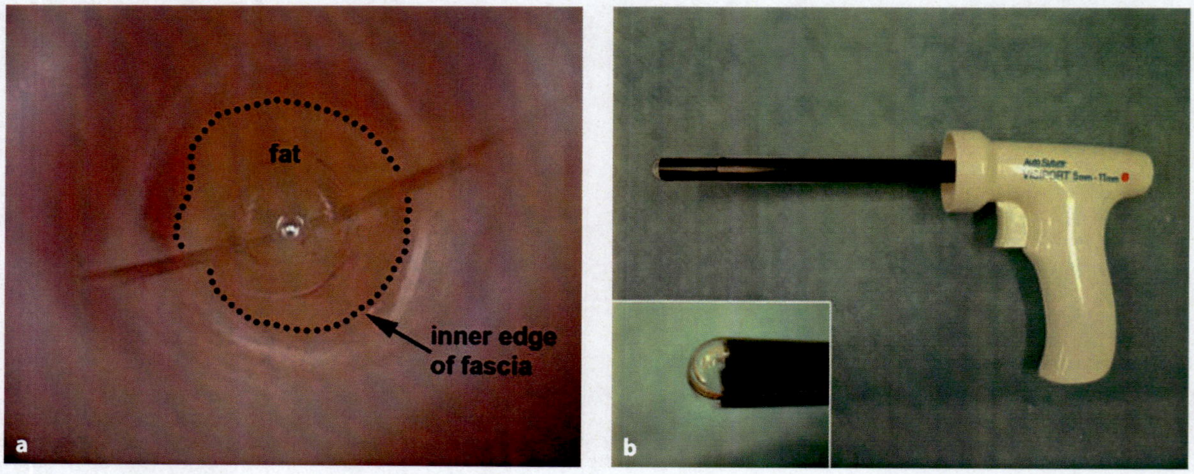

The patient position is described fully in Sect. 1.1. In this case, we used the Visiport optical trocar insertion device to enter the retroperitoneum (Step 1b). A small skin incision is made 5 cm below the costal margin on the mid-axillary line. The insertion technique is fully described in Sect. 1.2.1. It is important not to make the skin incision too large since there is no peritoneum to grip the port and help prevent gas leakage. As the tip of the trocar advances through the final, inner, layer of the muscle, fat will appear (Step 1a). The trocar is advanced slightly farther to the full width of the port and then removed.

Step 2: Establishing the retroperitoneal space

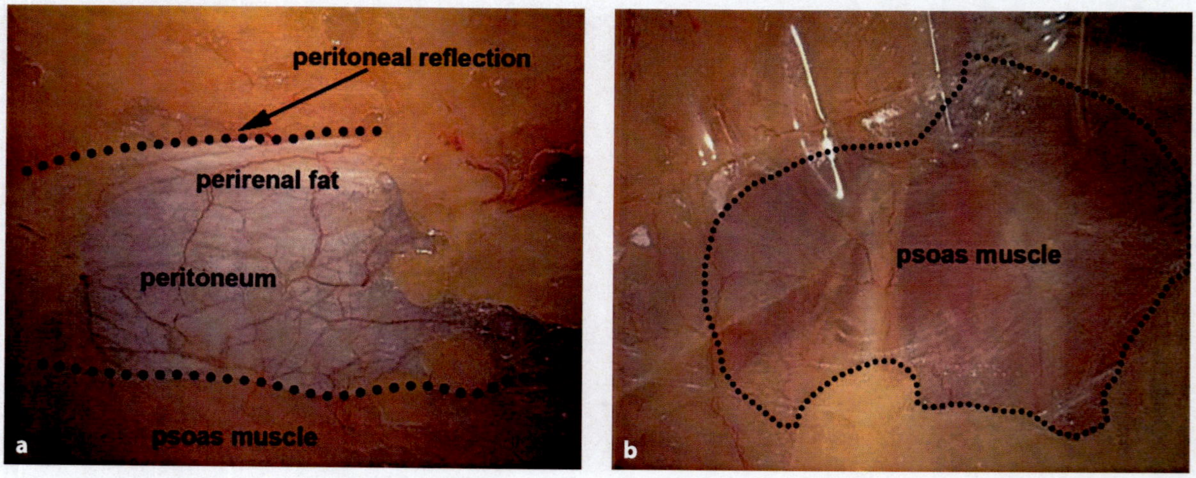

A balloon trocar is then inserted through the muscle layers, ensuring the shoulders of the balloon are beneath the muscle before inflation. The camera is returned to the balloon and inflation is started. The psoas muscle should be identified at the base of the picture (Step 2a). The edge of the peritoneum should be seen towards the top of the balloon and this will slowly peel as the balloon inflates (Step 2b). Once the balloon is inflated, the position of the anterior port should be confirmed by gentle pressure on the skin at the proposed site of the port. The balloon may need to be further inflated to create more space for the next trocar.

Step 3: Trocar placement

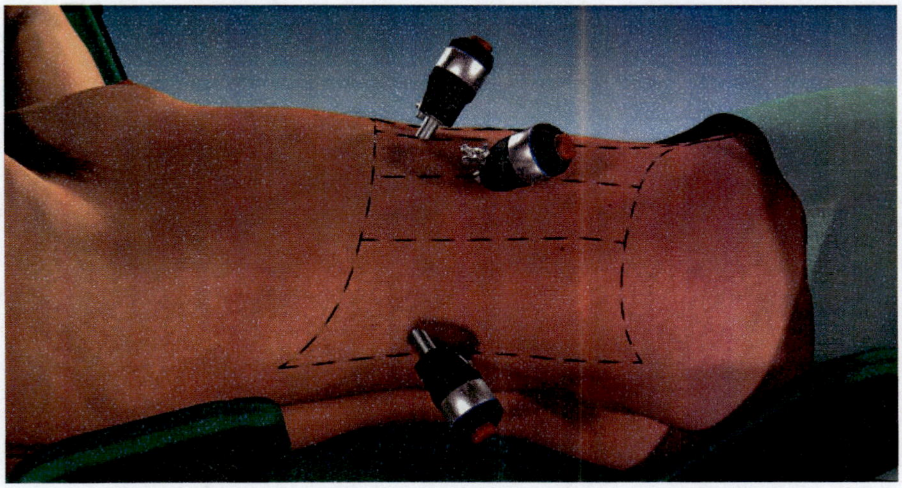

Following deflation of the balloon, the camera port is re-inserted and the gas switched on to fill the space. The anterior and posterior ports can then be placed under direct vision. The anterior port should be placed in the anterior axillary line. The posterior port should be placed lateral to the paraspinal musculature. The gas flow can then be transferred to either the anterior or posterior port. We prefer to use 12-mmHg high-flow pressure.

Step 4: Dissection of the retroperitoneal space

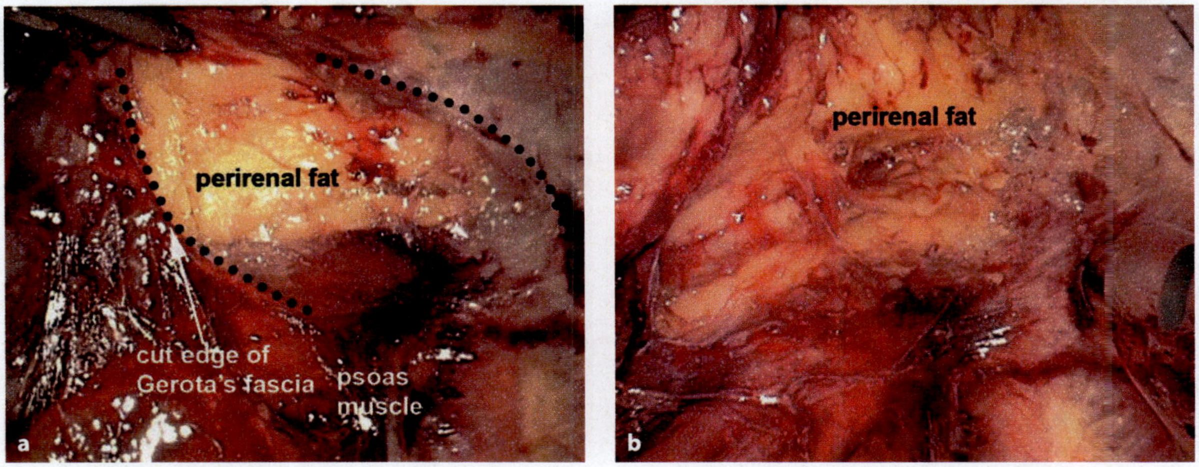

For orientation, the psoas muscle should be across the inferior aspect of the view and should be kept horizontal in the field of view. Looking slightly cephalad, the Gerota fascia will be seen and this is incised to reveal characteristic wispy perinephric tissue. Staying close to the psoas muscle, the plain between the kidney, surrounded by perinephric fat, and the psoas can be developed. Upward traction must be placed on the kidney to allow blunt dissection using a sucker.

Step 5: Dissection of the renal hilum

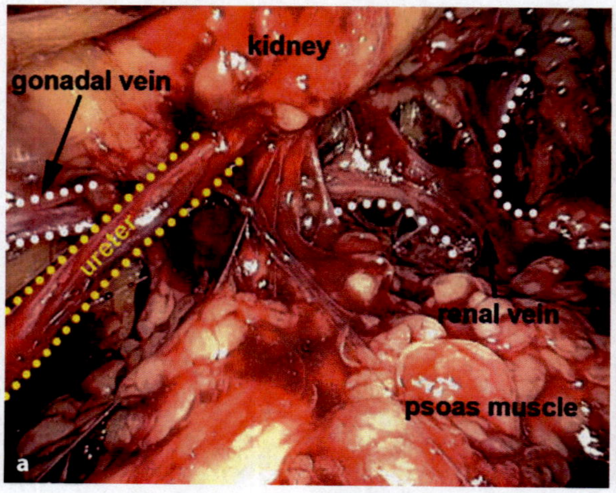

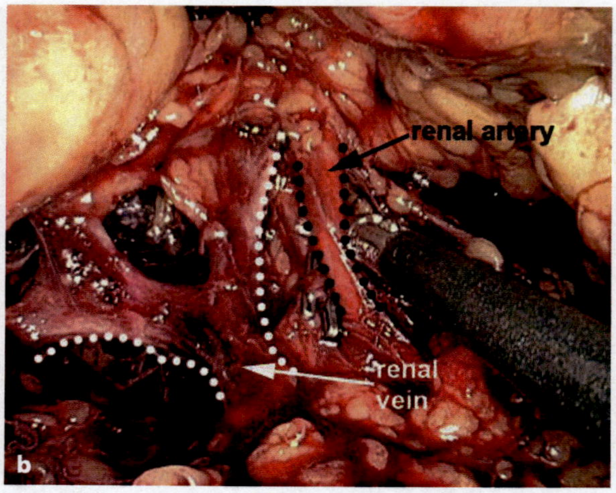

If the anatomy does not easily reveal itself, attention should move caudally and the ureter and/or the gonadal vein can be identified on the psoas and traced cranially to assist with orientation (Step 5a). Continued gentle dissection in a medial direction will lead to the renal hilum. The vein will be encountered first, and the artery will lie cranial to the vein. Good upward traction on the kidney must be maintained at all times and frequent repositioning may be required.

Step 6: Ligation of hilar vessels

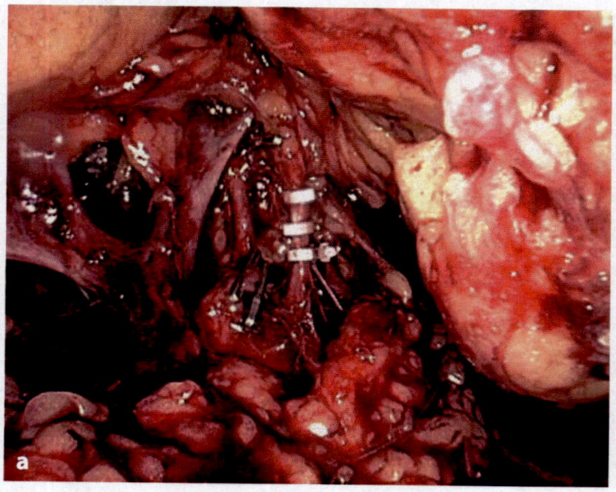

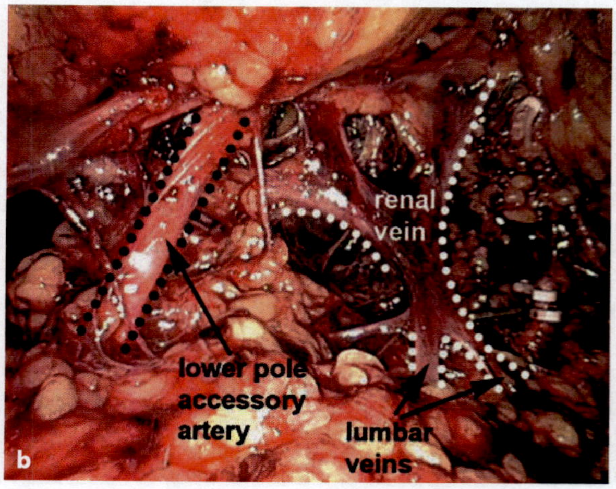

The artery can then be skeletonised, clipped and divided (in this case with Hem-o-lok clips) as demonstrated in Step 6a. The renal vein must be sufficiently mobilised. Caution must be observed at this stage because not uncommonly tributaries to the main renal vein such as the lumbar veins are encountered and must be divided before the main vein can be sufficiently exposed. In this case, a lower pole accessory artery is also present and must always be considered; it may not always be reported on preoperative imaging (Step 6b).

1

Step 7: Ligation of hilar vessels

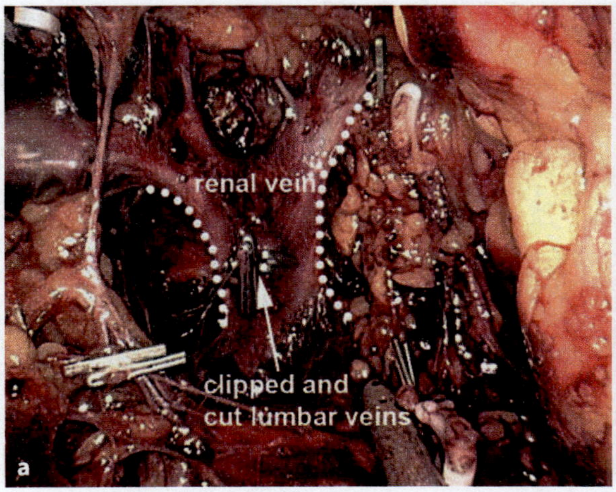

Step 7a demonstrates the lumbar veins, which have been clipped with titanium clips proximally and distally. They are then divided in preparation for exposure of the main vein. Often these lumbar vessels cannot be visualised.

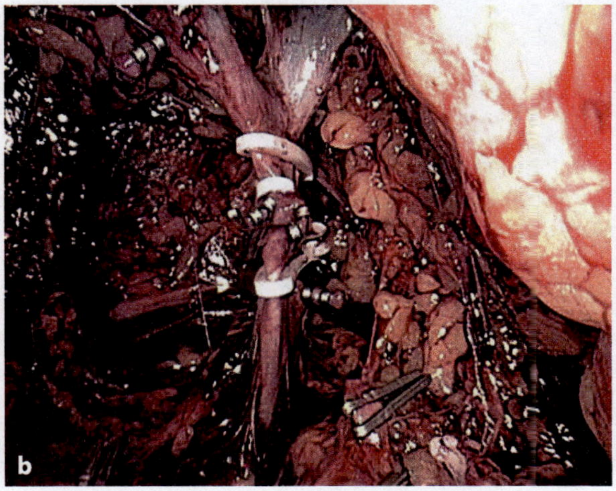

Once the vein is exposed, a minimum of three Hem-o-lok clips (two clips towards the cava, one clip towards the kidney) are applied prior to division.

Step 8: Renal mobilisation

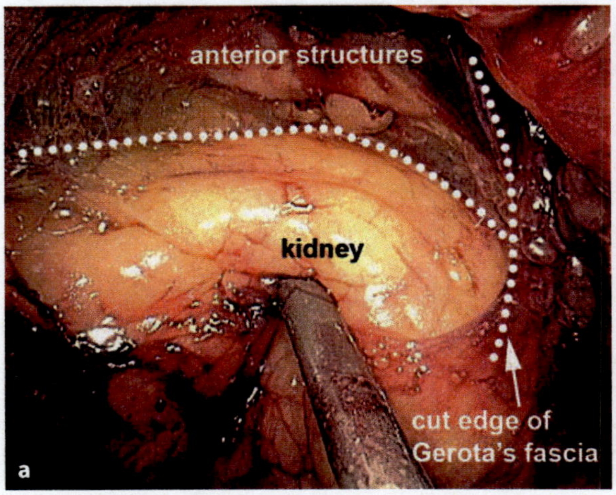

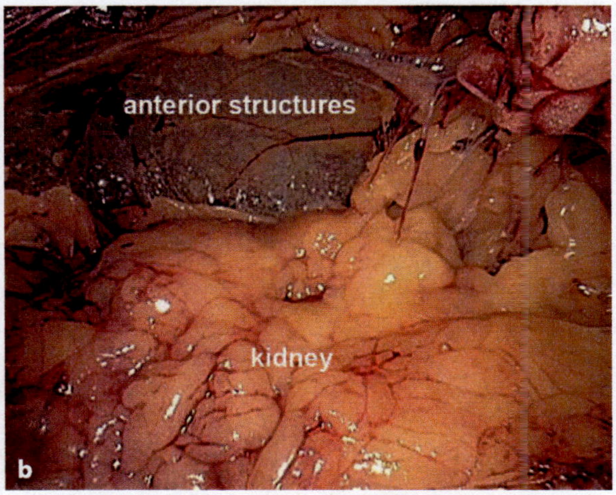

Now that the vessels are secure, mobilisation of the kidney can begin. If the adrenal is to be taken, the dissection continues along the psoas, dividing the adrenal vessels when encountered. If the adrenal gland is to be preserved, the fat can be peeled from the kidney at the hilum, leaving the adrenal to drop down away from the specimen. The dissection continues cranially to the upper pole. Good traction remains vital, and in the absence of perirenal inflammation, the tissues will separate out with gentle blunt dissection. However, the presence of scarring or inflammation may necessitate the use of sharp dissection.

Step 9: Completion of kidney mobilisation and delivery of kidney

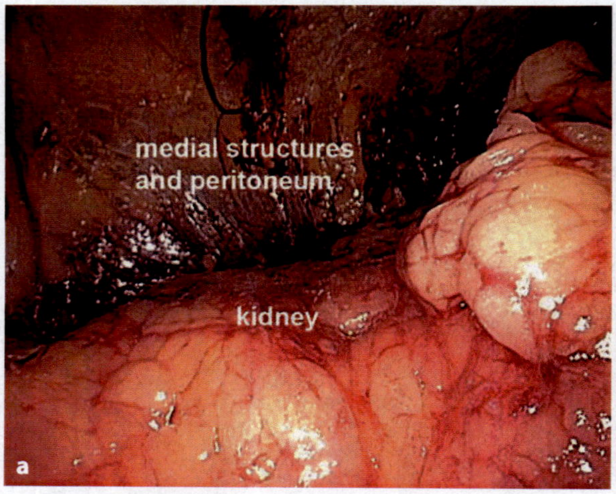

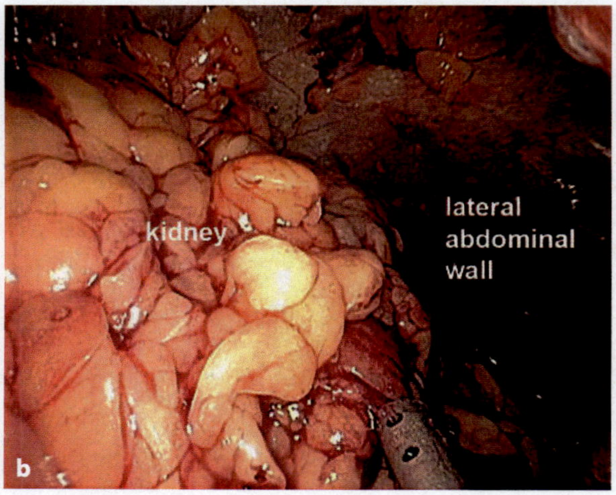

Once the medial border and upper pole are freed, the dissection moves to the anterior surface of the kidney. By removing the traction, the kidney will rest back onto the psoas. In a radical nephrectomy, the plane between the anterior surface of Gerota fascia and the perirenal fat is developed over the front of the kidney, until the hilar structures are encountered. Dissection then continues laterally towards the upper pole. The ureter is then divided. The specimen is finally placed superiorly and laterally, and the hilum can be inspected for haemostasis. A specimen bag is inserted through the anterior port. The hilum is inspected before closure. The specimen is removed through the anterior port incision. It is not usually necessary to leave a drain.

Postoperative Management

- Catheter removal 1st postoperative day
- Eat and drink same day
- Mobilise same day

References

1. Dunn MD, Portis AJ, Shalhav AL, Elbahnasy AM, Heidorn C, McDougall EM et al (2000) Laparoscopic versus open radical nephrectomy: a 9-year experience. J Urol 164:1153–1159
2. Berger A, Brandina R, Atall MA, Herati AS, Kamoi K, Aron M, Haber GP, Stein RJ, Desai MM, Kavoussi LR, Gill IS (2009) Laparoscopic radical nephrectomy for renal cell carcinoma: oncological outcomes at 10 years or more. J Urol 182:2172–2176
3. Desai MM Strzempowski B, Matin SF, Steinberg AP, Ng C, Meran M, Kauok JD, Gill IS (2005) Prospective randomised comparison of transperitoneal versus retroperitoneal laparoscopic radical nephrectomy. J Urol 173:38–41

1.9 Nephroureterectomy (Ureter and Bladder Cuff)

Jens Rassweiler, Ali Serdar Gözen, Levent Gürkan, Jan Thorsten Klein, Giovannalberto Pini, Michael Schulze, Dogu Teber

Introduction

Management of the distal ureter as part of radical nephroureterectomy is one of the most controversial areas in laparoscopic surgery for urological malignancies [1–3]. Today there is still no universally accepted gold standard. Laparoscopic nephrectomy and removal of the distal ureter can be achieved transperitoneally, retroperitoneally, hand-assisted and by open surgery. Initially, we started with a transurethral circumcision of the ureter followed by transperitoneal nephroureterectomy with antegrade stripping of the ureter [1]. However, due to the criticism of the pluck-off-technique (i.e. spillage of tumour cells) as well as morcellation of the specimen, we have changed to a retroperitoneal approach with open ureterectomy using the suprainguinal incision for en-bloc removal of the specimen as well as for the dissection of the distal ureter. The retroperitoneal approach allows the surgeon to work in an anatomical environment that is familiar from open surgery, and this space drains better if urine extravasation or bleeding occurs.

Technically, different transperitoneal techniques to perform complete ureterectomy including a bladder cuff have been described using stapling devices, tissue sealing and endoscopic suturing [4]. This section includes the demonstration of trans- and retroperitoneal dissection of the distal ureter, including three main techniques to approach the intramural part of the ureter.

Indications

- TCC of the upper urinary tract
- Nonfunction reflux nephropathy

Contra-indications

- Bleeding disorders
- Pluck technique and pure endoscopic resection methods are contraindicated in high-grade tumours of the distal ureter
- Any active disease in the bladder is a contraindication to laparoscopic management of intramural ureter

Relative Contra-indications

- Abdominal wall infections
- Aorta aneurysm
- Pregnancy
- Open dissection of the most distal and intramural ureter is recommended in cases with previous pelvic surgery or pelvic radiotherapy

Preoperative Preparation

- Single-shot broad-spectrum antibiotics
- Antiembolic stockings and low-molecular-weight heparin
- Preoperative cystoscopic evaluation of bladder for any active disease
- Sterile urinary catheter attached to sterile urine bag should be available for intraoperative manipulation

Step 1: Patient position and trocar placement (transperitoneal access)

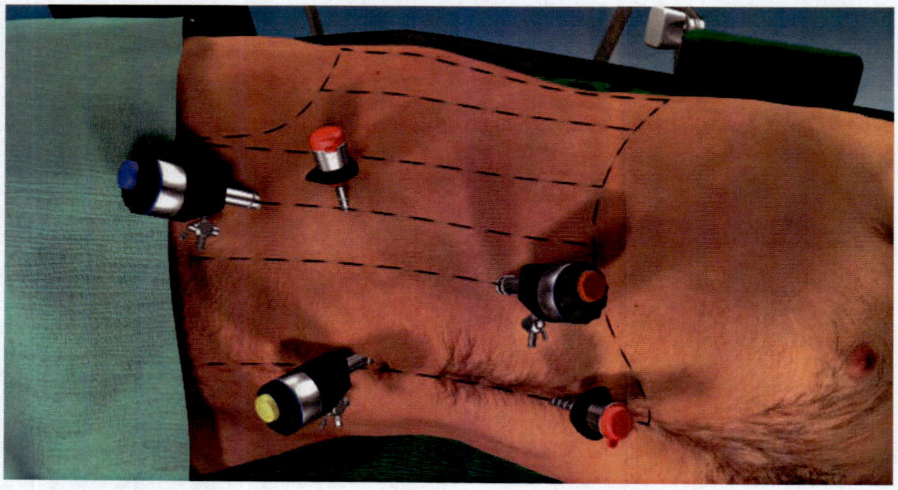

Oblique patient positioning allows medial rotation of the OR table (i.e. flank position) during the nephrectomy part and lateral rotation for dissection of the distal ureter without time-consuming repositioning. Only the transperitoneal access allows safe laparoscopic dissection of the distal ureter down to the bladder. Placing the patient in a 10–20° Trendelenburg position will ease dissection in the deep pelvis. A Veress needle is inserted paraumbilically to create a pneumoperitoneum. For the first port, we prefer a safety trocar for the telescope (11/12 mm). Two working trocars (10 mm and 5 mm) are placed under visual control pararectally.

Step 2: Dissection of the retroperitoneum and trocar placement (retroperitoneal access)

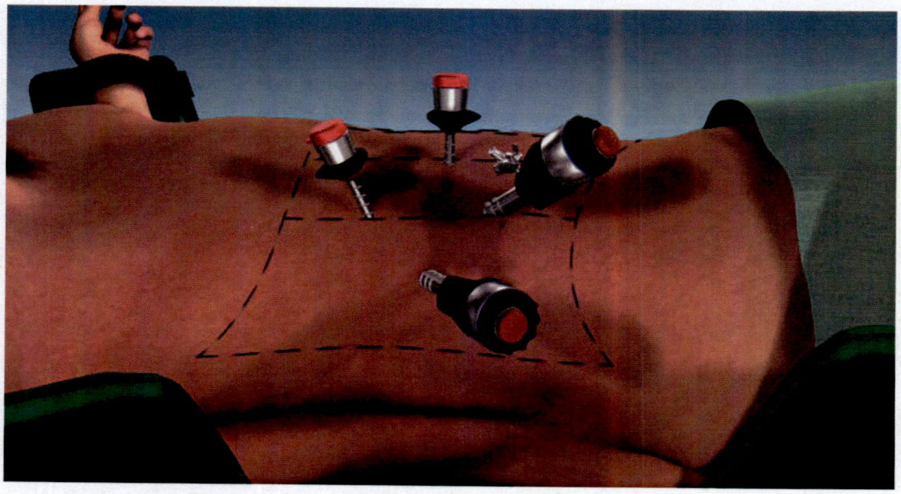

The dissection of the retroperitoneal space is described in detail in Sects. 1.3. and 1.13. After a 15-mm skin incision on the lumbar triangle (Petit triangle), a tunnel to the retroperitoneal space is created bluntly using Overholt forceps and dilated with the index finger and/or using a balloon-trocar system. Two working trocars (10 mm and 5 mm) are placed under control by the index finger and the optical trocar (10 mm) through the primary access site. Another 5-mm working trocar is placed under direct visual control. All the trocars are shown in the drawing.

Step 3: Dissection of the ureter (retroperitoneal)

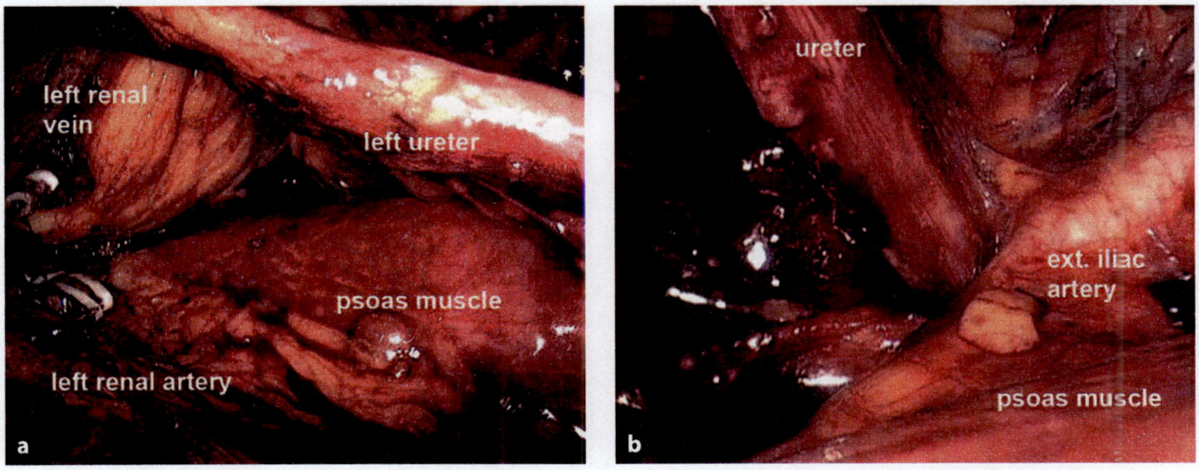

After trocar placement, the pneumoretroperitoneum is established using a maximum carbon dioxide pressure of 12 mmHg (children, 10 mmHg) and a flow of 3.5 l/min. A fourth 5-mm trocar is inserted as described in the previous step. The ureter is dissected (Step 3a) along the psoas muscle up to the crossing of the external iliac artery. The retroperitoneal access allows the dissection of the distal ureter just below its crossing with the iliac vessels (Step 3b). The renal pedicle is dissected, clipped and divided as described in the previous nephrectomy chapters.

Step 4: Dissection of the ureter (transperitoneal)

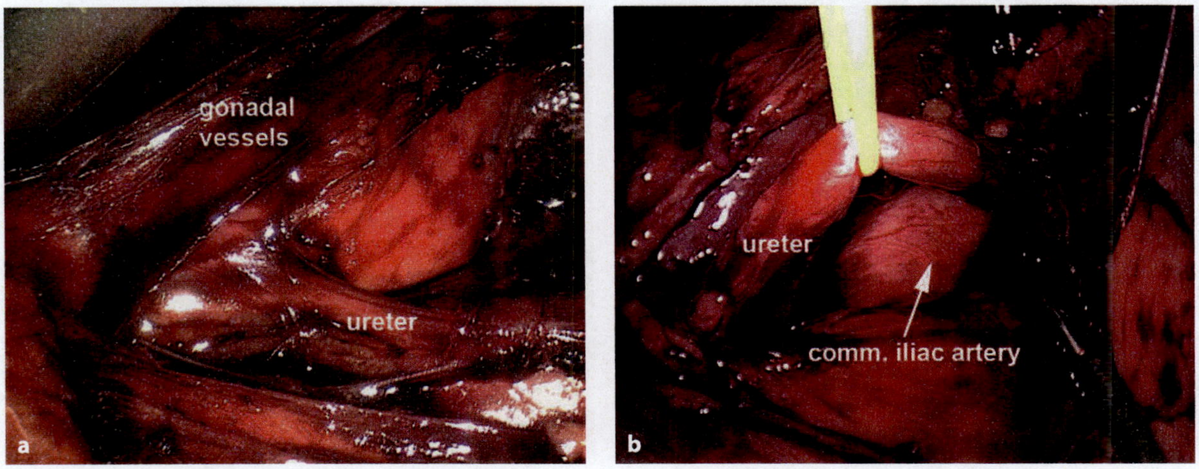

Following the laterocolic incision along the white line of Toldt, the colon is freed medially. After identification of the psoas muscle and the ureter, the ureter is dissected down to the iliac vessels to the bladder. The ureter crosses four important anatomic structures: the gonadal vein (Step 4a), common iliac artery (Step 4b), the umbilical artery (i.e. lateral umbilical ligament) (Step 5a) and the vas deferens or uterine artery (Step 5b). In close proximity to these vessels, the superior vesicle artery, the vas deferens or round ligament and the medial umbilical ligament are identified in that order and mobilised.

Step 5: Dissection of the ureter (transperitoneal)

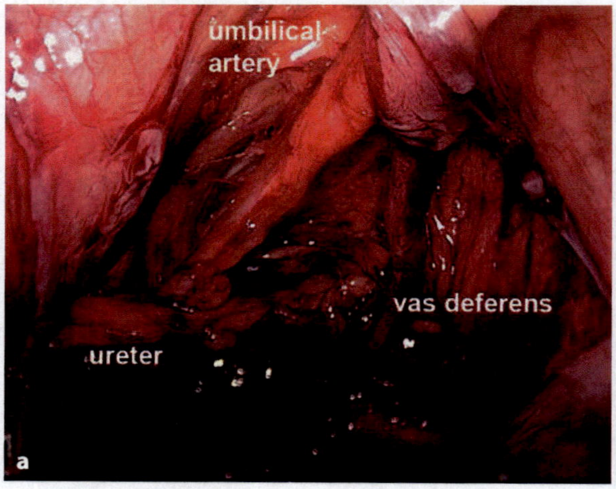

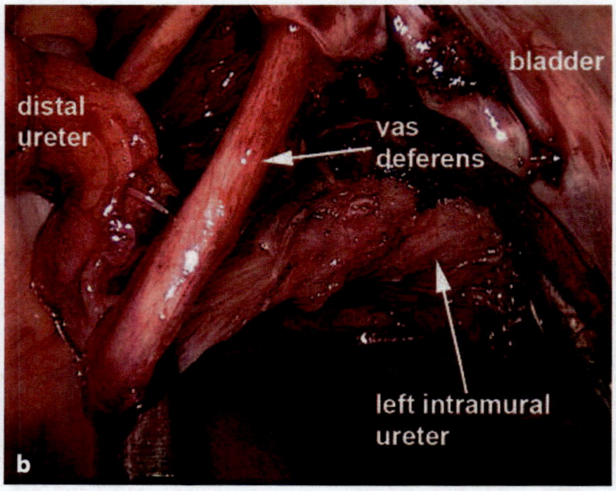

All these structures can be clipped and transected using Hem-o-lok clips, in case they hinder ureteral mobilisation. Dissection proceeds along the ureter until the detrusor muscle is identified (Step 5b). The transperitoneal route allows performing a completely laparoscopic nephroureterectomy, removing the bladder cuff using stapler or sealing devices (see Step 9). For this purpose, an additional 10- or 13-mm trocar at the midline in the lower abdomen is needed (see Step 1) to guarantee the proper instrument angle for dissection and excision of the bladder cuff.

Step 6: Clipping of distal ureter (retroperitoneal)

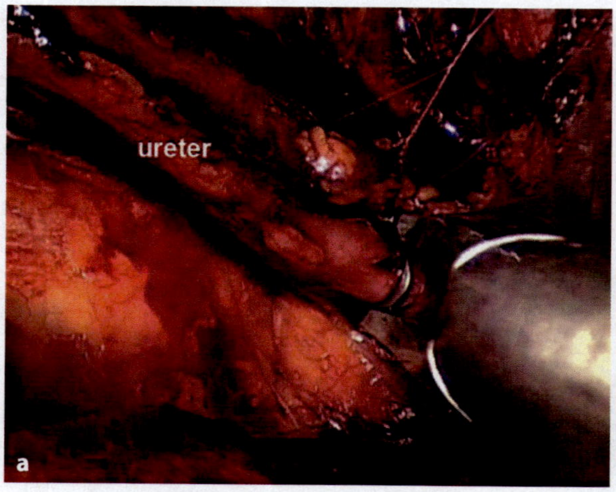

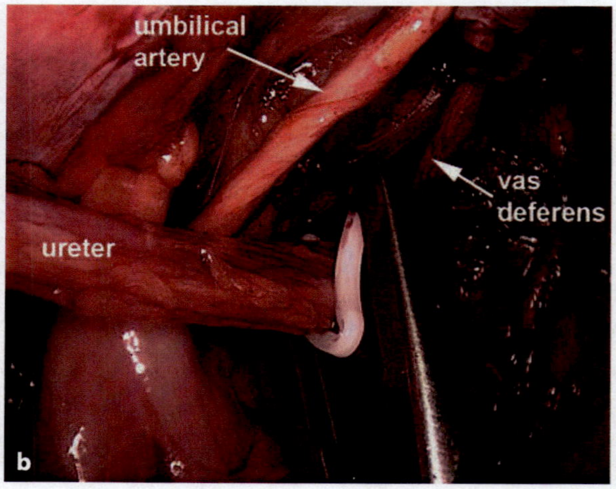

Before proceeding to the distal ureteral resection, the renal specimen within the Gerota fascia is dissected completely from its attachments to the retroperitoneum, leaving the ureter as the only attached structure. At this stage, early clipping of the ureter is advised to minimise the risk of tumour spillage. As an alternative, recently fibrin glue was injected transurethrally to seal the distal ureter [5]. Gentle cephalad traction is applied to the ureter and it is freed from the surrounding tissue. As the dissection proceeds caudally, the iliac vessels should be identified as a landmark followed by the other crossing structures as shown in the previous steps.

Step 7: Management of intramural ureter and bladder cuff (open resection)

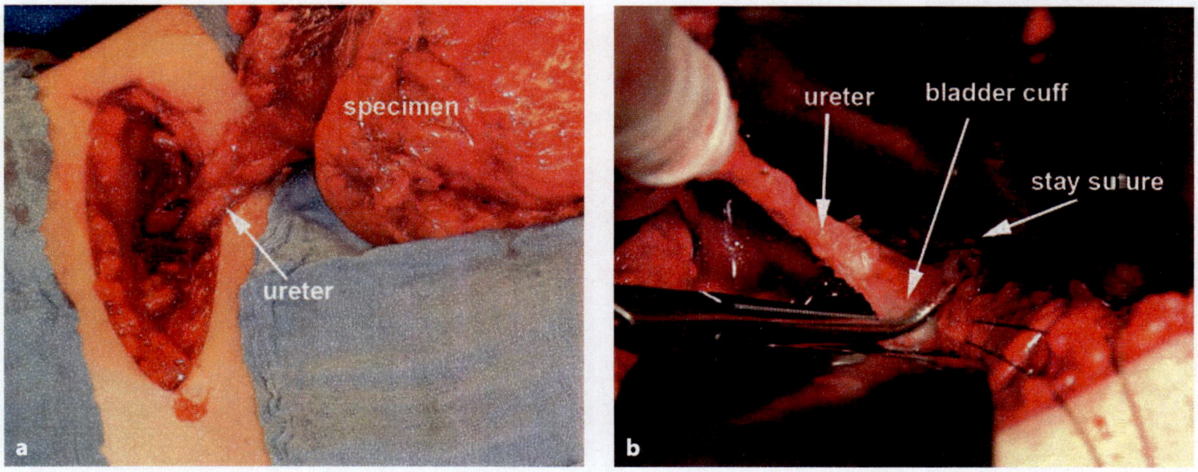

Since a complete removal of the specimen is highly recommended in oncological cases, a Gibson or Pfannenstiel incision is made (Step 7a). The specimen needs to be extracted inside an organ bag to minimise the risk of tumour cell spillage. The same incision can be used for distal ureterectomy and cuff excision. Distal ureterectomy can be performed if the patient is placed in the modified decubitus position with lateral rotation of the OR table. After the specimen is removed in a retrieval bag, it is checked for integrity outside the body and covered with a towel. The ureter is dissected caudally until the detrusor fibres can be identified. A cuff resection with a 2-cm margin is done and the bladder is closed using 3/0 Vicryl suture (Step 7b).

Step 8: Management of intramural ureter and bladder cuff (pluck technique, Step 1)

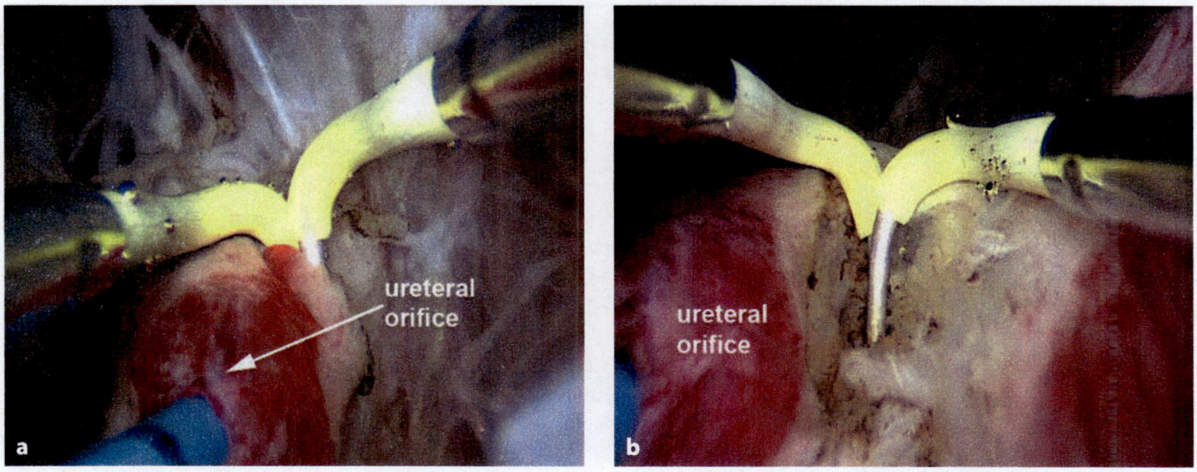

The pluck technique consists of two steps: intravesical resection of the intramural ureter and extravesical dissection of the distal ureter. Prior to patient positioning for nephrectomy, the patient is placed in the dorsal lithotomy position and the ureteral orifice and intramural ureter are resected transurethrally using a Collin knife attached to standard resectoscope. It is important to continue the resection until the ureter is fully detached from the bladder. Care must be taken in female patients for the course of the uterine artery.

Step 9: Management of intramural ureter and bladder cuff (pluck technique, Step 2)

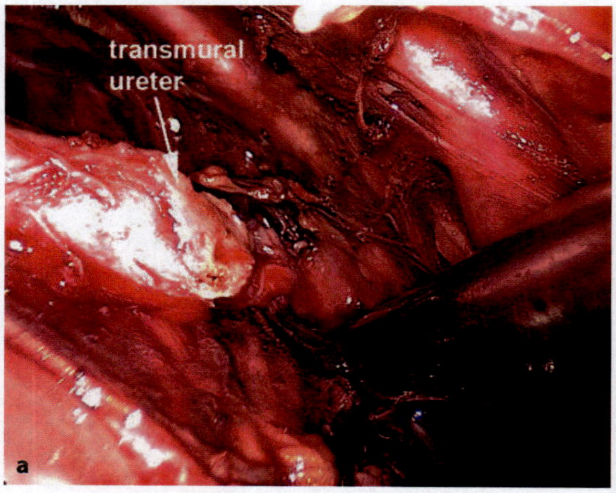

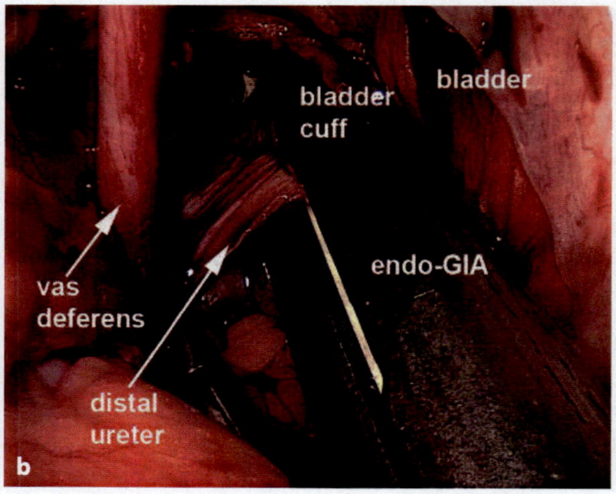

Dissection of the distal ureter is continued caudally under moderate tension on the ureter until the previously detached ureter plucks off (Step 9a). The bladder is left open under indwelling catheter drainage. Extravesically, the ureter is dissected caudally until detrusor fibres are identified [6]. A reticulated laparoscopic tissue stapler is placed cranially to caudally and medially to laterally on the bladder with precautions taken not to harm the unaffected ureteral orifice (Step 9b). After the bladder is transected, the specimen is retrieved and port sites are closed. Stone formation at the stapling clips migrating into the bladder has been observed [1].

Postoperative Management

- For open resection and the pluck technique
  - Confirm bladder integrity by cystography after 5–7 days
  - Remove indwelling urethral catheter if there is no extravasation at cystography
- For laparoscopic stapling technique
  - Remove indwelling urethral catheter if the urine is clear
  - A cystography is not mandatory

References

1. Rassweiler JJ, Schulze M, Marrero R, Frede T, Palou Redorta J, Bassi P (2004) Laparoscopic nephroureterectomy for upper urinary tract transitional cell carcinoma: is it better than open surgery? Eur Urol 46:690–697
2. Srirangam SJ, van Cleynenbreugel B, van Poppel H (2009) Laparoscopic nephroureterectomy: the distal ureteral dilemma. Adv Urol doi:10.1155/2009/316807
3. Tan BJ, Ost MC, Lee BR (2005) Laparoscopic nephroureterectomy with bladder-cuff resection: techniques and outcomes. J Endourol 19:664–676
4. El Fettouh HA, Rassweiler JJ, Schulze M, Salomon L, Allan J, Ramakumar S, Jarrett T, Abbou CC, Tolley DA, Kavoussi LR, Gill IS (2010) Laparoscopic radical nephroureterectomy: results of an international multicenter study. Eur Urol 42:447–452
5. Mueller TJ, DaJusta DG, Cha DY, Kim IY, Ankem MK (2010) Ureteral fibrin sealant injection of the distal ureter during laparoscopic nephroureterectomy – a novel and simple modification of the pluck technique. Urology 75:187–192
6. Shalhav AL, Dunn MD, Portis AJ, Elbahnasy AM, McDougall EM, Clayman RV (2000) Laparoscopic nephroureterectomy for upper tract transitional cell cancer: the Washington University experience. J Urol 163:1100–1104

1.10 Transperitoneal Partial Nephrectomy

1.10.1 Laparoscopic Transperitoneal Partial Nephrectomy

Günter Janetschek, Reinhold Zimmermann

Introduction

The first case of laparoscopic nephron-sparing surgery (LPNE) for benign disease was published in 1993. Since then, laparoscopic radical nephrectomy has become a standard procedure for treatment of renal cell cancer (RCC) [1]. LPNE provides cancer control which is comparable to total nephrectomy (TN). Several studies show that elective partial nephrectomy (PN) can achieve similar oncological outcome as RN in the treatment of T1b tumours. Recently, for 474 PN procedures an estimated cancer-specific survival (CSS) rate of 97.9% and 95.8% at 5 years, and 94.9% and 95.8% at 10 years after PN for small (≤ 4 cm) and large tumours (> 4 cm) was reported [2]

TN has to be considered an overtreatment in many if not the majority of renal cell carcinoma (RCC) cases. PN has widened its indications from imperative cases to selected small and mid-sized tumours due to comparable survival and recurrence rates with partial and radical nephrectomy for RCCs up to 7 cm [3]. Complication rates of LPNE are comparable to open surgery (21–33%) [4, 5]. Many surgeons perform laparoscopic radical nephrectomy (RN), but are unable to perform LPNE. Consecutively, the majority of PNs for smaller tumours are still done by open surgery. Establishing reproducible surgical techniques in order to implement LPNE as a standard operation procedure is urgently needed. It is necessary to:

- Avoid blood loss
- Treat the renal parenchyma as atraumatically as possible in order to avoid damage to the renal parenchyma
- Preserve renal function by excising the tumour precisely
- Keep time of ischaemia as short as possible and therefore

Choose the most appropriate method to reach this aim or to avoid ischaemia at all

Indications

- Elective indication: normal contra-lateral kidney
  a. Less than 4 cm whenever possible
  b. Up to 7 cm in synopsis of patient parameters (localisation in the kidney, age, general performance status)
- Imperative indication:
  a. Solitary kidney
  b. Impaired renal function (only feasible in cases where ischaemia time < 20 min is guaranteed)

Contra-indications

- Bleeding disorders
- Severe atherosclerosis
- Expected ischaemia time > 30 min (exception: cold ischaemia)

Preoperative Evaluation

Exact declination of the tumour to understand its exact location, depth of invasion, topographic anatomy in relation to the kidney (relationship to the collecting system, hilum and vascular anatomy). Also, additional tumours have to be ruled out. A CT scan with contrast (and 3D reconstruction) and/or angio-MRI provide precise information. In addition, an intraoperative ultrasound may provide additional information.

Preoperative Preparation

- Clear liquid diet day 1 preoperatively
- Enema
- Single-shot broad-spectrum antibiotics

Step 1: Operative setup

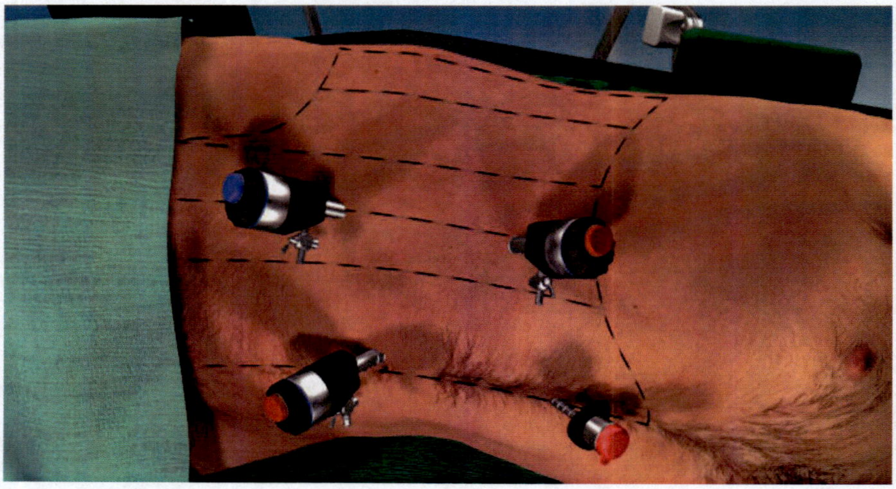

The patient is placed in the lateral decubitus position as already described for nephrectomy. The positions of the surgeon and assistant are also similar. The assistant operates the camera and an additional instrument, usually an Ellis clamp. The ports for lower-pole tumours are similar to those used for nephrectomy. The camera trocar is placed at the umbilicus. A 12-mm working trocar helps to rapidly insert and remove the tourniquets and suture materials. Obesity changes the relative position of the umbilicus. The trocar position must allow for this. Therefore, the trocar for the camera has to be moved laterally at least to the border of the rectus muscle, and the position of the other trocars adapted accordingly. For upper pole tumours, the camera is placed pararectally, above the umbilicus, and the working trocars just below the costal arch.

Step 2: Preparation of tourniquets

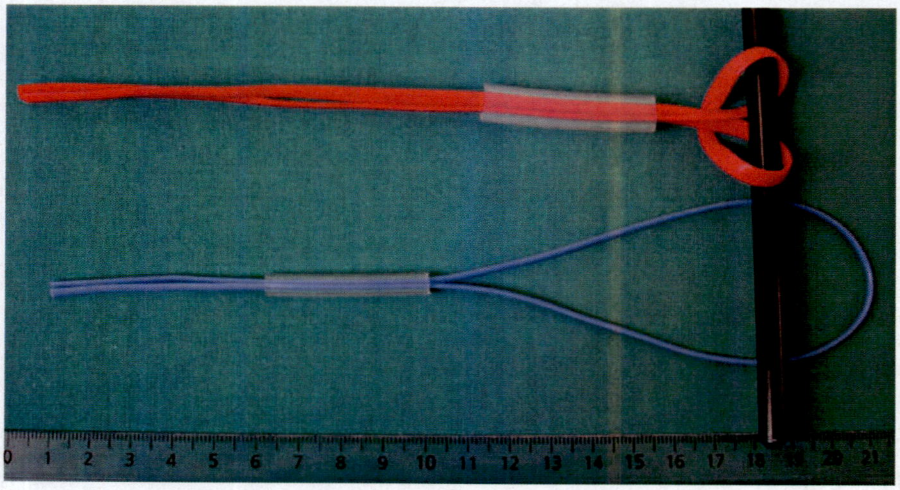

At the beginning of the procedure, the tourniquets are prepared as follows. Two vessel loops, one red (artery: Web sil loop maxi + 10-mm silicone tube) and one blue (vein: vascular silicone ties mini + 6-mm silicone tube) are required. The loops are folded, passed through the tubes, and then passed through a 12-mm trocar. The looped end of the vessel loop is passed around the vessel, and back over the end and tube (like attaching a luggage tag). The free ends of the vessel loops are then fixed with a large (purple) Hem-o-lok clip so that they cannot fall apart. Traction on the end of the vessel loop, with application of a second XL (gold) Hem-o-lok firmly against the end of the tube, causes vessel occlusion.

Step 3: Mobilisation of renal pedicle

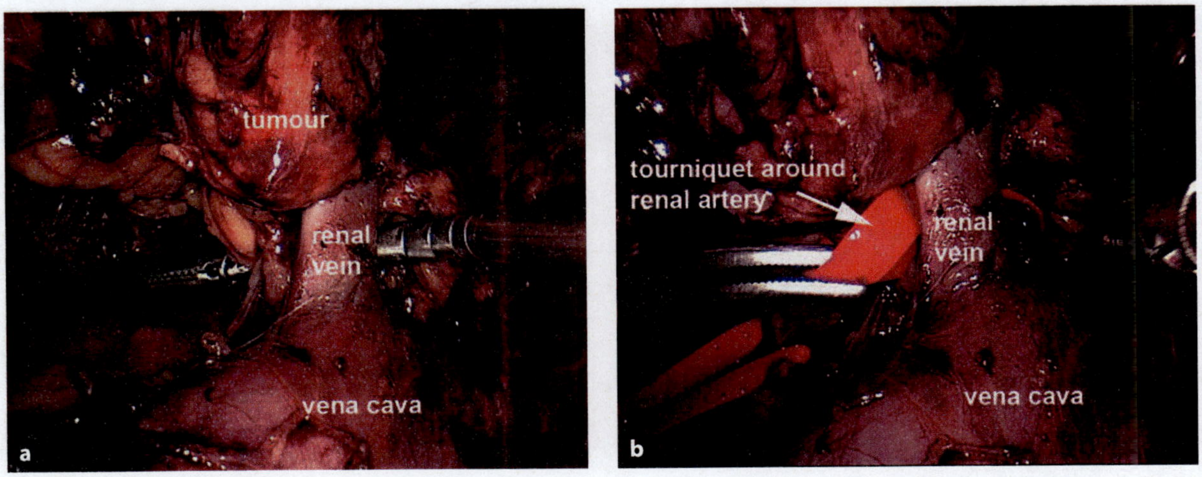

Following exposure of the retroperitoneum, the lower pole of the kidney is elevated (assistant via lateral port). The pedicle is freed from surrounding structures, without skeletalising. The artery is left undissected within the surrounding connective tissue to reduce the chance of injury. A window is made between the pedicle and adrenal gland, through which a right-angle clamp is passed around the pedicle. We use a deflectable clamp (Snowden-Pencer, CareFusion, San Diego, CA, USA). With this clamp, a self-made tourniquet folded over once to form a U-loop (vessel loop through 10-F silicon tube) is brought around the dorsal aspect of the pedicle.

Step 4: Placement of tourniquets

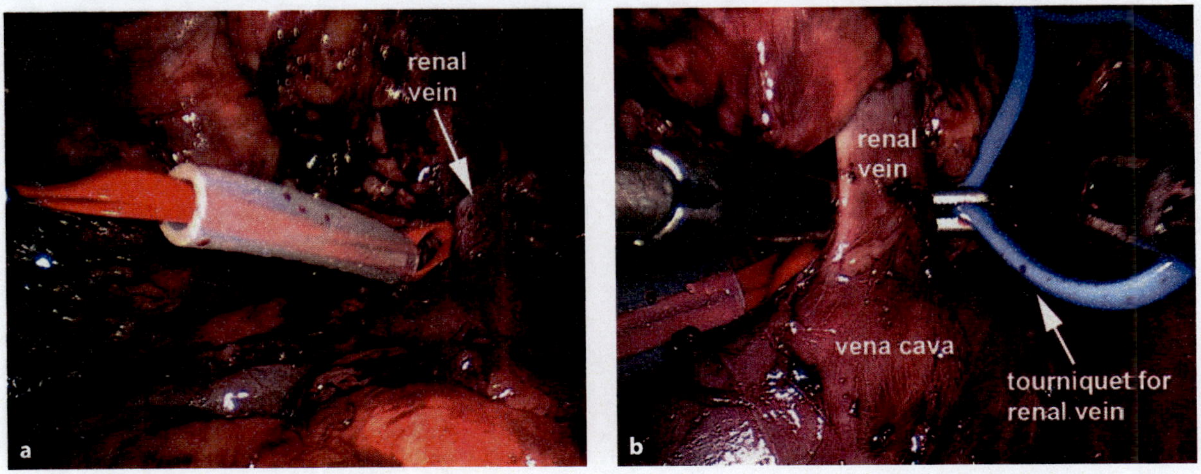

Next, the tourniquet is passed between the pedicle and the renal vein, therefore containing only the artery. The second tourniquet is placed around the renal vein. Both tourniquets are left loose at this time, but are secured with a Hem-o-lok clip to prevent the free ends slipping down the tube. The tourniquets remain in position, until the very end of the procedure, permitting vascular control at any time if necessary. The kidney is now mobilised completely outside the Gerota fascia. This facilitates renal manipulation into the optimal position for tumour excision and reconstruction.

Step 5: Removal of Gerota fascia and induction of ischaemia

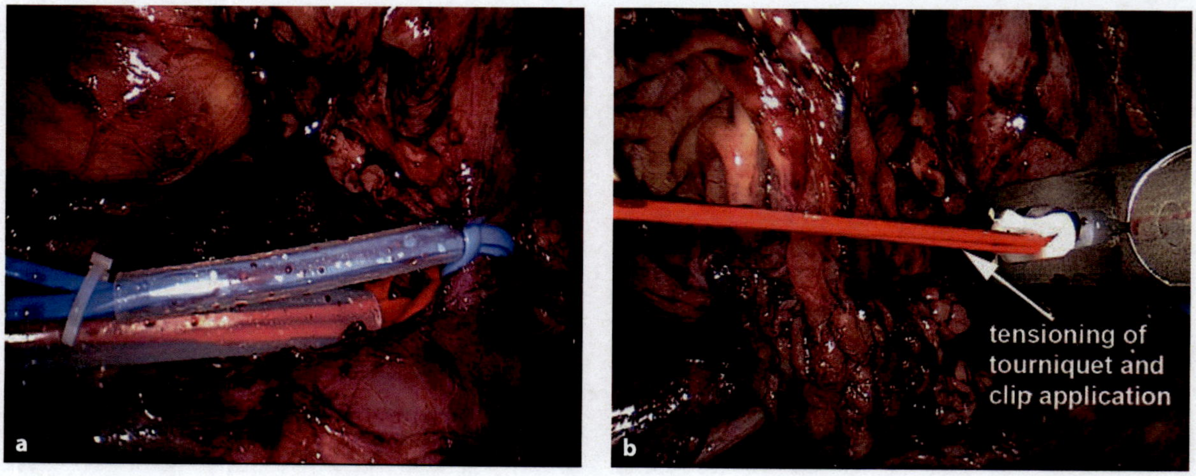

Next, the Gerota fascia is removed from the kidney, so that a broad margin of renal parenchyma adjacent to the tumour is exposed. If the fat is sclerotic and adherent, this may be difficult and slow. Ideally, the Gerota fascia overlying the tumour is left intact. Intravenous mannitol (15%, 250 ml) is administered prior to the onset of ischaemia. Then the arterial tourniquet is tightened and secured with a large Hem-o-lok clip. This clip is removed later to terminate ischaemia by means of an ultrasonic scalpel. The venous tourniquet is occluded only if venous backflow occurs.

Step 6: Tumour excision

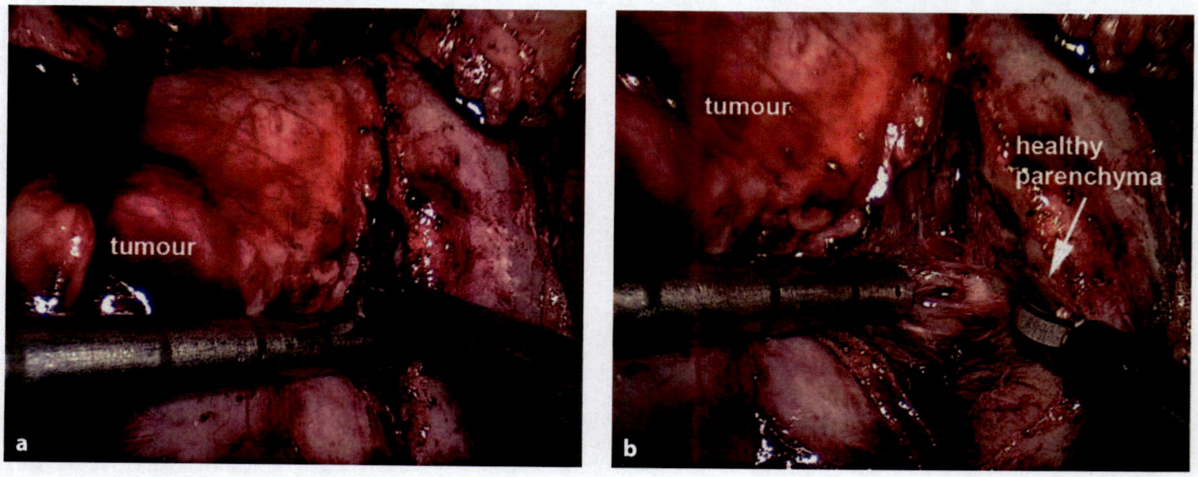

The renal capsule is incised about 5 mm away from the tumour by diathermy. The tumour is excised in a bloodless field, using cold Metzenbaum scissors to achieve a perpendicular incision through the whole layer of parenchyma. Continuous close inspection of the cut surface helps distinguish between normal parenchyma and tumour. If tumour tissue becomes visible, excision of the specimen is continued within healthy tissue. Strict observance of this technique makes random biopsies of the excision bed unnecessary. As excision proceeds, vessels may be identified and clipped. An endoscopic bag is used for specimen removal.

Step 7: uture of collecting system and interstitial tissue

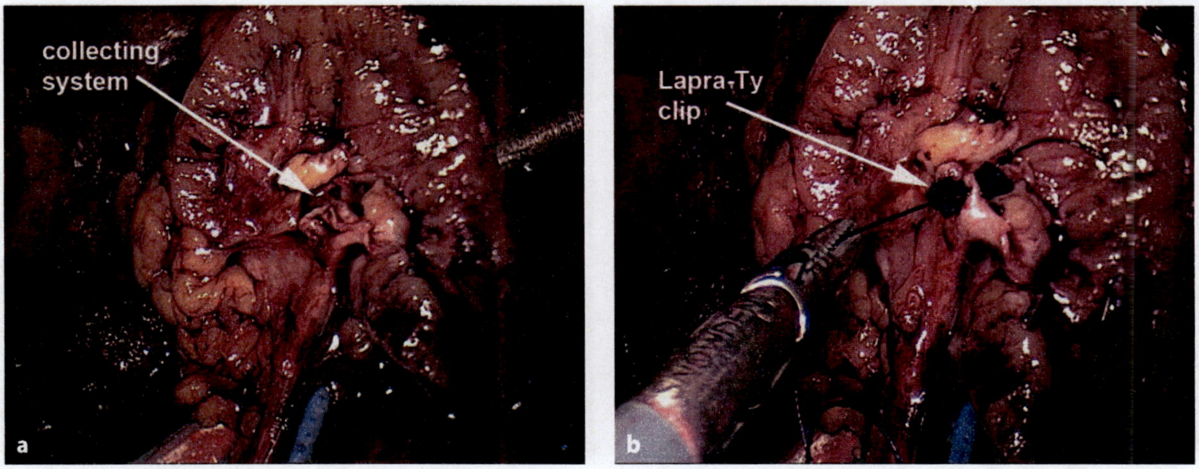

In this case, the lower pole of the kidney has been removed completely. Reconstruction is performed in two layers. It is started by closing the defect in the collecting system and by approximating the interstitial tissue using a running suture (2× 3/0 Vicryl 15 cm Lapra-Ty + knot at end of suture, 26.4 mm 5/8 needle). This suture, which is secured on both sides with a resorbable Lapra-Ty clip to avoid time-consuming knotting, is started at the opposite edge of the resection bed. It includes arteries and veins, thereby providing haemostasis. Care must be taken to avoid injury of large central vessels. Therefore the stitches are made superficially only.

Step 8: Parenchymal suture I

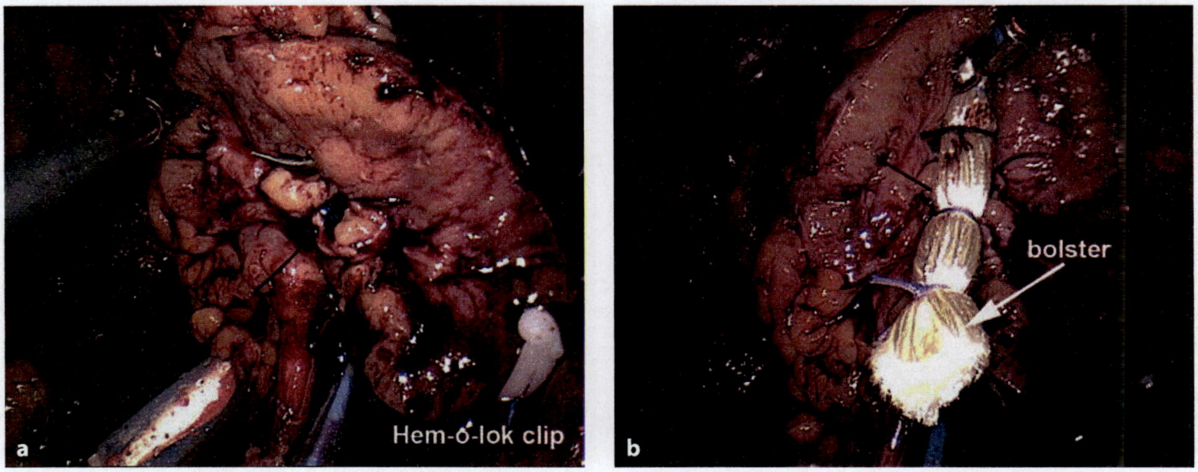

The second running suture (Vicryl 1, M04 needle, 15 cm + 20 cm) is applied through the whole thickness of the renal parenchyma. This running suture is secured with a large Hem-o-lok clip on the end of the thread. A knot behind the clip prevents it from slipping off. Underneath the suture, a bolster of oxidized regenerated cellulose (Tabotamp/Surgicel) is placed. This bolster is haemostatic by itself, but also provides haemostasis by pressure on the vessels underneath in the interstitial layer. This suture is secured after each stitch with a large Hem-o-lok clip. These clips aid compression of the renal parenchyma, resulting in efficient haemostasis, and reduce the chance of the suture cutting through the parenchyma.

Step 9: Parenchymal suture II

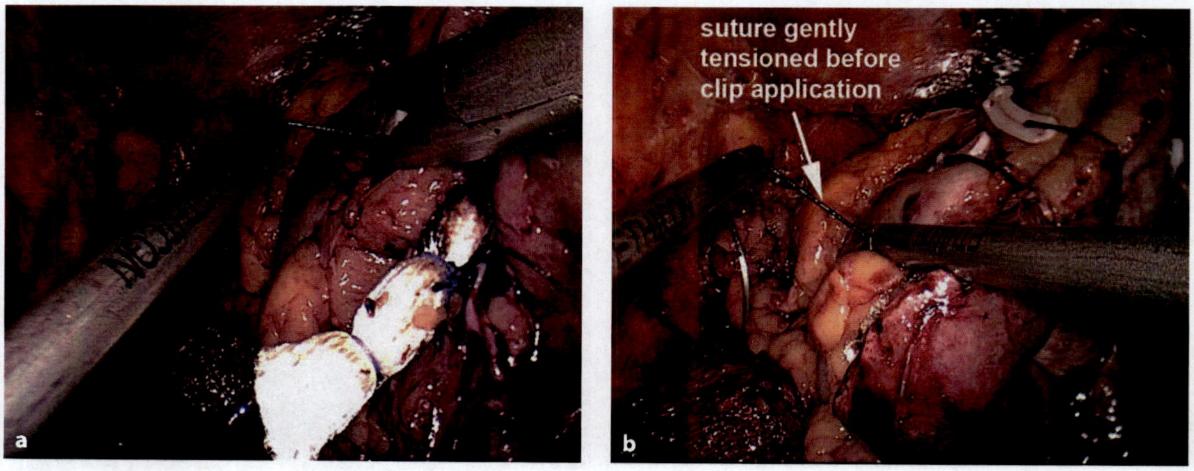

Ischaemia is terminated after the first stitch and placement of the Tabotamp roll by releasing the tourniquet (which remains in position). The Hem-o-lok clip is cut by means of an ultrasonic scalpel. This early declamping reduces ischaemia time is by about 10 min. It is never a problem to continue the parenchymal suture without ischaemia. As an alternative, an interrupted suture may allow more parenchymal compression than a running suture. However, it is more time-consuming. Therefore, we use it only exceptionally if bleeding persists or if we are concerned that the running suture may cut through the parenchyma.

Step 10: Sealing of the resection area

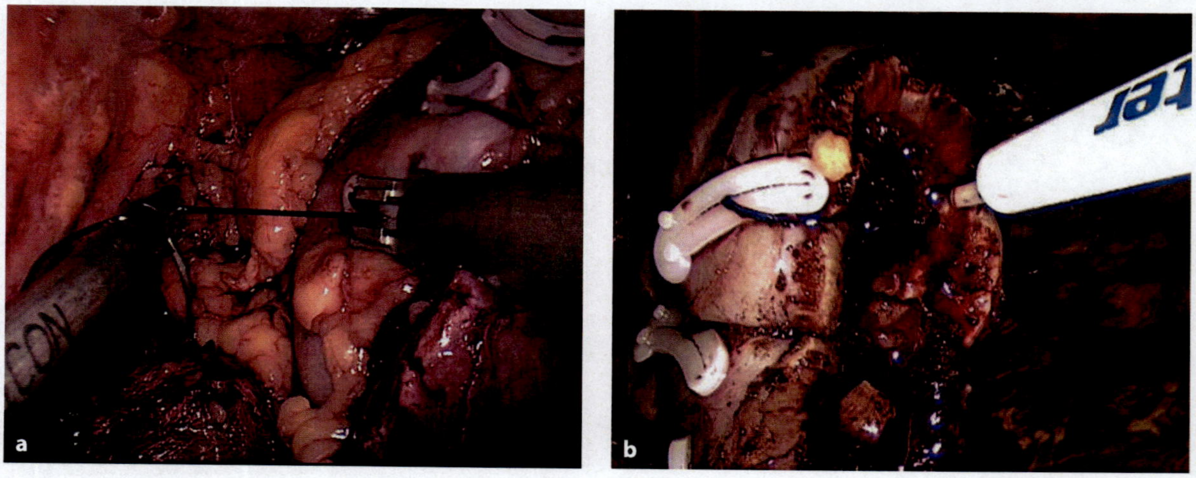

The end of the running suture is secured with a Lapra-Ty clip in addition to the Hem-o-lok clip so that the suture cannot loosen. Fibrin glue (Tissucol Duo S Immuno, Baxter, Deerfield, IL, USA) is applied over the suture line and between the approximated edges of the parenchyma to avoid delayed bleeding. A double-lumen laparoscopic applicator (Duplocath 180, Baxter) is designed for this purpose. To reinforce the repair, a stripe of Tabotamp may be added to cover the suture. Finally, the remnants of the Gerota fascia are reapproximated over the repair. The kidney is brought back into its normal position and attached to the lateral abdominal wall with one suture to avoid torsion. A drain is placed through the most lateral port. The specimen is removed through an extension of the lower abdominal port site incision.

Postoperative Management

- Monitoring of RBC/CREA postoperative day 1/day 5
- Analgesics as required
- No heparin injection on day of surgery
- Mobilisation on day 1
- Drainage removal on day 2 or 3 according to output
- No specific diet
- Discharge on day 4 or 5
- Ultrasonography before discharge

References

1. Janetschek G, Jeschke K, Peschel R, Strohmeyer D, Henning K, Bartsch G (2000) Laparoscopic surgery for stage T1 renal cell carcinoma: radical nephrectomy and wedge resection. Eur Urol 38:131–138
2. Crispen PL, Boorjian SA, Lohse CM, Sebo TS, Cheville JC, Blute ML, Leibovich BC (2008) Outcomes following partial nephrectomy by tumor size. J Urol 180:1912–1917
3. Albqami N, Janetschek G (2006) Indications and contraindications for the use of laparoscopic surgery for renal cell carcinoma. Nat Clin Pract Urol 3:32–37
4. Zimmermann R, Janetschek G (2008) Complications of laparoscopic partial nephrectomy. World J Urol 26:531–537
5. Janetschek G (2007) Laparoscopic partial nephrectomy for RCC: how can we avoid ischemic damage of the renal parenchyma? Eur Urol 52:1303–1305

1.10.2 Robot-Assisted Transperitoneal Partial Nephrectomy

Ingolf A. Tuerk, Rowan Casey, Evangelos Liatsikos, Jens-Uwe Stolzenburg

Introduction

The management of renal masses has changed significantly in the past 20 years with the improvement in imaging modalities for detecting and staging of renal lesions. This allows many more patients to be considered for partial nephrectomy. Further improvements in haemostatic agents such as fibrin glue allow the procedure to be performed safely with minimally invasive techniques.

Robotic surgery provides the same benefits as laparoscopic surgery, in terms of less postoperative pain, shorter hospital stay, improved cosmetic result and faster return to normal activities, compared to open surgery [1, 2]. In comparison to laparoscopic surgery, the robot offers further advantages of a shorter learning curve, three-dimensional stereoscopic vision, 7° of wrist motion, movement scale-down and tremor filtration [3]. Robotic surgery also permits more rapid intracorporeal suturing and application of haemostatic agents within the allowable warm ischaemia period [4].

Indications

- Mainly exophytic renal tumours smaller than 4 cm
- Patients with solitary kidneys
- Bilateral renal tumours

Contra-indications

- Endophytic or central renal lesions
- Severe cardiorespiratory co-morbidity
- Multiple prior abdominal surgeries

Preoperative Preparation

- Broad-spectrum antibiotic prophylaxis
- Thromboprophylaxis (as per local protocols)
- Informed consent (including risk of conversion)
- Retrograde ureteric stenting in selected cases

Step 1: Patient and robot position

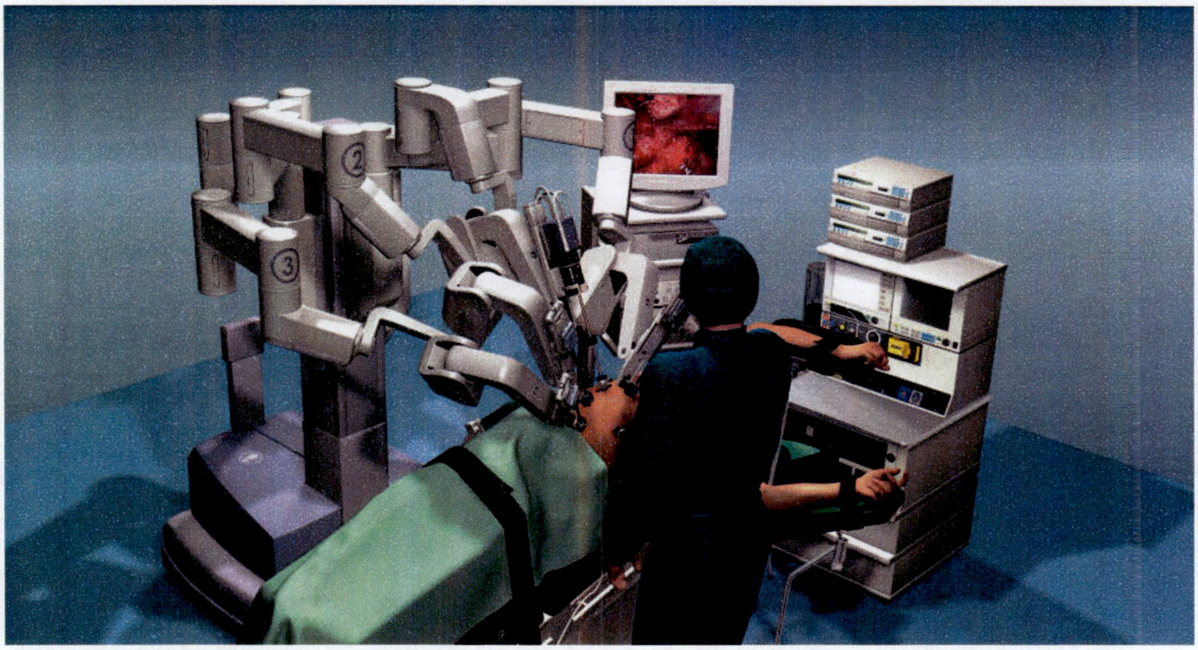

In all robot-assisted laparoscopic procedures, patient positioning and port placement are very important considerations in order to ensure that the operation can be completed successfully. The requirement for the robot is that it can be docked properly with the patient and laparoscopic instruments and that the instruments or robot arms do not clash either outside or inside the patient. The patient is placed in a modified lateral decubitus position with 20–30° rotation of the shoulder and hip away from the surgeon. The robot is positioned at the patient's back and is docked from here. The operating table is flexed at the level of the umbilicus (see Sect. 1.4).

Step 2: Trocar placement: left side

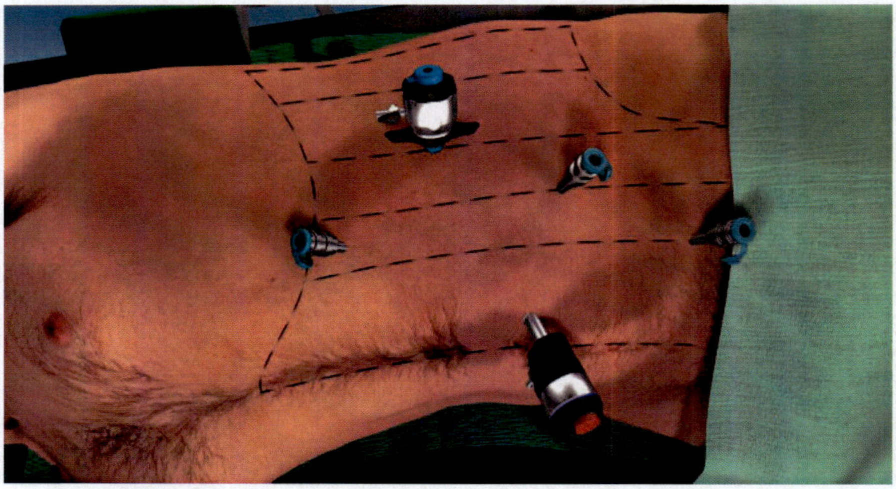

The 12-mm camera port is placed on the anterior axillary line on the same level as the umbilicus. The two 8-mm robotic arms are placed in the midclavicular line triangulating with the optic, allowing a minimum distance between them to prevent clashing of the robot arms. We favour positioning of the assistant 12-mm port paraumbilically rather than in a pararectal position between umbilicus and pubic bone. The fourth robot trocar is placed along a pararectal line below the iliac crest. Port placements can be moved upwards and rotated in cases of an upper pole tumour and must be shifted laterally in obese patients [5]. The transperitoneal approach offers more port placement and working space options.

Step 3: Trocar placement: right side

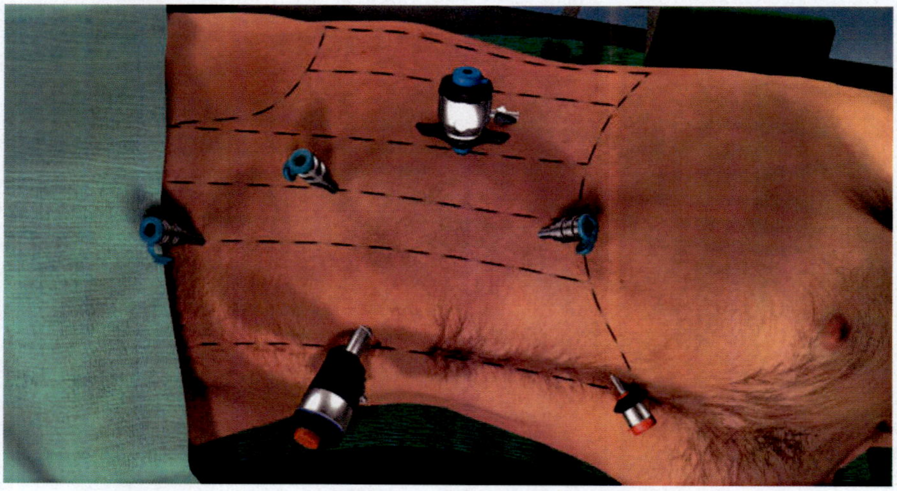

On the right side, the 12-mm camera trocar is placed on the anterior axillary line at a point midway between the costal margin and umbilicus. The 8-mm robotic arms are placed along the midclavicular line triangulating with the optical trocar. The fourth robot arm is placed medial to the pararectal line below the iliac crest level. The assistant 12-mm trocar is then placed periumbilically and the assistant 5-mm retractor, which is usually employed for liver retraction, is placed below the costal margin close to the xiphisternum.

Step 4: Colon mobilisation (left side)

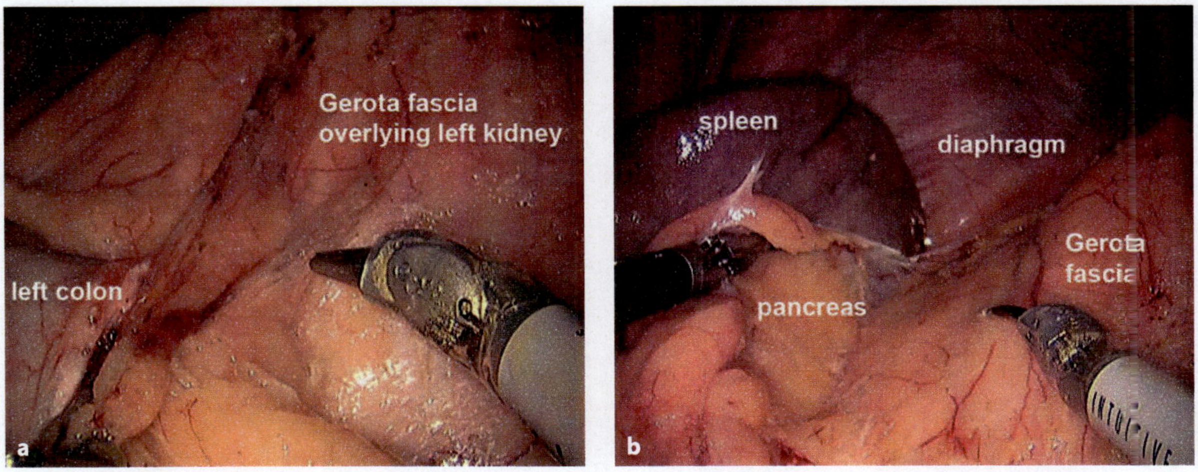

Using a dissecting forceps and monopolar scissors, a lateral incision is made along the line of Toldt to mobilise the left colon (Step 4a). Continued mobilisation of the left colon is made up to level of the spleen and superior pole of the kidney. Transection of the phrenicolienal ligament and pancreas tail mobilisation is performed in order to allow the colon to retract medially and the hilum to be exposed more completely. This also allows the spleen to be mobilised cranially to facilitate access to the upper pole of the kidney or adrenal gland, as in Step 4b.

Step 5: Renal hilum dissection

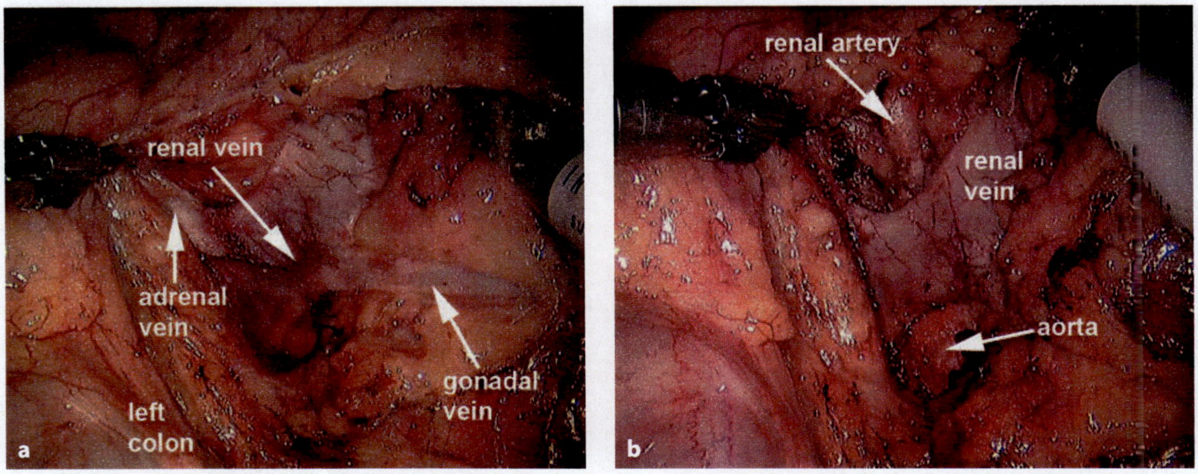

Attention now focuses on dissection of the renal hilum. The kidney is retracted laterally out of the renal fossa by the side surgeon in order to allow dissection of the hilum. The robotic grasping forceps allow dissection of the fatty and perirenal layers over the hilar area until the main renal vessels are identified. Step 5a demonstrates the gonadal and adrenal veins arising feeding into the renal vein. Further dissection of the left renal vein reveals the aorta and left renal artery, which in this case is located superior to the renal vein, as seen in Step 5b. Full dissection of the renal artery and vein are required to allow passage of a laparoscopic bulldog or Satinsky clamp around the vein and/or artery later in the procedure.

Step 6: Perirenal fat mobilisation and tumour identification

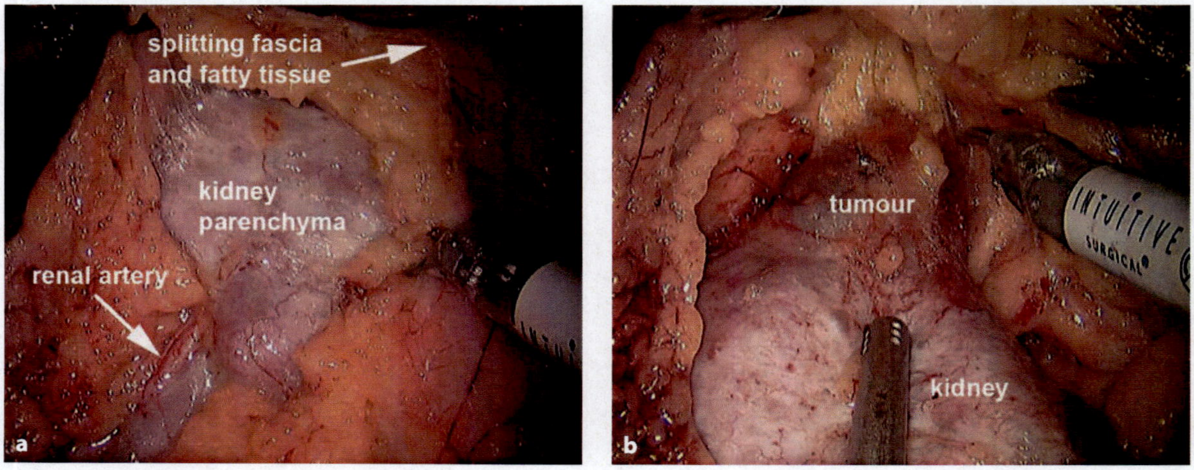

The Gerota fascia and the perirenal fatty tissue over the renal vein are split laterally in the direction of the kidney and this is continued over the kidney capsule. This step preserves the fat and Gerota fascia, as will be required later to close over the kidney for reconstruction. Mobilisation of the lower pole of the left kidney, identification of the ureter and lateral and posterior mobilisation of the kidney are now performed in order to allow the kidney to be rotated as necessary. Continue dissection of the Gerota fascia off the kidney to the renal tumour is reached. Here a cap of perinephric fat can be retained on the surface of the tumour as part of the final resection specimen, and this also allows traction with graspers.

Step 7: Renal clamping

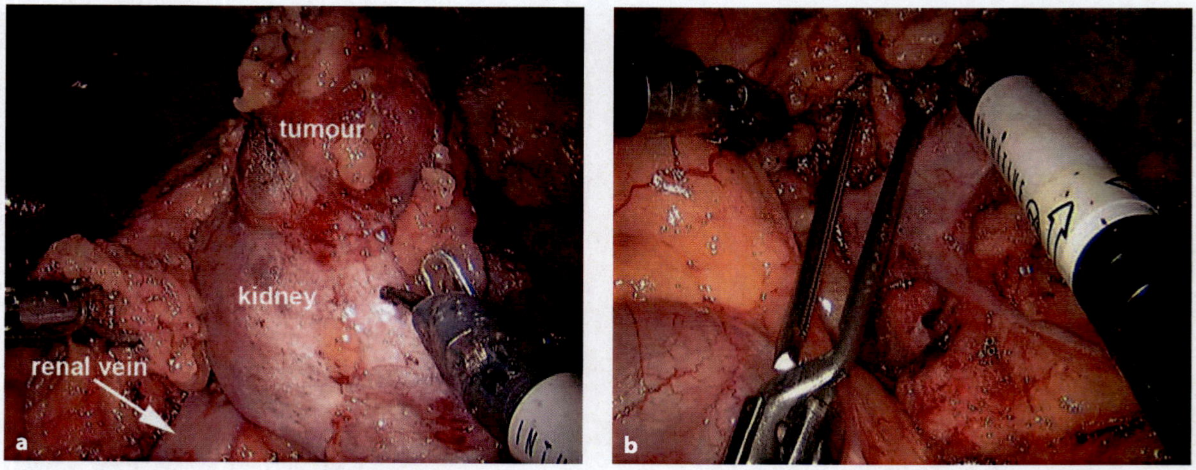

The dissected tumour is now further exposed on the renal capsule while slightly rotating the mobilised kidney. The margin of the tumour on the renal surface for incision is scored with monopolar scissors and prior to renal artery clamping, one or two surgical bolsters and 2/0 Monocryl suture material are placed inside the abdomen by the assistant in order to facilitate quick access for haemostasis once the kidney capsule has been incised. In this case, the assistant clamps the renal artery with a laparoscopic bulldog clamp through the assistant 12-mm port. The use of a laparoscopic Satinsky clamp is also described and allows en-bloc renal artery and vein occlusion.

Step 8: Tumour resection and collecting system closure

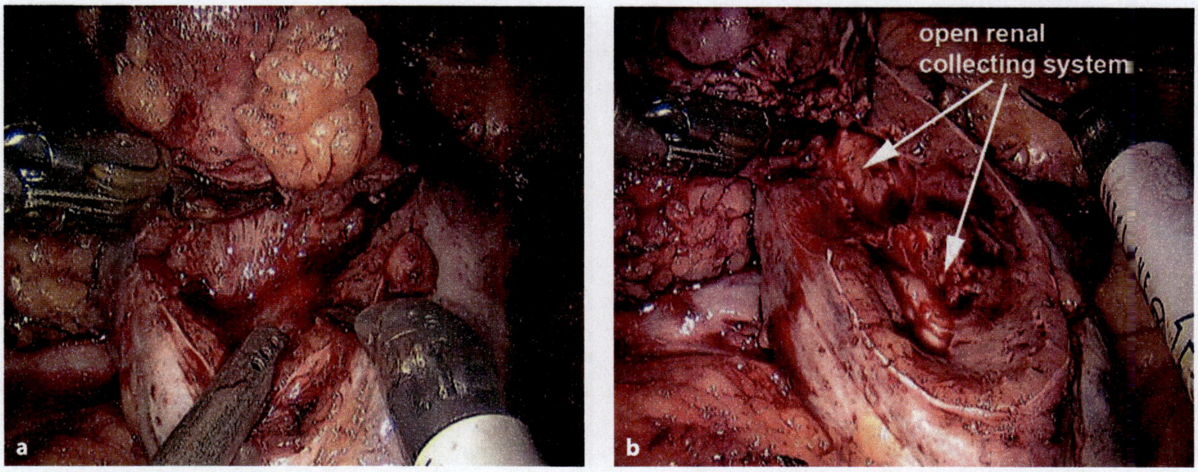

The tumour is resected with cold scissors while the assistant utilises the suction to keep the resection field bloodless and to assist with counter-traction. Step 8b illustrates the final resection of the tumour with the exposed collecting system. If a positive margin is suspected deeper resection can be carried out using cold scissors. Similarly, frozen section biopsies of the tumour base can be sent for immediate analysis in order to determine microscopic margin clearance. The collecting system of the kidney has been opened during dissection and should be readily identified by the console surgeon. At this stage, some surgeons instill methylene blue via a ureteric catheter inserted preoperatively in order to ensure complete closure of the collecting system.

Step 9: Collecting system closure

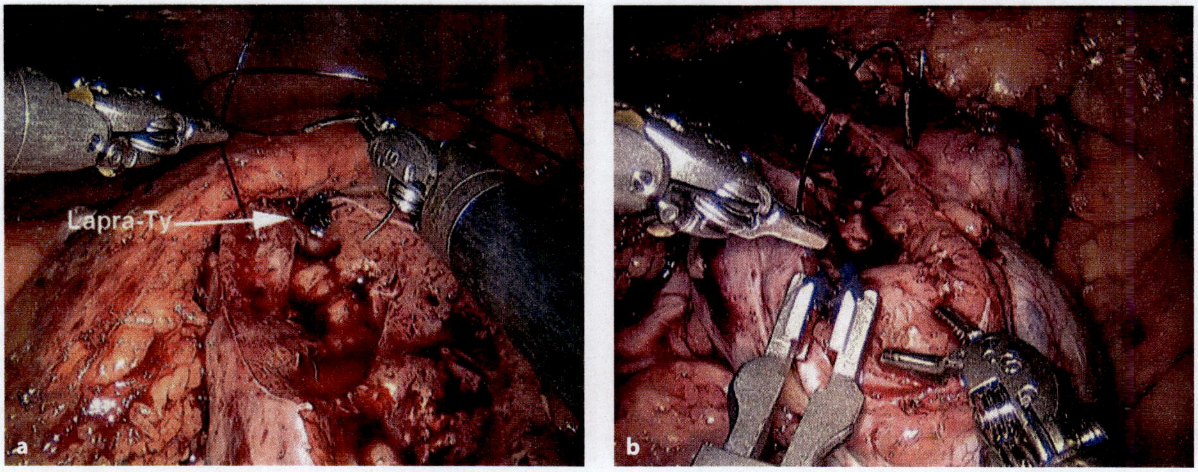

The tumour bed and the collecting system are now sutured closed with a 2/0 Monocryl running suture, on an SH needle, secured on the starting end with a Lapra-Ty clip, as in Step 9a. The advantage of robot-assisted laparoscopic surgery is that it allows a greater degree of magnification, which aids detection of defects in the collecting system. This running suture is continued along the tumour bed and collecting system to achieve closure of the collecting system and haemostasis. Once the running suture is completed, the other end of the tumour bed suture can be secured with a Lapra-Ty clip, which grasps the suture very well and does not slip. Step 9b demonstrates this Lapra-Ty being applied to the proximal end of the tensioned suture.

Step 10: Renorrhaphy

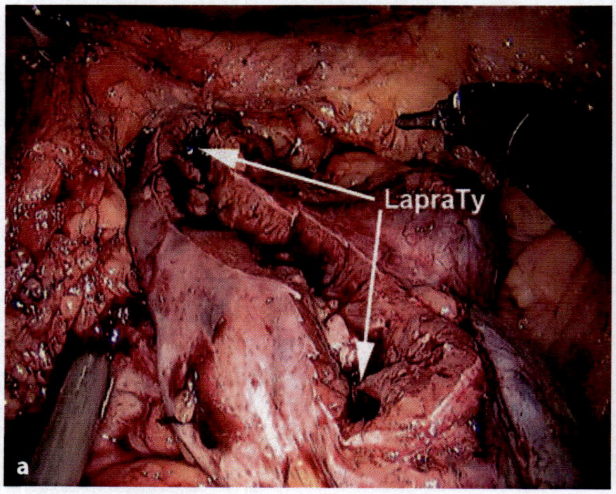

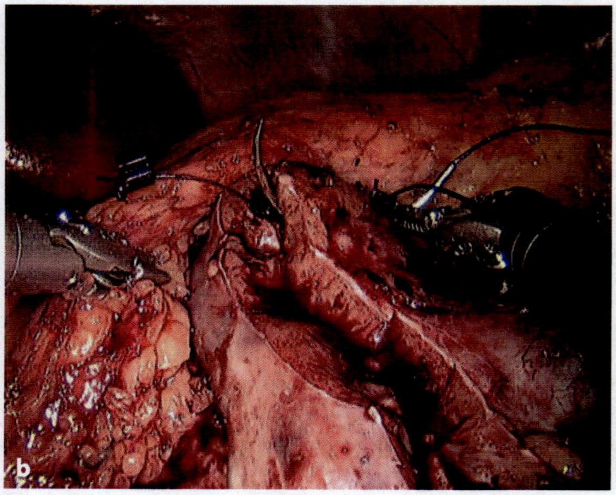

The finished tumour bed running suture is demonstrated in Step 10a using Lapra-Ty clips at both ends. This provides significant haemostasis and collecting system closure. The bulldog clamp is released by the side surgeon at this stage to check whether there are any large perforating vessels in the kidney parenchyma that require individual interrupted suturing to achieve further haemostasis. In this case, it can be seen that the Lapra-Ty suture provides very good approximation of the edges of the defect. Vertical mattress suturing is now commenced with 0 Monocryl on a CT-1 needle. These sutures are placed deep in the renal cortex and secured on one end with a Lapra-Ty clip initially, as can be seen in Step 10b.

Step 11: Renorrhaphy and haemostatic agents

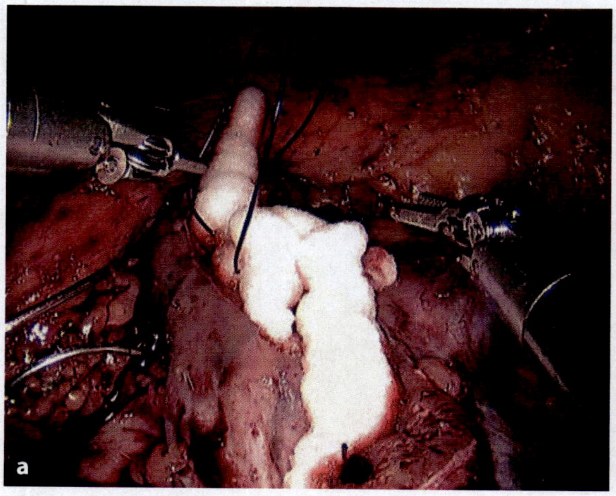

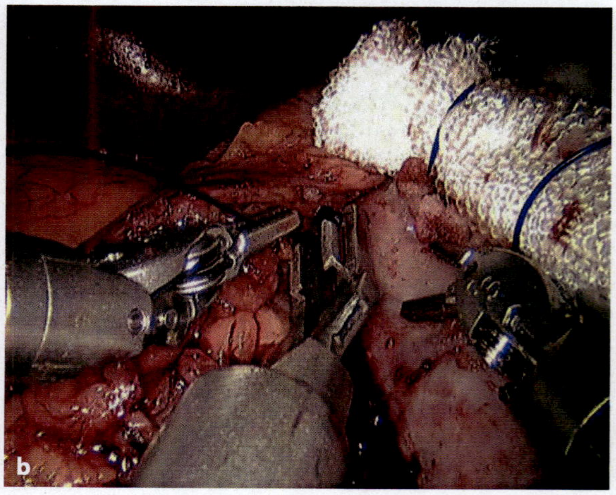

After two to four preplaced mattress sutures, FloSeal is applied to the exposed renal cortical surface for additional haemostasis (Step 11a). One or two Surgicel bolsters can then be placed under the mattress sutures, which are then tightened and on the other end secured with a Lapra-Ty clip. The side surgeon elevates the kidney laterally at this point in order to assess the haemostatic control. The gas pressure can also be reduced as a further check of haemostasis.

Step 12: Final result and specimen bagging

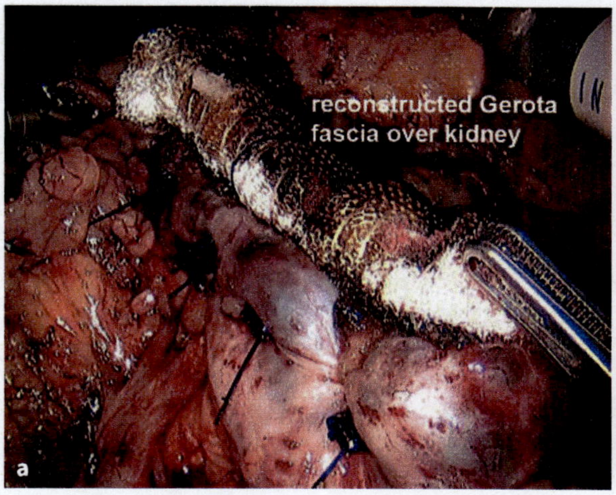

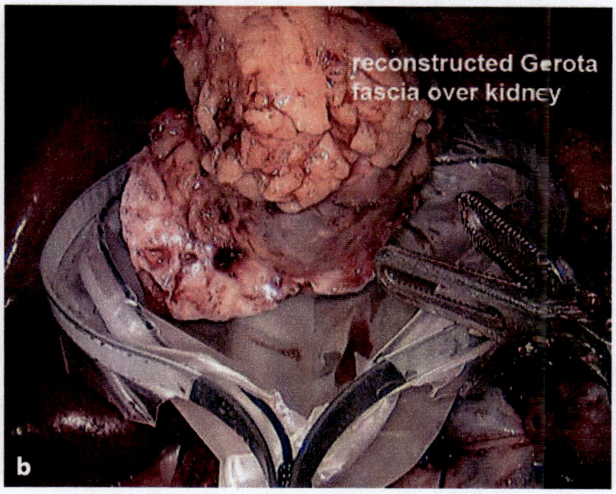

The finished procedure demonstrates the final kidney resection closure. Four mattress sutures have been placed deep in the parenchyma and have secured a large Surgicel bolster to the exposed renal surface. These sutures have been secured with Lapra-Ty clips. The specimen is now bagged using an EndoCatch bag, as in Step 12b. It is stored above the spleen during reconstruction of the perirenal fat and Gerota fascia or is sent immediately for frozen section.

Step 13: Kidney reconstruction and specimen removal

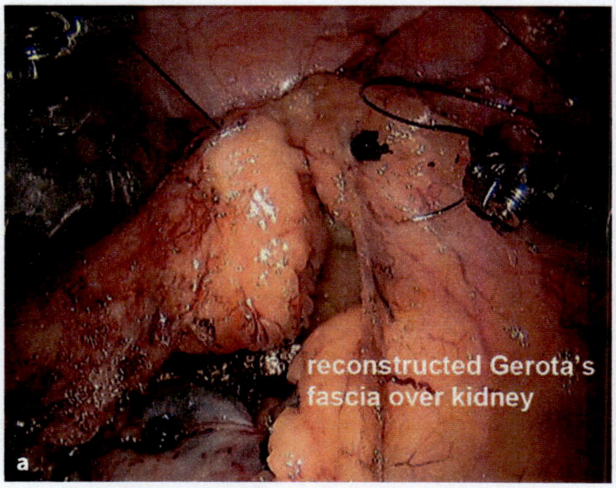

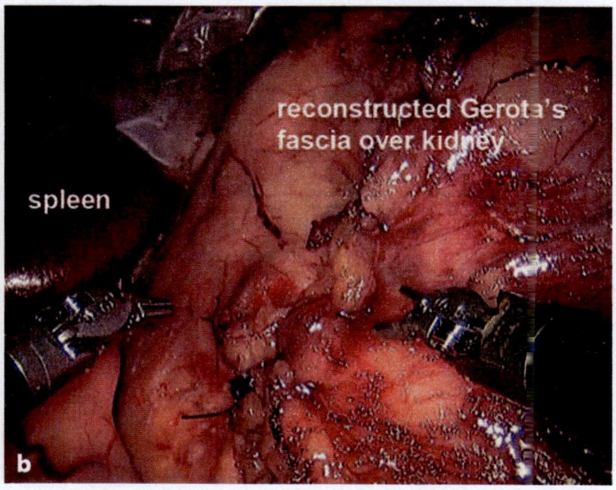

The Gerota fascia and the perirenal fat are brought together and closed over the kidney with a running suture of 2/0 Monocryl. Both ends are secured by Lapra-Ty clips in this case. A drain is inserted near the resection site or hilum, in most cases through one of the lateral 8-mm trocar ports. In small exophytic tumours or straightforward cases, this may not be necessary. The robot is now undocked from the patient, and the specimen, which had been placed above the spleen, is removed via one the 12-mm port sites. The 10-mm port site fascial closure is now performed and subcuticular sutures are used for skin closure.

Postoperative Management

- Early mobilisation
- Oral intake on day of surgery
- Full diet on day 2
- Urinary catheter removed on day 1–2
- Drain removal on day prior to discharge (if no bleeding or leak)

References

1. Guillonneau B, Jayet C, Tewari A, Vallancien G (2001) Robotic assisted laparoscopic nephrectomy. J Urol 166:200–201
2. Hoznek A, Hubert J, Antiphon P et al (2004) Robotic renal surgery. Urol CLin North Am. 31:731–736
3. Shapiro E, Benway BM, Wang AJ, Bhayani SB (2009) The role of nephron-sparing robotic surgery in the management of renal malignancy. Curr Opin Urol 19:76–80
4. JA Smith, AK Tewari (2008) Robotics in Urologic Surgery. Saunders Elsevier, Philadelphia
5. Fazeli-Matin S, Gill IS, Hsu TH et al (1999) Laparoscopic renal and adrenal surgery in obese patients: comparison to open surgery. J Urol 162:665–669

1.11 Retroperitoneal Partial Nephrectomy

Jens-Uwe Stolzenburg, Christopher Anderson, Rowan Casey, Minh Do, Anja Dietel, Andreas Gonsior, Evangelos Liatsikos

Introduction

The widespread use of contemporary imaging techniques has resulted in an increased detection of incidental small renal tumours. Many centres have published their experience with laparoscopic partial nephrectomy and with increasing experience, larger, infiltrating tumours have been amenable to this technique [1].

Laparoscopic partial nephrectomy is considerably more technically challenging than performing radical nephrectomy and requires a higher level of laparoscopic skill to perform renal parenchymal haemostasis, pelvicalyceal reconstruction, and parenchymal renorrhaphy [2–6]. In principle, transperitoneal and retroperitoneal access is feasible depending on the tumour location. We recommend transperitoneal access for anterior, anterolateral, and lateral tumours. Retroperitoneal access is more suitable for posterior, posteromedial, and posterolateral tumours. Today, depending on the surgeon's experience, nearly every kidney tumour which is suitable for partial nephrectomy can be removed laparoscopically or by a robot-assisted procedure.

Absolute Indications

- Anatomical or functional solitary kidney
- Bilateral renal cell carcinoma

Relative Indications

- Kidney failure (creatinine significantly increased)
- Hereditary forms of renal cell tumours with known risk of contra-lateral kidney tumour in future (tuberous sclerosis, Hippel-Lindau disease)
- Selected patients with an associated disease compromising the contra-lateral kidney

Elective Indications

- Unilateral tumour and normal functioning contra-lateral kidney
- Tumour < 4 cm
- Central tumours and > 4cm only for experienced surgeons

Contra-indications

- Interpolar or a completely intrarenal tumour
- Vena cava tumour thrombus
- Morbid obesity (relative)
- History of ipsilateral renal surgery (relative)

Preoperative Preparation

- Complete physical examination
- Full blood count, blood chemistry, including liver and renal function tests
- Preoperative computed tomographic staging (abdominal/pelvic CT)
- Chest radiography, thoracic CT for patients with x-ray findings
- Bone scans in case of elevated serum alkaline phosphatase or bone pain
- Empty urinary bladder (bladder catheterisation)
- Antibiotic prophylaxis

Step 1: Patient position and trocar placement

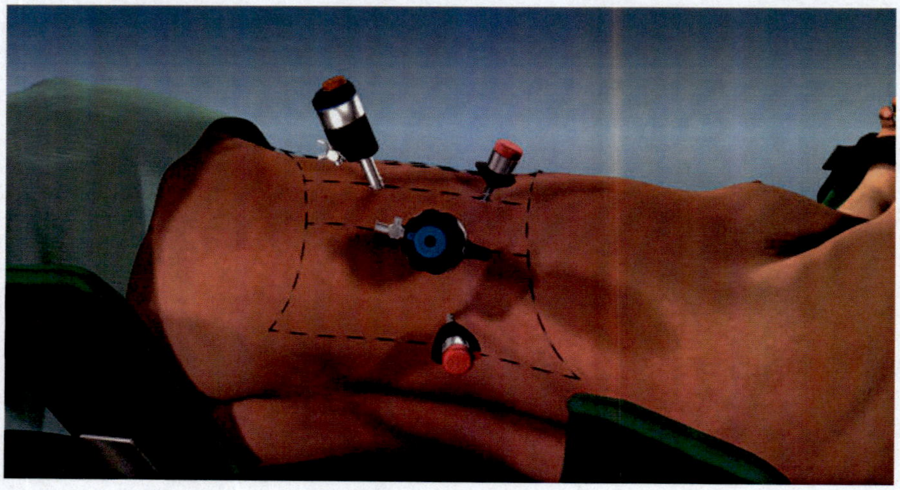

A 2-cm incision is made in the posterior axillary line, 1–2 cm below the 12th rib. The abdominal wall and transversalis fascia are incised sharply with the scissors and the blades are separated periodically to aid progression. The tract is widened bluntly with a finger, which also develops the retroperitoneal space slightly and the lower pole of the kidney may be felt. A balloon-dilating trocar is inserted and insufflation is commenced with the camera in the trocar to confirm correct position and expansion of the retroperitoneal space. The optical trocar is then inserted into the tract and gas insufflation is commenced. A second 10- to 12-mm trocar is placed lateral to the peritoneal reflection under direct vision in the midaxillary line. Two additional 5-mm trocars are placed, as shown in Step 1.

Step 2: External landmarks and trocar placement

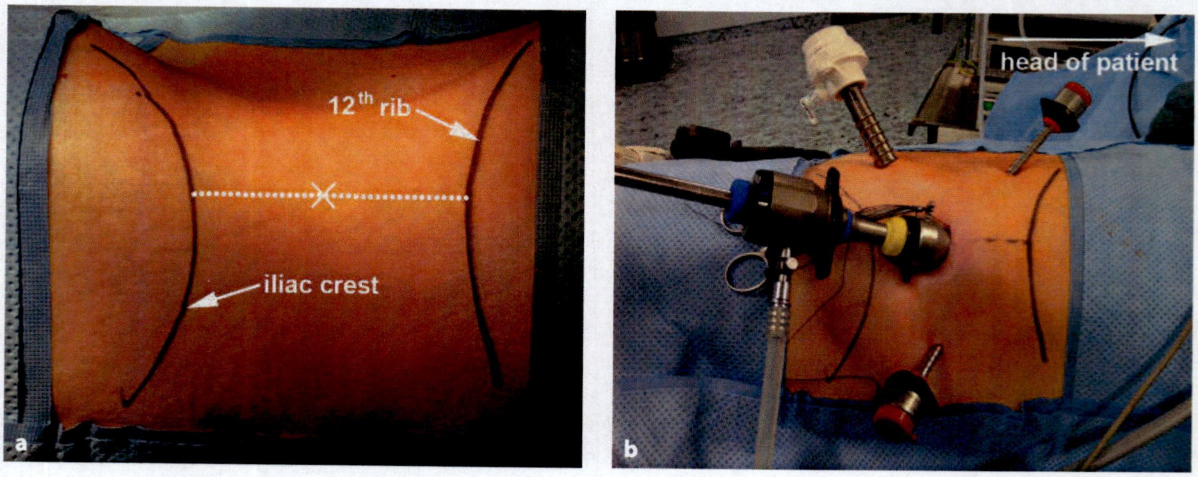

Step 2a shows the external landmarks during a real procedure. The patient is in the lateral position, which allows the bowel and peritoneum to fall away from the flank once the retroperitoneal space has been created. As can be seen, there is sufficient space for port placement for both surgeon and assistant (Step 2b). In a patient with a large kidney and/or much perinephric fat, a fan retractor might be necessary to allow access to the kidney tumour and the hilum of the kidney. It can be placed through the 10- to 12-mm port. Very rarely, an extra port is necessary for retraction and this can be placed caudally between the camera and the left- or right-hand port.

Step 3: Dissection of the retroperitoneal space and identification of the hilar vessels

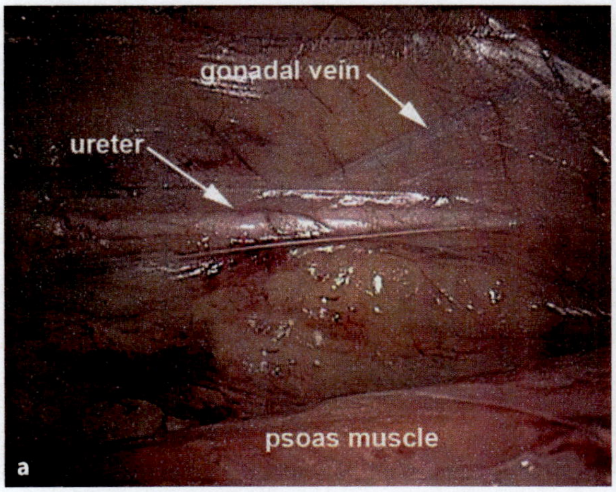

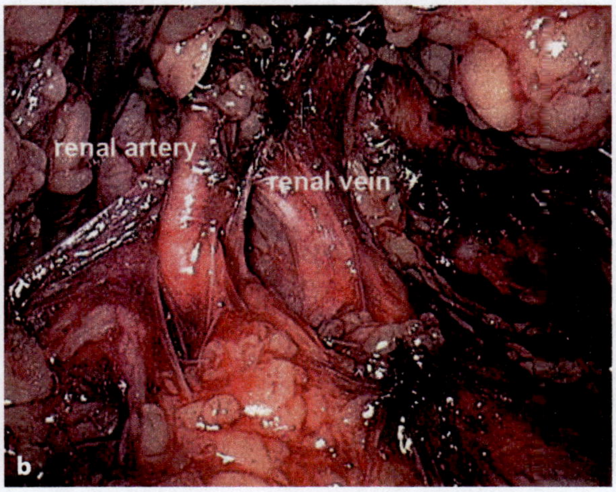

The psoas muscle is kept horizontal at the base of the picture. The dissection of the posterior perirenal space is commenced by incising the Gerota fascia. On the left side, the ureter or gonadal vein is seen first superior to the psoas muscle (Step 3a). On the right side, the inferior vena cava is the first landmark encountered and the ureter and gonadal vein should be seen subsequently. On the left side, progress is made along the anterior aspect of the psoas adjacent to the ureter towards the renal pedicle. The renal artery and vein are then seen (Step 3b) after dissection and mobilisation.

Step 4: Identification of the tumour

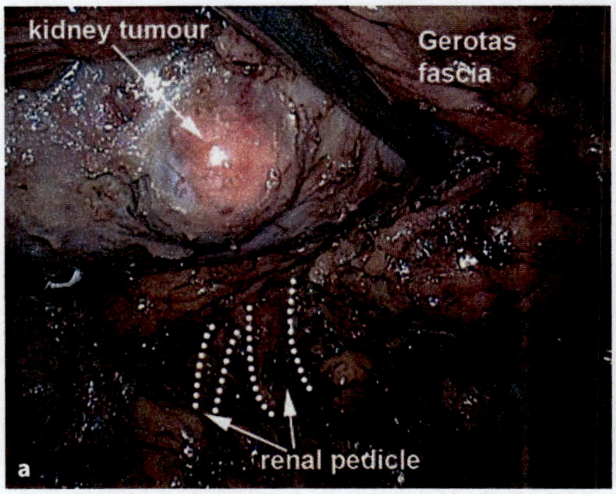

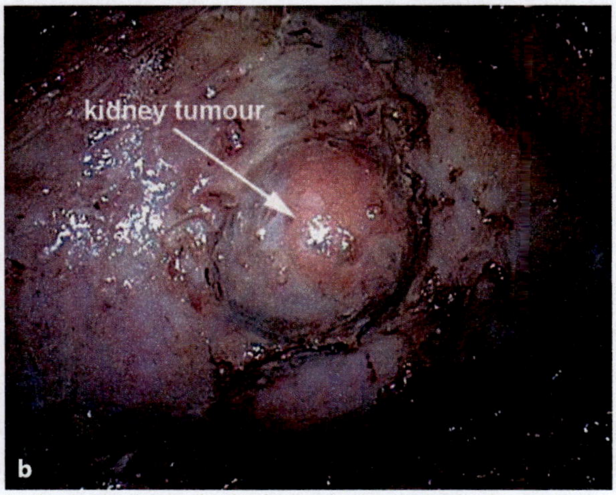

Full or partial mobilisation of the kidney is performed depending on the location of the tumour, to visualise the tumour and facilitate the subsequent reconstruction by making the kidney mobile so that it can be rotated to improve on difficult angles. Prior CT scan provides information regarding the size and location of the tumour, parenchymal infiltration, proximity to the renal sinus and renal hilum, and the number and location of renal vessels. Intraoperative laparoscopic ultrasonography, if available, can also be used to delineate the tumour location and characteristics.

Step 5: Control of the vascular pedicle

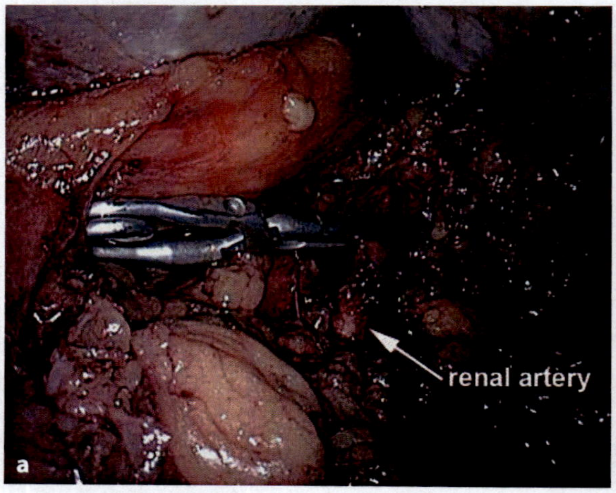

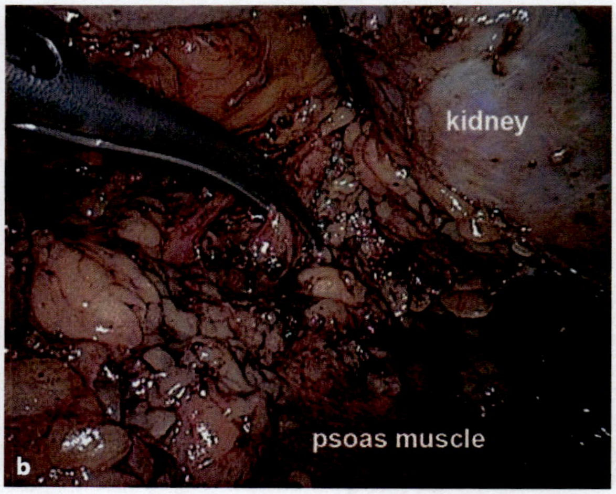

The stretched hilar vessels are cleared of loose areolar tissue and fascia to facilitate subsequent clamping (do not skeletonise the vessels completely to prevent intimal damage during clamping). The renal artery can be occluded with bulldog clamps, as seen in Step 5a. A laparoscopic Satinsky clamp is an alternative but might further limit the restricted working space, especially during a retroperitoneal approach (Step 5b). Smaller exophytic tumours might be excised without clamping, but it is essential that the artery has been mobilised in case urgent clamping is required.

Step 6: Tumour excision

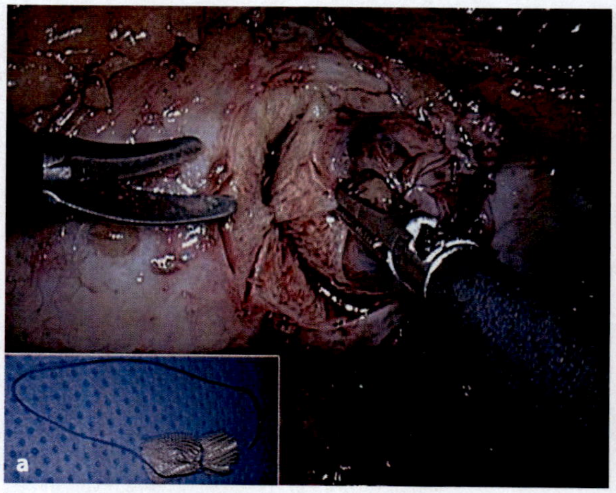

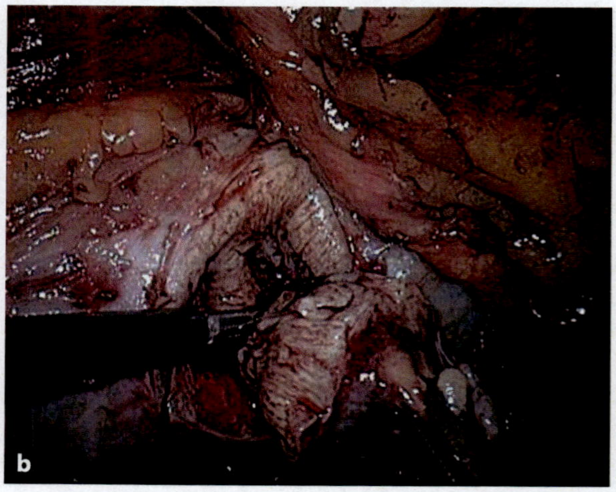

Immediately prior to tumour excision and renal hilar clamping, the suture (2/0 Vicryl) and with a Surgicel bolster at the end (alternatively a Lapra-Ty clip), required for subsequent reconstruction and haemostasis, are placed inside the retroperitoneal space available for rapid use (inlay). Targeted dissection of the perinephric fat isolates the tumour. The renal parenchyma is scored circumferentially around the tumour with electrocautery (Step 6a). With a nontraumatic grasper firmly holding a cap of fat over the tumour, the tumour is excised by sharp dissection and removed with a rim of normal parenchyma. Tumour excision is completed by circumferential dissection (Step 6b). If there is an obvious and significant calyceal defect, this can be sutured precisely intracorporally.

Step 7: Renorrhaphy

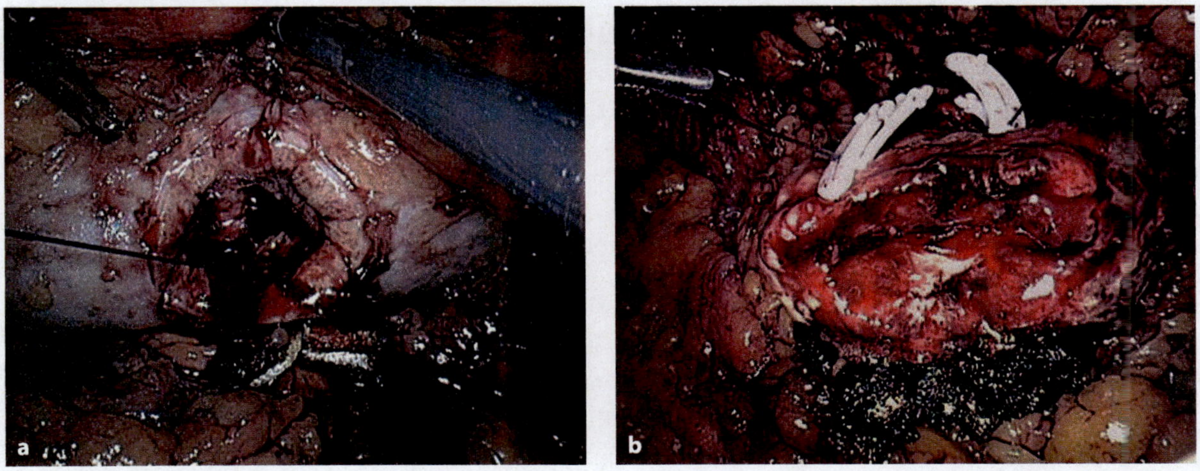

The suture (with bolster attached), which has been placed inside the retroperitoneal space, is used now. The suture is directed through the depths of the parenchymal defect on one side and exits on the opposite side of the defect. It is secured with Lapra-Ty clips. Alternatively, Hem-o-lok clips (minimum of two) can be used to secure under moderate tension, as shown in Step 7b. FloSeal may be inserted into the defect for further haemostasis. The vascular clamps are now released and the area is inspected for further bleeding. A drain is placed through a 5-mm trocar.

Postoperative Management

- Early mobilisation
- Oral intake on day of surgery
- Full diet on day 2
- Urinary catheter removed on day 1–2
- Drain removal on day prior to discharge (if no bleeding or leak)

References

1. Gill IS, Matin SF, Desai MM et al (2003) Comparative analysis of laparoscopic versus open partial nephrectomy for renal tumors in 200 patients. J Urol 170:64–68
2. Beasley KA, Omar MA, Shaikh A et al (2000) Laparoscopic versus open partial nephrectomy. Urology 64:458–461
3. Ramani AP, Desai MM, Steinberg AP et al (2005) Complications of laparoscopic partial nephrectomy in 200 cases. J Urol 173:42–47
4. Johnston WK, Wolf JS (2006) Laparoscopic partial nephrectomy: technique, oncologic efficacy, and safety. Curr Urol Rep 6:19–28
5. Allaf ME, Bhayani SB, Rogers C et al (2004) Laparoscopic partial nephrectomy: evaluation of long-term oncological outcome. J Urol 172:871–873
6. Gill IS, Kamoi K, Aron M, Desai MM (2010) 800 Laparoscopic partial nephrectomies: a single surgeon series. J Urol 183:34–41

1.12 Donor Nephrectomy

1.12.1 Retroperitoneal Donor Nephrectomy

Alexander Bachmann, Stephen Wyler, Svetozar Subotic

Introduction

The first open donor nephrectomy was described in 1956 by Merril et al. in a transplantation for siblings [1]. Improvements in immunosuppressive therapy allowed tolerance of transplanted organs and made modern transplantation possible. For end-stage renal insufficiency, kidney transplantation became the therapy of choice. To meet the increasing need for donor kidneys, living donor nephrectomy was performed laparoscopically for the first time in 1995 [2]. This work had been pioneered by the first laparoscopic nephrectomy performed by Clayman in 1991 [3]. Since then, laparoscopic living-donor nephrectomy has been established in various centres worldwide for transplantation.

Gill described the retroperitoneal access for laparoscopic living donor nephrectomy in 2000 [4]. The advantage of the retroperitoneal access is the rapid and safe control of the renal pedicle. The colon does not need to be dissected, leading to fewer bowel problems. Furthermore, post-operative accumulation of lymphatic fluid and blood is limited to the retroperitoneal space.

Indications

- End-stage renal insufficiency

Absolute Contra-indications

- Significant restrictive or obstructive pulmonary disease
- Solitary kidney
- Lesion of other (remaining) kidney

Relative Contra-indications

- Previous retroperitoneal surgery
- Previous retroperitoneal trauma

Preoperative Preparation

- Transurethral catheterisation
- Single-shot broad-spectrum antibiotic

1

Step 1: Patient position, trocar placement and initial dissection of retroperitoneal space

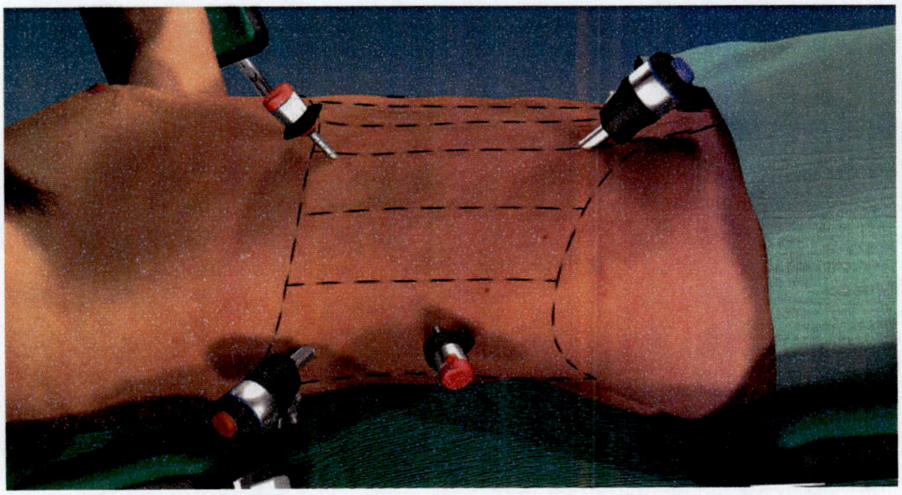

The patient is placed in the 45° lateral position with the operating table slightly flexed (see also Sect. 1.1). The retroperitoneal access is described fully in Sect. 1.3. After establishing a pneumoretroperitoneum with a pressure of 14 mmHg, retroperitoneoscopy is performed. Three additional trocars are placed under direct visual control, as shown in Step 1a. The Gerota fascia and the border of the psoas muscle are identified. These are the reference structures of the retroperitoneal space (see Step 2a).

Step 2: Initial exposure of the hilum

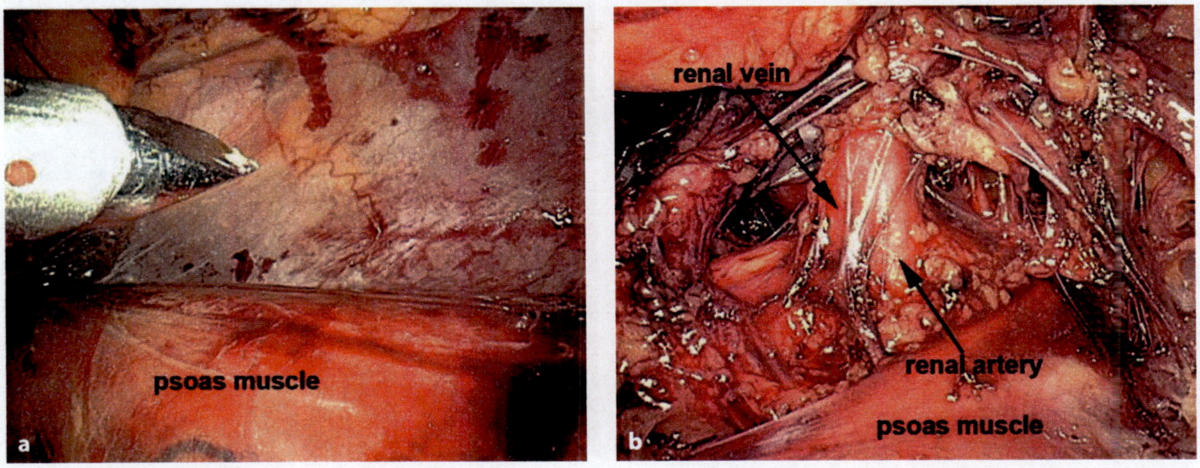

The psoas muscle is freed completely, leaving the perirenal fat untouched. Identification of the hilar vessels (Step 2a, Step 2b) can be difficult in cases of abundant renal hilar fatty tissue. It is critical to perform the dissection of the hilum carefully in order not to risk haemorrhage. The ventral aspect of the kidney is freed at the end of this stage, as tears of the fragile peritoneum can occur, which can make the operative space very small. A fourth trocar can be inserted if needed to further retract the Gerota fascia.

Step 3: Renal artery isolation

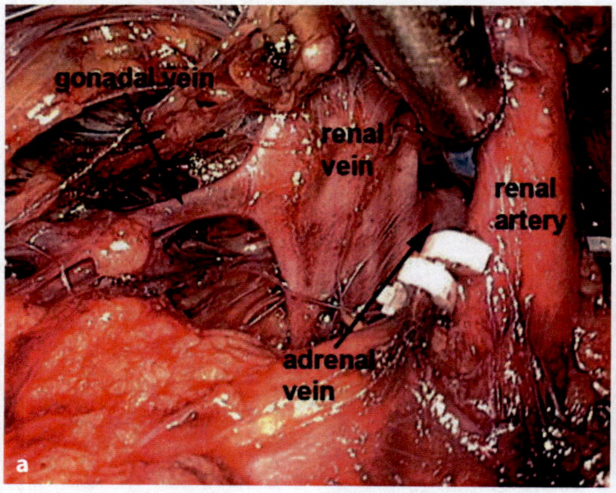

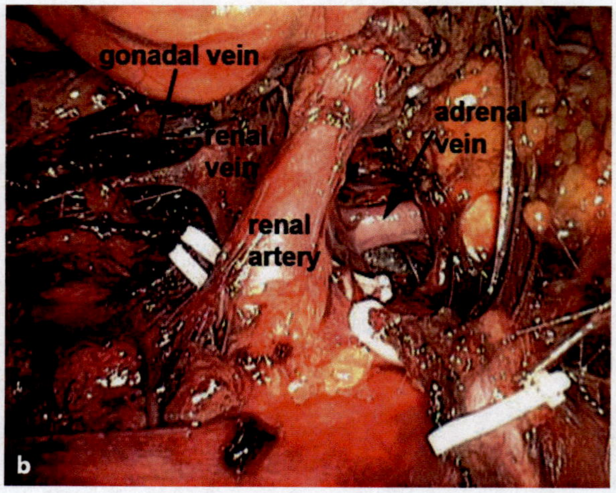

When preparing the renal hilum, search for the pulsations of the renal artery and then the renal artery can be freed completely. It is critically important to release the vessel completely from surrounding tissue and vessels with sufficient arterial length to enable a safe clip or Endo-GIA application. The preparation can be done with a right-angle endo-dissector or the tip of the suction device. For coagulation of small vessels, bipolar electrocautery or the SonoSurg (Olympus, Hamburg, Germany) device is recommended.

Step 4: Further venous dissection

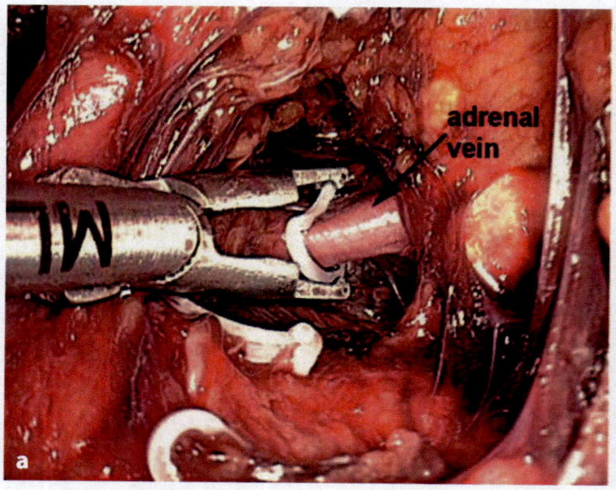

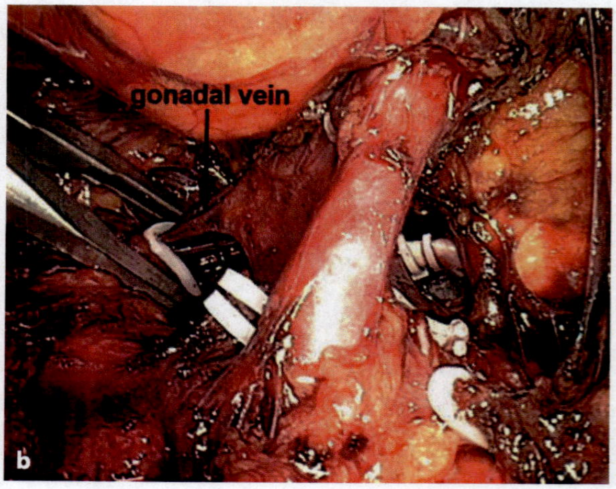

The adrenal vein can be identified joining the renal vein cranially (Step 4a). The gonadal vein can aid in identifying the renal vein if it cannot be identified initially (Step 4b). Extensive lymphatic tissue is often found on the left side. Special care should be taken to identify the para-aortal lymph nodes, as they drain to the cisterna chyli and severe lymphatic fistula can occur in case of damage. After having freed the renal artery and vein completely, the adrenal vein is clipped with 5-mm Hem-o-lok clips and divided. The gonadal vein is then clipped and divided.

Step 5: Freeing the kidney capsule

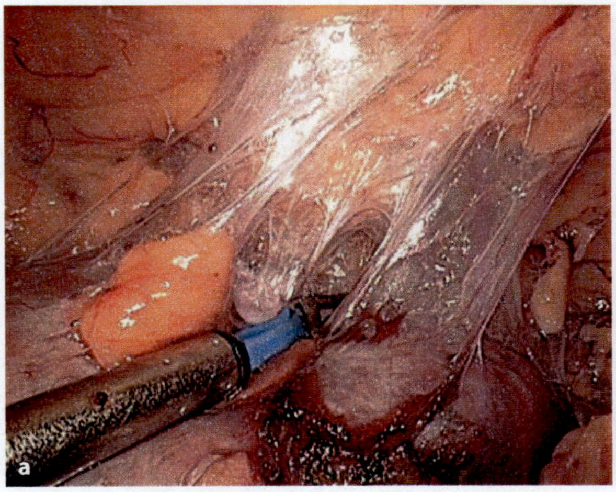

a

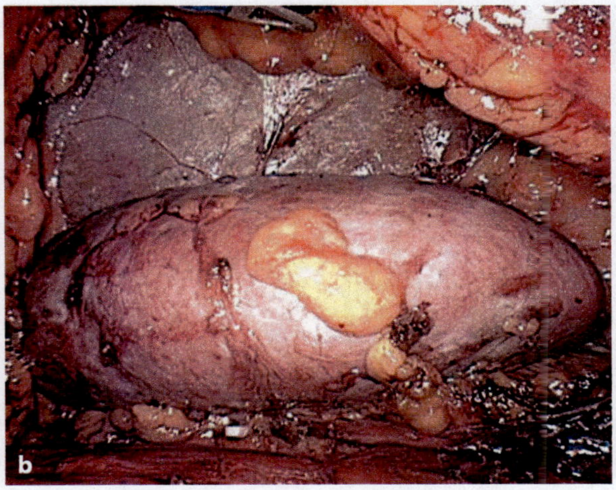

b

In the case of retroperitoneal donor nephrectomy, the next steps are different from simple nephrectomies or tumour nephrectomies. The perinephric fat is now completely removed from the kidney, as shown in Step 5a and Step 5b. Furthermore, the renal pelvis and the proximal ureter are freed from surrounding tissue. Care has to be taken not to injure the renal capsule. Most of the dissection is done bluntly. Minor bleeding can be controlled using bipolar forceps.

Step 6: Ureteric mobilisation and division

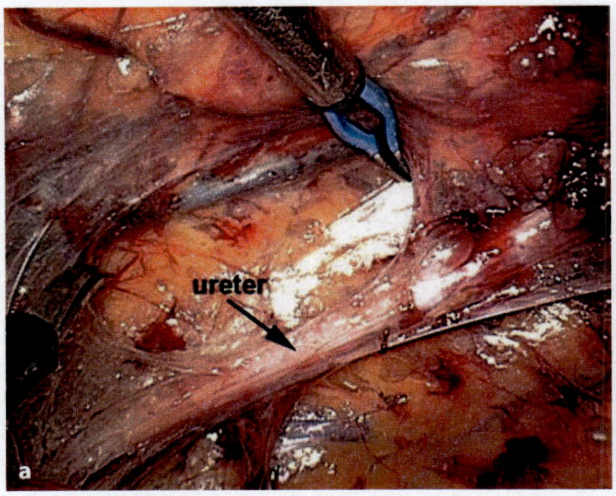

a

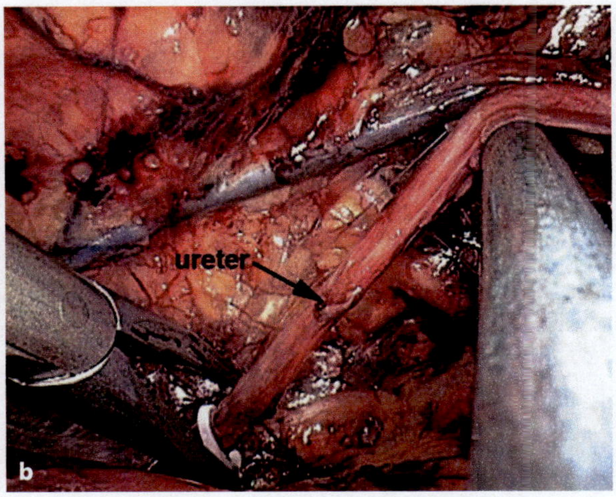

b

The ureter must be carefully mobilised, leaving plenty of periureteral tissue on it in the case of transplantation. Skeletonising the ureter can result in later necrosis of the ureteral wall. The ureter must be mobilised as far as possible to the pelvis to provide sufficient length. Only the distal end of the ureter requires clipping for transplantation purposes. The ureter is clipped and dissected as low as possible (minimum below the level where it crosses the iliac vessels).

Step 7: Vessel mobilisation and division

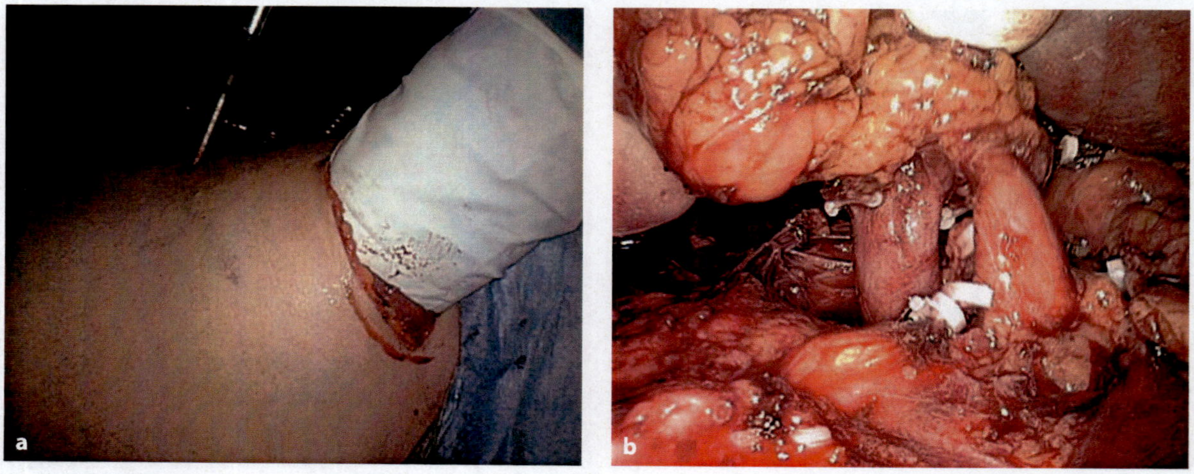

For reasons of safety and time, we prefer to manually extract the kidney (short warm ischaemia time). The incision of the caudal working trocar is broadened to 9 cm. The muscles are split and the surgeon's hand is inserted (Step 7a). After insertion of the surgeon's hand, the pneumoretroperitoneum is established again. The kidney is elevated and the pedicle is stretched carefully to identify the renal artery and vein (Step 7b).

Step 8: Vessel division

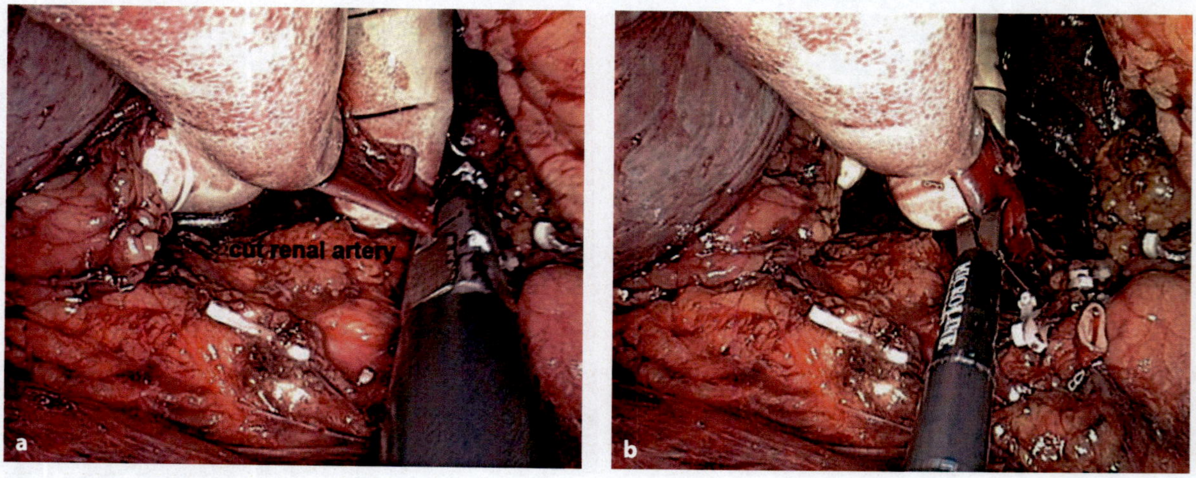

The remaining lymphatic vessels are transected to allow maximum length of renal vessels. After final preparation of the vessels, transection is possible. With a TA-30 vascular stapler (Autosuture) the renal artery is secured. The artery is transected just distal of the stapler line. The renal vein is stretched carefully with the index and middle fingers to obtain maximal length and is secured with the TA-30 stapler (Step 8a). Using the TA-30 stapler, maximum length of the vessels is gained, as compared to the GIA stapler, as the TA stapler only staples on the donor side in contrast to the GIA stapler. The vein is then cut above the staple line (Step 8b).

Step 9: Kidney extraction

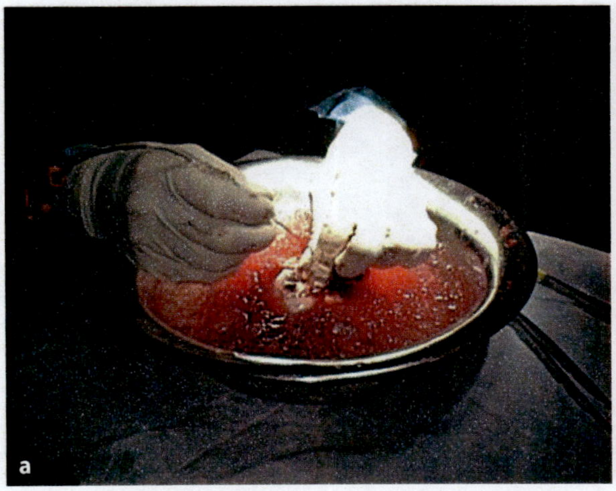

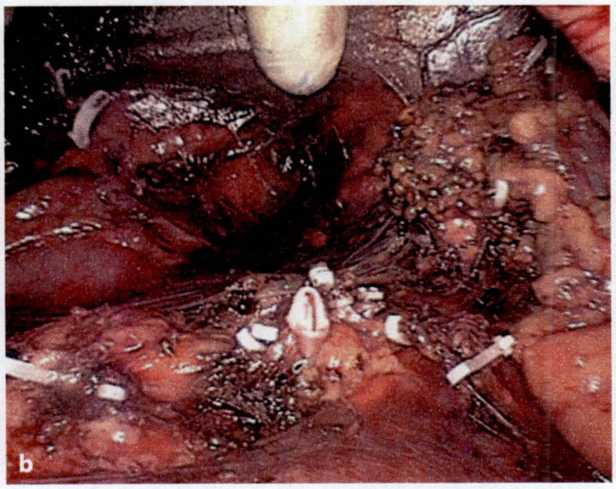

The kidney is immediately removed either manually or in an EndoCatch bag. It is then perfused and cooled on a back table. The fascial incision used for the hand-assisted port is now closed, the pneumoretroperitoneum re-established and the retroperitoneal space is checked for haemostasis. After extraction of the specimen, the retroperitoneal space is checked for haemorrhage and the insertion of a drainage is assessed. The insertion of a drainage is not necessary in all cases.

Step 10: Renal artery division (alternative in tumour nephrectomy)

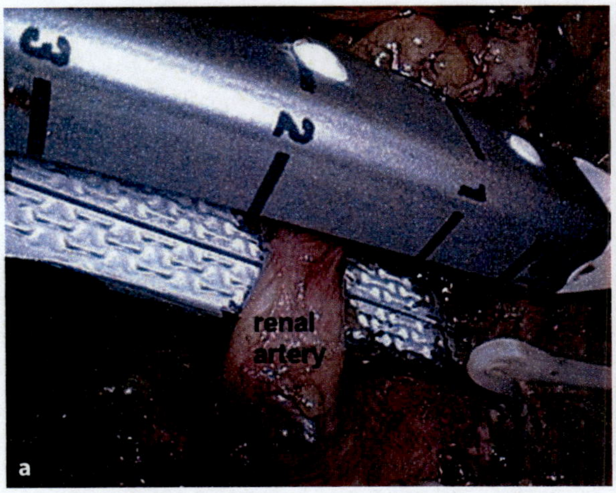

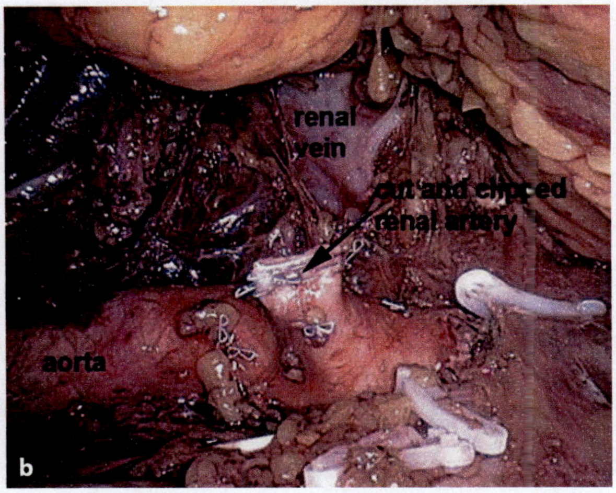

The renal artery is clipped and dissected with either Hem-o-lok-clips or an Endo-GIA stapler (no TA-30 stapler) in cases of simple nephrectomies or tumour nephrectomies before mobilisation of the whole kidney package, as shown in Step 10a. It is vital that the stapler can be placed completely around the artery without any other vessel or tissue interposing between the ends. Cutting the artery now enables the further identification and dissection of the renal vein behind it (Step 10b).

Step 11: Renal vein division (alternative in tumour nephrectomy)

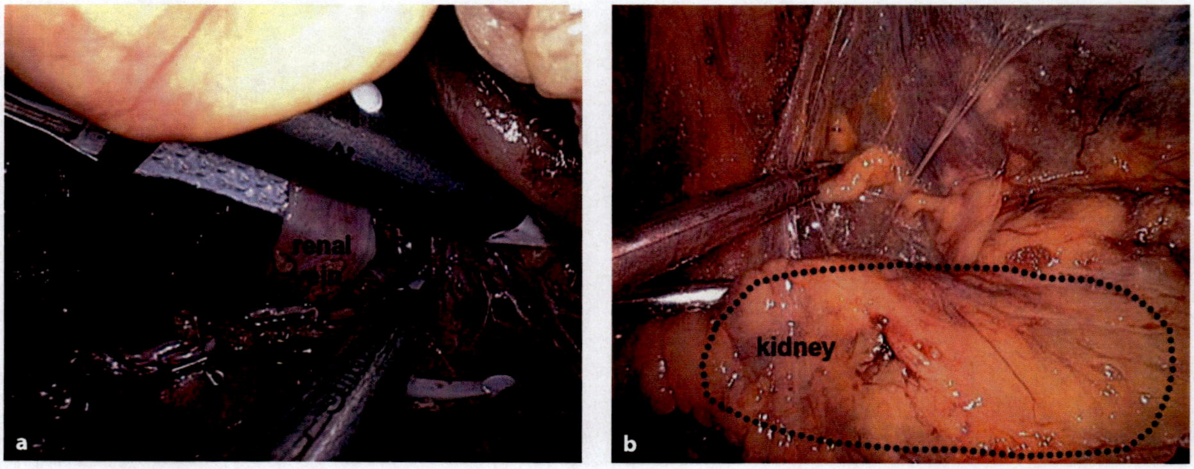

After preparation of the renal vein, it is dissected with an Endo-GIA stapler (Step 11a). Dysfunction of the stapler because of previously placed obstructing clips rarely occurs. In contrast to donor nephrectomy, the kidney including the Gerota fascia is completely mobilised after division of the renal pedicle, as shown in Step 11b. If possible, one should dissect along the psoas muscle from caudally to cranially. In case of an upper pole tumour, the adrenal gland is part of the specimen.

Step 12: Removing the kidney in a laparoscopic harvesting bag

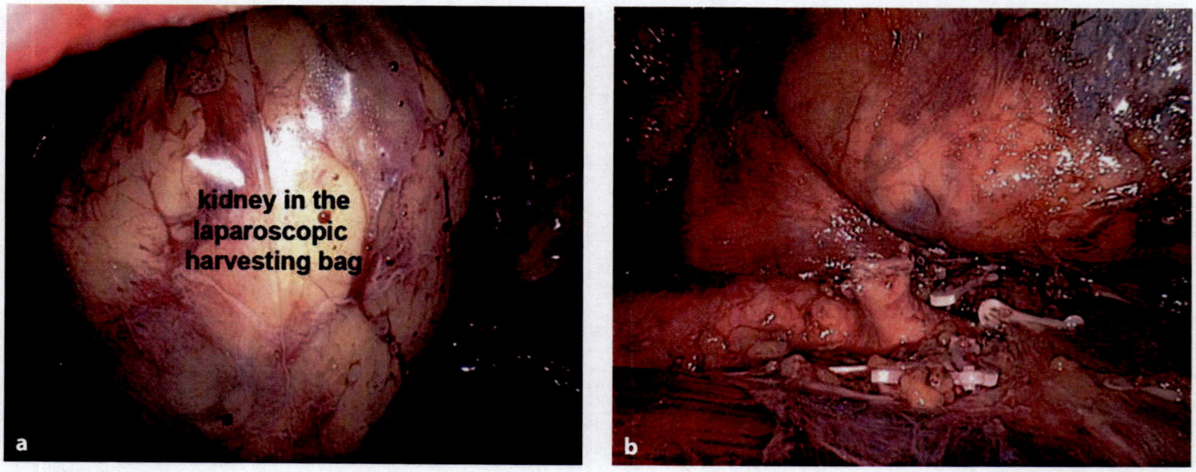

The specimen is placed in a laparoscopic harvesting bag before removing the package. After extraction of the specimen, the retroperitoneal space is checked for haemorrhage and the insertion of drainage is optional. Minor bleeding can be carefully coagulated using bipolar forceps.

Step 13: Final inspection and skin suture

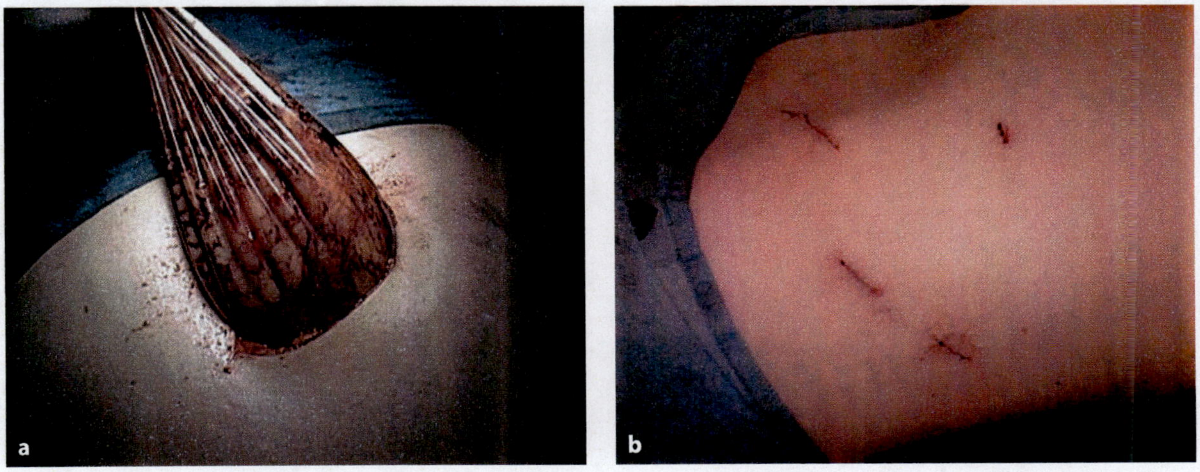

To remove the whole specimen, the skin incision of the first trocar is enlarged. Another option for removal of the specimen is to create an oblique muscle-splitting incision above and medial to the anterior superior iliac crest if sufficient space has been created and the peritoneum mobilised in the retroperitoneal approach. Alternatively, the specimen can be extracted through a hockey stick incision in the lower abdomen or classical transverse incision (see Sect. 1.13).

Postoperative Management

- Removal of the transurethral catheter on the 1st postoperative day
- Ambulation and oral intake immediately
- Analgesia according to pain
- Creatinine monitoring

References

1. Merrill JP, Murray JE, Harrison JH, Guild WR (1956) Successful homotransplantation of the human kidney between identical twins. JAMA 160:277
2. Ratner LE, Ciseck LJ, Moore RG, Cigarroa FG, Kaufmann HS, Kavoussi LR (1995) Laparoscopic live donor nephrectomy. Transplantation 60:1047–1049
3. Clayman RV, Kavoussi LR, Soper NJ, Dierks SM, Meretyk S, Darcy MD, Roemer FD, Pingleton ED, Thomson PG, Long SR (1991) Laparoscopic nephrectomy: initial case report. J Urol 146:278–282
4. Gill IS, Uzzo RG, Hobart MG, Streem SB, Goldfarb DA, Noble MJ (2000) Laparoscopic retroperitoneal live donor right nephrectomy for purposes of allotransplantation and autotransplantation. J Urol 164:1500–1504

1.12.2 Transperitoneal Donor Nephrectomy

Serdar Deger

Introduction

As increasing numbers of patients with end-stage renal failure are considered candidates for kidney transplantation, a significant organ shortage in the number of cadaveric kidneys available for donation has become a problem. Therefore, expanding the donor pool remains one of the central issues in kidney transplantation [1]. Compared with cadaveric transplantation, live-donor transplants are associated with fewer technical graft failures and better short-term and long-term renal function [2]. Since the outcome of living donor kidneys is better than cadaveric kidneys and the recipient waiting time can be reduced significantly, laparoscopic procedures are being increasingly introduced into the operative spectrum of many transplant centres [1, 3]. The laparoscopic organ harvesting technique may increase the number of donors [4].

Indications

- Criteria for kidney donation were specified by the consensus of an International Forum on the care of the Live Kidney Donor held in Amsterdam, The Netherlands, April 1–4, 2004 [5] The conference participants highlighted the following aspects of informed consent as essential for competent individuals to decide to donate: understanding, disclosure, voluntary nature (freedom to choose to proceed with donation or decline), and documentation of consent

Contra-indications

- All legal regulations of countries regarding living donor criteria have to be considered
- Body mass index, previous surgeries, vascular anomalies and surgeon's laparoscopic experience can be relative but not absolute contra-indications [6]

Preoperative Preparation

- No specific bowel preparation is necessary
- Rectal enema is administered in the evening
- Third-generation cephalosporin as a single shot during surgery

Step 1: Patient position

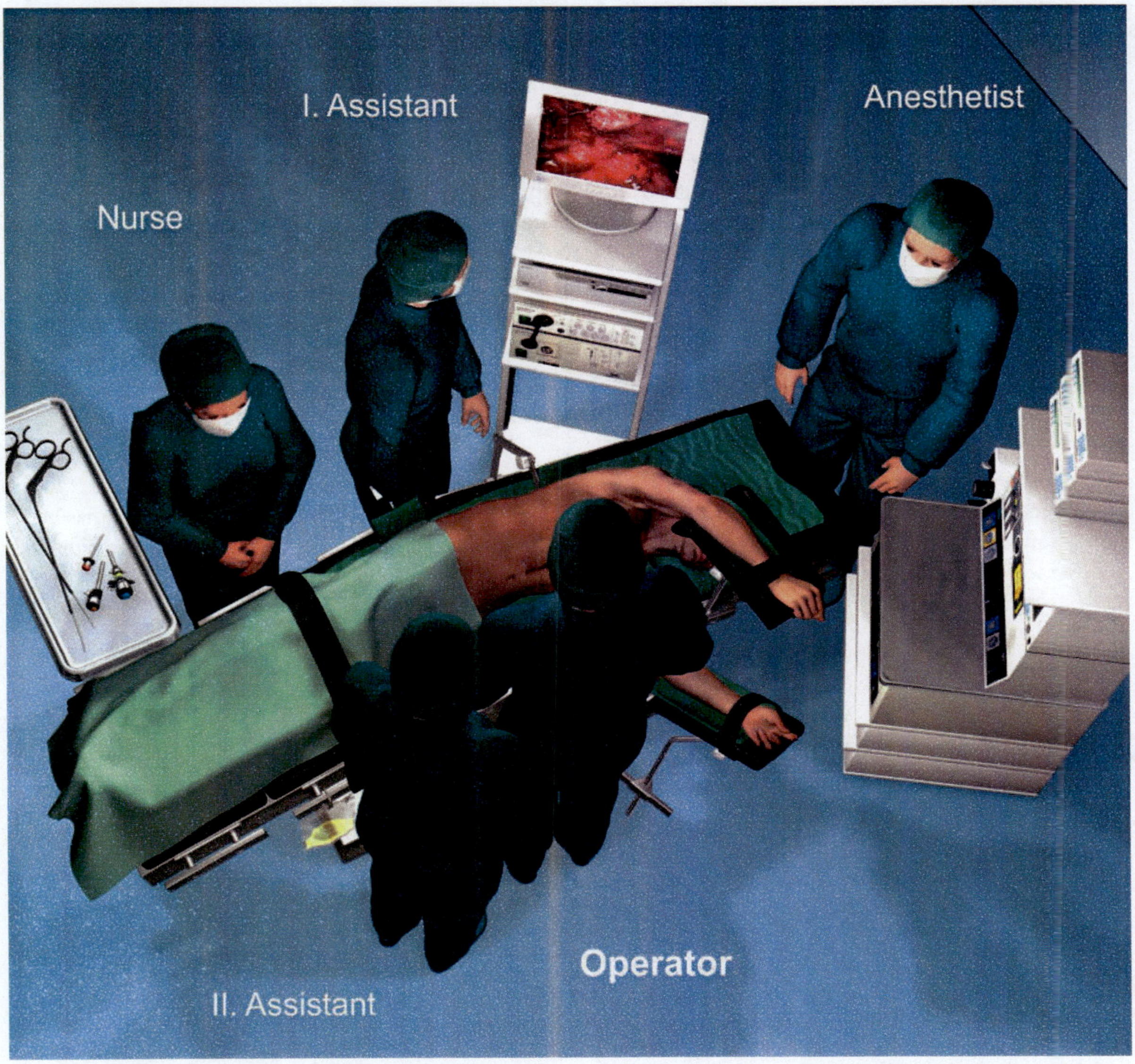

A urinary catheter is inserted while the patient is supine. The patient is then positioned in a lateral decubitus position at a 45° angle and the operating table is flexed at the umbilical level. This figure shows the position of the entire operative team. The surgeon and the second assistant are facing the front of the patient. The nurse and first assistant are on the opposite side.

Step 2: Trocar placement

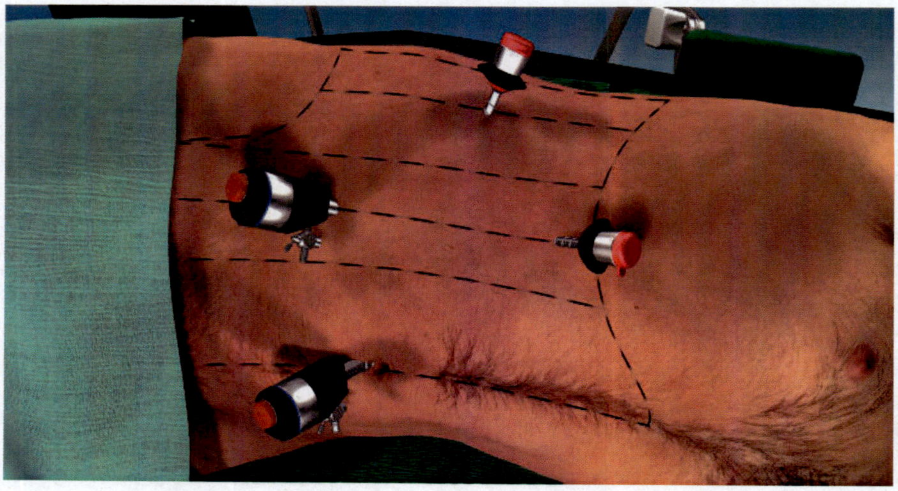

Pneumoperitoneum has to be established and a 10-mm optical trocar can be placed using a Veress needle or the Hasson technique through a paraumbilical incision. A 5-mm working trocar in the upper midclavicular line and a 12-mm trocar, for introducing instruments, such as a vascular stapler or clip applier to control vessels, is needed in the midclavicular line also. The lateral 5- or 10-mm trocar is usually placed after the colon has been extensively mobilised to retract the liver on the right and the colon flexure on the left side. A 30° laparoscope is used.

Step 3: Kidney preparation (left side)

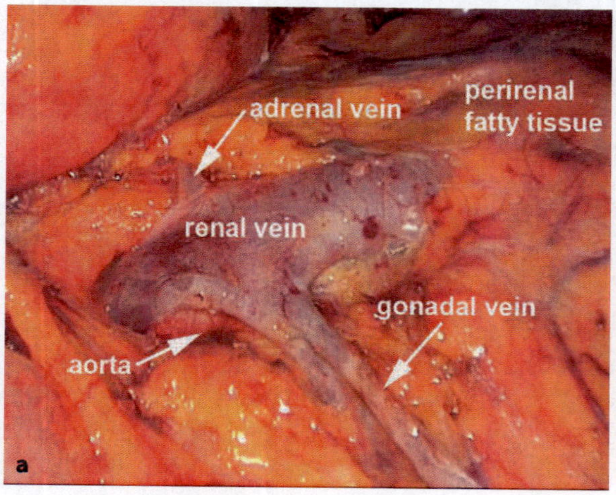

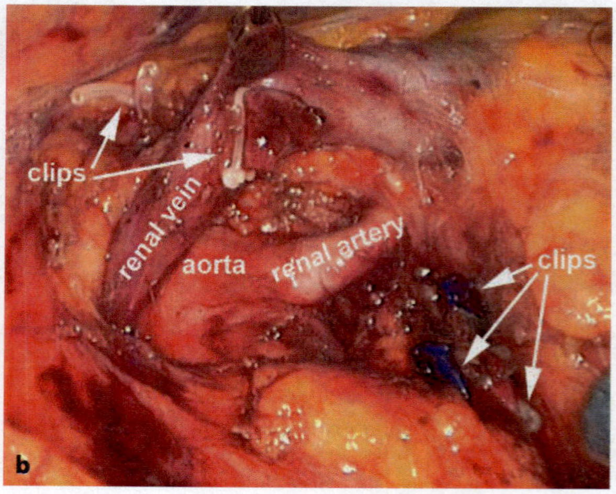

First, extensive mobilisation of the descending colon is required. The left renal vein has to be dissected completely. The gonadal, suprarenal and lumbar veins must also be cleared as shown in Step 3a. They are double-clipped and divided. All clips should be removed during the in vitro preparation of the donated kidney later. Therefore, enough length should be provided during clipping. After the complete mobilisation of the left renal vein, the aorta and left renal artery can be identified easily. They are mobilised from the aorta until enough space for a central double clipping is possible, as shown in Step 3b.

Step 4: Kidney preparation (right side)

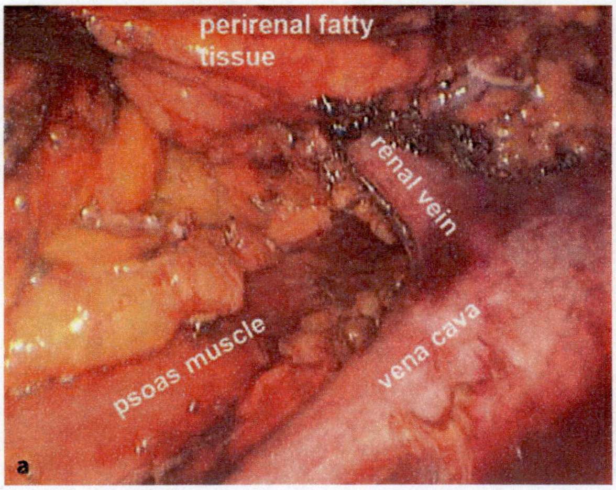

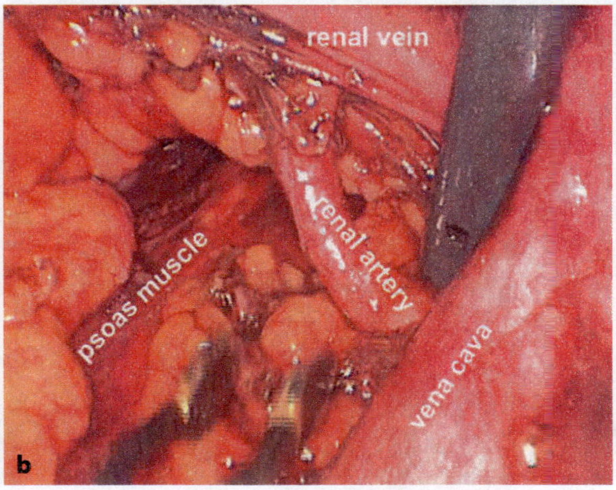

After mobilisation of the ascending colon and duodenum, the inferior vena cava must be mobilised 2 cm above the renal vein and down to the gonadal vein. The renal vein has to be dissected from the cava up to the renal hilum (Step 4a). The ureter can be identified close to the gonadal vein and the latter vein can be further prepared to identify the renal vein more easily. The cava can be slightly rotated in order to prepare the renal artery from behind, as in Step 4b. In these cases, the renal artery can be clipped under the cava. If necessary, interaortocaval preparation can be done to achieve a maximum arterial length, especially when multiple arteries or an early bifurcation are present.

Step 5: Ureteral preparation and packing the kidney

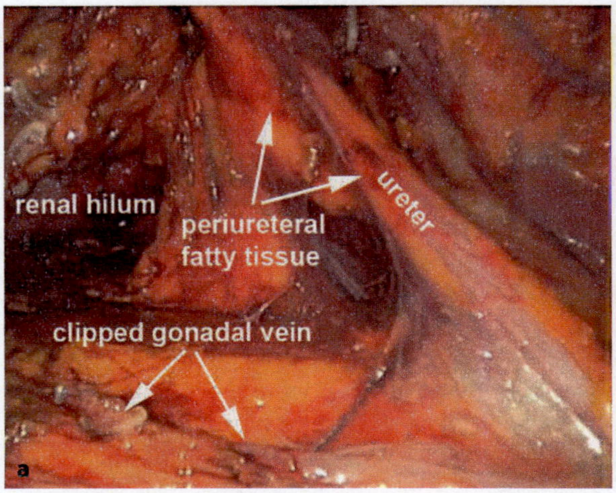

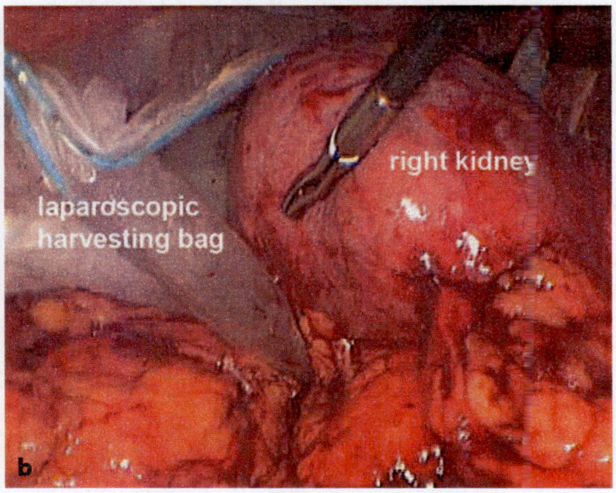

The ureter should be mobilised using a no-touch technique. The fatty tissue around the ureter should not be stripped (Step 5a) completely. The small vessels to the ureter must be clipped as thermal damage caused by coagulation must be avoided. The ureter should be mobilised to below the level where it crosses the iliac vessels. The kidney has to be mobilised completely until it is only attached to its renal vessels. A laparoscopic harvesting specimen bag is placed through the 12-mm port and then the kidney is placed completely inside (Step 5b).

Step 6: ascular inspection prior to clipping (right and left side)

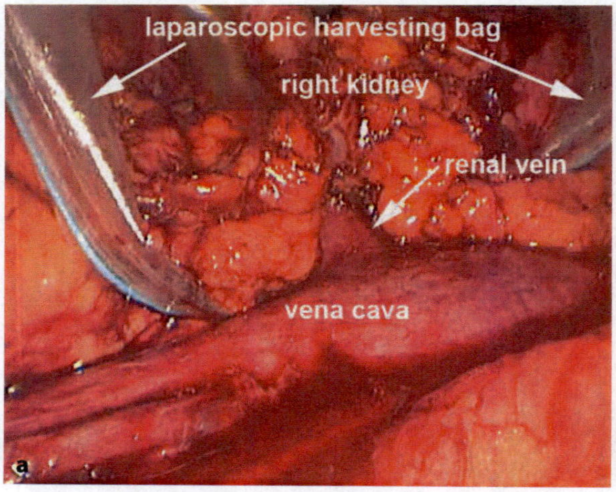

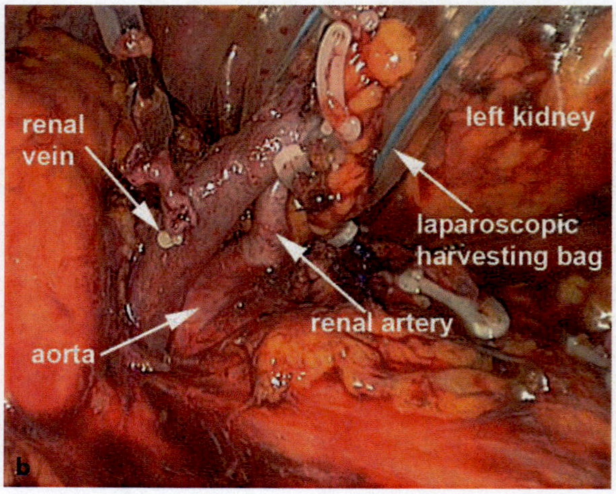

After the kidney has been securely packed in the bag, the vessels are inspected to ensure that they can be clipped with sufficient length and without any tissue interposition. Step 6a and 6b show the packed kidney in different cases on the right and left side. The renal artery and veins have been dissected back to the aorta and vena cava, respectively. The lateral trocar incision is then enlarged up to 5 cm for organ extraction. The fascia and muscle layers are divided, but the peritoneum is left intact to maintain the pneumoperitoneum.

Step 7: Vessel control (left side)

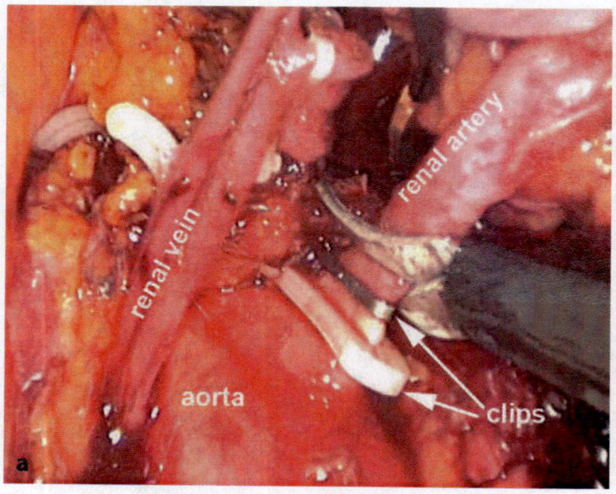

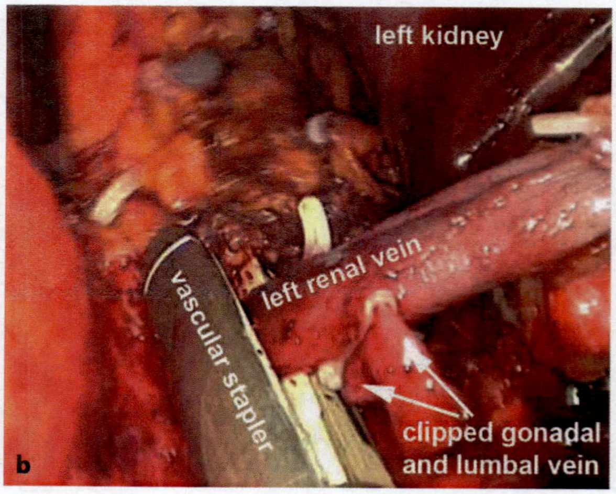

It is important to place two central clips and leave the kidney side unclipped in order to reduce warm ischaemia time, for easier access to the artery during perfusion and to prevent crushing of the arterial intima on the kidney side (Step 7a). The left vein is divided using a vascular stapler (Step 7b). The row of staples on the kidney side has to be removed afterwards by the perfusion team prior to transportation. Alternatively, large Hem-o-lok clips can be used for the vein.

1

Step 8: Vessel control (right side)

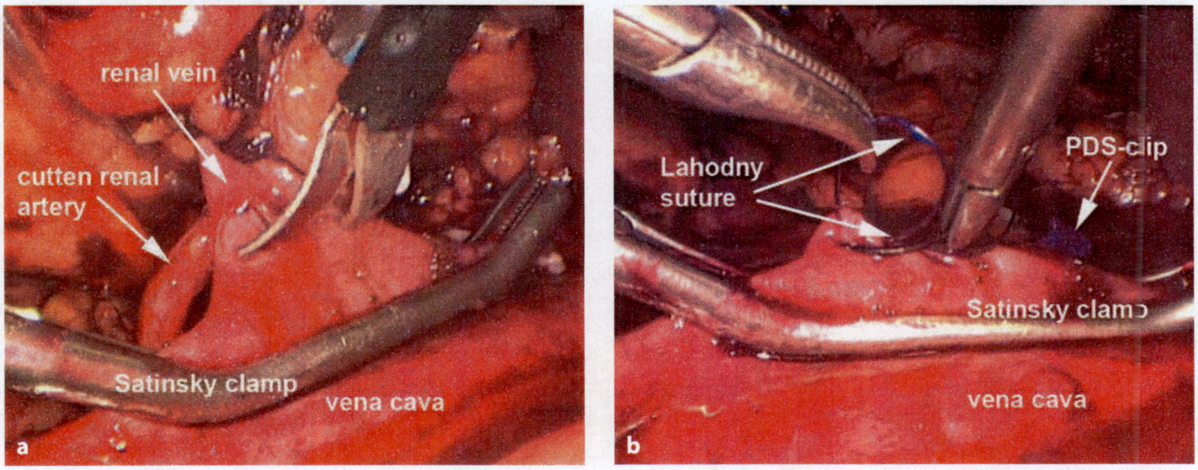

A small incision is made medial to the right anterior superior iliac spine, and a laparoscopic Satinsky clamp is inserted under direct vision directly through the skin at a suitable angle to the cava. After central double clipping and division of the renal artery, the cava can be clamped and the renal vein is transected sharply close to the cava (Step 8a). Then the endobag is closed, the peritoneum opened, and the bag removed with the kidney and provided to the perfusion team. The warm ischaemia time is reduced because no staples needing removal are present. The donor extraction site is closed with absorbable sutures, and the pneumoperitoneum is re-established. The cavotomy is closed with a laparoscopic running 3-0 PDS suture (Step 8b).

Postoperative Management

- Fluid intake 2 h after surgery
- Light diet 4 h after surgery
- Mobilisation on the evening of surgery
- Urinary catheter for 24 h after surgery

References

1. Giessing M, Reuter S, Deger S, Tüllmann M, Hirte I, Budde K, Fritsche L, Slowinski T, Dragun D, Neumayer HH, Loening SA (2005) Laparoscopic versus open donor nephrectomy in Germany: impact on donor health-related quality of life and willingness to donate. Transplant Proc 37:2011–2015
2. Thiel G (1998) Living kidney transplantation – new dimensions. Transplant Int 11:50–56
3. Ratner LE, Hiller J, Sroka M et al (1997) Laparoscopic live donor nephrectomy removes disincentives to live donation. Transplant Proc 29:3402–3403
4. Kuo PC, Johnson LB (2000) Laparoscopic donor nephrectomy increases the supply of living donor kidneys: a center-specific microeconomic analysis. Transplantation 69:211–213
5. Delmonico F (2005) A Report of the Amsterdam Forum On the care of the live kidney donor: care and medical guidelines. Transplantation 79:S51–S66
6. Alston C, Spaliviero M, Gill IS (2005) Laparoscopic donor nephrectomy. Urology 65:833–839

1.12.3 LESS: Donor Nephrectomy

Mihir Desai, Pascal Zehnder, Ricardo Brandina, Inderbir S. Gill

Introduction

Laparoscopic donor nephrectomy has become the technique of choice for allograft procurement for living renal transplantation. Laparoscopic renal allograft retrieval results in comparable recipient functional outcomes while resulting in shorter hospital stay, rapid convalescence and improved cosmesis. Despite this reduction in perioperative morbidity, donor kidneys remain in short supply. Surgery on an otherwise healthy donor population is certainly challenging, with little room for error. Efforts are ongoing to further reduce morbidity and improve cosmetic outcomes of laparoscopic surgery. Laparoendoscopic single-site surgery (LESS) is a recently coined term that encompasses a group of procedures that aims to perform laparoscopic surgery through a single skin incision. Within a short time, a variety of urological procedures have been performed using the LESS approach. Even though living-donor nephrectomy is a high-stakes operation, the healthy altruistic donor pool is likely to be desirous of cosmetically superior outcome. We initially reported the technical feasibility of LESS donor nephrectomy and retrospectively demonstrated a lower postoperative morbidity compared to conventional laparoscopic donor nephrectomy.

Indications

- Living renal donors that meet criteria for kidney donation

Relative Contra-indications

- Prior extensive abdominal surgery
- BMI greater than 30
- Right-sided kidney

Preoperative Preparation

- Mechanical bowel preparation
- Low-molecular-weight heparin and antibiotic prophylaxis at induction

Instruments

Even though we typically use standard straight laparoscopic instruments, rigid-curved (Olympus Medical, Tokyo, Japan) or articulating systems (CambridgeEndo, Framingham, MA, USA; Novarre Medical Systems, Cupertino, CA, USA) are available in the operating room and used as necessary.

- Conventional laparoscopic instruments:
  - Small bowel grasper
  - Straight dissector
  - Right-angle dissector
  - Curved Maryland dissector
  - Hem-o-lok clip applier
  - Multiple clip applier with titanium clips
  - Endo-GIA stapler (vessels, ureter)
  - 2-mm needlescopic grasper
- LESS:
  - Certain access ports such as the QuadPort (Advanced Surgical Concepts, Wicklow, Ireland) and Gelport (Applied Medical, Rancho Santa Margarita, CA, USA) as well as multiple conventional trocars can be used with a relatively longer skin and fascial incision and in our opinion are preferred for LESS donor nephrectomy
  - Rigid 5-mm 30° or flexible-tip digital video-laparoscope (EndoEye, Olympus Medical, Hamburg, Germany) with a coaxial light and video cable is particularly helpful for LESS surgery
  - 15-mm retrieval bag

Step 1: Patient position and trocar placement

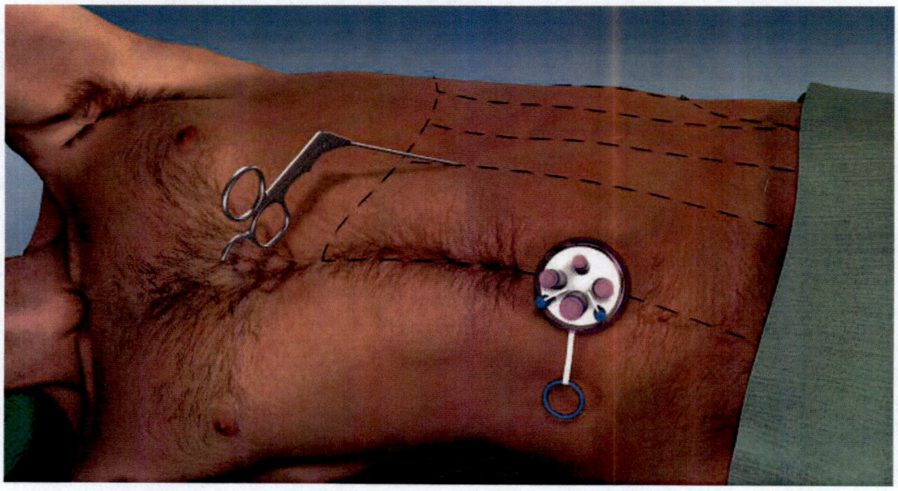

With the patient in a 45° flank position, pneumoperitoneum is established either using a transumbilical open Hasson technique or via a Veress needle puncture in the left hypochondrium. The length of the incision depends upon the type of single-port access device used. However, since an approximately 4.5-cm vertical intra-umbilical skin incision and a 6-cm fascial incision is eventually needed for allograft extraction, it is desirable to make the full extent of the incision upfront in order to improve the working space and to avoid any unnecessary delay. We have typically used the four-channel R-port (QuadPort). Additionally, we routinely applied a needlescopic (trocar free) 2-mm grasper, directly put into the abdominal cavity lateral to the rectus muscle and about two finger-widths under the costal margin to facilitate the procedure.

Step 2: Colon mobilisation, incision for parietal peritoneum, identification of ureter and gonadal vessels

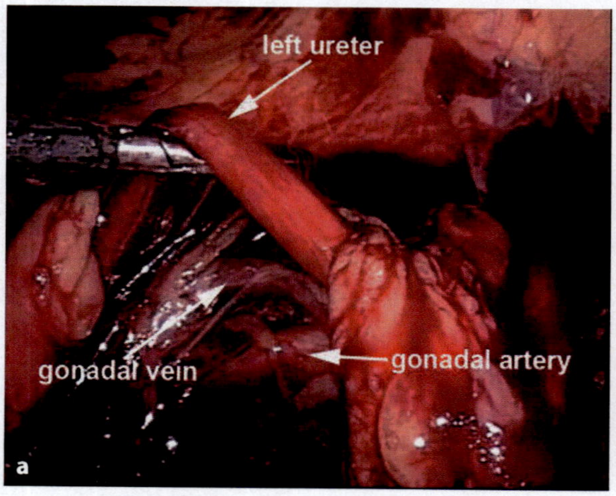

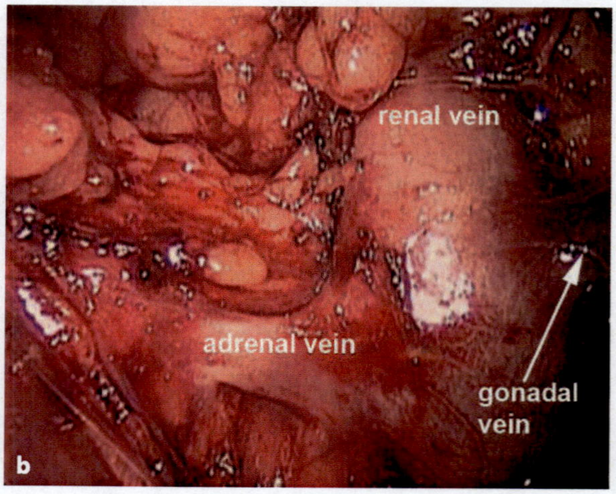

The LESS donor nephrectomy technique duplicates all the steps of standard laparoscopic donor nephrectomy. Descending colon, spleen and tail of pancreas are widely mobilised from the Gerota fascia so that they fall off the kidney medially without the need for constant retraction. Caudally to the lower pole of the kidney, the ureter and gonadal packet are lifted off the psoas muscle and the lateral border of the aorta, taking care to preserve the surrounding periureteral fibroareolar tissue. To facilitate exposure, the Gerota fascia may be fixed to the abdominal side wall with an internal stay suture of 2-0 Vicryl if necessary. The left adrenal vein typically enters the superior border of the renal vein at or medial to the level of insertion of the gonadal vessel.

1

Step 3: Adrenal mobilisation and upper pole dissection

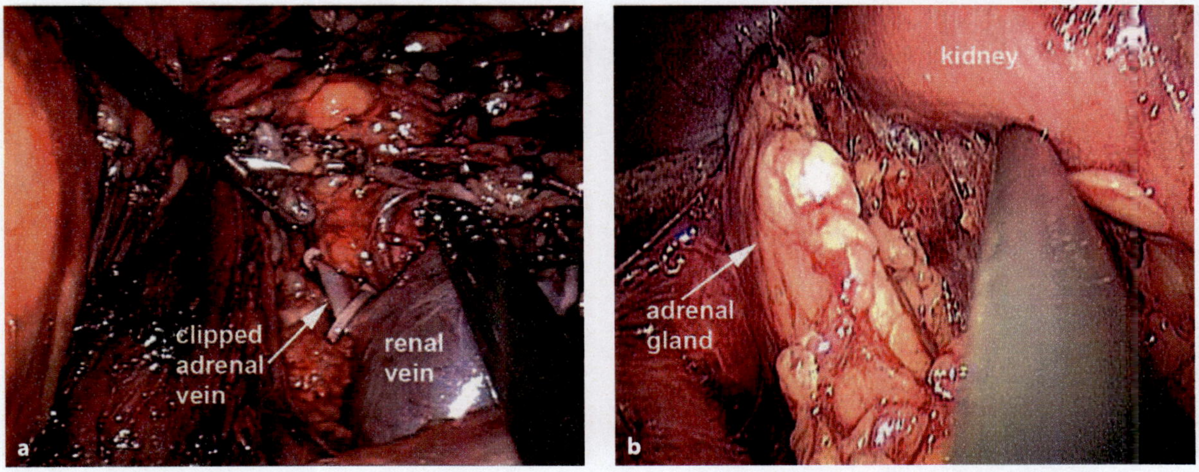

The adrenal vein is carefully dissected to obtain adequate length for secure clipping and division. This maneuver enables mobilisation of the adrenal gland from the upper pole. Care is taken to avoid fracturing the adrenal gland. Once the adrenal gland has been completely released, the upper pole of the kidney is completely freed and lifted off the psoas muscle. Dissection along the gonadal vein brings us to its junction into the renal vein. The renal vein is skeletonised to the interaortocaval region.

Step 4: Preparation up to the hilum

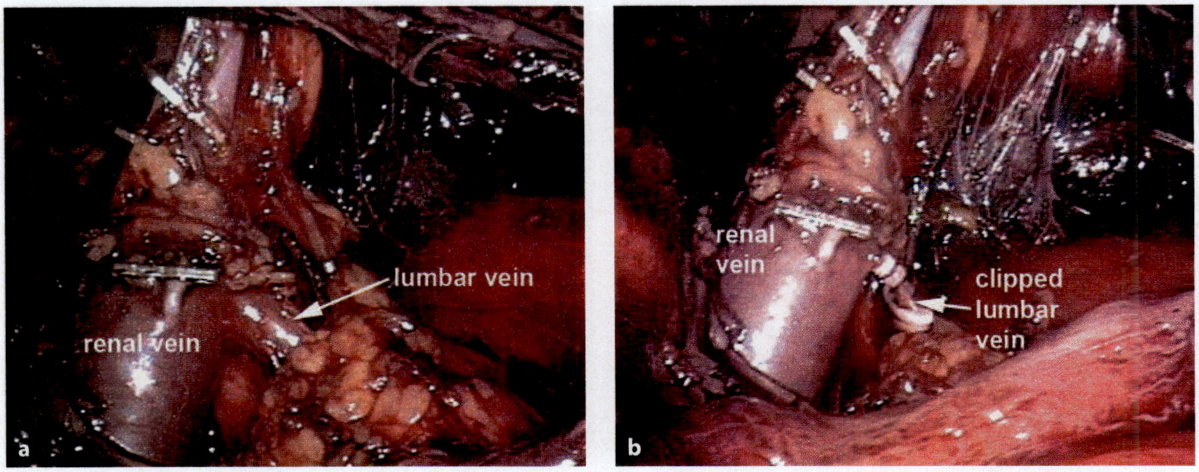

Dissecting the vessels' inferior margin identifies the lumbar venous branches that are carefully exposed for an adequate length, then clipped and divided. The division of the lumbar veins opens the space to the root of the renal artery as it originates from the aorta. We mobilise approximately 1–2 cm of the renal artery stump to enable subsequent secure placement of clips. It is unnecessary to dissect additional length and in fact doing so may induce arterial spasm. Therefore, this is best done on the bench after allograft retrieval. Occasionally, the main trunk of the artery may be more cephalad and eventually necessitates gentle retraction of the renal vein. This maneuver is best done with a 5-mm grasper inserted through the single port device and preferably not with the 2-mm grasper that has a sharp tip and may be traumatic.

Step 5: Ureter transection, complete kidney mobilisation

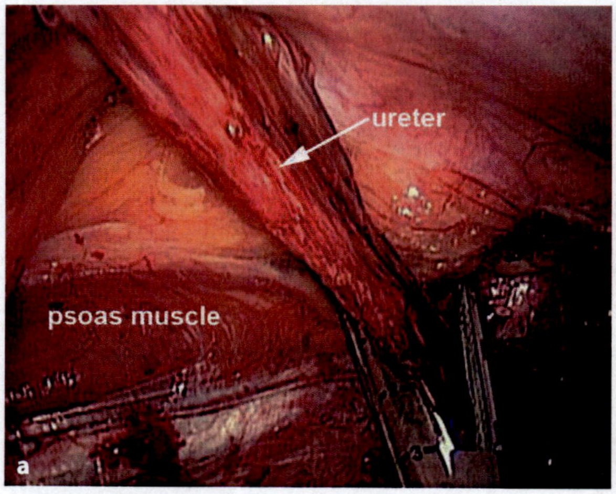

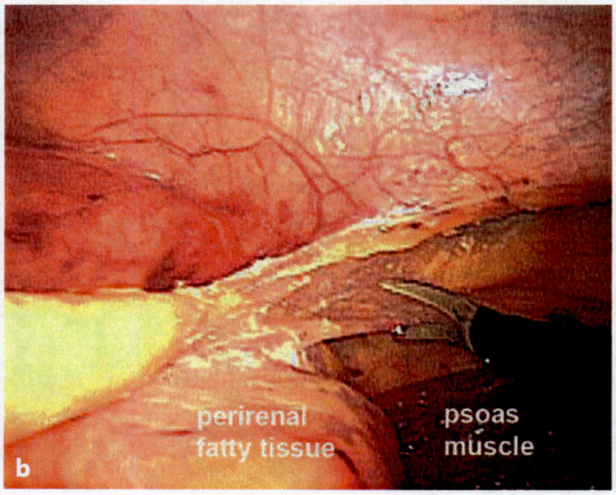

It is important that lateral kidney attachments are left untouched until hilar preparation is complete. After perfusion with mannitol (250 ml, 20%), the ureter is divided (stapler or Hem-o-lok) inferiorly to the iliac vessels. The kidney is circumferentially mobilised while leaving its perirenal fat intact.

Step 6: Vascular control

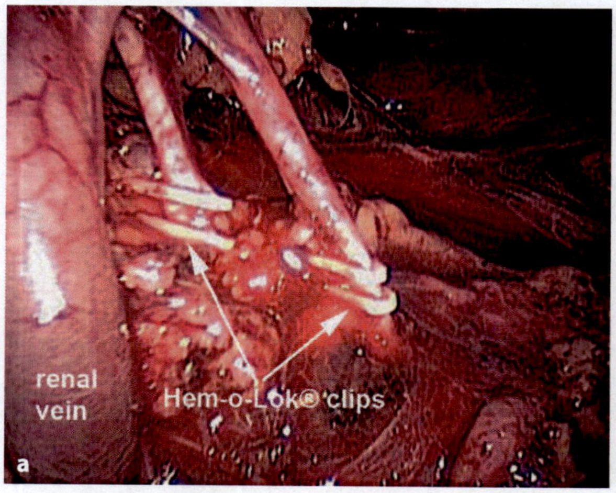

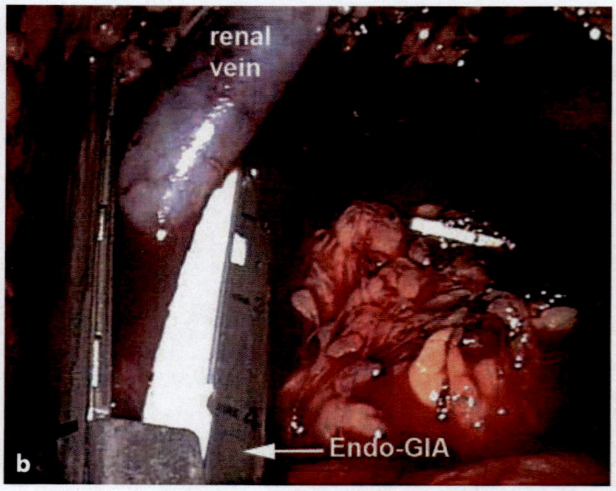

After placing two central Hem-o-lok clips and one titanium clip on the stay side (Step 6a), the renal artery is divided. The artery is clipped as close as possible to the aorta and care is taken to leave a 1- to 2-mm cuff after the most proximal clip. The renal vein is secured with a 12-mm vascular Endo-GIA stapler (Covidien, Dublin, Ireland). Since the dissection takes place in the inter-aortocaval region, one has to be careful not to injure the superior mesenteric artery.

Step 7: Vascular control

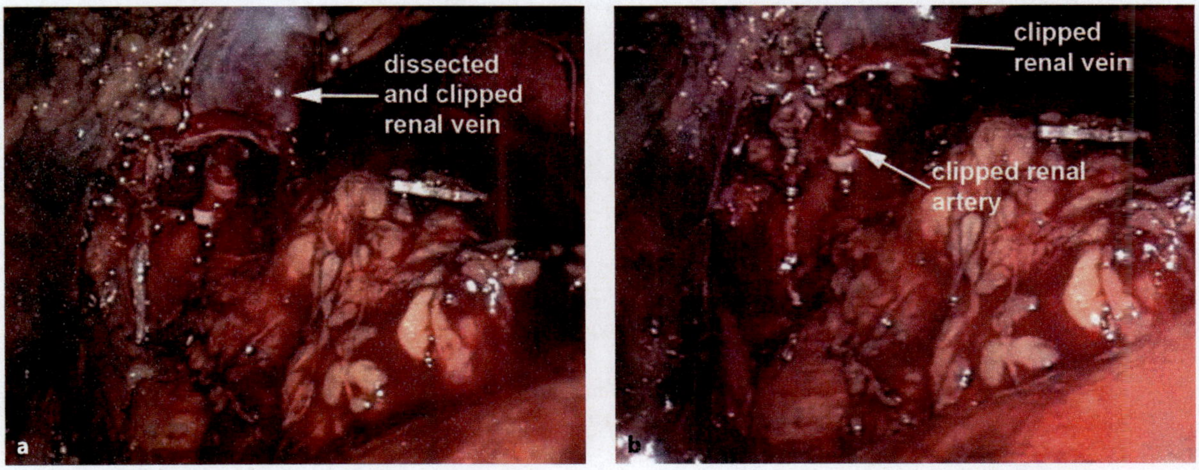

The remaining proximal tissue (vessel wall plus perivascular tissue) prevents retraction of the vein into the interaortocaval region in case of stapler misfire and is divided after placing clips (Step 7a). Occasionally, the stapler line on the stay side may be reinforced with additional titanium clips. Any residual perihilar attachments are carefully clipped and divided to completely free the allograft (Step 7b).

Step 8: Specimen extraction

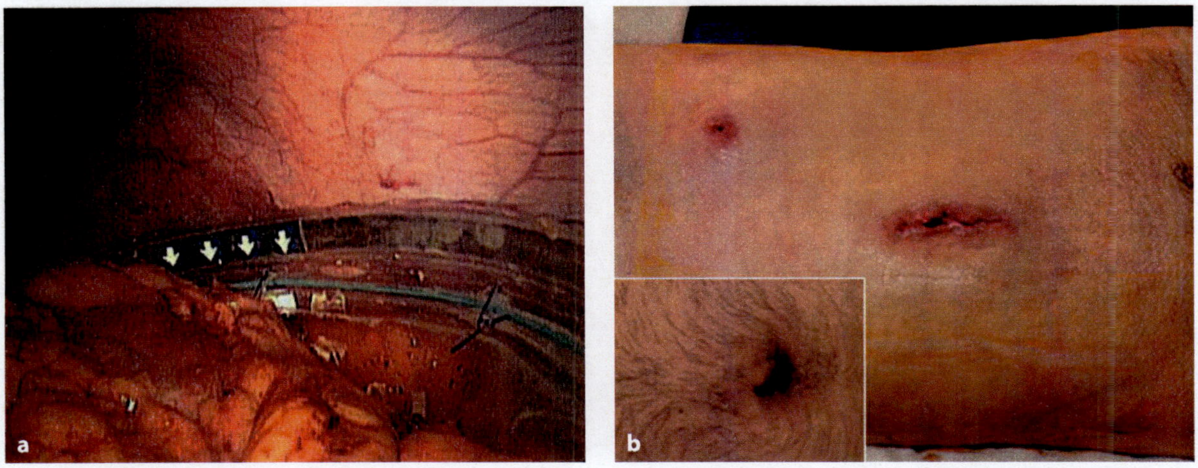

Through the 15-mm port of the QuadPort, a 15-mm specimen retrieval bag (Endocath II, Covidien) is introduced and the kidney entrapped. After removing the single port, the bagged allograft is gently extracted through the initially performed 4.5-cm skin incision and approximately 6-cm rectus fasciotomy and thereafter handed to the recipient surgeon for perfusion and subsequent transplantation. The port is then re-inserted to re-inspect the surgical area and confirm haemostasis. Step 8b shows the incision site immediately after port removal and 1 month postoperatively.

Postoperative Management

- Check complete blood count and basic metabolic panel in recovery area and next day
- Progressive ambulation and advancement of diet
- Patients are advised not to lift weights heavier than 5 kg for 6 weeks

References

1. Canes D, Berger A, Aron M et al (2010) Laparo-endoscopic single site (LESS) versus standard laparoscopic left donor nephrectomy: matched-pair comparison. Euro Urol 57:95–101
2. Canes D, Desai MM, Aron M et al (2008) Transumbilical single port surgery: evolution and current status. Eur Urol 54:1020–1030
3. Hadjianastassiou VG, Johnson RJ, Rudge CJ, Masmode N (2007) 2509 living donor nephrectomies, morbidity and mortality, including the UK introduction of laparoscopic donor surgery. Am J Transplant 7:2532–2537

1.12.4 Robot-Assisted Donor Nephrectomy

Alberto Breda

Introduction

Robotic surgery has exploded into the realm of urologists. Nevertheless, robotic nephrectomy has not gained popularity yet, probably due to the high costs of the robot and the minimal benefits over the standard laparoscopic approach. Robotic nephrectomy may offer some advantages to the patient in selected cases. Specifically, laparoscopic living-donor nephrectomy (LLDN) has become the standard of care for kidney procurement and subsequent kidney transplantation [1]. A robotic procedure may in fact offer an advantage over the laparoscopic approach due to the extreme precision needed to manipulate and dissect the renal vessels and ureter. There are two approaches to a robotic nephrectomy, as for the laparoscopic technique: transperitoneal and retroperitoneal. Although it has been shown that no difference exists between the two approaches during a laparoscopic procedure [2], in robotic surgery the transperitoneal approach is preferred over the retroperitoneal approach due to the larger surgical field.

Indications

Patients candidates for:

- Live donor nephrectomy
- Radical nephrectomy
- Simple nephrectomy

Contra-indications

- Previous major abdominal surgery on the side of the nephrectomy
- Large renal vein thrombus
- Large (>12 cm) renal tumour

Preoperative Preparation

- Orogastric tube placement, urinary catheter (Foley, 18 F)

Single shot of first-generation cephalosporin 30 min before starting surgery

Step 1: Port placement for three-arm robotic system

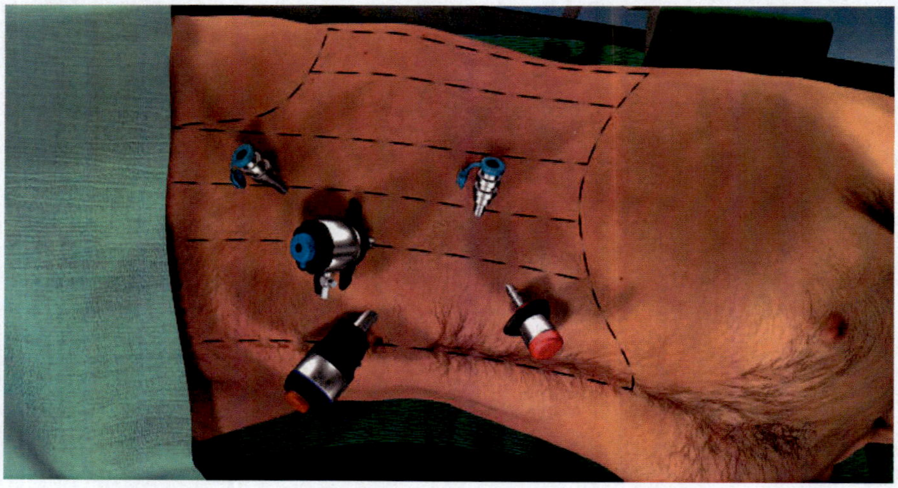

The patient is placed in a 60° flank and 10° Trendelenburg position. Trocar positioning is operator-dependent. The majority of surgeons adopt a classical diamond-shaped configuration with the camera port in the middle at the level of the lateral margin of the rectus sheath. The procedure starts with the placement of the 12-mm trocar for the robotic camera. Then two 8-mm robotic trocars are placed on midclavicular line. Trocar positioning of the remaining trocars varies according to the number of the robotic arms available. Step 1 shows the configuration for a three-arm robotic system. A 12-mm assistant trocar is placed in the midline parallel to the camera trocar, while a 5-mm trocar is placed in the midline parallel to the most cephalic robotic port.

Step 2: Port placement for four-arm robotic system

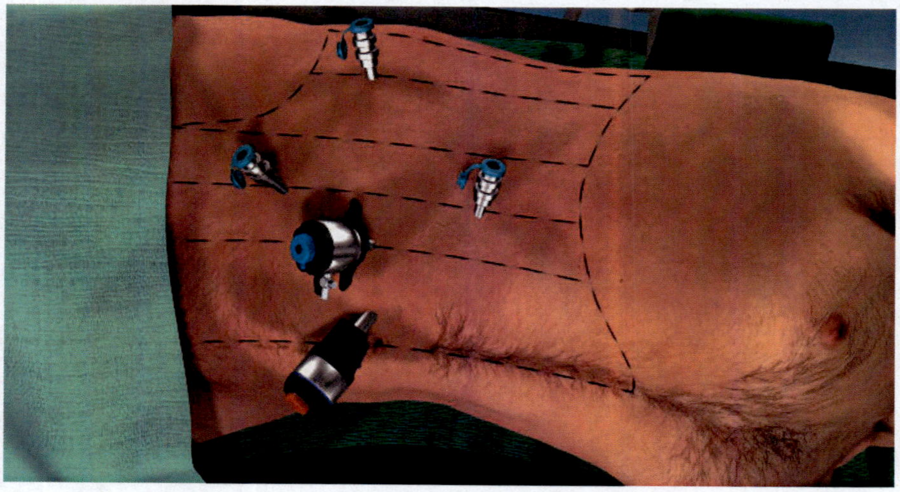

The positioning of the trocars for the use of a four-arm robotic system is different from the three-arm system. The positioning of camera and first robotic trocars is the same as for the three-arm configuration. An additional fourth robotic port (8 mm) is placed at the same level as the camera trocar on the midaxillary line. An assistant trocar is placed medially at the same level as the camera trocar. Port placement is the same both for a right and a left nephrectomy. All trocars except for the camera port, which is positioned by open Hasson technique, should be placed under direct vision after the introduction of the pneumoperitoneum in order to prevent any abdominal organ injuries.

Step 3: Mobilisation of the colon

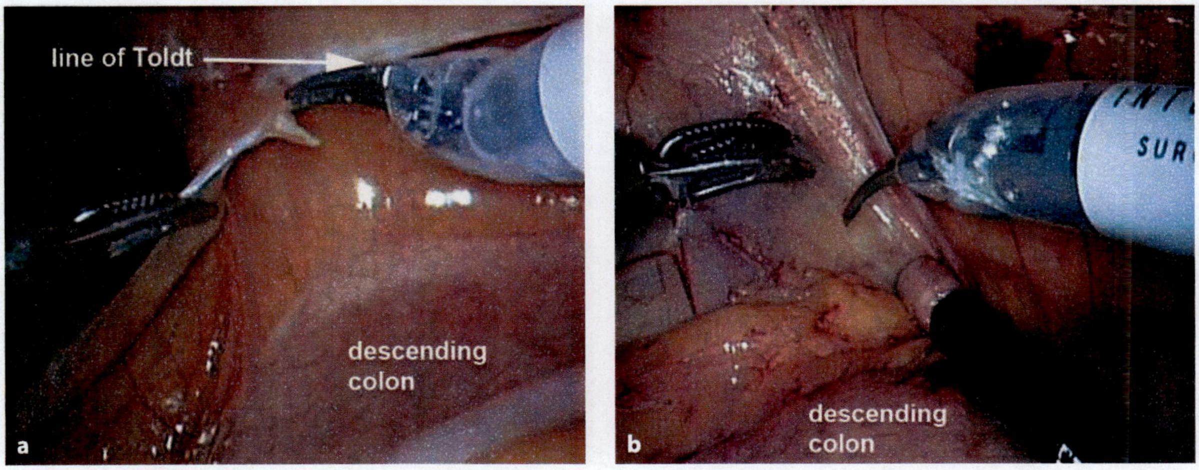

Once the access has been correctly obtained and all the ports are placed, the robot is connected. The robot is positioned posterior to the patient and perpendicular to the patient's kidney. This is crucial to allow the device to work appropriately. Thereafter the procedure starts with mobilisation of the colon. Although the colon is usually mobilised to the level of the common iliac artery, the dissection could start at the level of the left or right colonic flexures. Step 3a shows the initiation of the dissection of the white line of Toldt at the level of the splenic flexure. A combination of robotic graspers and scissors is used while sharp and blunt dissection takes place. The dissection continues along the line (Step 3b).

Step4: Mobilisation of spleen and adrenal gland

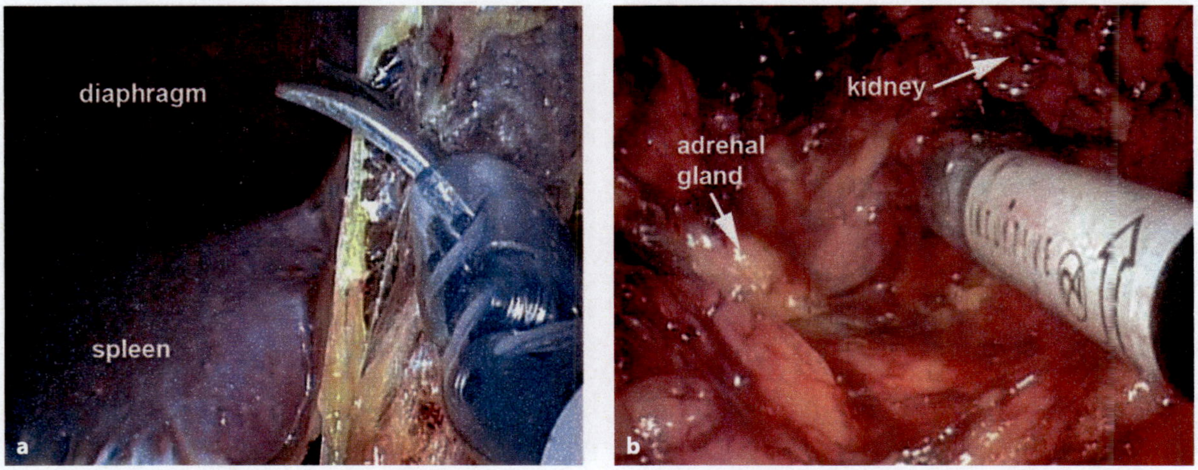

Mobilisation of the upper pole of the kidney follows. In order to facilitate this part of the procedure, mobilisation of the spleen or liver depending on the side is recommended. For a left nephrectomy, the posterior peritoneum is incised to the level of the crus of the diaphragm, thus obtaining a complete reflection of the spleen (Step 4a). For a right nephrectomy, the triangular ligament of the liver is incised allowing elevation of the liver with the help of the 5-mm assistant trocar. At this point, the renal vein is identified and the plain between the adrenal gland and the upper pole of the kidney is meticulously dissected to completely expose the upper pole (Step 4b). In case of a radical nephrectomy, this step is avoided and the adrenal gland is taken with the specimen.

Step5: Gonadal vein and ureter dissection

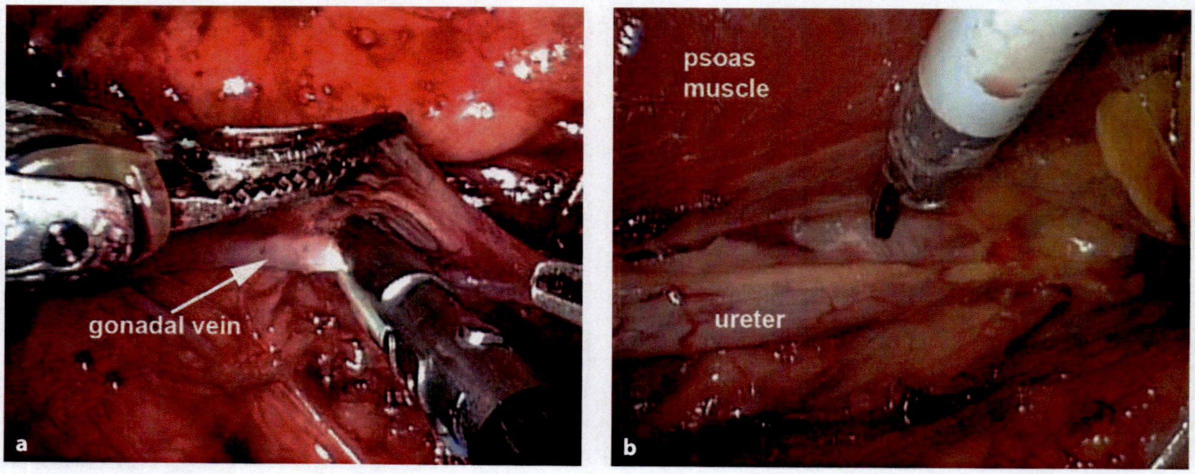

Attention is then moved to the lower pole of the kidney. The gonadal vein and the ureter are identified. At this point, the procedure varies depending on the type of the surgery. In left donor nephrectomy, the majority of cases are in fact left-sided due to the longer renal vein. Recent data clearly shows that the gonadal vein can safely be taken at 2–3 cm from the renal vein with dissection between the ureter and the gonadal vein itself [3] (Step 5a). The advantage of this technique is the easier elevation of the kidney and access to the lumbar vein. Dissection of the ureter to the level of the iliac vessels follows (Step 5b). A less extensive dissection of the ureter is adequate for radical nephrectomy.

Step 6: Renal artery identification and dissection to the aorta

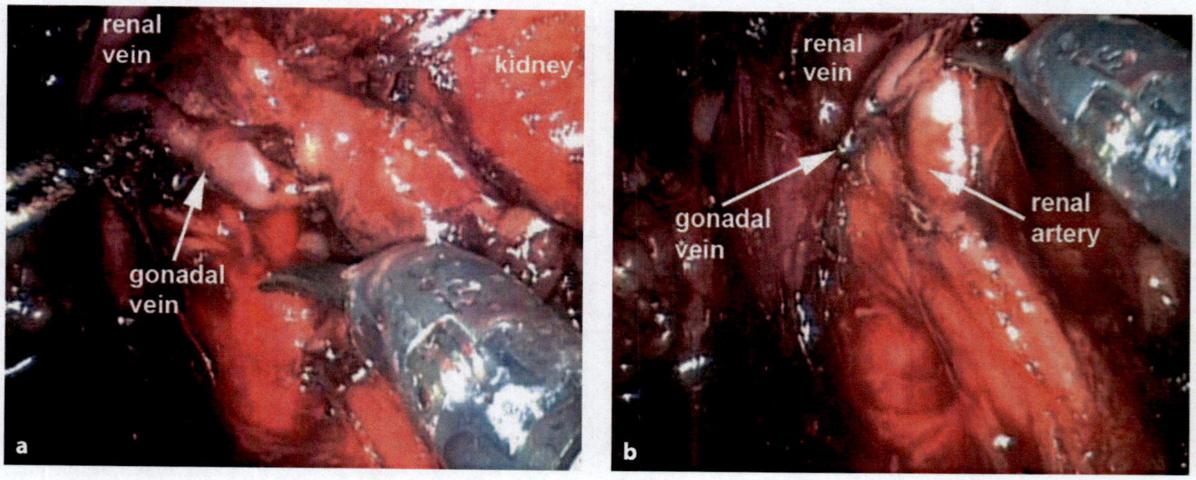

The ureter is elevated by the assistant or the fourth arm and dissection of the posterior attachments of the kidney is bluntly performed. Thus, the renal hilum is exposed. The dissection is then initiated inferior to the gonadal vein stump and continues upwards to the renal vein (Step 6a). If a lumbar vein is identified it is clipped by the first assistant and transected. Meticulous dissection is performed at the level of the renal hilum. The renal artery is carefully prepared to the level of the aorta (Step 6b). The whole length should be visible so as to perform the ligation as proximal as possible to the aorta and to eventually provide sufficient renal artery stump for transplantation (such extensive preparation is not necessary in radical nephrectomy).

Step 7: Adrenal vein identification and dissection

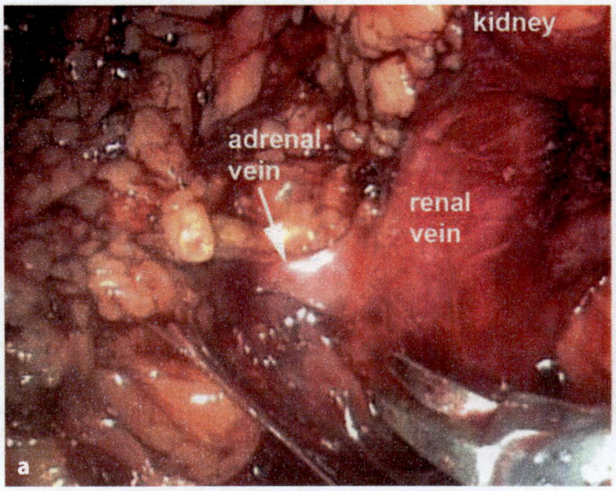

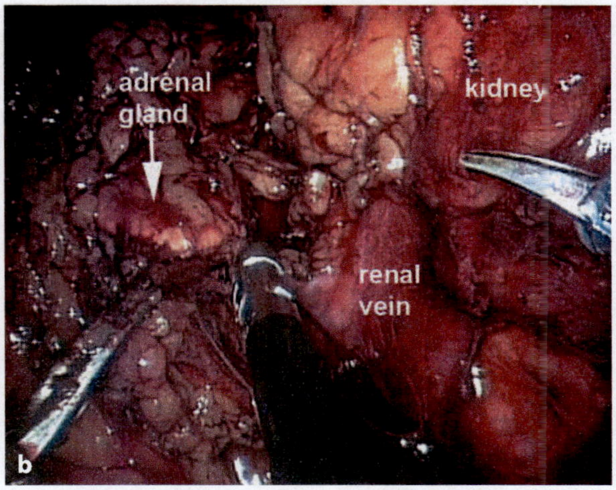

Careful dissection of the renal vein exposes the adrenal vein. Step 7a shows the adrenal vein prepared from the surrounding fatty tissue. The vessel is ligated by clips and scissors or with the help of ultrasonic scissors in an attempt to obtain adequate length of the renal vein (Step 7b). The kidney is fully mobilised from its lateral attachments and the only site that remains attached is the renal hilum. A fourth robotic arm facilitates dissection by lifting the kidney. At this point the robotic system is disconnected and the procedure continues laparoscopically. The conversion to laparoscopy is not necessary but the author considers that it is safer to retrieve the organ without the presence of the robotic arms in the field.

Step 8: Stapling of the renal artery and vein separately

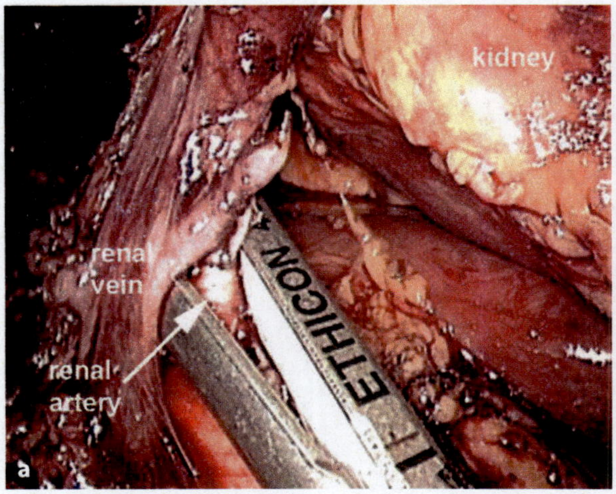

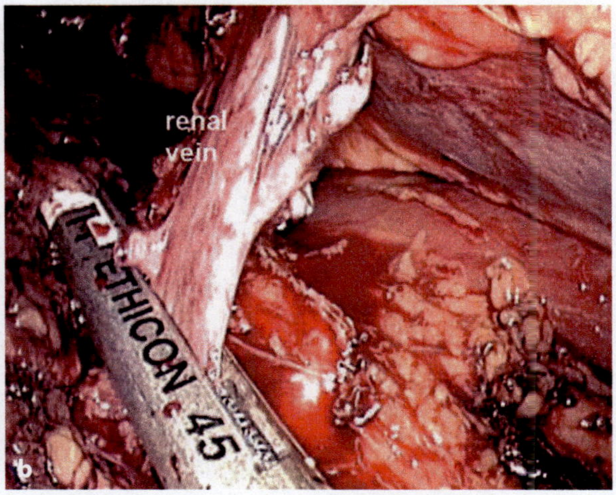

A vertical incision of the fascia is performed to the level of the umbilicus. A 15-mm trocar is inserted as close as possible to the umbilicus. The latter port is inserted to fit the vascular stapler and the 15-mm endobag for organ extraction. The ureter is transected at the level of the iliac vessels. The kidney is fully elevated by the first assistant to obtain length and tension on the renal hilum while the renal artery is ligated first with the use of the vascular stapler (Step 8a). The separate ligation of the renal vein by the same method follows (Step 8b). The organ is than placed into an endobag and a midline or a Pfannenstiel incision is performed. Once the organ has been extracted it is placed in ice and flushed with cool solution or sent for pathology evaluation.

Postoperative Management

- No drain is left in place (usually)
- Remove Foley catheter on postoperative day 1
- Start regular diet on postoperative day 1
- Discharge from the hospital on postoperative day 2
- Resumption of normal activities in 10–15 days

References

1. Lam JS, Breda A, Schulam PG (2007) Is laparoscopic donor nephrectomy the new standard? Nat Clin Pract Urol 4:186–187
2. Desai MM, Strzempkowski B, Matin SF, Steinberg AP, Ng C, Meraney AM, Kaouk JH, Gill IS (2005) Prospective randomized comparison of transperitoneal versus retroperitoneal laparoscopic radical nephrectomy. J Urol 173:38–41
3. Breda A, Bui MH, Liao JC, Gritsch HA, Schulam PG (2006) Incidence of ureteral strictures after laparoscopic donor nephrectomy. J Urol 176:1065–1068

1.13 Recommended Incisions for Kidney Removal

Jens-Uwe Stolzenburg, Rowan Casey, Minh Do, Anja Dietel, Ho Thi Phuc, Andreas Gonsior, Thilo Schwalenberg, Evangelos Liatsikos

Morcellation of the specimen in kidney cancer surgery is not the advised because of the inability to perform pathological analysis and the risk of tumour seeding if the bag ruptures. For this reason, the specimen must be removed intact. Renal cancer surgery can employ many different port placements, as seen in the chapters of this book. As a result, there is more than one option for the skin incision for the specimen removal. The following figures will demonstrate a number of possibilities when siting the skin and fascial incision. These same incisions can be used for donor nephrectomy and other noncancerous renal procedures.

Before inserting the first port, consideration should be given to where one plans to remove the specimen. Usually the site of specimen removal is through one of the port entry sites and this can be extended in either direction. Other factors to be considered are the body habitus, patient position, the patient's wishes and the surgeon's preference.

Option 1: Specimen removal during transperitoneal nephrectomy

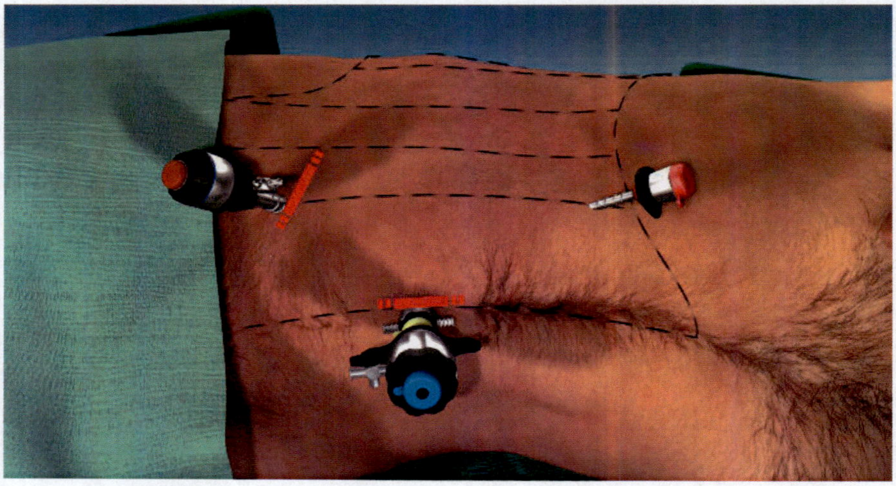

Many surgeons use the camera port at the umbilicus as shown in the figure. For specimen removal, an EndoCatch bag can be inserted through this port whilst using the camera through the caudal 10-mm port. The specimen is then bagged and removed through a midline laparotomy incision (4–6 cm depending on the size of the kidney) directly through the umbilicus. The same technique is used for single-port surgery. Alternatively, the EndoCatch bag is inserted through the 10-mm caudal port and removed via an oblique muscle-splitting incision (grid-iron incision) extending the skin incision at the port site.

Option 2: Specimen removal during transperitoneal nephrectomy

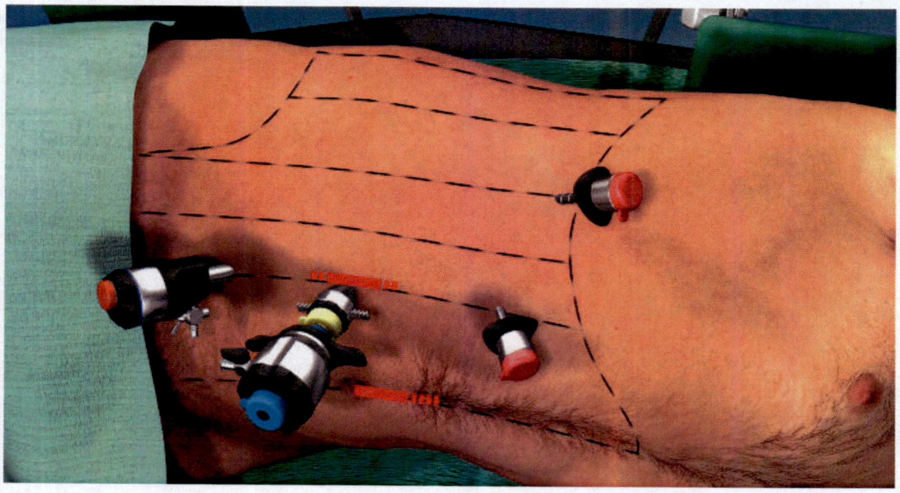

If the camera port is placed paraumbilically on the pararectal line the specimen can be removed through a laparotomy performed on the pararectal line, as indicated in the figure. This has the advantage of avoiding muscle cutting. We prefer this specimen removal incision during LESS surgery in obese patients when the Quad-Port is placed paraumbilically. Alternatively, an EndoCatch bag can be separately inserted directly through the umbilicus (without a port), and when the kidney is bagged, this incision can be enlarged in a cranial direction as a laparotomy, as also shown in the figure. It can also be extended periumbilically as shown in Option 1.

Option 3: Specimen removal during transperitoneal nephrectomy

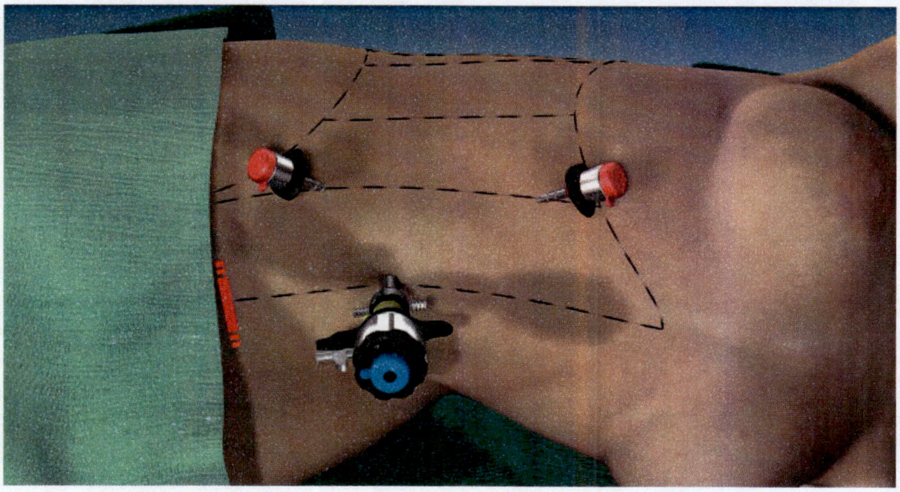

Especially for cosmetic reasons, the specimen can be removed via a Pfannenstiel incision. To perform this, an EndoCatch bag must be inserted suprapubically through a small trocarless incision. Alternatively, the bag can be inserted via the 10- or 12-mm ports and once the specimen has been placed in the bag, it can be brought out through the Pfannenstiel incision. This technique is rarely used, except in younger women. All the other techniques provide inferior cosmetic results.

Option 4: Specimen removal during retroperitoneal nephrectomy

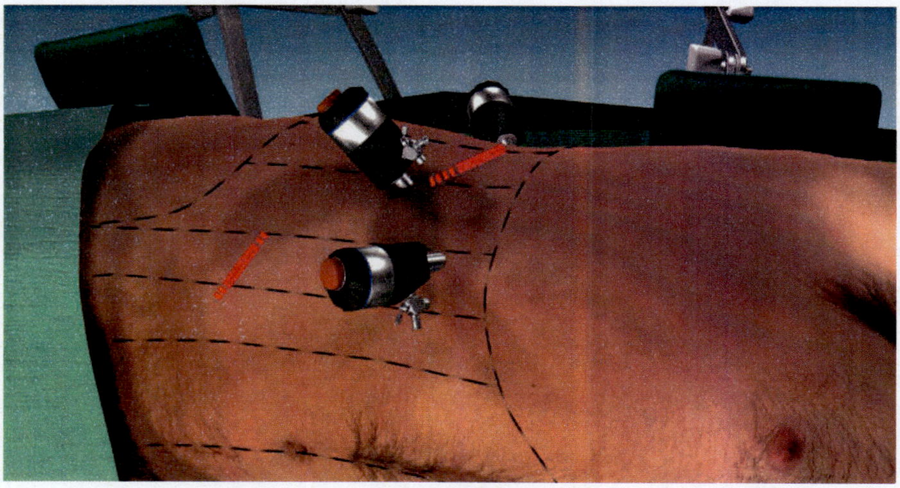

The figure demonstrates the standard port placements for a retroperitoneal procedure. One option for removal of the specimen is to create an oblique muscle-splitting incision above and medial to the anterior superior iliac crest if sufficient space has been created and the peritoneum mobilised in the retroperitoneal approach. An alternative approach would be to make an incision between the most lateral port and the camera port. This incision is commonly used despite the disadvantage of requiring incision through deep muscle layers.

1.14 Transperitoneal Pyeloplasty

1.14.1 Laparoscopic Pyeloplasty

Niklas Kreutzer, Sherif Abulsorour, Rowan Casey, Jens-Uwe Stolzenburg, Michael C. Truß

Introduction

Pyeloplasty has become one of the most frequent reconstructive procedures in urology. Since the first reports in the early 1990s, the repair of the obstructed ureteropelvic junction (UPJ) with laparoscopic procedures (transperitoneal or retroperitoneal) is nowadays broadly accepted [1, 2]. The advantages of the laparoscopic approach (good vision, less postoperative pain and small scars) and good functional results similar to the results obtained with open procedures, even in young children, have been demonstrated [3, 4]. Laparoscopic pyeloplasty series recently showed a success rate greater than 95% [5], with failure being mostly the result of poor technical quality, particularly in the earlier cases of reported series [6]. Laparoscopic pyeloplasty is also a safe and successful alternative to open surgery for management of secondary UPJ obstruction, like revision pyeloplasty with similar success rates [6, 7]. The described dismembered technique is an adoption of the classic operation.

Indications

- Impaired tracer elimination on MAG-3 renogram
- Persistent loin pain based on hydronephrosis and impaired MAG-3 renogram
- Combination of UPJ obstruction and calculi

Contra-indications

- Pregnancy
- Kidney function below 15%
- Large calculi

Preoperative Preparation

- Ultrasound, renal scintigraphy, (intravenous urogram), retrograde pyelogram
- Single-dose broad-spectrum antibiotic
- If stented pyeloplasty is planned, a double-J stent is inserted
- Urinary catheter

Step 1: Patient position and trocar placement

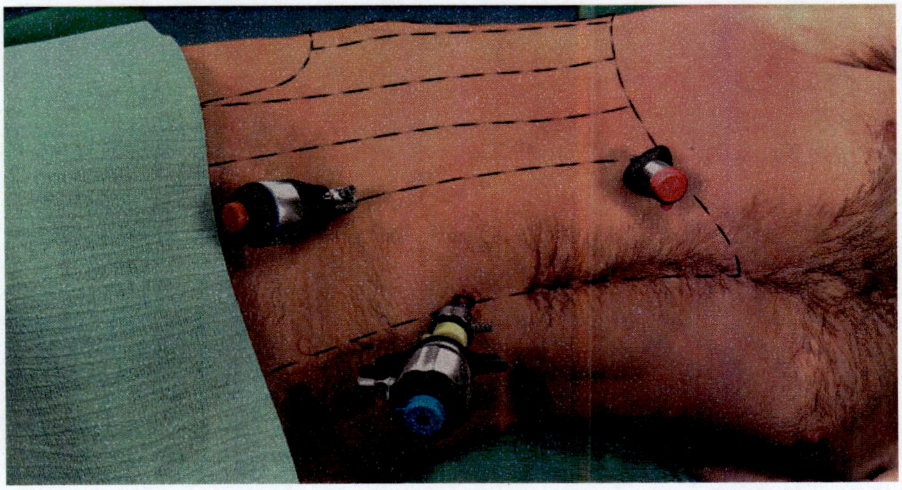

The patient position is detailed in Sect. 1.1. A Veress needle is inserted supraumbilically to create a pneumoperitoneum, as described in Sect. 1.2.1. Alternatively, a minilaparotomy is possible, especially in previously operated patients. The 10-mm camera trocar is inserted and inspection is made for trocar-induced injury. The second trocar is placed lateral to the rectus muscle beneath the costal margin. The third trocar is placed lateral to the rectus muscle at the level of the anterior superior iliac spine, as shown in the figure. The trocar size depends on the instruments used. In a patient with a large liver disturbing visualisation of the right kidney, another small trocar near the xiphoid process can be used to retract the liver.

Step 2: View of the colonic flexure and Gerota fascia after colon dissection

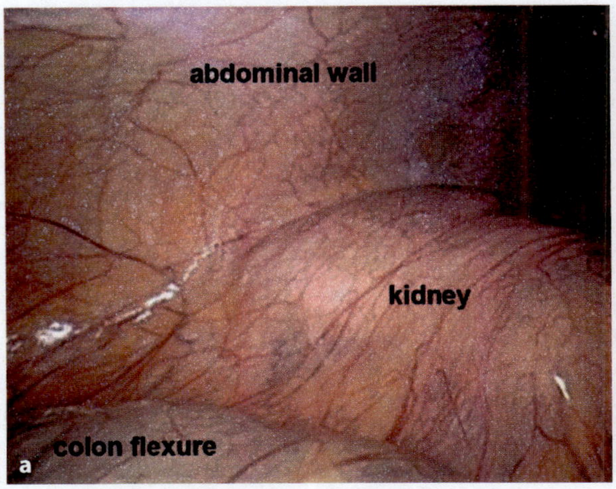

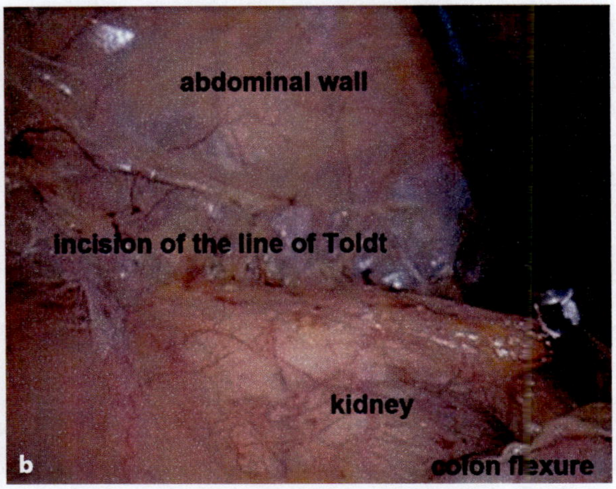

Make an incision at the white line of Toldt from the level of the colonic flexure to the iliac vessels (Step 2b). Bluntly dissect the colon medially to access the ureter and renal pelvis. Beware on the right side: the duodenum might be adherent to the renal pelvis and must always be identified, dissected and reflected medially. The ureter and the renal pelvis are identified next. These structures may be more easily located when stented, although stenting will result in the loss of a large dilated obstructed pelvis, which is often useful as a guide. The kidney does not usually require mobilisation.

Step 3: Stay suture in the ureter and renal pelvis

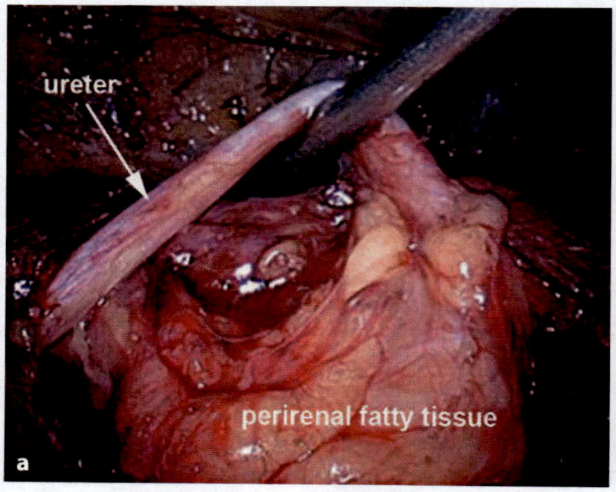

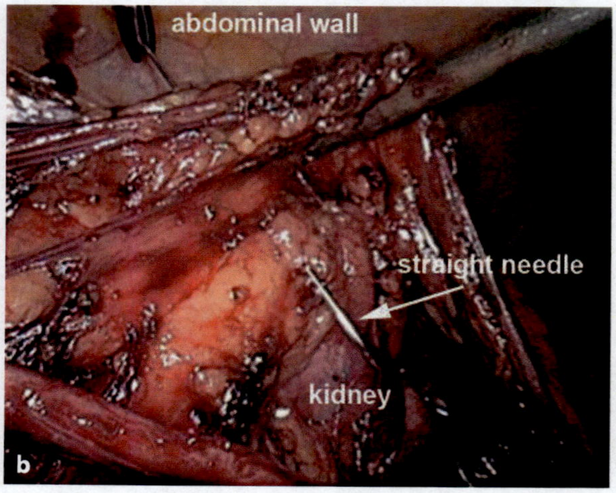

A suture around the ureter with its end passing through the abdominal wall and secured on the skin can help dissecting the ureter and the renal pelvis (Step 3a). However, one must avoid too much traction. Furthermore, electrocautery or other energy sources must not be used near the ureter. If present, a lower pole vessel must be dissected from the ureter; damage of this lower pole artery can cause partial renal ischaemia. Free the renal pelvis from adherent tissues by blunt and sharp dissection. If the surrounding fat is troublesome, another stay suture from outside the abdomen can be used with a straight needle to hold it out of the way (Step 3b).

Step 4: Ureteric stay suture distally and opened renal pelvis

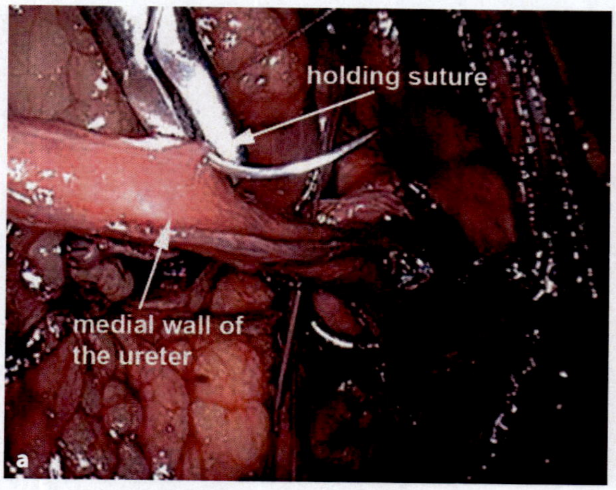

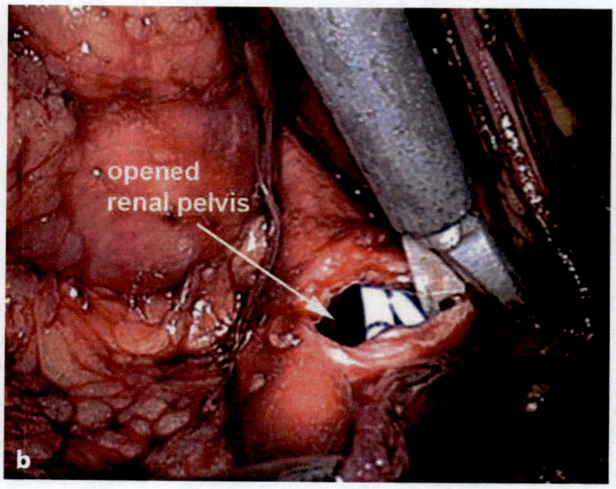

A stay suture is placed in the ureter medially and distally to the UPJ (Step 4a). This suture serves two purposes. Firstly, it helps avoid rotation during dismembering. Secondly, it also serves as traction during pelviureteric anastomosis. The renal pelvis is opened (Step 4b) and the stenotic part is resected with scissors (e.g. Potts scissors). Be careful that the renal pelvis is not excised too cranially as this may injure the renal calices. A further stay suture (4/0 Vicryl) can also be placed on the anterior aspect of the renal pelvis medially in the upper part to separate the two layers of the renal pelvis; this allows easier suturing without the need for additional instruments.

Step 5: Spatulated ureter and placement of the first stitch

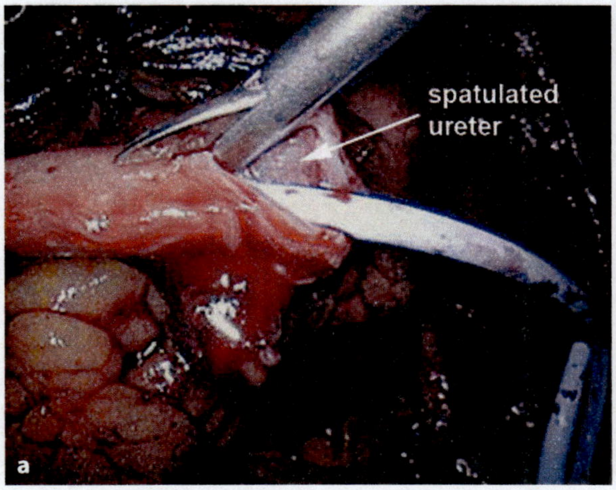

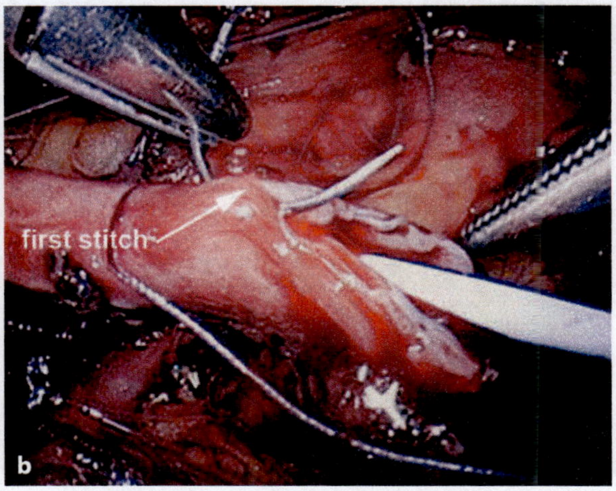

The ureter is then spatulated laterally for a distance of 1–1.5 cm (Step 5a). Make sure that the ureter does not rotate using the traction suture placed earlier. Beware of damaging its blood supply. It should be allowed to bleed freely after spatulation. Diathermy should not be used for haemostasis. The first stitch is made from the lowest point of the V-shaped spatulated ureter (stitch out-in) to the lowest point of the opened renal pelvis (stitch in-out) with Vicryl 4/0 on an Rb1 needle. The magnification of the optical trocar helps ensure that ureteral mucosa is taken with each suture (Step 5b).

Step 6: Ureteropelvic anastomosis

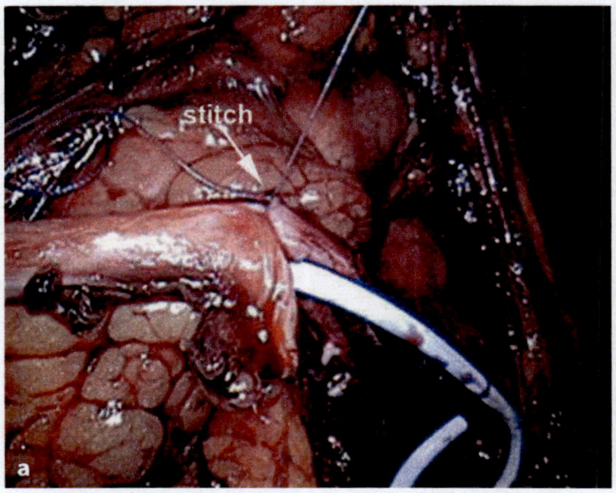

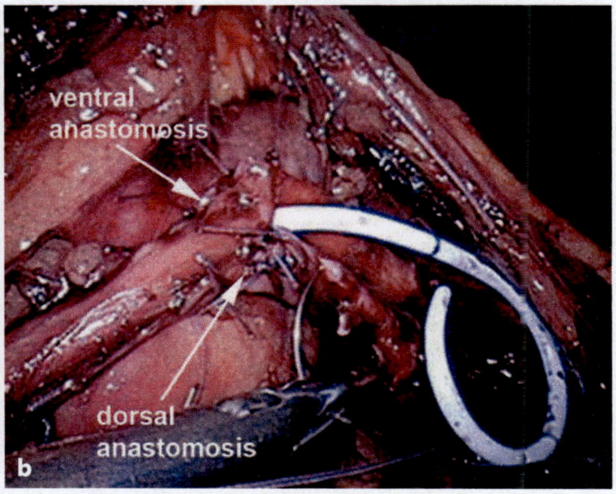

The first suture is carefully tied to ensure good apposition. If there is too much tension, the ureter and/or the kidney have to be mobilised to allow a tension-free anastomosis. It can be helpful to suture the two terminal ends of the ureter to the renal pelvis first. Then the front and back wall of the anastomosis can be sutured by simple interrupted sutures (spaced 3 mm apart). If a stent has not been inserted preoperatively one is inserted now. The technique for on-table stent insertion is described in Sect. 1.14.2.

Step 7: Renal pelvis closure and drain insertion

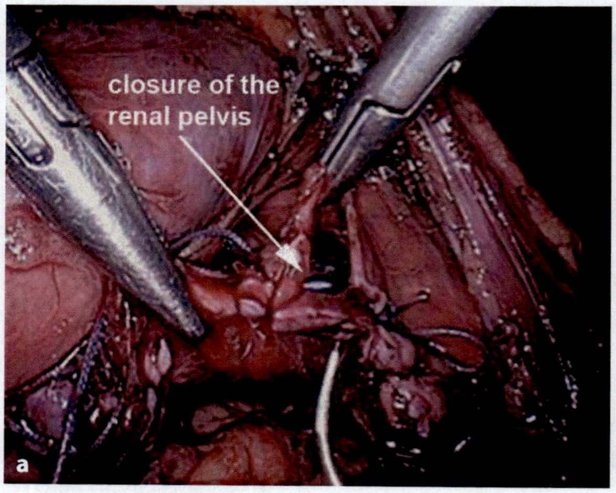

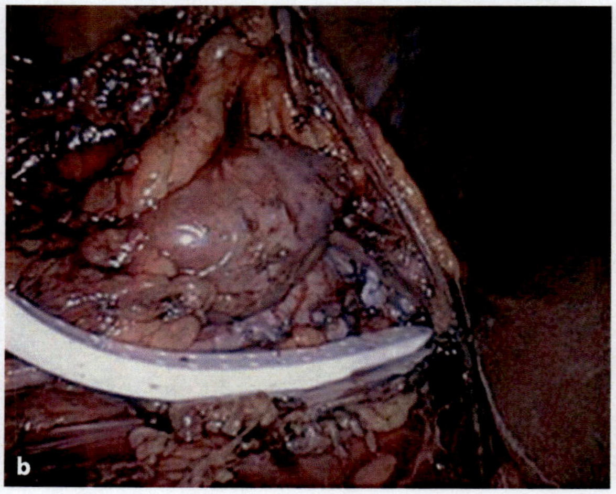

Check the double-J stent for possible obstruction by clots by filling the bladder with irrigation fluid and allowing it to reflux up the ureter and stent. The rest of the renal pelvis is now closed with a running suture beginning at the cranial point (Step 7a). To close the triangular gap between the ureter and the renal pelvis, make a three-point suture (renal pelvis out-in, ureter in-out-in, renal pelvis in-out). Check for anastomotic leakage by filling the bladder until the renal pelvis distends. Place a 16-Ch drain medially near the anastomosis (Step 7b). If possible, cover the anastomosis with perirenal fatty tissue. Make a final inspection for bleeding and bowel injury and remove the trocars under vision.

Postoperative Management

- Check for diuresis
- Ultrasound on 1st day after surgery
- Cystography with reflux through double-J stent after 3 days and Foley catheter removal if there is no leakage at anastomosis
- Double-J stent removal after 4 weeks
- Evaluation by ultrasound on day 1, after Foley catheter removal and after double-J stent removal

References

1. Kavoussi LR, Peters CA (1993) Laparoscopic pyeloplasty. J Urol 150:1891–1894
2. Schuessler WW, Grune MT, Tecuanhuey LV, Preminger GM (1993) Laparoscopic dismembered pyeloplasty. J Urol 150:1795–1799
3. Metzelder ML, Schier F, Petersen C, Truss M, Ure BM (2006) Laparoscopic transabdominal pyeloplasty in children is feasible irrespective of age. J Urol 175:688–691
4. Inagaki T, Rha KH, Ong AM, Kavoussi LR, Jarrett TW (2005) Laparoscopic pyeloplasty: current status. BJU 95 (Suppl 2):102–105
5. Jarrett TW, Chan DY, Charambura TC, Fugita O, Kavoussi LR (2002) Laparoscopic pyeloplasty: the first 100 cases. J Urol 167:1253–1256
6. Basiri A, Behjati S, Zand S, Moghaddam SM (2007) Laparoscopic pyeloplasty in secondary uretero-pelvic junction obstruction after failed open surgery. J Endourol 21:1045–1052
7. Sundaram CP, Grubb RL 3rd, Rehman J, Yan Y, Chen C, Landman J, McDougall EM, Clayman RV (2003) Laparoscopic pyeloplasty for secondary ureteropelvic junction obstruction. J Urol 169:2037–2040

1.14.2 Robot-Assisted Pyeloplasty

H. P. Beerlage, Rowan Casey, Panagiotis Kallidonis, Evangelos Liatsikos, Jens-Uwe Stolzenburg

Introduction

The first operative repair of ureteropelvic junction obstruction (UPJO) was described by Trendelenburg in 1886. Anderson and Hynes [1] described the open dismembered pyeloplasty in 1949 and the Anderson Hynes pyeloplasty became the gold standard in the treatment of UPJO in the following decades. The procedure is considered safe and the results are excellent [2]. In the era before laparoscopy, a large flank incision was necessary in order to perform pyeloplasty successfully. Therefore less invasive alternatives were developed. Davis et al. popularised the first open incision and stenting of the ureter in the 1940s [3]. Endourologists advanced these techniques with minimally invasive access such as endopyelotomy and balloon dilation, with and without incision of the UPJ. Nevertheless, the outcomes could not match the results of dismembered pyeloplasty (the overall success rate of endoscopic procedures for UPJO is 10–20% lower) and reports of severe bleeding from crossing vessels surfaced. In an attempt to combine the good results of the dismembered pyeloplasty with the minimally invasive nature of endopyelotomy, laparoscopic dismembered pyeloplasty was introduced by Schuessler et al. in 1993 [4].

A further development of laparoscopic dismembered pyeloplasty is the robot-assisted pyeloplasty. The initial perioperative results and intermediate follow-up of cases of UPJO repair with robot-assisted pyeloplasty appear to be favourable and comparable to that of open pyeloplasty. The current literature contains 25 published series of 740 cases with mean operative time, estimated blood loss, hospital stay, perioperative complication rate and follow-up duration of 194 min, 50 ml, 2.3 days, 6% and 14.9 months, respectively [5].

Step 1: Patient position

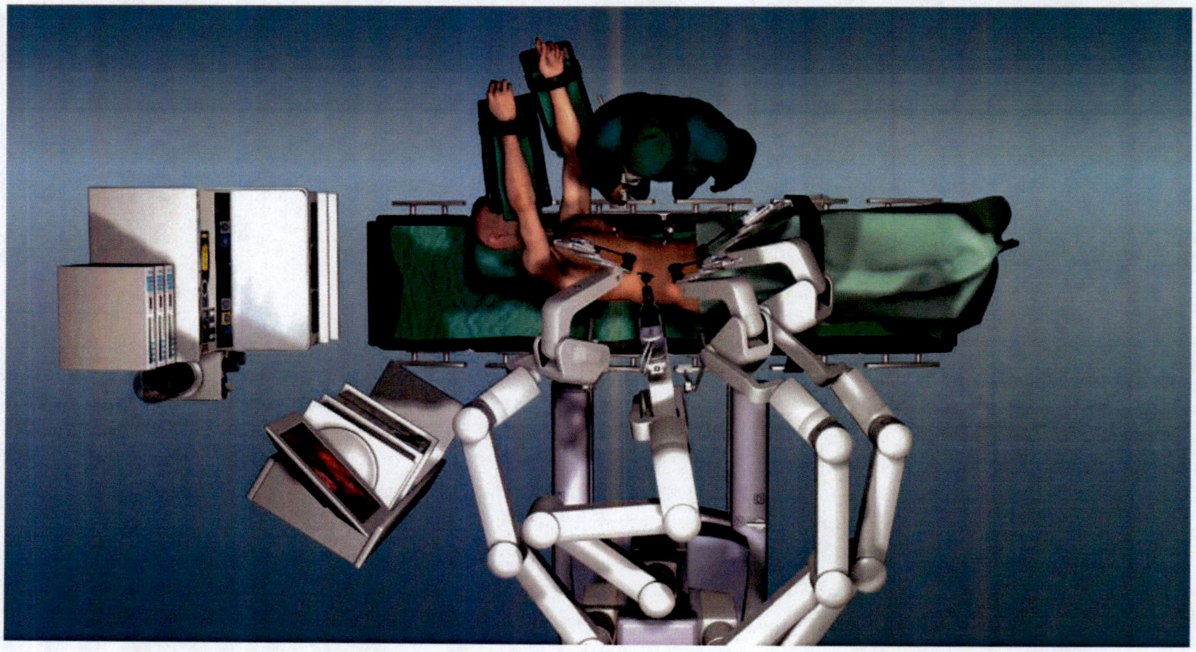

The patient is placed in the lateral decubitus position, as described in Sect. 1.1. After the skin has been prepared using standard antiseptic solution, drapes are applied. The da Vinci robotic arms are then covered by sterile plastic bags. Then it is docked step by step, as described in Sect. 1.4. The surgical assistant stands (or sits) opposite the da Vinci. The laparoscopic stack including monitor, gas insufflator, etc. can be placed either on the right or left side of the robot arms. The optimal operating theatre set-up is a combination of complex integrated operating systems such as the Endo-Alpha OR (Olympus, Hamburg, Germany) and da Vinci system, where the necessary equipment is suspended from the ceiling.

Step 2: Trocar placement

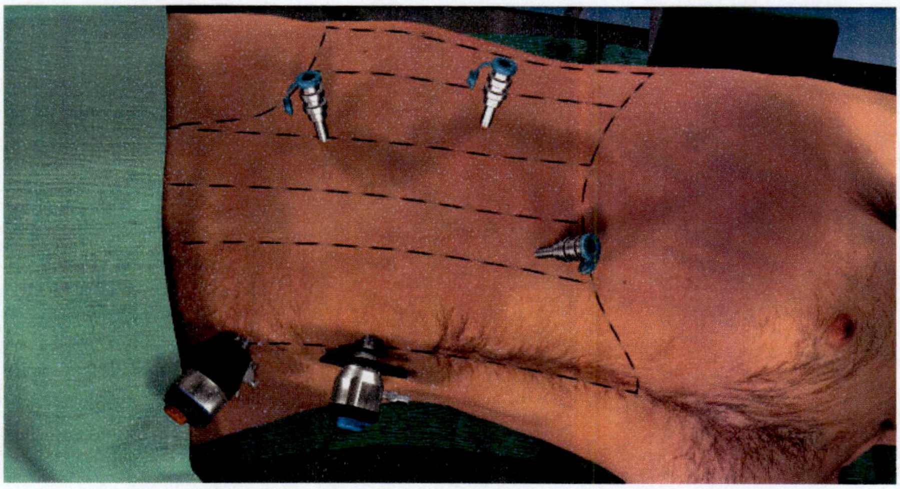

A 12-mm camera trocar is inserted using the Hasson technique through the umbilicus in slim patients and more laterally in obese patients (pararectal line). Two 8-mm robotic trocars are placed along the anterior axillary line. The third 8-mm robotic trocar is placed on the midclavicular line below the costal margin. A conventional laparoscopic trocar could be placed on the lateral margin of the rectus muscle near the pubic bone. A 30° optic is used. Insufflation pressure is set at 12 mmHg.

Step 3: Access to the retroperitoneum and identification of the ureter

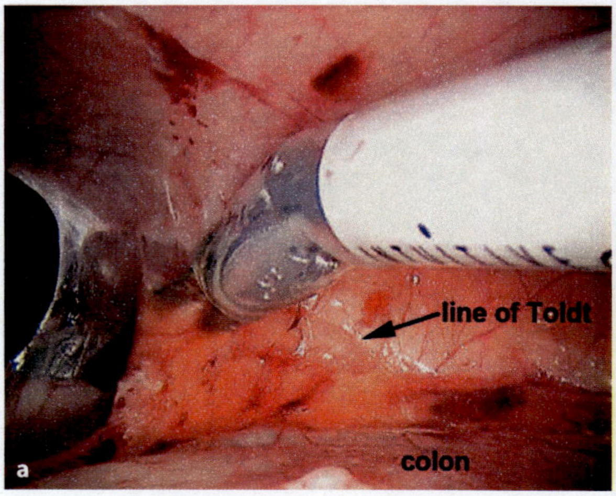

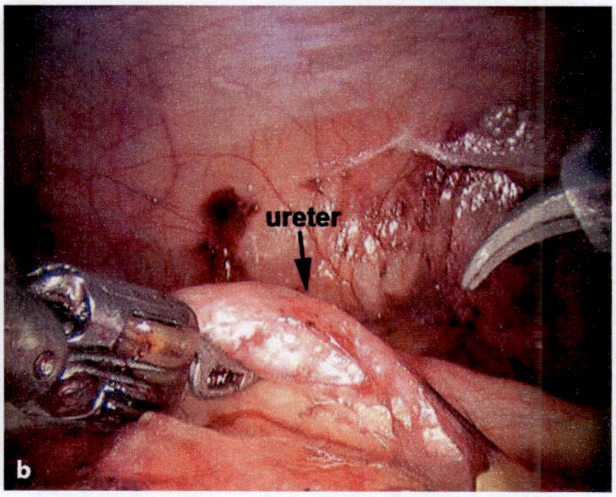

The dissection of the white line of Toldt is necessary for the mobilisation of the colon (Step 3a). The use of forceps and cutting scissors is appropriate for mobilisation, which is performed in sharp and blunt fashion. The identification of the psoas muscle should follow and the ureter is located on the medial aspect of the psoas. The gonadal vein can easily be mistaken for the ureter which is confirmed by the presence of peristalsis. The ureter is elevated with robotic graspers in an atraumatic fashion (Step 3b). The fourth robotic arm could be used for the continuous retraction of the ureter while the other two aforementioned robotic instruments mobilise the ureter towards the renal pelvis. It is important to avoid stripping the ureter of its adventitia.

Step 4: Visualisation of the renal pelvis and UPJ

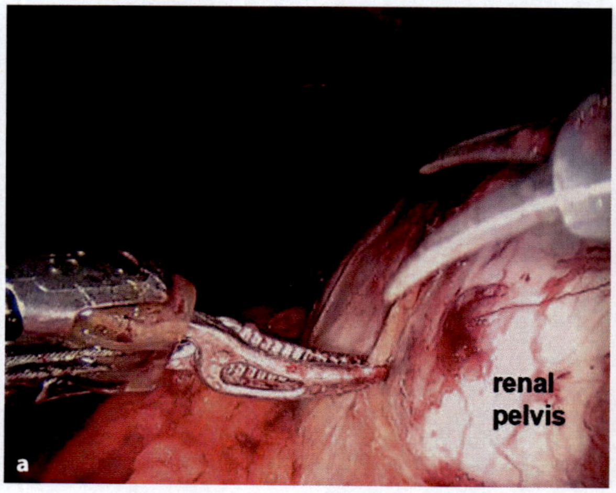

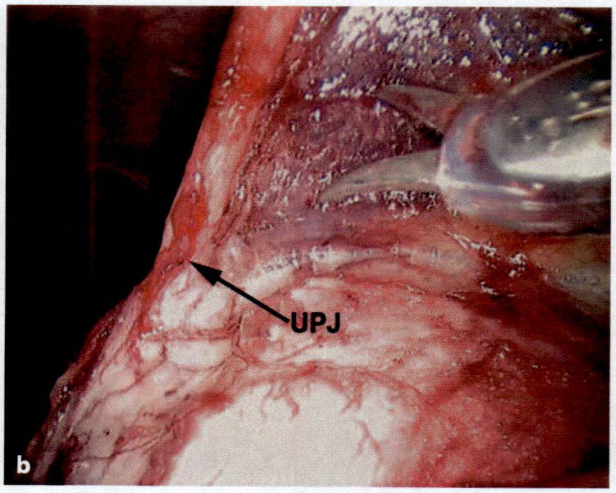

During the mobilisation of the ureter proximally towards the renal pelvis, care should be taken for the prompt detection of crossing lower pole vessels in an attempt to avoid injuring them during the dissection. The renal pelvis is mobilised along with the lower pole and the ureteropelvic junction (UPJ) is visualised (Step 4a). When the dissection of the ureter has been completed, the fourth robotic arm allows elevation and traction on the renal pelvis in an attempt to facilitate the dissection of the UPJ as well as to identify and prepare any crossing vessel. When a crossing vessel is present, the general idea of the pyeloplasty procedure is to transect the UPJ and transpose the ureter anteriorly, leaving the crossing artery to the dorsal aspect of the subsequent anastomosis.

Step 5: Transection of the UPJ and excision of the stenotic segment

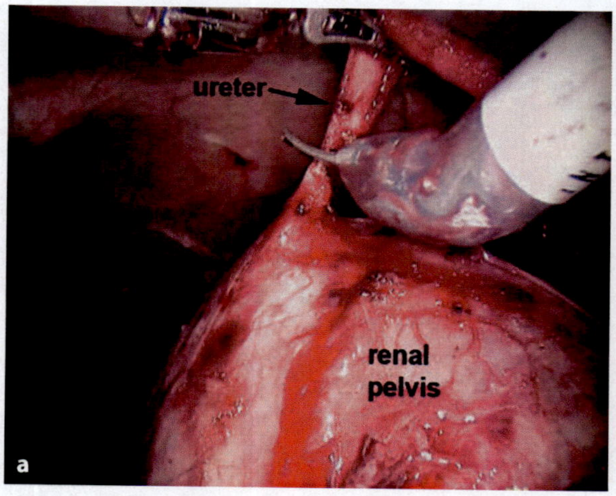

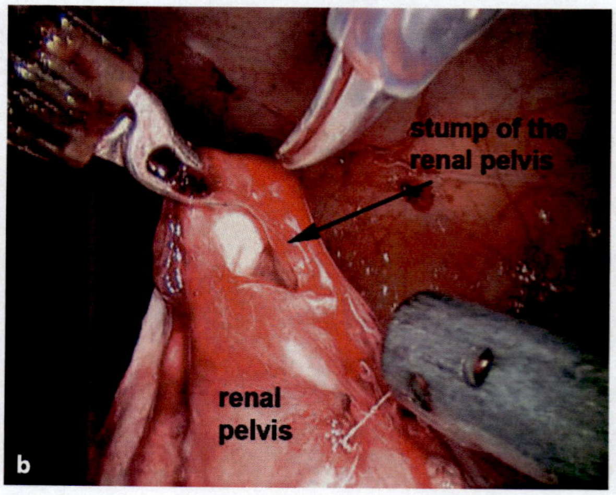

The ureter is transected at the UPJ distal to the stenotic segment (Step 5a). When a dismembered pyeloplasty is selected, the stenotic segment could be longer than 2 cm. In that case, a long ureteral segment must be excised. Moreover, a large dilated renal pelvis could be managed efficiently using this technique. After the excision of the ureter, the stenotic segment is retracted by the fourth arm and is excised proximally. Robotic scissors and graspers are appropriate for making the excision. Step 5b shows the stump of the renal pelvis after the stenotic segment is removed. At this point, the surgeon should consider excising redundant renal pelvic tissue.

Step 6: Trimming of the renal pelvis

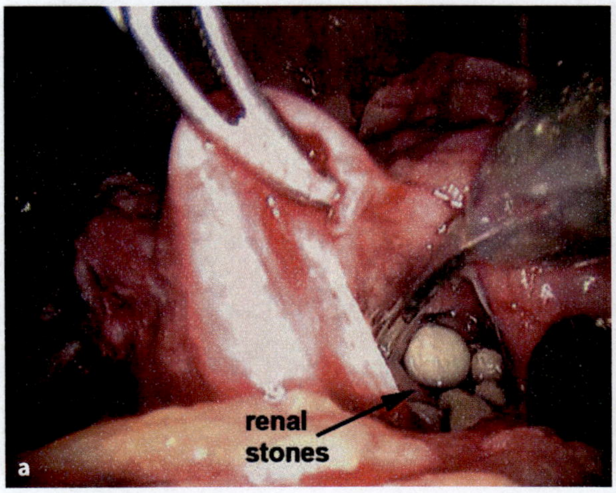

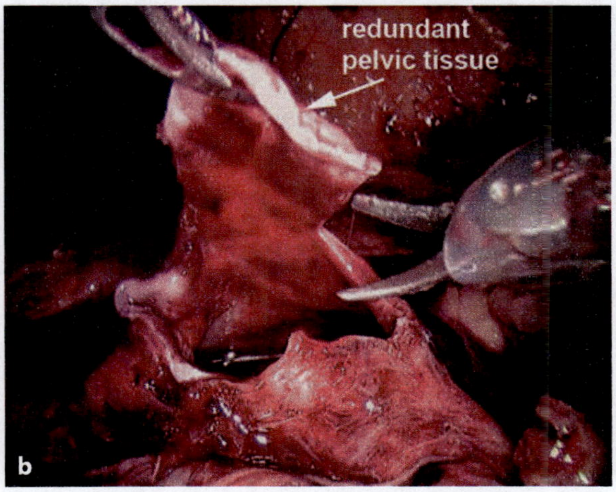

When the excision of the stenotic segment has been completed, access to the lumen of the renal pelvis is gained. Renal stones are sometimes present (Step 6a) and can be easily removed by introducing a flexible cystoscope with forceps or basket through one of the ports. Step 6b shows the renal pelvis being trimmed and any redundant tissue removed (Step 6b). Care should be taken not to remove too much pelvic tissue since the calices may end up very close to the subsequent anastomosis and may be at risk of obstruction. A combination of scissors and graspers is adequate for the performance of the above manoeuvres. The fourth robotic arm could be used for the retraction of the renal pelvis if deemed necessary.

Step 7: Spatulisation of the ureter

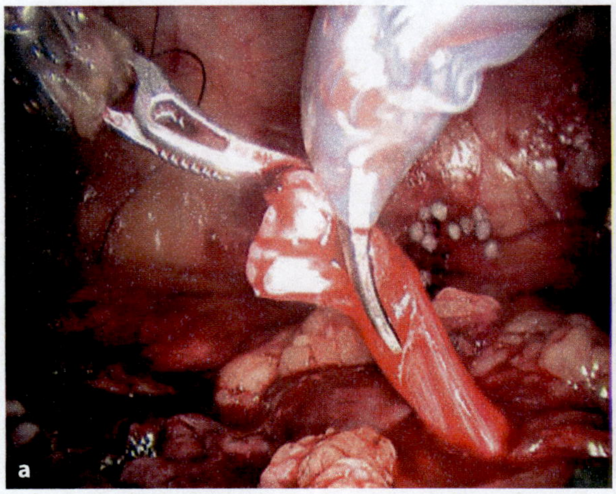

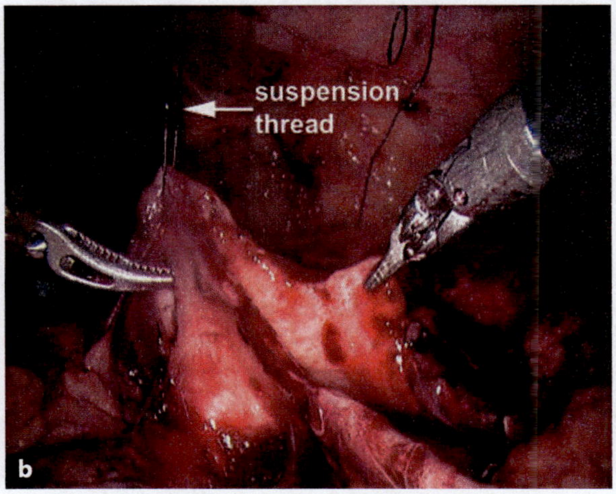

The ureter should be spatulated for approximately 2 cm in order to obtain a patent anastomosis. The ureter is spatulated on its lateral aspect with care taken not to spiral the incision. Thus, the ureter is lifted by the robotic graspers and spatulated with the help of robotic scissors (Step 7a). It is very helpful to use a suture on a straight needle through the anterior abdominal wall to suspend the upper corner of the renal pelvis (Step 7b). This facilitates the closure of the pelvis during the next step. The latter manoeuvre is performed if a three-arm robotic system is available. Otherwise, a grasper inserted through the fourth robotic arm could be used to retract the renal pelvis.

Step 8: Partial pelvis closure and antegrade insertion of a double-J stent

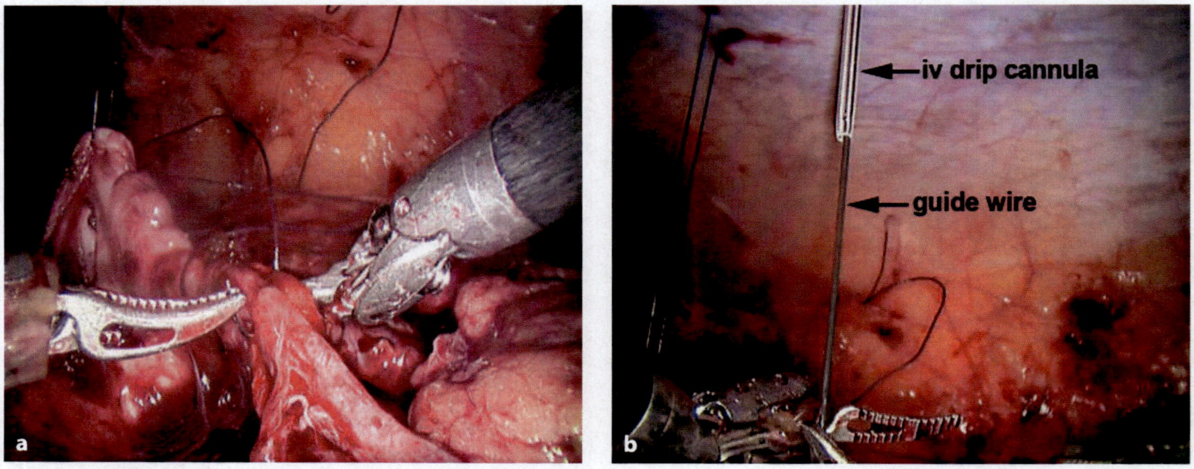

The renal pelvis is closed with a continuous suture from the cranial end, leaving a large enough opening for pelviureteral anastomosis (Step 8a). A large-bore intravenous cannula is inserted through the abdominal wall. A guidewire can be inserted through the cannula and guided with robotic forceps into the ureter distally towards the bladder (Step 8b). The cannula is removed and the double-J stent is placed percutaneously over the guidewire into the ureter and bladder, leaving a few centimetres outside of the ureter. The fourth robotic arm could be used for the continuous retraction of the spatulated ureter while the other two robotic instruments are used for the insertion of the double-J stent.

Step 9: Ureteral stent insertion

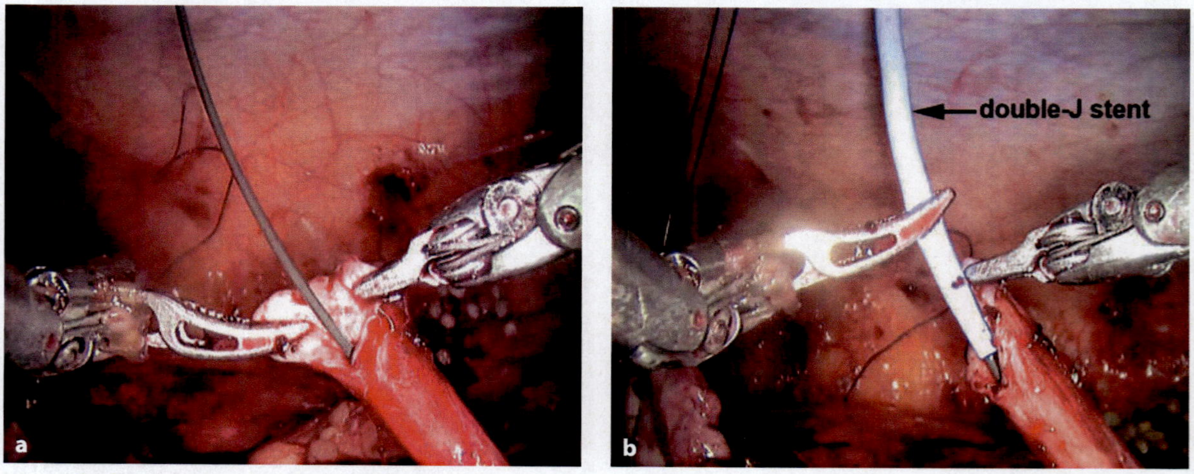

Step 9a shows the ureter with the guidewire inserted while Step 9b demonstrates the insertion of the double-J stent over the guidewire in the ureter. The point of insertion of the ureteral stent depends on the surgeon's preference. Some surgeons insert the double-J preoperatively and carefully dissect the stenotic segment and ureter to avoid cutting the stent. Others insert the stent right after the transaction of the ureter. Ureteral spatulisation takes place with the double-J in place in both methods. The authors prefer the insertion method described in this section because the possibility of damaging the double-J stent is minimal. Moreover, the presence of the fourth robotic arm, which provides continuous retraction, minimises the need to stabilise the ureter with an indwelling stent.

Step 10: Anastomosis between the renal pelvis and ureter

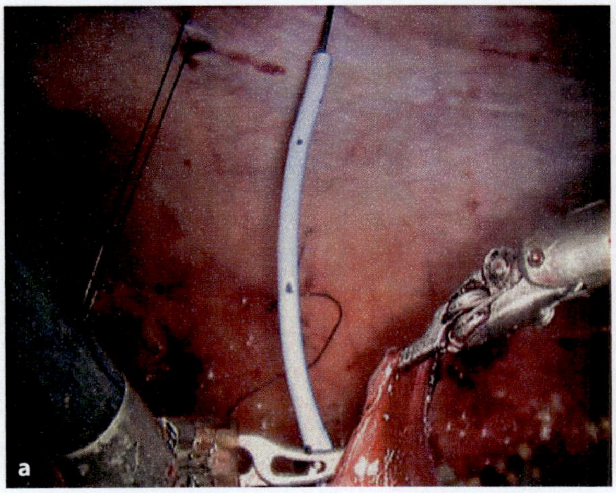

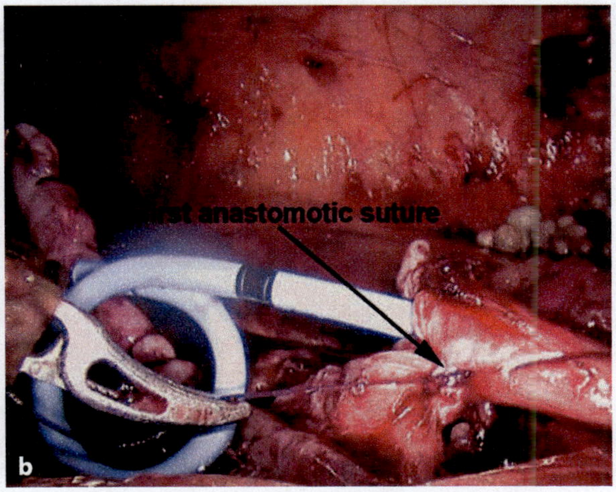

Step 10a demonstrates the removal of the guidewire. Adequate length of the proximal segment of the stent should be protruding out of the ureter as the stent needs to be inserted in the renal pelvis. With either interrupted or running 3/0 Vicryl sutures, a tension-free anastomosis is performed between the ureter at the spatulated end and the aforementioned opening in the renal pelvis. The first suture approximates the lower end of the spatulated ureter to the lower edge of the trimmed renal pelvis (Step 10b). The anastomosis requires careful handling to avoid tension. If the stenotic segment is too long and tension in the anastomosis is high, the lower pole of the kidney could be mobilised to reduce tension.

Step11: Anastomosis between renal pelvis and ureter

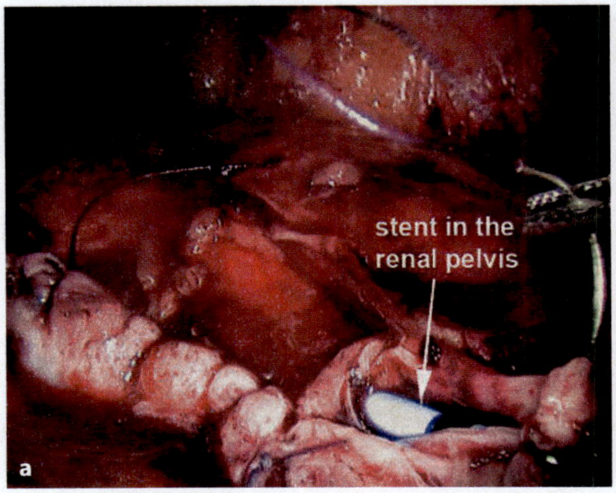

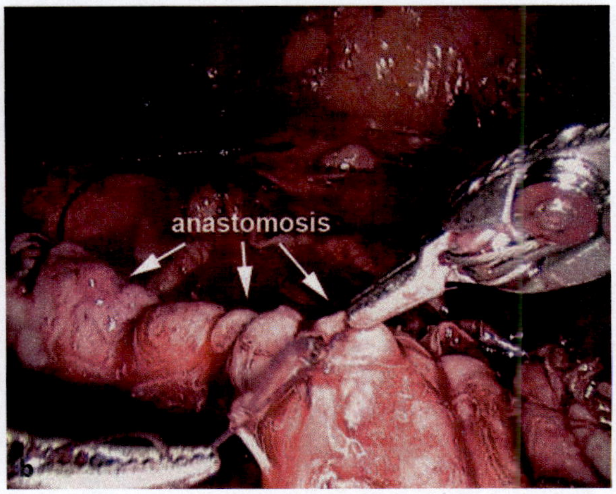

The proximal end of the double-J stent is placed in the pelvis after completion of the first suture and the remaining anastomosis is then done (Step 11a). The posterior side of the anastomosis is performed first and the anterior portion follows. Running sutures are performed. Step 11b shows the final appearance of the pelviureteral anastomosis. The robotic system facilitates suturing by the high degree of freedom of the robotic needle holder. The fourth arm provides continuous traction where it is deemed necessary. A drain is left in place (no or low vacuum) through one of the robotic 8-mm ports. Port sites should be checked for bleeding. Fascia of the 10- to 12-mm port sites should be closed with either a J-needle or a Carter-Thompson closure device.

Postoperative Management

- Full diet on postoperative day 1
- Urethral catheter is removed on postoperative day 2 if the drain output ist not high
- If the drain output is minimal, then remove it on postoperative day 3

References

1. Anderson JC, Hynes W (1949) Retrocaval ureter: case diagnosed preoperatively and treated successfully by a plastic operation. Br J Urol 21:209
2. Scardino PT, Scardino PL (1981) Obstruction at the ureteropelvic junction. In: Bergman H (ed) The Ureter. Springer Verlag, New York, pp. 697–716
3. Davis DM, Strong GH, Drake WM (1948) Intubated ureterotomy: experimental work and clinical results. J Urol 56:851–862
4. Schuessler WW, Grune MT, Tecuanhuey LV, Preminger GM (1993) Laparoscopic dismembered pyeloplasty. J Urol 150:1795–1799
5. Singh I, Hemal AK (2010) Robot-assisted pyeloplasty: review of the current literature, technique and outcome. Can J Urol 17:5099–5108

1.15 Retroperitoneal Pyeloplasty (Conventional Laparoscopy and SMART Technique)

Jens Rassweiler, Marcel Hruza, Ali Serdar Gozen, Giovannalberto Pini, Dogu Teber

Introduction

Ureteropelvic junction (UPJ) obstruction is defined as an impaired urine flow from the renal pelvis to the proximal ureter with subsequent dilatation of renal pelvis and collecting system and a potential loss of kidney function.

Two types of UPJ obstruction can be distinguished. Extrinsic obstructions are caused by lower pole vessels or fibrous bands crossing the UPJ leading to hydronephrosis. In most of these cases, UPJ remains at the deepest part of the renal pelvis. Intrinsic obstructions are characterised by a loss of viscoelastic properties of the proximal ureter through an increase in collagen deposition due to an adynamic segment or a scar within the ureter often associated with high insertion of the ureter.

UPJ obstruction can cause flank pain or recurrent infections of the urinary tract, but may also be asymptomatic in some patients. It is diagnosed using ultrasound, diuretic urogram and renogram.

Open pyeloplasty as described by Anderson and Hynes in 1949 [1] is still the gold standard in the treatment of UPJ obstruction. However, laparoscopic pyeloplasty has gained increasing importance since its first description by Schuessler in 1993 [2]. The dismembered Anderson-Hynes technique as well as nondismembered techniques (i.e. YV-plasty) can be carried out laparoscopically. Several studies summarising more than 1,000 patients reported high success rates of 88–100% after laparoscopic pyeloplasty equivalent to the excellent results of open pyeloplasty [3]. Complication and conversion rates are low and occurred mostly in an early stage of the personal and institutional learning curves [4]. In patients with concomitant urolithiasis, stones can be simultaneously removed during laparoscopic pyeloplasty. In experienced hands, laparoscopic pyeloplasty can successfully be performed not only in adults with an abnormal renal anatomy, but also in children [5] and in patients with anatomical variations such as horseshoe kidneys or crossed fused ectopia [6].

There are also reports on laparoscopic pyeloplasty for secondary UPJ obstruction after failure of a previous open, laparoscopic or endourological procedure: these cases are more challenging because of fibrosis and adhesions. The success rates are lower compared to primary laparoscopic treatment, but comparable to secondary open pyeloplasty [7]. Recently, the introduction of high-definition video technology allowed the use of smaller (i.e. 5-mm) telescopes together with especially developed 3-mm instruments, thereby further reducing the access trauma (i.e. SMART, mini-laparoscopy).

According to the available short-term data, robot-assisted laparoscopic pyeloplasty seems to provide results similar to the conventional laparoscopic technique.

Indications

- The indication is ureteropelvic junction (UPJ) obstruction in adults as well as in children. In very small children, in patients with abnormal anatomy of the kidney and in cases having undergone prior kidney surgery, the procedure should be performed only in centres with laparoscopic excellence.

Absolute Contraindications

- Malignancies of the kidney, ureter or urinary bladder
- Total loss of kidney function
- Bleeding disorders
- Pregnancy

Relative Contraindications

- Acute infections of kidney or urinary tract
- Relative loss of kidney function (less than 15% in the diuretic renogram)

Preoperative Preparation

- Single-shot broad-spectrum antibiotics
- Antiembolic stockings and low-molecular-weight heparin
- Preoperative cystoscopy and retrograde stenting of the ureter (double-J stent): some authors advocate intraoperative antegrade stenting, but we prefer preoperative retrograde stenting: It is technically less difficult and less time-consuming compared to antegrade stenting during laparoscopy and the indwelling stent can help to identify the ureter during retroperitoneoscopy. Additionally, preoperative cystoscopy may detect disorders of the bladder or distal ureter that could affect the indication for pyeloplasty
- Urinary catheter

Step 1: Retroperitoneoscopic access to the renal pelvis

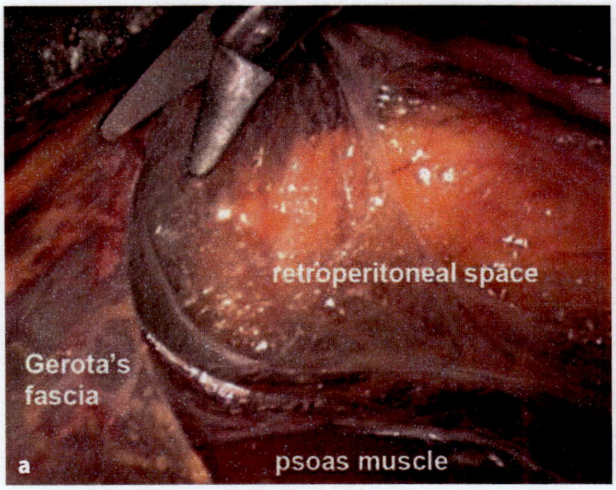

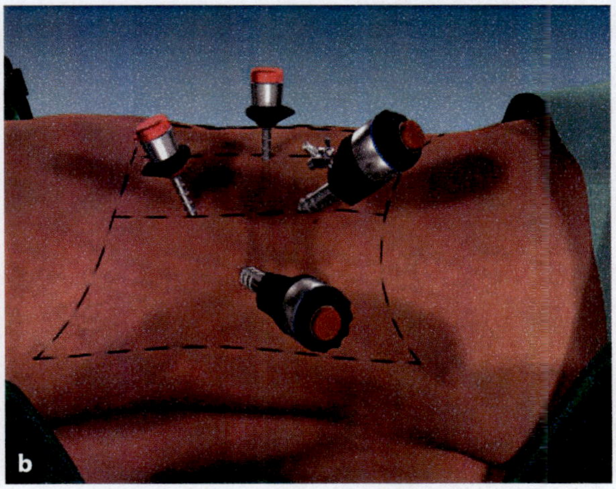

The patient is positioned in the flank position with 20° Trendelenburg decline. A 15-mm skin incision is made in the lumbar triangle (Petit triangle) between the 12th rib and the iliac crest. After creating a tunnel to the retroperitoneal space using an Overholt forceps for blunt dissection, the tunnel is dilated using the index finger. The peritoneum is pushed forwards from the aponeurosis lumbodorsalis and the retroperitoneal cavity is developed. Optionally, a balloon-trocar system can be used. Controlled by the index finger, two (optionally three) trocars are placed, as shown in Step 1b. Then pneumoretroperitoneum is established (pressure, 12 mmHg; children, 10 mmHg; flow, 3.5 l/min).

Step 2: Small incision access retroperitoneoscopic technique

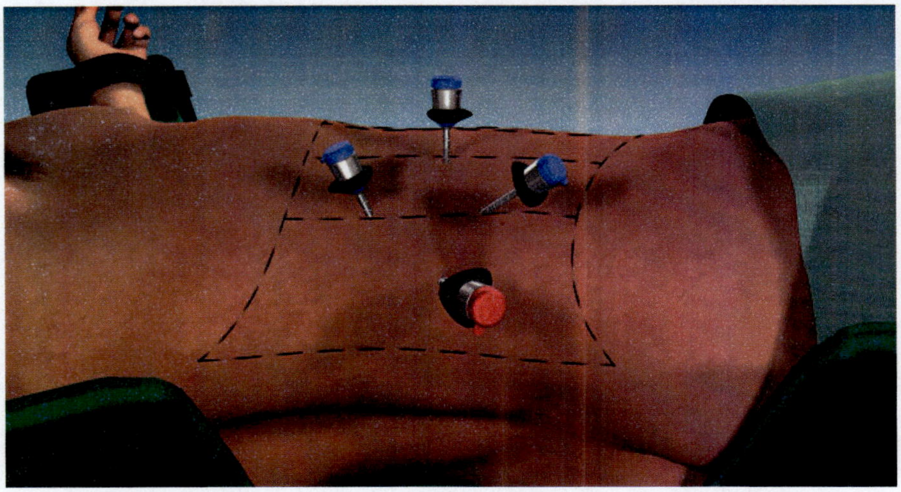

We have recently developed the small incision access retroperitoneoscopic technique (SMART) to further reduce surgical morbidity and improve cosmetic results. In this technique, a tunnel is created via a 5-mm incision bluntly to the retroperitoneal space using a haemostatic clamp. The retroperitoneal space is developed with a specially designed 6-mm balloon trocar. An improved 5-mm 30° telescope together with a HD wide-view camera system, a 6-mm port, two 3.5-mm working ports and specially developed 3-mm instruments (Karl Storz, Tuttlingen, Germany) are used. The ports are triangulated as in a standard retroperitoneal technique.

Step 3: Creation of the retroperitoneal space

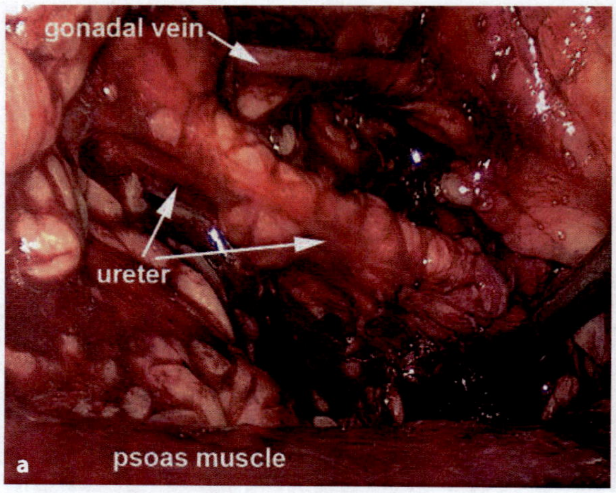

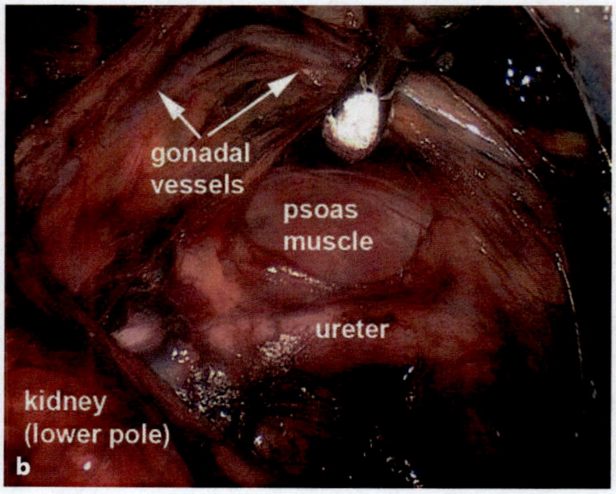

In the first surgical step, the Gerota fascia is incised completely. The psoas muscle is exposed as the most important anatomical landmark. Now, all further anatomical structures such as the ureter, renal pelvis and vessels can be exposed. We favour the retroperitoneal approach because of the direct and rapid access to the renal pelvis, less risk of damage to the intraperitoneal organs and less risk of ileus.

Step 4: Exposure of the ureter and the renal pelvis

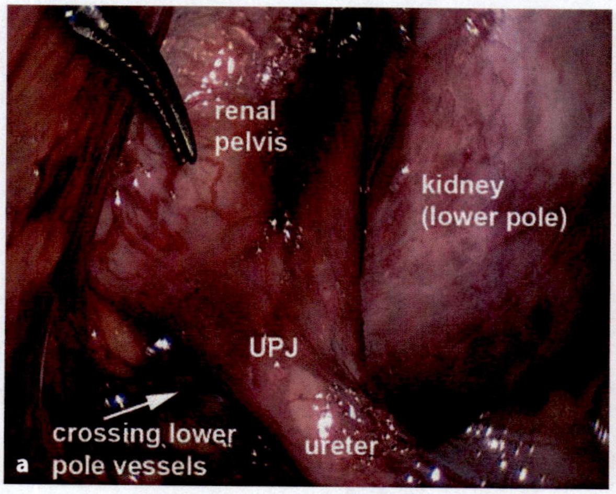

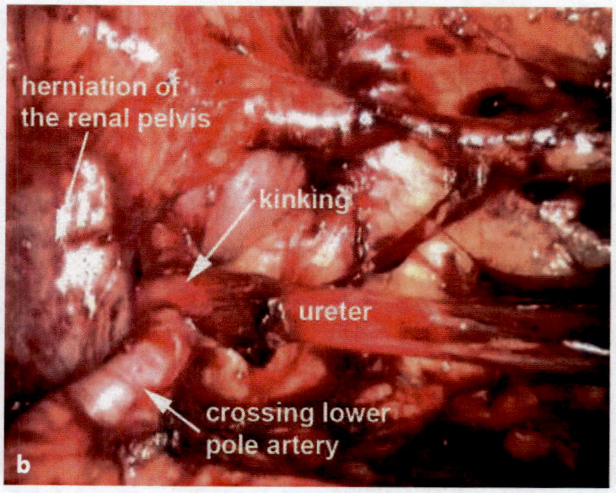

When the renal pelvis and the proximal ureter are exposed (Step 4a), care must be taken not to injure an aberrant artery if present. In most cases, crossing lower pole vessels are found anteriorly to the ureter (Step 4b), sometimes associated with herniation of the renal pelvis.

A complete ureterolysis has to be done in all cases. Small aberrant veins or fibrous bands can be transected. Lower arteries require complete dissection to accomplish maximal cranial translocation of the vessel from the UPJ.

Step 5: Exposure of the ureter and the renal pelvis

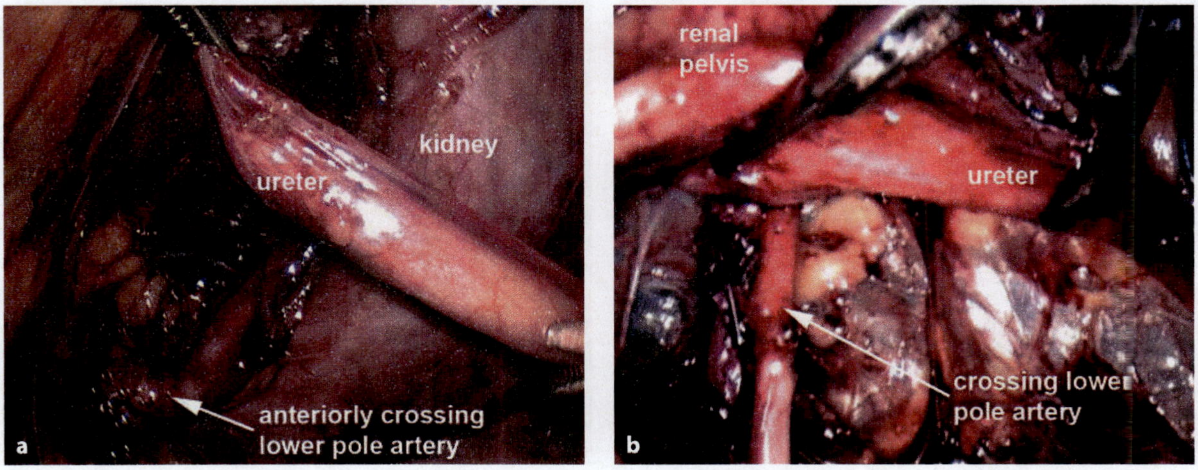

If there is no need to transpose the ureter or to reduce the size of a redundant pelvis, we perform a nondismembered YV-pyeloplasty. The renal pelvis is incised at the UPJ to create a V-shaped flap (see Step 6). Thereafter, we incise the stenotic UPJ followed by a 2-cm longitudinal posterior spatulation of the ureter. Hence, the whole incision is Y-shaped. The V-shaped flap is sutured to the proximal ureter using a running monofilament (4/0 PDS, Rb1 needle). It is important to start the suture at the distal end of the V instead of adapting the apex of the V to the end of the spatulated ureter first. Thereby, both ends (i.e. renal pelvis and ureter) are optimally exposed, gradually decreasing the tension on the suture line.

Step 6: YV-pyeloplasty

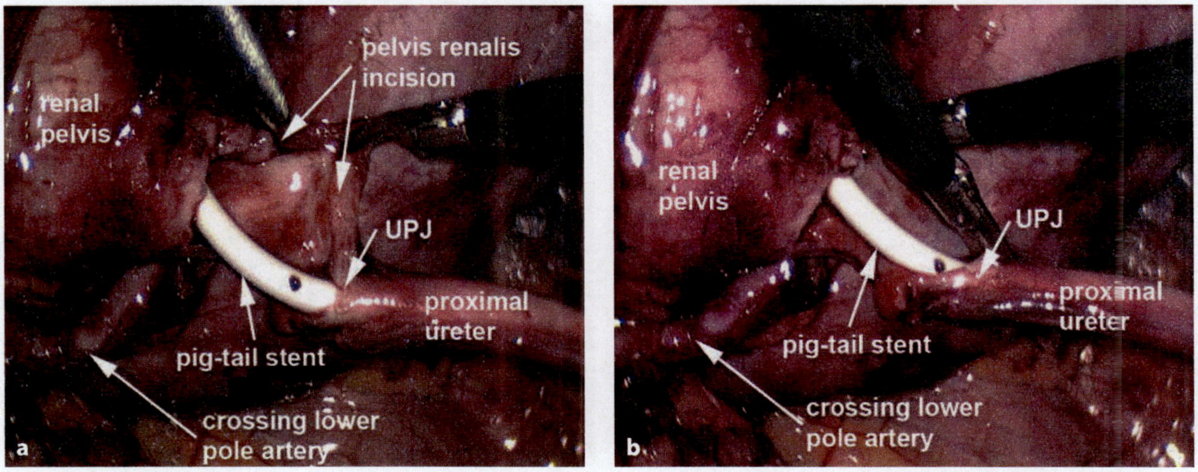

The YV-pyeloplasty applies the same principle as the Anderson-Hynes technique: spatulation of the ureter with caudal transposition of the UPJ. However, the stenotic part is included in the renal pelvis. Therefore, we do not recommend other nondismembered technique (only incising the narrow segment and closing it transversally in a Heineke-Mikulicz fashion (i.e. Fenger-plasty)). The dismembered laparoscopic pyeloplasty is performed according to the technique described by Anderson and Hynes: the ureter is separated completely from the renal pelvis. The narrow segment of the proximal ureter is resected and the ureter is spatulated. Now an anterior crossing vessel, when present, can be transposed posteriorly.

Step 7: Ureteropelvic anastomosis

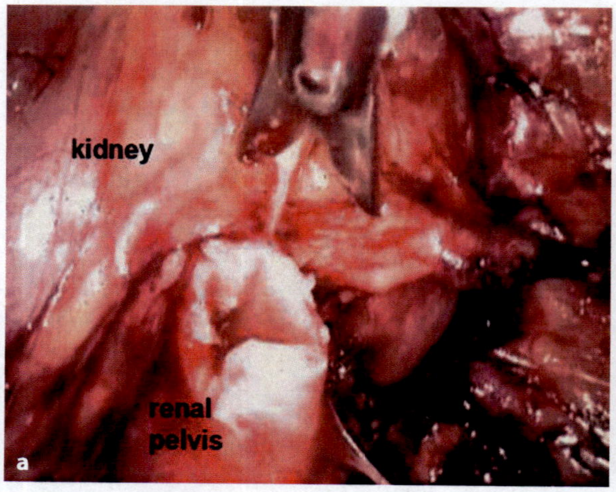

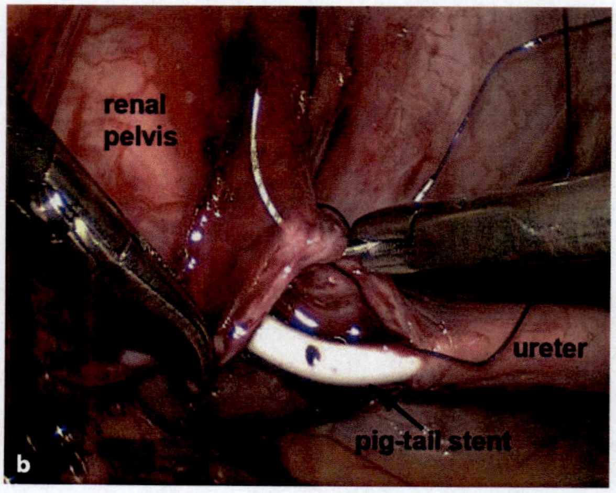

The renal pelvis may be reduced if necessary (Step 7a). After trimming, the renal pelvis should be reconstructed before performing the ureteropelvic re-anastomosis to shorten the distance to be bridged. For the anastomosis, we use a continuous suture technique comparable to the Van-Velthoven anastomosis in laparoscopic radical prostatectomy (Step 7b): two needle-armed sutures (4/0 PDS, Rb1 needle) were knotted extracorporally. One of the sutures is used for the posterior, one for the anterior wall of the anastomosis. At the end, an intracorporal knot is performed. The anastomosis may also be performed in a single knot technique using 4/0 PDS, Rb1 needle.

Step 8: Stone extraction and drain placement

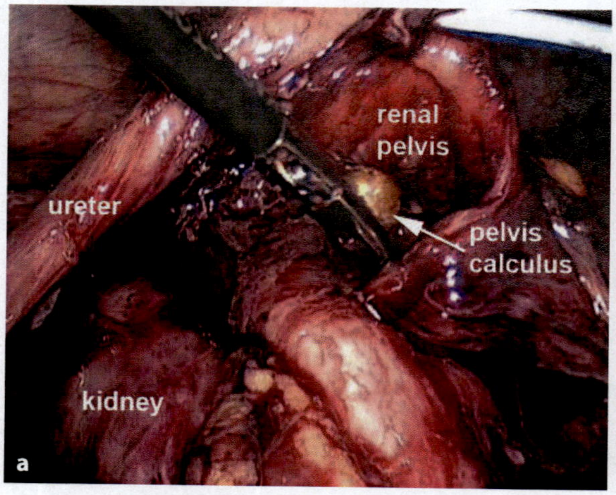

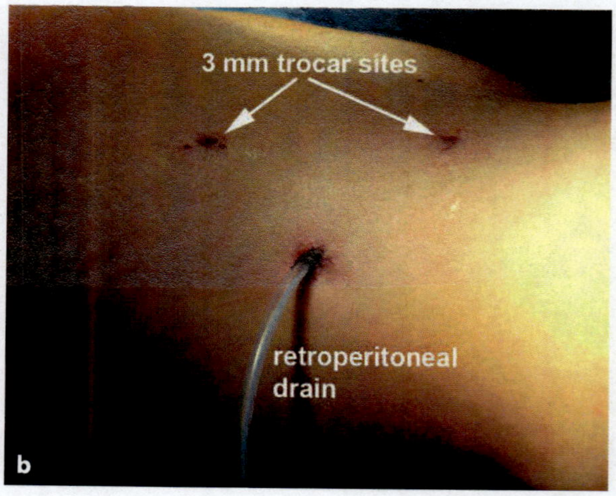

In patients with calculi in the collecting system, grasping forceps can now be used to extract them (Step 8a). If a stone cannot be reached, a flexible cystoscope passed down a 10-mm or 13-mm trocar may be used. At the end of the operation, a perinephric drain is placed.

A nonsuction drain is placed via the trocar side into the retroperitoneal space. After having released the pneumoretroperitoneum, the trocars are removed and the incisions are closed in layers.

Postoperative Management

- Removal of the indwelling urethral catheter 3–4 days after surgery
- Removal of the indwelling drain half a day or 1 day after removal of the urethral catheter when no liquids are leaking through the drain
- Removal of the double-J stent 4–6 weeks after surgery. We do a retrograde ureterography during removal of the stent and sonographic verification on the following day
- Patients should be followed up using ultrasound at least twice a year. The Doppler Ultrasound Resistance Index may help discriminate between a hydronephrosis due to an obstructed UPJ and a wide renal pelvis without urodynamically relevant obstruction. Another diuretic renogram may be performed at 6 months after surgery, but is not mandatory in asymptomatic patients. Most failures of pyeloplasty occur within 2 years after surgery, but they may also appear years later. Therefore, the optimal duration of follow-up remains unclear

References

1. Anderson JC, Hynes W (1949) Retrocaval ureter: case diagnosed preoperatively and treated successfully by a plastic operation. Br J Urol 21:209
2. Schuessler WW, Grune MT, Tecuanhuey LV, Preminger GM (1993) Laparoscopic dismembered pyeloplasty. J Urol 150:1795–1799
3. Symons SJ, Bhirud PS, Jain V, Shetty AS, Desai MR (2009) Laparoscopic pyeloplasty: our new gold standard. J Endourol 23:463–467
4. Rassweiler JJ, Teber D, Frede T (2008) Complications of laparoscopic pyeloplasty. World J Urol 26:539–547
5. Rassweiler JJ, Subotic S, Feist-Schwenk M, Sugiono M, Schulze M, Teber D, Frede T (2007) Minimally invasive treatment of ureteropelvic junction obstruction: long-term experience with an algorithm for laser endopyelotomy and laparoscopic retroperitoneal pyeloplasty. J Urol 177:1000–1005
6. Janetschek G, Peschel R, Frauscher F (2000) Laparoscopic pyeloplasty. Urol Clin N Am 27:695–704
7. Sundaram CP, Grubb RL, Rehman J, Yan Y, Chen C, Landman J, McDougall EM, Clayman RV (2003) Laparoscopic pyeloplasty for secondary ureteropelvic junction obstruction. J Urol 169:2037–2040

1.16 Transperitoneal Left Adrenalectomy

Evangelos Liatsikos, Panagiotis Kallidonis, Minh Do, Jens-Uwe Stolzenburg

Introduction

The transperitoneal approach to laparoscopic adrenalectomy (LA) is an alternative to the retroperitoneal approach. Transperitoneal LA could be performed by an anterior or lateral approach. The former approach has the advantage of performing bilateral adrenalectomy without repositioning the patient. Nevertheless, the working space is not as wide as the lateral transperitoneal approach where gravity retracts intra-abdominal organs away from the operative field. The lateral transperitoneal approach is the surgical approach characterised by the widest operative field and is suited for excision of adrenal masses regardless of their size. The side of adrenalectomy is important due to the different anatomical structures that interfere with the operative field. The excision of the right adrenal requires the retraction of the liver to achieve a clear operative field, while the adrenal vein drains directly to the vena cava. On the left side, the spleen should be mobilised for the excision of the adrenal, while the adrenal vein is related to left renal vein.

Indications and Contra-indications

- The indications and contra-indications of the procedure are similar to those for the retroperitoneal approach [1, 2] (see Sect. 1.17)

Preoperative Preparation

- Preparation of patients for transperitoneal adrenalectomy varies depending on the tumour to be treated. Nevertheless, the preparation remains identical to the retroperitoneal approach (see Sect. 1.17)

Step 1: Patient position and trocar placement

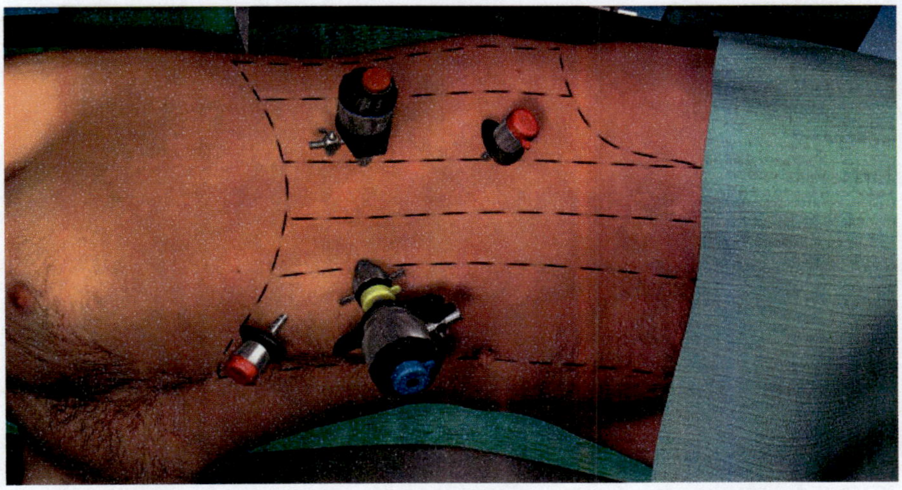

A modified flank position is used (see Sect. 1.1). The latter position prevents the interference of the intra-abdominal organs with the operative field. The arrangement of trocars for laparoscopic adrenalectomy is different from the one used for laparoscopic renal surgery. In the former, the primary trocar (camera trocar) is inserted at the lateral margin of the ipsilateral rectus muscle in a site cranially to the level of the umbilicus (10-mm trocar), while one working trocar is placed in the midaxillary line near the costal margin and the other approximately 2 cm caudally to the xiphoid. A fourth port for retraction purposes is usually not necessary and could be placed superior to the iliac crest in the midaxillary line.

Step 2: Dissection of the line of Toldt

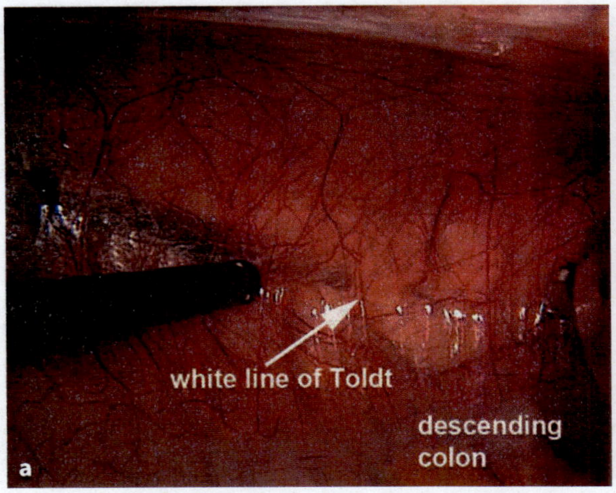

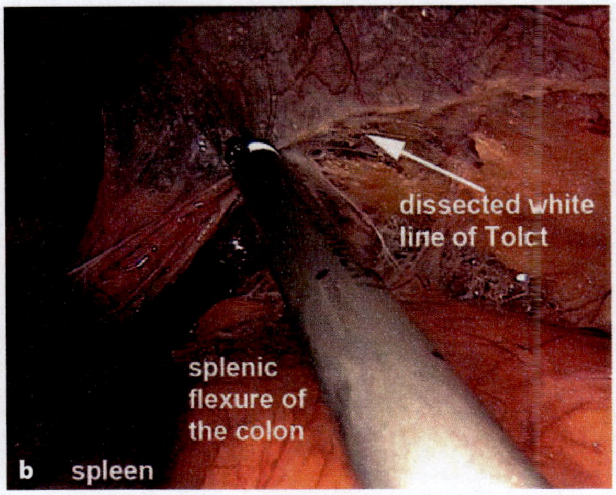

Step 2a presents the landmarks for the dissection of the white line of Toldt. The incision of the line of Toldt is made using a combination of sharp and blunt dissection with 5-mm instruments such as ultrasound or electrosurgical scissors for dissection and atraumatic grasper or suction–irrigation instrument for medial retraction of the colon medially (Step 2b). The splenic flexure and the descending colon are mobilised medially. The splenocolic and lienorenal ligaments are divided allowing the mobilisation of the spleen. It is important to note that the medial mobilisation of the spleen is possible without retraction if there is adequate mobilisation of the organ by its surrounding ligaments.

Step 3: Access to the adrenal

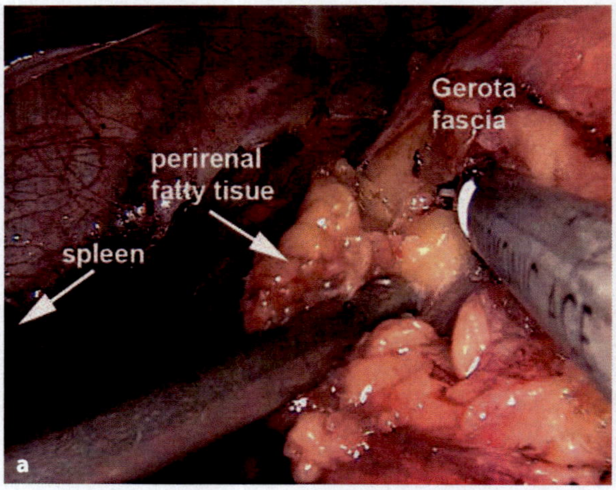

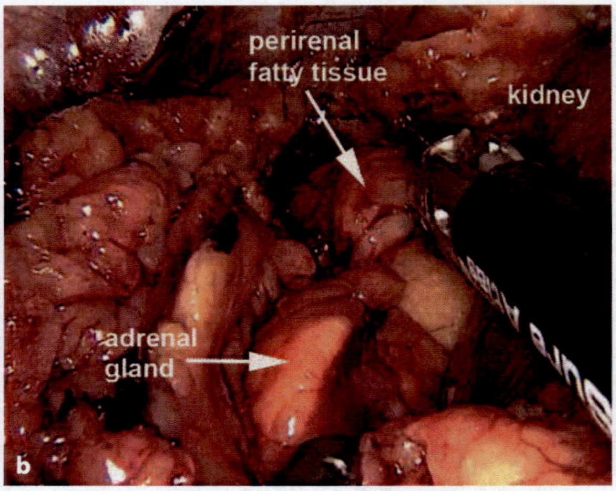

Access to the retroperitoneal space and identification of the Gerota fascia has been achieved and the fascia is opened using the harmonic scalpel (Step 3a). The use of coagulation or scissors is also indicated. The renal artery is visualised. The latter landmark is very important for continuing the dissection as the major adrenal vessels are related to the renal artery and vein. Thus, the dissection to a caudal direction provides access to the adrenal and its blood supply. Moreover, the risk of injury to major renal vessels is minimised. The gradual development of the plane between the tail of pancreas and renal hilum reveals the adrenal gland (Step 3b).

Step 4: Identification of the adrenal

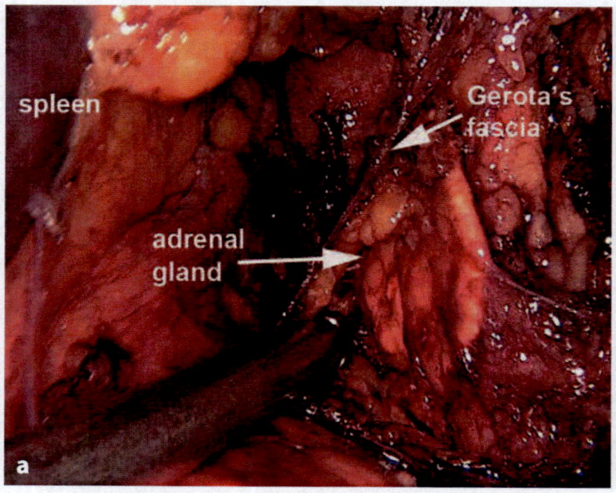

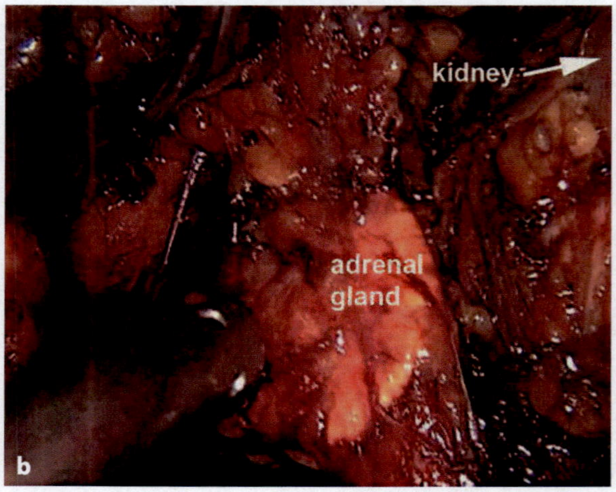

Careful preparation of the adrenal gland from its surrounding attachments and vascular supply follows. The left adrenal arterial supply originates from small branches of the left inferior phrenic artery, middle suprarenal artery (aorta) and the inferior suprarenal artery (renal artery). The left adrenal vein drains into the ipsilateral renal vein. Step 4a shows the adrenal within the perirenal fat, which is enclosed by the Gerota fascia. Step 4b shows the close relation of the adrenal to the ipsilateral kidney. In the case of a pheochromocytoma, the vascular supply and especially the adrenal vein should be identified and clipped before performing any manipulations of the adrenal as there is risk for releasing catecholamines into the blood circulation [3].

Step 5: Identification and ligation of the adrenal vein

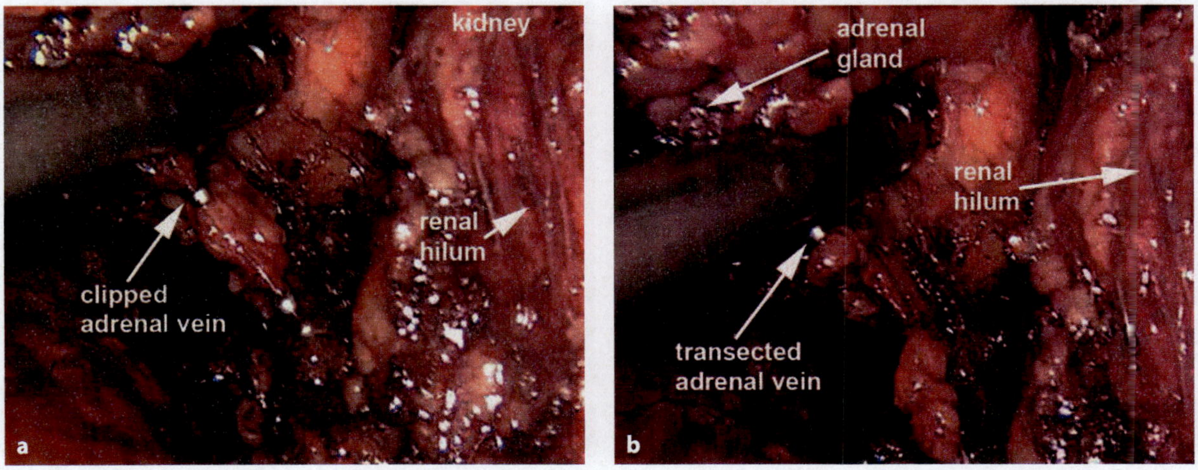

Retraction of the adrenal laterally facilitates the visualisation of the blood supply. The inferior adrenal vein providing drainage to the renal vein is identified and clipped. The identification of the inferior adrenal vein is possible by dissecting the superior border of the renal vein. Metal clips can be used on the vessel proximally and distally to its connection to the major vessel (Step 5a). Transection of the vessel between the clips takes place. Care should be taken to avoid any injury of the renal artery, which can be located immediately posterior to the main adrenal gland (Step 5b). Smaller arteries arising from the renal artery should also be considered during the dissection.

Step 6: Mobilisation of the medial border of the adrenal

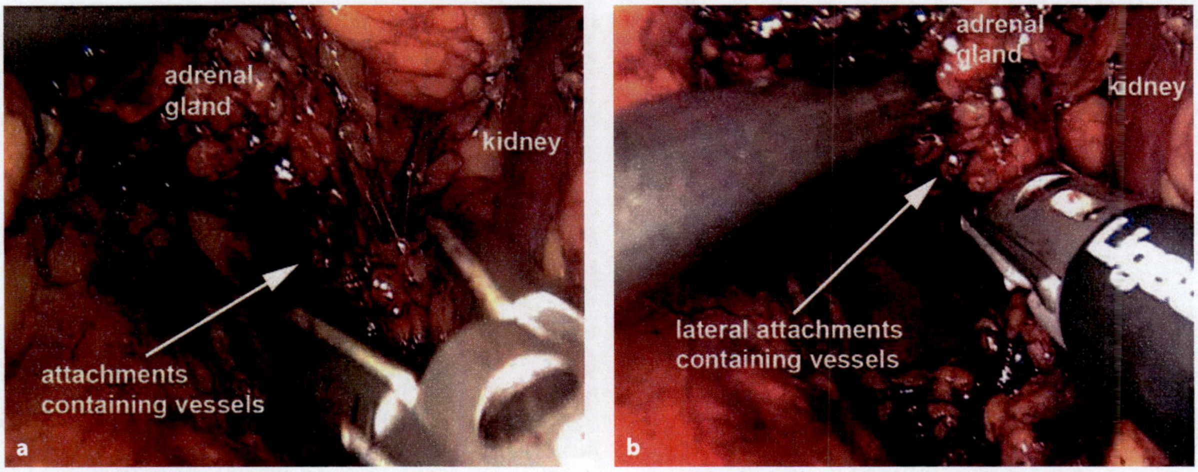

The medial border of the adrenal gland is carefully dissected to reveal adrenal vessels (Step 6a). Coagulation, clips or the ultrasonic scalpel are used for ligation of these vessels and the dissection proceeds until the medial portion of the adrenal has been mobilised (Step 6b). The use of clips is advisable for all vessels of adequate size as it provides additional safety to the ligation. The dissection of the plane is extended until the psoas muscle is revealed and the adrenal is completely mobilised from its medial attachments. The mobilisation of the medial border of the adrenal requires special care due to the close relation of major blood vessels to the organs.

Step 7: Mobilisation of the lateral border of the adrenal

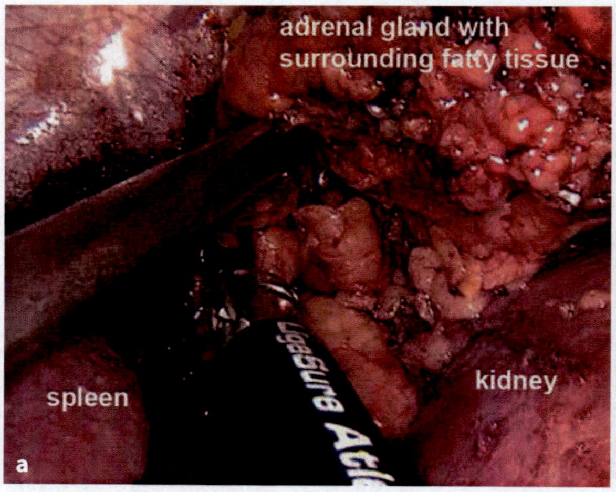

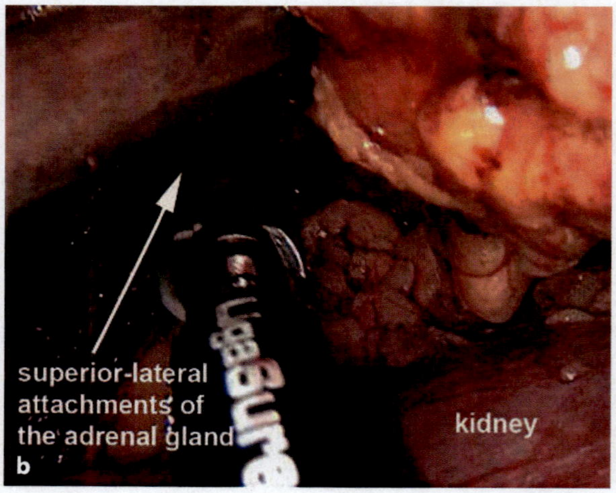

The superio lateral mobilisation of the adrenal should be performed by ligating the inferior phrenic vessels with clips, coagulation or the ultrasonic scalpel (Step 7a). The inferolateral border of the adrenal gland is dissected from the upper pole of the kidney by ligating vessels included in the attachments (Step 7b). The upper polar renal artery may be close to the infero- and superolateral dissection planes and care should be taken to avoid injury. It should be noted that the lateral mobilisation of the adrenal is a step that should be performed at this stage of the procedure as the early mobilisation of the lateral attachments may result in difficult mobilisation of the medial border of the organ.

Step 8: Complete mobilisation of the adrenal and removal

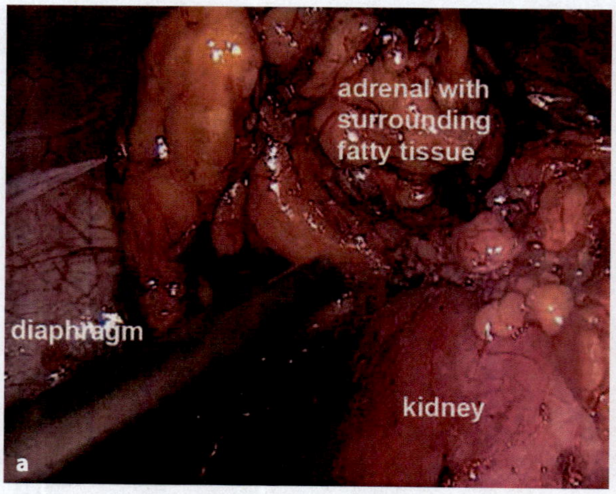

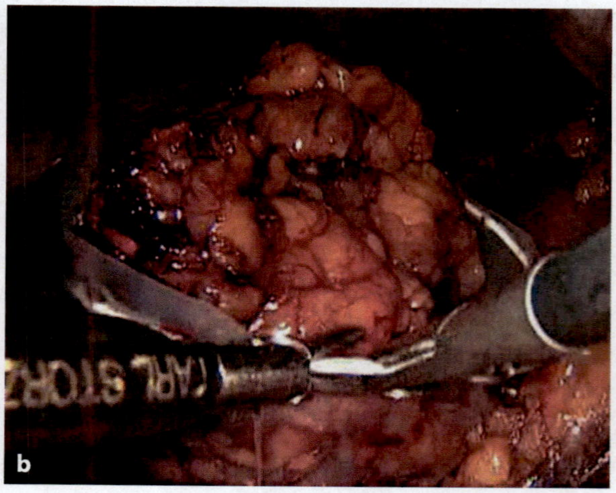

Step 8a presents the final division of the all attachments of the adrenal gland. It is not uncommon to excise the gland along with its surrounding fatty tissue. Then the gland is inserted in one piece in an endoscopic bag (Step 8b) and left in the abdomen. An EndoCatch bag or an inexpensive sterile urinary catheter bag could be used for specimen extraction. The small size of the adrenal does not require morcellation or cutting of the specimen. Careful inspection for haemostasis should always take place. Haemostatics can be used for the management of venous oozing on the site of adrenal excision.

Step 9: Final inspection and trocar removal

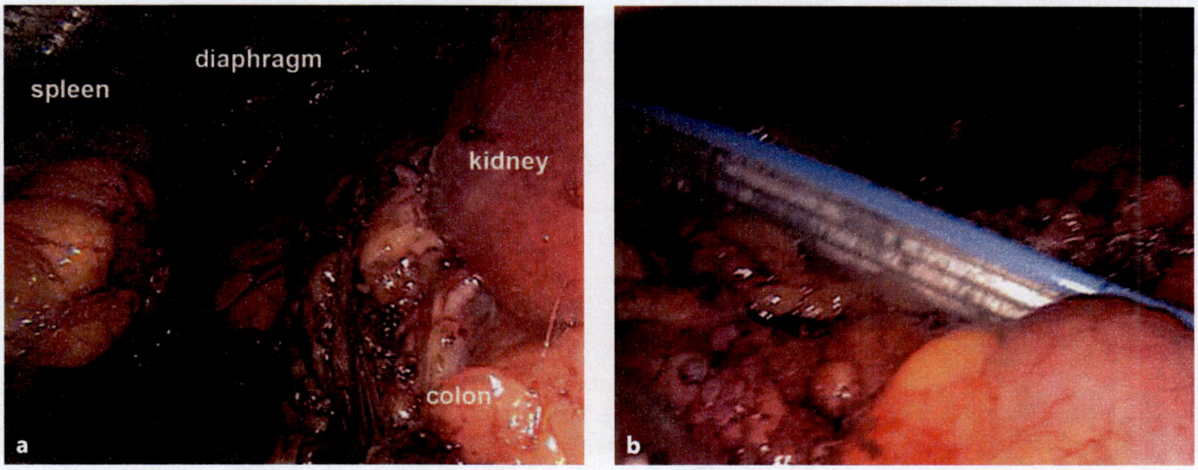

Step 9a shows all landmarks that should be inspected before the removal of the trocars. Careful inspection of the surgical field includes the reduction of gas pressure to less than 5 mmHg in order to check for any venous bleeding. A nonsuction drainage tube is inserted in an anterior 10-mm port in the site of the procedure (Step 9b). Trocars should be removed under direct vision as these sites are among the most common sites for bleeding. The specimen can be extracted through a small incision at a trocar site (usually the supraumbilical trocar). Fascial closure takes place at the specimen extraction and the 10-mm trocar sites.

Postoperative Management

- Oral or intramuscular analgesia is sufficient
- Drain removal on day 1 postoperatively in case of minimal output
- Normal diet and mobilisation of the patient from day 1 postoperatively
- Urinary catheter removed on day 2 postoperatively
- Discharge home on day 3 postoperatively
- Resume normal activities on day 7 postoperatively

References

1. Tanaka M, Ono Y, Matsuda T, Terachi T, Suzuki K, Baba S, Hara I, Hirao Y; Urological Laparoscopic Surgery Guideline Committee, Japanese Society of Endourology and ESWL(2009) Guidelines for urological laparoscopic surgery. Int J Uro 16:115–125
2. Saunders BD, Doherty GM (2004) Laparoscopic adrenalectomy for malignant disease. Lancet Oncol 5:718–726
3. Gagner M, Lacroix A, Bolte E (1992) Laparoscopic adrenalectomy in Cushing's syndrome and pheochromocytoma. New Engl J Med 327:1033

1.17 Retroperitoneal Right Adrenalectomy

Jens-Uwe Stolzenburg, Panagiotis Kallidonis, Minh Do, Rowan Casey, Anja Dietel, Andreas Gonsior, Evangelos Liatsikos

Introduction

Snow et al. [1] were the first to perform retroperitoneal right adrenalectomy in 1991 for a benign lesion and Gagner et al. [2] further documented the technique of laparoscopic adrenalectomy (LA) for neoplasia in 1992. As the surgical technique and instrumentation have been refined, laparoscopic adrenalectomy has become the standard of care for the majority of adrenal tumours [3, 4].

Since the introduction of laparoscopic adrenalectomy, it is difficult to find another approach for an ablative surgical operation that provides, so completely, such a clear discrepancy between the extended incision in traditional adrenalectomy and the smaller size of the targeted organ. Today there are several approaches described in the literature to perform adrenalectomy: the lateral transperitoneal, anterior transperitoneal, lateral retroperitoneal, and posterior retroperitoneal techniques. The lateral transperitoneal approach is the technique most often used for laparoscopic adrenalectomy. However, for right-side adrenalectomy we favour the retroperitoneal access as described in this section.

Indications

- Functional benign lesions (aldosteronoma, Cushing's syndrome, pheochromocytoma, adrenal hyperandrogenism)
- Nonfunctioning lesions ganglioneuroma, adenoma, myelolipoma and cyst)
- Suspected malignant lesions (primary adrenal carcinoma, 3- to 4-cm lesion with serial growth or suspicious character on MRI/CT imaging, isolated metastases to the adrenal gland, or >5-cm lesion)

Absolute Contraindications

- Benign adrenal tumours greater than 10–12 cm in diameter, due to the increased malignant risk
- Malignant tumours with local invasion, venous thrombus, regional nodal involvement
- Uncontrolled pheochromocytoma
- Severe cardiorespiratory disorders, coagulopathy and cranial hypertension
- Symptomatic pheochromocytomas during pregnancy
- Active retroperitoneal fibrosis (morbus Ormond)

Relative Contraindications

- Morbid obesity
- Malignant tumours due to high risk of tumour spillage
- Prior abdominal surgery associated with the presence of adhesions

Preoperative Preparation

- Antiplatelet/anticoagulant therapy held for at least 8 days
- Metabolic abnormalities due to functional tumours should be addressed
- Aldosteronomas: spirolactone to manage hypertension and hypokalaemia
- Cortisol-secreting adenomas: normoglycemic status and stress dose steroid administration
- Pheochromocytomas: phenoxybenzamine for 14 days to control blood pressure, additional blockade for arrhythmias if necessary

Perioperative Pharmacological Management [5]

Pheochromocytoma

Phenoxybenzamine [α-adrenergic blocker]

- 10–14 days preoperatively
- Initial divided dose of 3 × 5 mg is given orally and is increased by 10–20 mg per day up to maximum of 1 mg/day/kg

Propanolol [β-adrenergic blocker] (never start before α-adrenergic blocker)

- Preoperative for patient with reflex tachycardia (tachycardia > 100/min)
- 10 mg two to four times daily

Cushing disease (unilateral adrenalectomy, bilateral subtotal adrenalectomy)

Hydrocortisone

- 200 mg / 24 h on day of operation
- Postoperatively continuous dose reduction: day 1, 150mg/day; day 2, 100 mg/day, down to 20–30 mg/day (+ 0.05–0.2 mg fludrocortisone), higher doses during stress situations
- Patients need hydrocortisone emergency card during time of substitution
- Substitutions stop after convalescence of hypophysis and contralateral adrenal gland (some months)

Conn disease (Aldosteronoma)

Spironolactone

- 2–3 weeks preoperatively to normalise blood pressure
- Start with low dose 25 mg/day, up to 300 mg/day
- Potassium substitution

Unilateral adrenal gland (contralateral gland removal in past)

- Postoperatively continuous hydrocortisone substitution: 20–30 mg/day (+ 0.05–0.2 mg fludrocortisone), higher doses during stress situations
- Patients need hydrocortisone emergency card

Step 1: Patient position and trocar placement

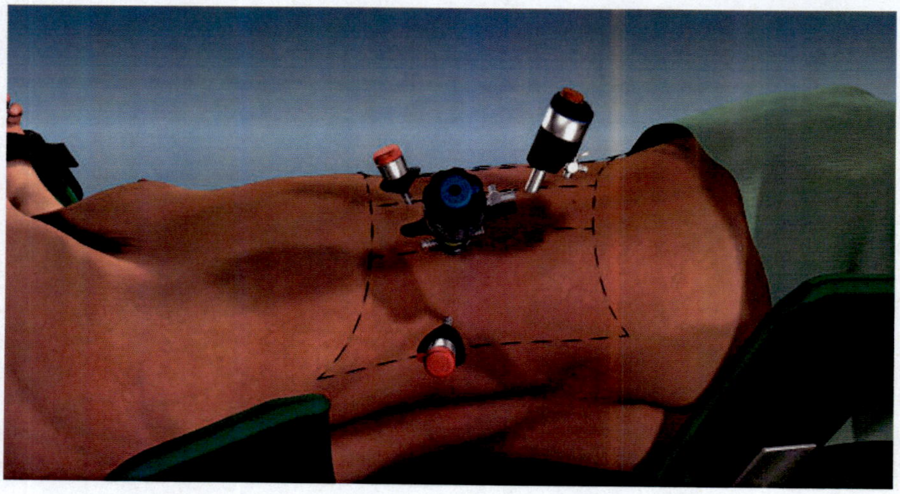

The patient is positioned in the flank position with the table flexed as described in Sect. 1.1. The procedure can be performed with either three or four trocars. We prefer a four-trocar technique as shown in the figure. A mini-lumbotomy (2-cm incision) is performed in the posterior axillary line 1–2 cm below the 12th rib. The abdominal wall and the transversalis fascia are incised. The retroperitoneal space is dissected with the finger and the balloon trocar followed by the placement of the optical trocar. A 5-mm trocar is inserted under visual guidance paravertebrally. The dissection of the retroperitoneal space is continued and two trocars (5 and 10–12 mm) are placed in the midaxillary line. In a three-trocar technique, the 10- to 12-mm trocar is placed paravertebrally.

Step 2: Dissection of the retroperitoneal space

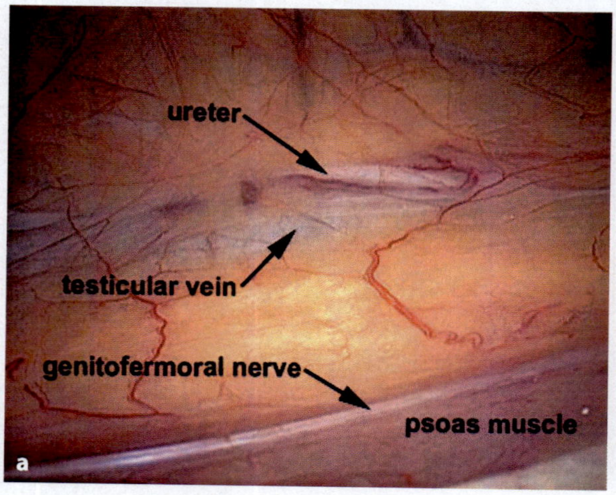

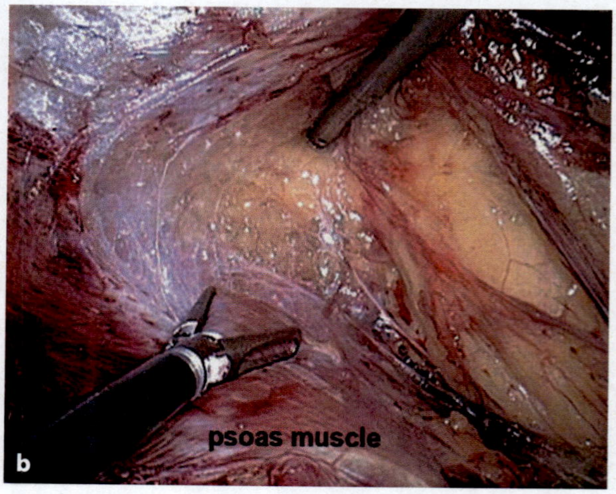

Step 2a shows the typical landmarks initially seen after balloon dissection of the retroperitoneal space, insufflation and insertion of the laparoscope. The psoas muscle is at the base. In most cases, the genitofemoral nerve can also be identified. The ureter and testicular vein, running together, can be identified medially to the psoas muscle. The dissection of the extraperitoneal space is continued in a cranial direction on top of the psoas muscle. The insufflated gas helps identify plans of cleavage as seen in Step 2b.

1

Step 3: Identification of the renal artery and adrenal tumour

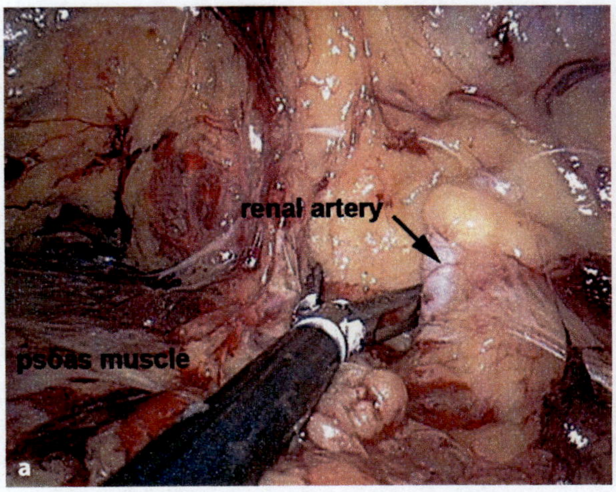

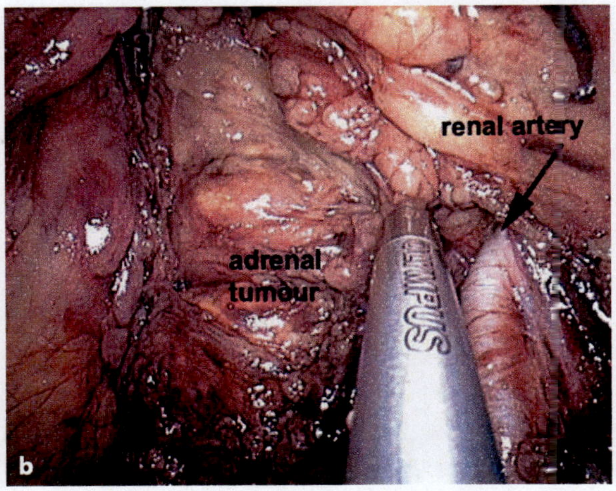

In adrenalectomy, there is no need to mobilise the ureter and testicular vein as in nephrectomy. The dissection should be focused in the identification of the renal hilum. Step 3a demonstrates blunt dissection of the renal artery. The artery is normally located in front of the renal vein during extraperitoneal dissection. The adrenal tumour can be identified just cranially to the artery. Before full mobilisation of the tumour, the renal vein must be identified.

Step 4: Renal vein and inferior adrenal vein mobilisation

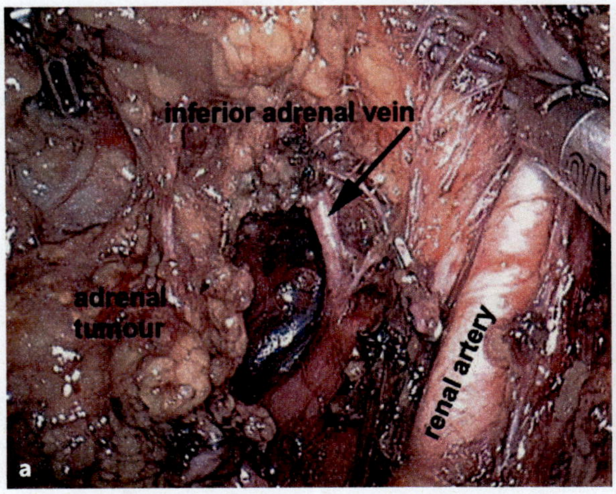

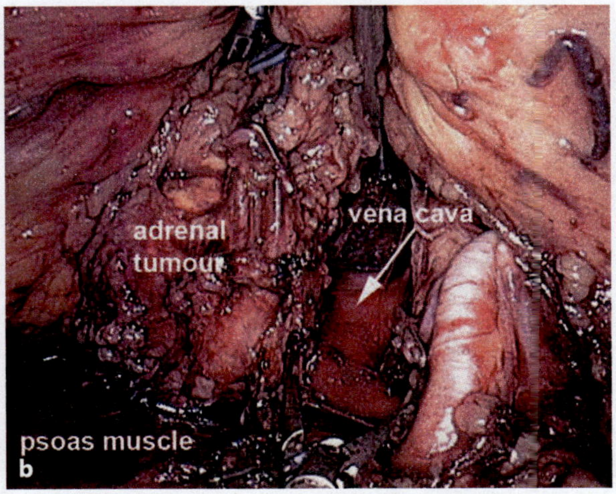

To identify the inferior adrenal vein, the renal vein must first be identified cranioposteriorly to the renal artery (Step 4a). Retraction of the adrenal gland laterally facilitates the visualisation of these vessels. For dissection, we prefer to use a bipolar forceps and the SonoSurg device. Any other kind of dissecting forceps can also be used. The use of the ligature device provides the advantage of dividing the adrenal vessels without the need for clips. When the inferior adrenal vein is divided, the vena cava can be easily identified (Step 4b).

Step 5: Identification of the medial adrenal vein

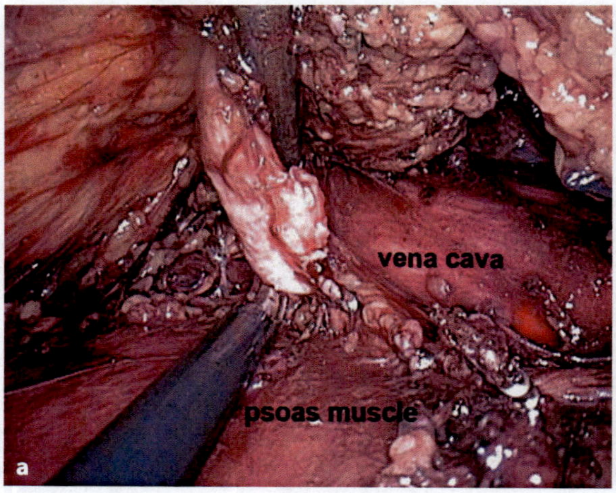

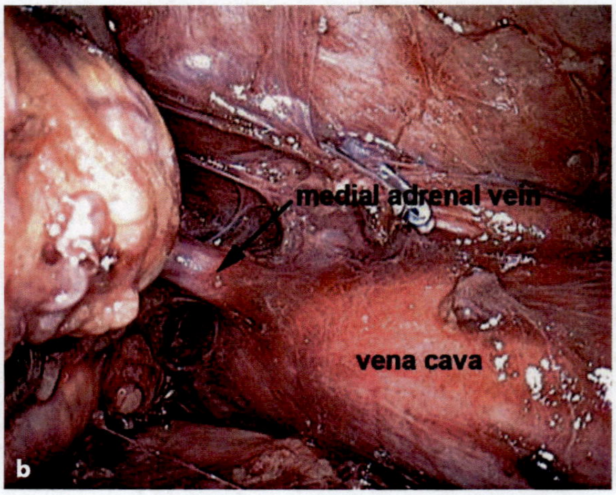

The dissection is continued on the surface of the vena cava. In this case, in order to expose the medial adrenal vein the medial aspect of the adrenal gland must be mobilised (Step 5a). The medial adrenal vein is exposed by a combination of blunt and sharp dissection and carefully prepared for ligation and division. On the right side, the medial adrenal vein (Step 5b), which drains directly in the vena cava, is the main venous drainage as opposed to the left side where the inferior adrenal vein is the main (thickest) vein. This is especially important in phaeochromocytoma as this vein should be divided first.

Step 6: Division of the medial adrenal vein

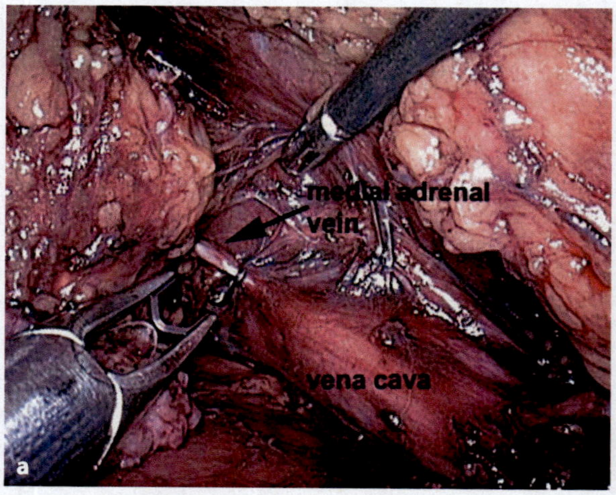

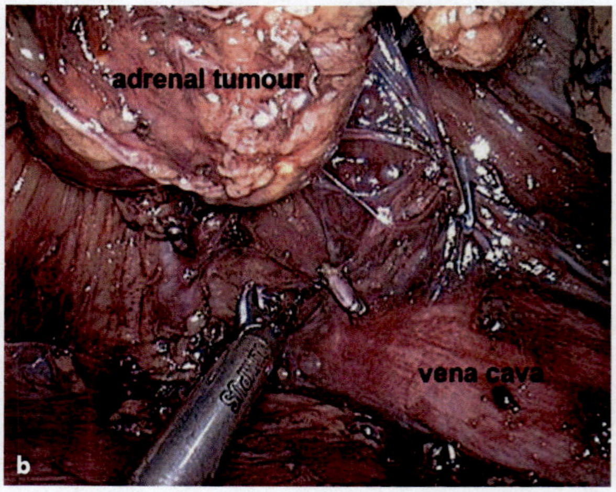

Metal clips can be used on these vessels proximally and distally. Proximally, two clips should always be placed to ensure secure closure of the vein. Alternatively, small-size Hem-o-lok clips can be used. Care should be taken to avoid any injury of the renal vein and vena cava. It is of paramount importance that orientation with the vena cava is maintained during the entire dissection and mobilisation. If an injury of the vena cava occurs, bleeding can be normally controlled laparoscopically. Because of the gas pressure, bleeding is not as pronounced as in open surgery. Pressure can be applied to the bleeding point with suction whilst another trocar is inserted to facilitate suturing of the defect. Clips should not be used for haemostasis on the cava.

Step 7: Mobilisation of the adrenal tumour

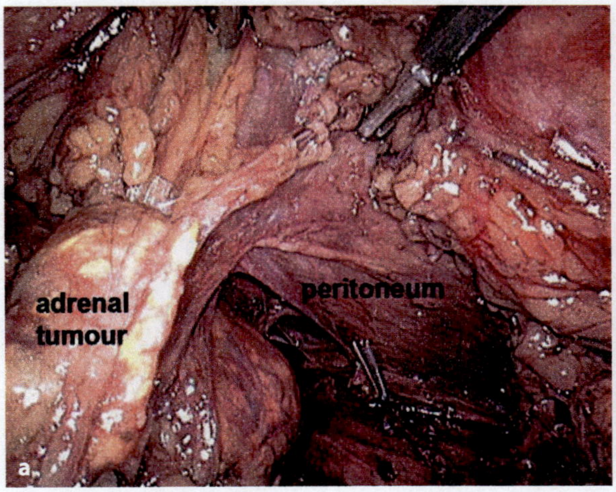

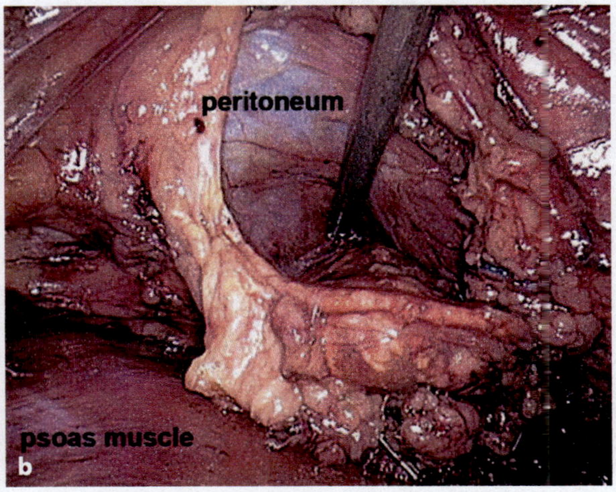

The adrenal tumour is now fully mobilised medially and cranially. Most of the dissection can be performed bluntly or using the SonoSurg device. The superior adrenal vein, which originated from the inferior phrenic vessel, is normally small and can also be dissected with the SonoSurg device. Care should be taken not to damage the tumour during mobilisation to avoid tumour spillage or, in the case of phaeochromocytoma, hypertensive crisis. It is also important to avoid opening the peritoneum, which can cause loss of the operative field.

Step 8: Removal of the specimen

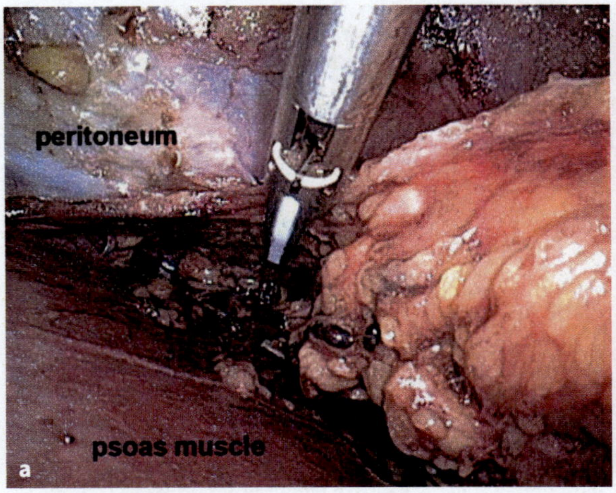

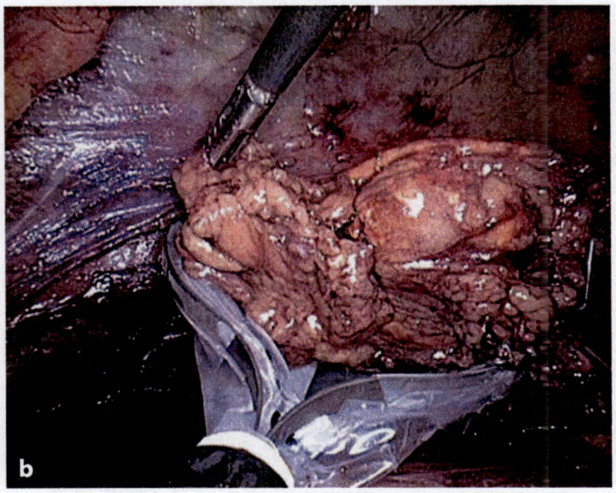

The final attachments of the adrenal tumour to the peritoneum are divided carefully. The adrenal tumour is then placed in an EndoCatch retrieval bag. The tumour should not be divided and removed through a trocar in pieces. Alternatively, a simple plastic bag (the bag from the drain or urinary catheter) can be used instead of the expensive EndoCatch bag. The bag can be removed immediately via an enlarged 12-mm trocar site or it can be placed in the lower aspect of the retroperitoneal space to check haemostasis before removal.

Step 9: Final inspection and drain placement

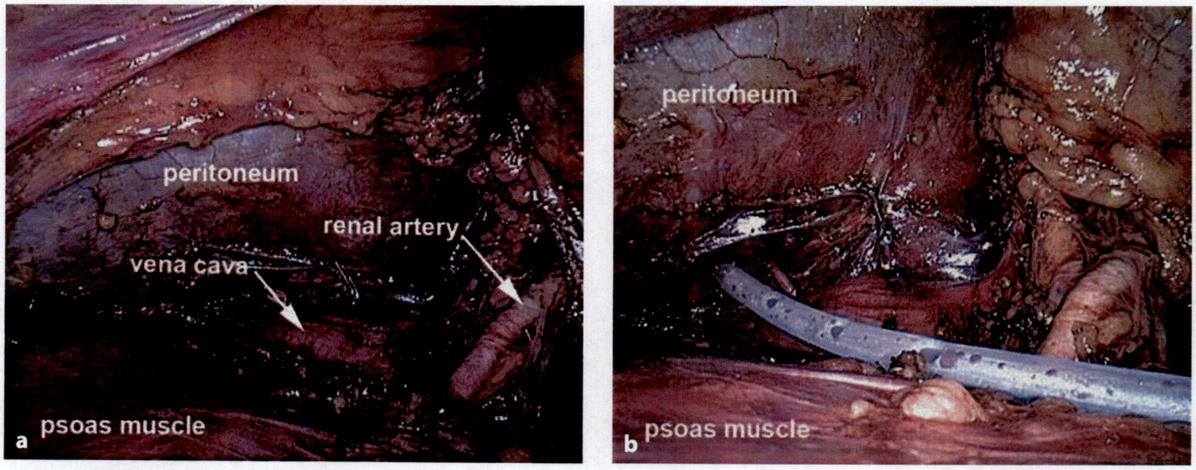

To check haemostasis, the gas pressure should be reduced to 5–6 mmHg because venous bleeding may not be apparent at high gas pressures. This prevents overlooking subtle venous oozing, which does not occur at higher gas pressures. It is optional to insert a nonsuction drainage tube through an anterior 5-mm port into the adrenal bed. Trocars are now removed under direct laparoscopic vision. Fascial closure is only necessary in 10-mm trocar sites. The skin is closed with intracutaneous sutures.

Postoperative Management

- Drain removal on day 1 if minimal output
- Normal diet and mobilisation from day 1
- Frequent electrolyte controls and volume substitution to prevent prerenal failure for patients with primary hyperaldosteronism or phaeochromocytoma
- Hydrocortisone replacement in descending dose within the next 7 days followed by continuous substitution for patients with primary hypercortisolism
- Frequent blood pressure measurements
- Genetic diagnosis for all patients with phaeochromocytoma, irrespective of uni- or bilateral gland disease or family history

References

1. Snow LL (1991) Endoscopic general surgery: an update. Laser Highlights 2:1–3
2. Gagner M, Lacroix A, Bolte E (1992) Laparoscopic adrenalectomy in Cushing's syndrome and pheochromocytoma. New Engl J Med 327:1033
3. Lal G, Duh Q-Y (2003) Laparoscopic adrenalectomy – indications and technique. Surg Oncol 12:105–123
4. Tanaka M, Ono Y, Matsuda T, Terachi T, Suzuki K, Baba S, Hara I, Hirao Y; Urological Laparoscopic Surgery Guideline Committee, Japanese Society of Endourology and ESWL (2009) Guidelines for urological laparoscopic surgery. Int J Urol 16 :115–125
5. ErlicZ, Rybicki L, Peczkowska M et al (2009) Clinical predictors and algorithm for the genetic diagnosis of pheochromocytoma patients. Clin Cancer Res 15:6378–6385

1.18 Retroperitoneal Ureterolithotomy

Minh Do, Peter Tenke, Rowan Casey, Evangelos Liatsikos, Phuc Ho Thi, Andreas Gonsior, Ian Dunn, Jens-Uwe Stolzenburg

Introduction

The management of ureteral stones has changed over the last two decades. Currently, the management of upper and middle ureteral stones is treatment with shock wave lithotripsy, ureteroscopic lithotripsy or percutaneous lithotripsy [1]. In rare cases, ureteral stones are treated with open surgery after failure of first-line treatments. Following Wickham's initial report of laparoscopic ureterolithotomy by a retroperitoneal approach in 1979, there were no major developments in laparoscopic therapy for a certain period of time [2, 3]. However, Gaur described the new balloon dissection technique of retroperitoneoscopy, which was recognised as a useful minimally invasive therapeutic advance [3, 4]. Therefore, laparoscopic ureterolithotomy is an alternative to open surgery for removing large stones where other minimally invasive treatments have failed and can achieve complete stone clearance in a single operative session. Upper and midureteral stones are safely approached retroperitoneally, but lower ureteral stones are better suited to transperitoneal techniques, albeit with less success than upper ureteric stones. The retroperitoneal approach has several advantages over the transperitoneal approach, including a low risk of visceral organ injury, no bowel mobilisation and a postoperative urinary leak does not interfere with the peritoneal cavity. The retroperitoneal technique is also associated with a shorter period of convalescence [5, 6].

Indications

- Large impacted ureteral stones
- Failure to localise or access the stone via endoscopic or percutaneous routes
- Inability to focus extracorporeal shock wave lithotripsy (ESWL) shock waves
- Failure to fragment the stone
- Stone that would require multiple settings and auxiliary procedures

Contra-indications

- Anaesthetic contra-indications
- Serious cardiorespiratory conditions
- Bleeding disorders, anticoagulation, antiplatelet therapy

Preoperative Preparation

- Radiological imaging to visualise the stone and ureter (CT or IVU or retrograde uretero-pyelography)
- Compression stockings and perioperative antibiotic treatment are advisable

Step 1: Radiological imaging and placement of double-J catheter

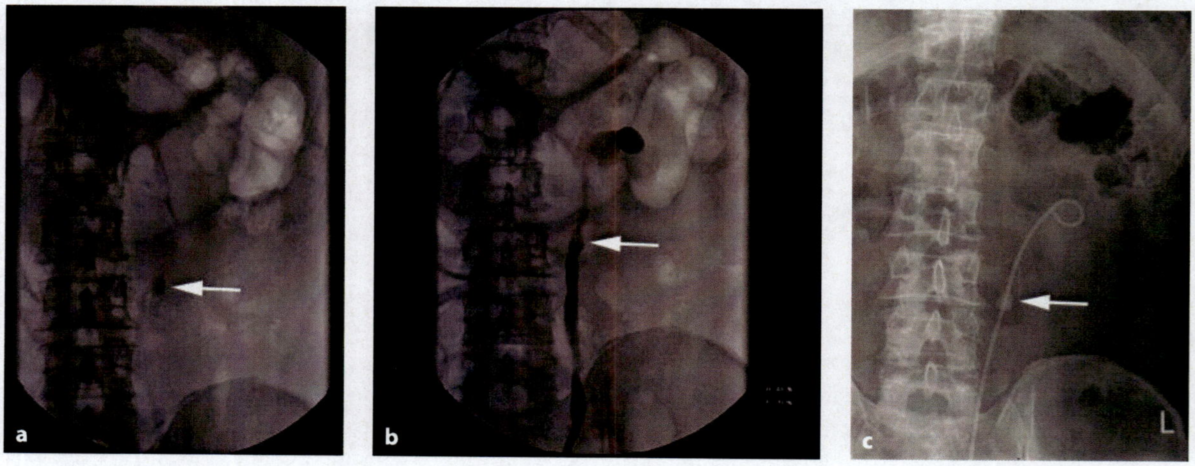

To visualise the stone, either a CT scan or IVU or retrograde ureteropyelography should be performed. A double-J stent is inserted after ureteropyelography and is in a good position across the stone, as in Step1c. Typically a 6-F double-J ureteral stent is placed. If you cannot insert a 6-F stent, attempt a narrower lumen stent via guidewire because it makes the procedure much more difficult to place a double stent during the lithotomy. This preplaced stent also helps identify the ureter. When the stone is impacted and the double-J stent cannot be placed, a guidewire or open-ended ureteral catheter is retrogradely placed distal to the stone in the ureter and fixed at the urethral catheter. Once the stone has been extracted, the stent is then advanced into the renal pelvis under laparoscopic guidance.

Step 2: Patient position and trocar placement

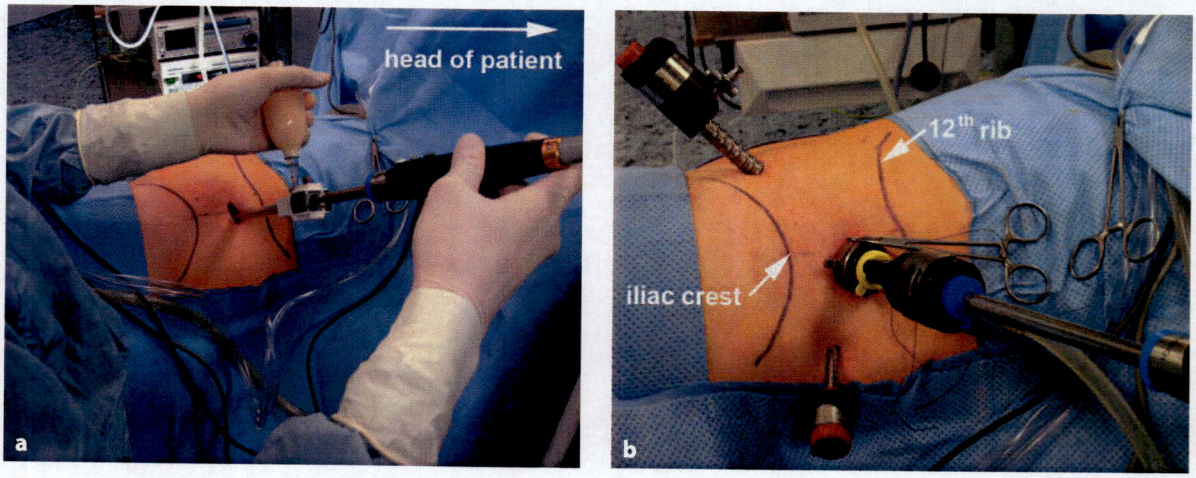

The patient is placed in the full flank position with the table flexed and the patient fully supported. A 1.5-cm incision is made at the midpoint between the 12th costal margin and iliac crest on the posterior axillary line. The transversalis fascia is incised, and the posterior pararenal space is developed bluntly. A balloon trocar is placed and develops the retroperitoneal space under direct visual control (Step 2a). A 10-mm trocar is inserted under direct laparoscopic guidance at the superior edge of the iliac crest and another 5-mm trocar is placed lateral to the lumbar muscles at the same level (Step 2b). A pneumoretroperitoneum is created at a pressure of 12 mmHg.

Step 3: Anatomical landmarks and stone localisation

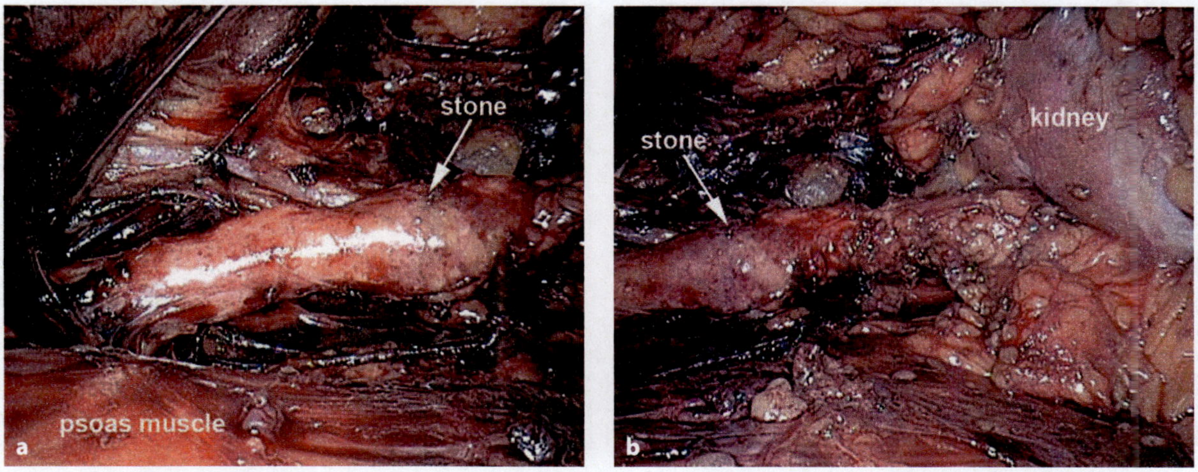

The retroperitoneal landmarks should be identifiable immediately: the psoas muscle, Gerota fascia, lateral peritoneal reflection, aortic pulsation (left side), and partially collapsed vena cava (right side). The ureter should be identified within its sheath of periureteric fat at a point below the stone (Step 3a). There is usually a great deal of periureteric fibrosis around and above the site of an impacted stone and this is not the best place to start dissection (Step 3b). Stone localisation is obviously the most important step in the procedure. In some cases, when the ureter is not markedly dilated, the stone can be seen bulging in the ureter. In cases where the stone is not seen prominently, it is sometimes difficult to localise the stone visually. In this situation, we pinch the ureter gently with forceps to locate the stone.

Step 4: Ureteric dissection, ureterotomy and stone extraction

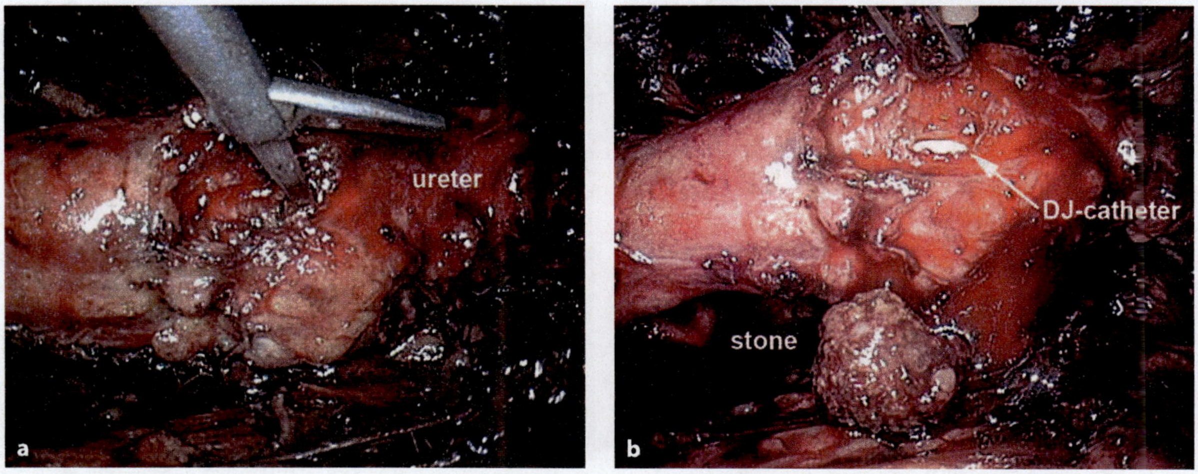

Usually, the calculus is large and the ureter can be easily dissected with blunt dissector or forceps in one port and an atraumatic clamp in the other. Stones in the upper ureter are more easily removed but there is a risk of their migration into the dilated pelvicaliceal system during dissection of the ureter. To prevent this, the proximal ureter should be first dissected from above and a rubber sling can be used to prevent the stone migration. We recommend the use of a straight laparoscopic scissors rather then curved in order to incised the ureter longitudinally (Step 4a). The length of the incision depends upon the stone size. A Maryland dissector is used to fish out the stone. Make sure that there is no inadvertent grasping of the mucosa together with the stone on removal.

Step 5: Stone removal and ureterotomy closure

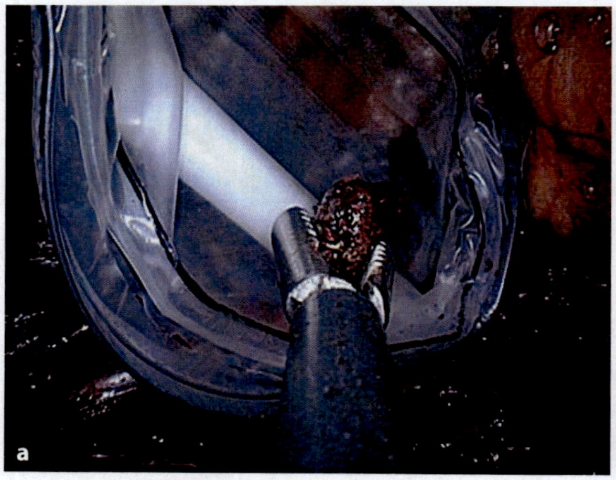
a

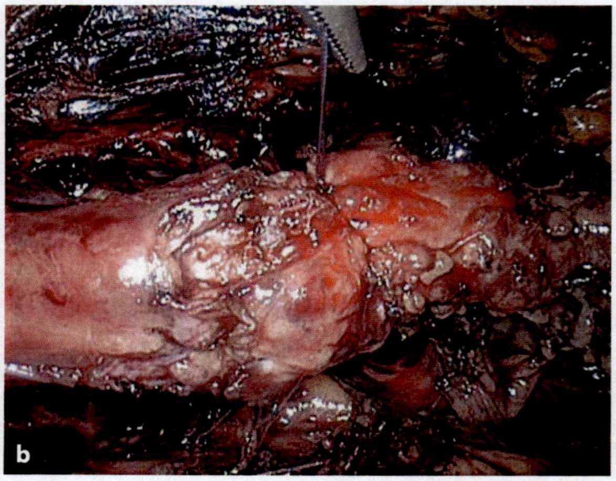
b

A dissector is used to grasp the stone. It may be possible to extract the stone through the 10- to 12-mm port. If not, it is entrapped in an EndoCatch bag and extracted through an enlarged port site (Step 5a). It is also possible to use the bag that the drain was in as an extraction bag. This step is monitored by the laparoscope. Losing the stone in the retroperitoneal space can create serious problems. In cases where the double-J stent could not be placed to the renal pelvis, the guidewire is now advanced under laparoscopic vision into the renal pelvis. The stent can now be placed over the guidewire. The ureterotomy can now be closed by interrupted sutures (Step 5b).

Step 6: Final ureterotomy closure and drain insertion

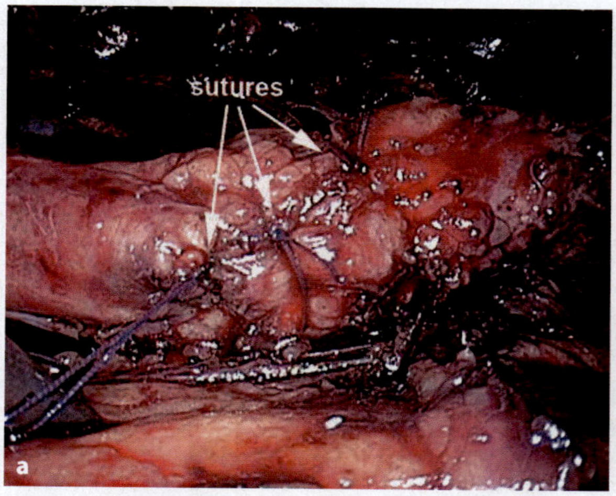

a

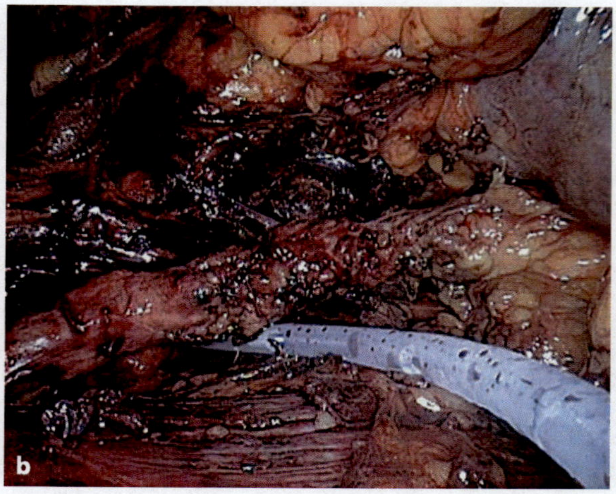
b

The ureterotomy is closed over the ureteral stent with interrupted 4/0 Vicryl sutures using intracorporeal suturing techniques. The interrupted sutures are spaced approximately 3–4 mm apart (Step 6a). Suturing should not include large portion of ureteral mucosa. Only if the incision is very small can the ureterotomy be left open to heal around the stent. One of the major complications of laparoscopic ureterolithotomy is stenosis, which may be due to local ureteral wall ischaemia. This can be due to inflammatory reaction or sutures that narrow the lumen of the ureter. After closing the ureterotomy, a nonsuction drain is inserted through one of the 5-mm ports to prevent urinoma or collection (Step 6b). The ports are removed under direct vision and the wounds are closed in the standard fashion.

Postoperative Management

- Urinary catheter removed day 2–3
- The drain is removed when volumes are insignificant (if there is persistent drainage check the fluid creatinine value to exclude urine leakage)
- Ureteral stent removed at week 2–3
- Parenteral antibiotics are continued for 24 h, and then the patient is switched to a prophylactic oral agent, which is continued until the stent is removed

References

1. Marberger M, Hofbauer J, Türk C, Höbarth K, Albrecht W (1994) Management of ureteric stones. Eur Urol 25:265–272
2. Wickham JEA (ed) (1979) Surgical treatment of renal lithiasis. In Urinary Calculus Disease. New York: Churchill Livingstone 145–198
3. Clayman RV, Kavaussi LR, Soper NJ et al (1991) Laparoscopic nephrectomy: initial case report. J Urol 146:278–281
4. Gaur DD (1992) Laparoscopic operative retroperitoneoscopy. Use of the new device. J Urol 148:1137–1139
5. Kiyota H, Ikemoto I, Asano K, Madarame J, Miki K, Yoshino Y, Hasegawa T, Ohishi Y (2001) Retroperitoneoscopic ureterolithotomy for impacted ureteral stone. Int J Urol 8:391–397
6. Keeley FX, Gialas I, Pillai M, Chrisofos M, Tolley DA (1999) Laparoscopic ureterolithotomy: the Edinburgh experience. BJU Int 84:765–769

Chapter 2

Lympadenectomy

CONTENTS

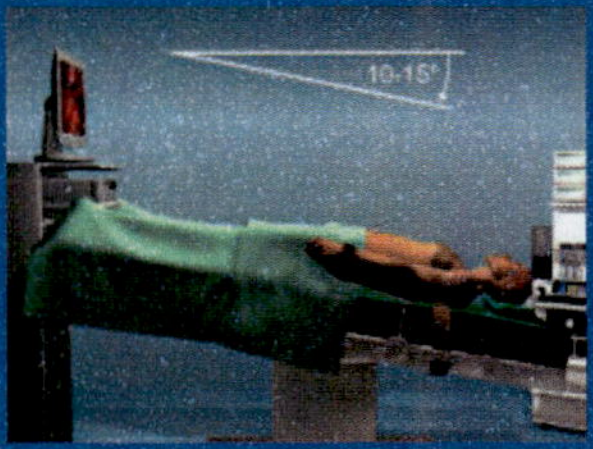

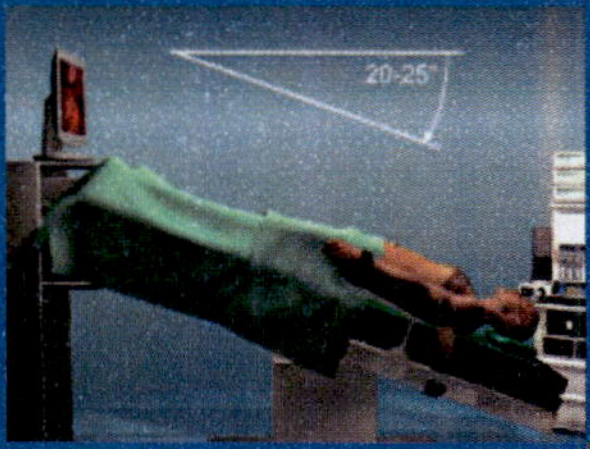

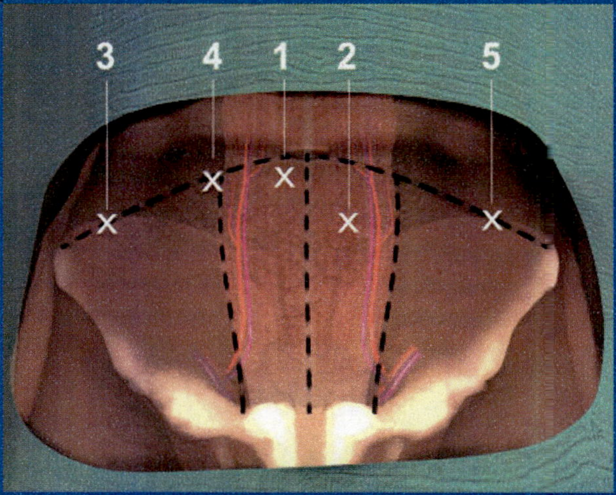

J.-U. Stolzenburg, I. Türk, E. Liatsikos: *Laparoscopic and Robot-Assisted Surgery in Urology*
DOI: 10.1007/978-3-642-00891-7_2, © Springer-Verlag Berlin Heidelberg 2011

2.1 Retroperitoneal Lymph Node Dissection

Ingolf A. Tuerk, Rowan Casey, Jens-Uwe Stolzenburg

Introduction

Current management options for low-stage malignant germ-cell testicular tumours after radical orchiectomy include surveillance, chemotherapy, or retroperitoneal lymph node dissection (RPLND). Open RPLND is the surgical gold standard but has a number of limitations. Firstly, approximately two-thirds of patients have either necrosis/fibrosis or pathologically negative nodes. Secondly, the operation results in a large scar and significant perioperative morbidity and convalescence. Laparoscopic retroperitoneal lymph node dissection has developed as a possible alternative to the open procedure.

Currently, laparoscopic retroperitoneal lymph node dissection (L-RPLND) is not recommended as a standard therapeutic option in the European Association of Urology (EAU) guidelines. L-RPLND has, however, proved to be an excellent staging tool ,which should be developed as a less invasive alternative to primary open RPLND. As a staging tool, L-RPLND is performed usually without retrocaval or retroaortic dissection and is used to determine pathological status. The therapeutic value of this more limited dissection is not known and currently trials are underway to establish the therapeutic benefits. L-RPLND has been reported as efficacious compared to open RPLND for staging of the retroperitoneum in patients with stage I nonseminomatous germ-cell testis tumours (NSGCT). The rate of tumour control after L-RPLND and the diagnostic accuracy of L-RPLND were equal to the open procedure, and the morbidity was significantly lower [1, 2]. Therefore, L-RPLND for stage I and low-volume retroperitoneal stage II disease may be performed at experienced urology centres as part of ongoing trials [3, 4].

Loss of antegrade ejaculation is the most common long-term problem that the young men who undergo this operation experience. In an attempt to minimise this problem, either a template dissection or nerve-sparing RPLND should be performed. In a right template dissection, the right postganglionic fibres are resected whilst the left side ones are left intact. This applies to the left side also. Complete unilateral resection of the nerves should not result in loss of antegrade ejaculation. Dissection of both sides is only required in bilateral RPLND.

Indications

- Staging patients pre- or postchemotherapy in clinical stage I nonseminomatous germ cell tumour (NSGCT)
- Stage IIa NSGCT (only experienced surgeons as part of a clinical trial)

Contra-indications

- Marked pulmonary fibrosis (secondary to bleomycin chemotherapy) because the patient may not tolerate pneumoperitoneum
- Bleeding diathesis
- Abnormal tumour markers

Preoperative Preparation

- Bowel preparation 2 days before surgery
- Antibiotic prophylaxis
- Group and cross-match 3 units of blood
- Low-fat diet 1 week and 2 weeks postoperatively
- Nasogastric tube and double-J stent insertion (optional)
- Urinary catheter after induction of anaesthesia

Step 1: Patient position and port placement (left-sided template RPLND)

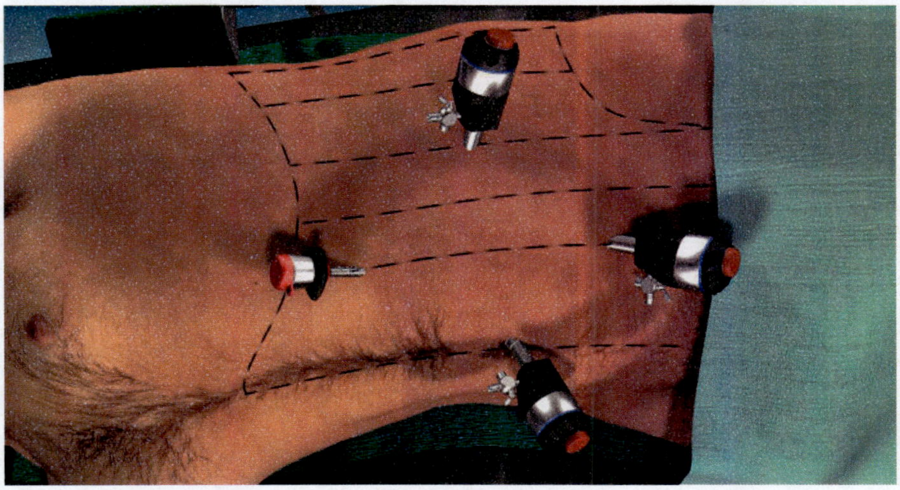

The patient is positioned on the operating table with the side elevated at 45° upwards. The patient is securely strapped to the table so the table can be tilted during the procedure. The table is flexed at the umbilicus and the patient is placed slightly head down. The procedure is performed transperitoneally. For a left-sided RPLND, we place the 12-mm optical trocar at the umbilicus. The 12-mm working trocar is placed on the pararectal line to the right of this and a 5-mm working trocar on the same line to the left. The assistant uses a 12-mm trocar placed at the midclavicular or anterior axillary line. On the right side, we add another 5-mm trocar below the costal margin for liver retraction.

Step 2: Peritoneal incision and colon mobilisation

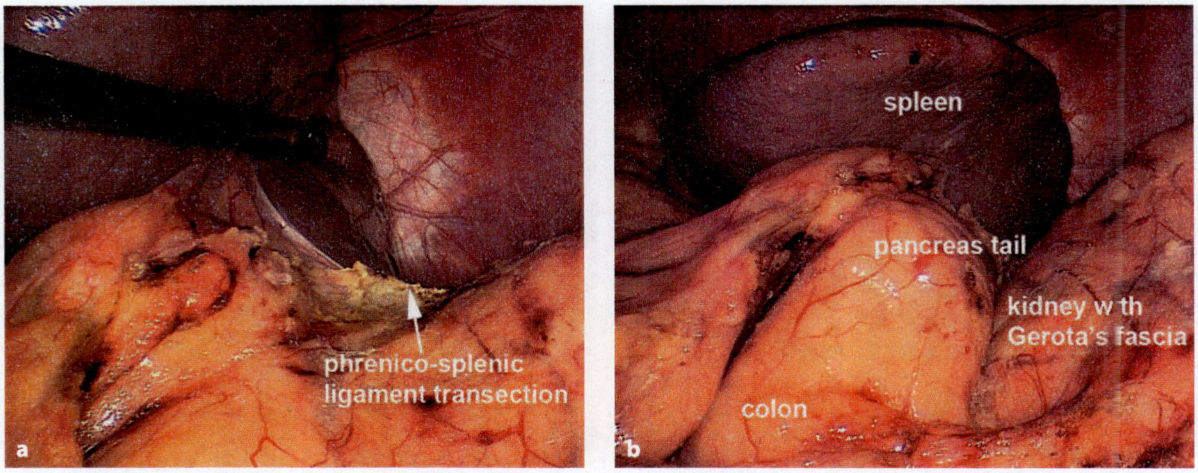

The peritoneum is incised along the line of Toldt from the left colonic flexure to the pelvic brim and distally along the spermatic vein to the internal inguinal ring. In a cranial direction, the splenicocolic ligament must be incised to allow the bowel and spleen to be retracted (Step 2a). If the exposure is not good the incision can be continued lateral to the spleen up to the diaphragm. This allows the spleen and the tail of the pancreas to be freed completely and rotated medially to allow access to the upper retroperitoneum (Step 2b) and complete exposure of the aorta and iliac vessels.

Step 3: Dissection of the left renal hilum

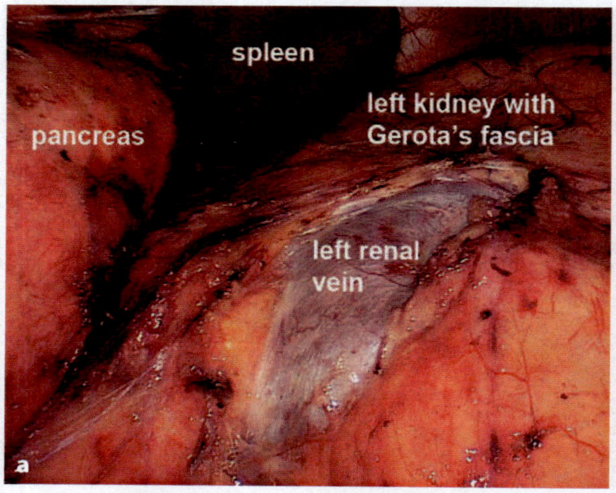

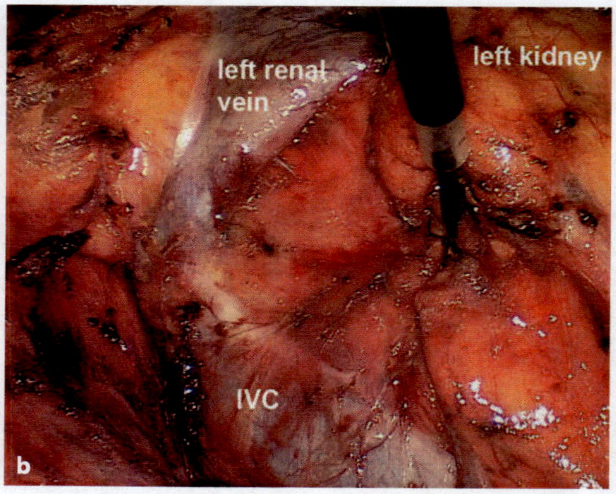

Mobilisation of the colon should allow the aorta and the inferior vena cava (IVC), with the overlying nodal packages, to come into view easily. The left renal vein is now identified. Further dissection of the left retroperitoneum defines the IVC and left renal vein junction. The lower pole of the kidney and ureter (not shown) should also be dissected. Now the surface of the aorta is completely exposed. Care should be taken when resecting the lumbar vein, which joins either the renal vein or spermatic vein dorsally on the left. The boundaries of the template dissection on the left side are the ureter laterally, the renal vessels superiorly, and all the preaortic and lateral aortic nodal tissue down to the inferior mesenteric artery.

Step 4: Interaortocaval lymph node dissection

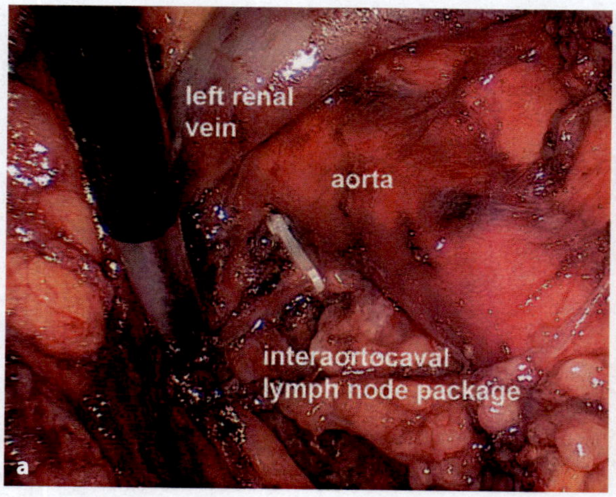

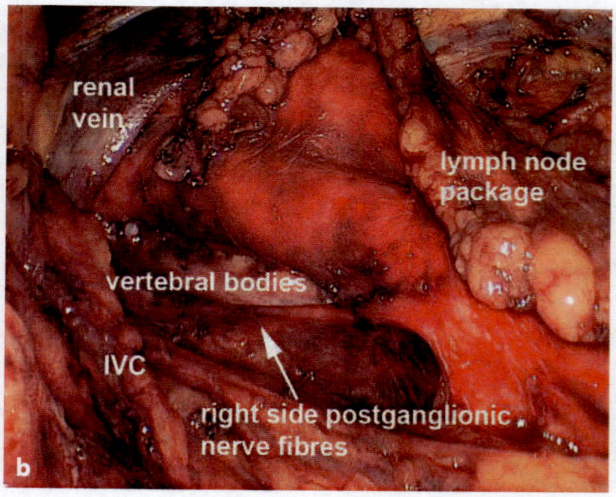

The ureter is identified and separated from lymphatic tissue and must not be skeletonised. The left renal vein, including its course ventral to the aorta, can be further freed then in order to access the inter aortocaval nodes (these nodes can be left if a modified template is used for staging purposes). The node package must be clipped liberally to avoid development of chylous ascites or a lymphocoele postoperatively. Step 4a and Step 4b demonstrate the major landmarks. The dissection continues down to the lumbar arteries without resecting them. (In a therapeutic L-RPLND the lumbar vessels must be divided to access the posterior aorta, IVC and spine in order to perform a complete split-and-roll technique.)

Step 5: Para-aortic lymph node dissection

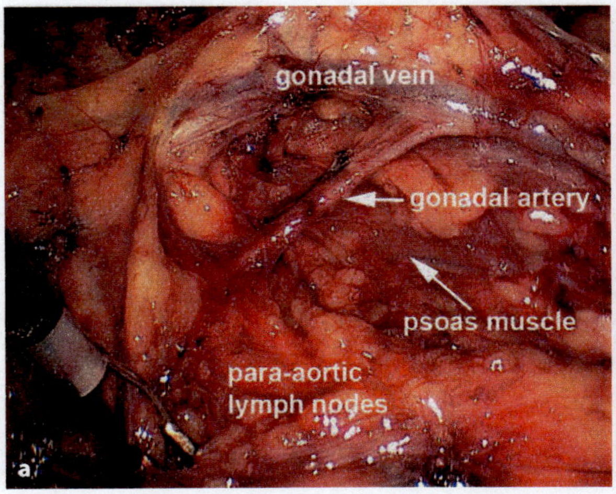

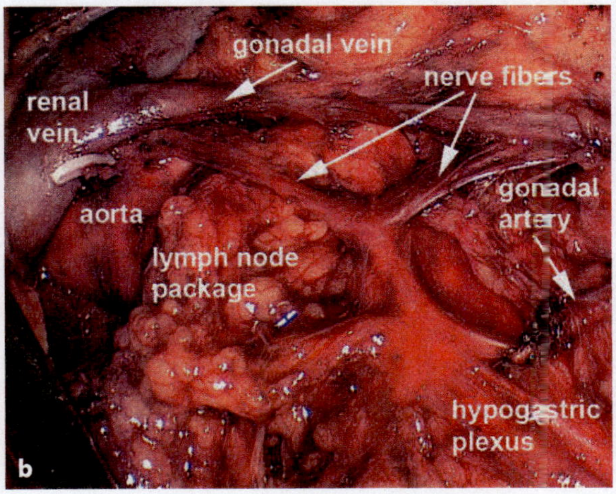

Further dissection now takes place of the interaortocaval and preaortic lymph node packages. After mobilising these lymph node packages, start dissection on the left lateral side of the aorta with identification of the sympathetic trunk and identification of the left postganglionic nerve fibres coming from the trunk. The ureter and psoas muscle form important landmarks to ensure complete dissection of nodes. The hypogastric plexus as seen in Step 5b caudally must be preserved by careful dissection. Step 5b also demonstrates further dissection of the para-aortic lymph nodes with preservation of the postganglionic nerve fibres. The gonadal artery insertion can be clipped and divided at this stage.

Step 6: Para-aortic lymph node dissection

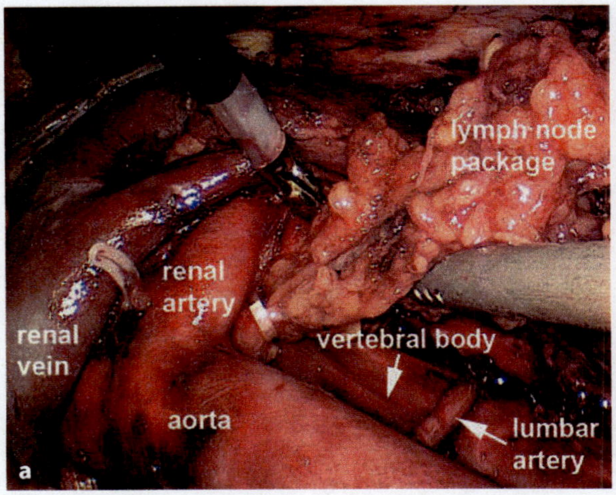

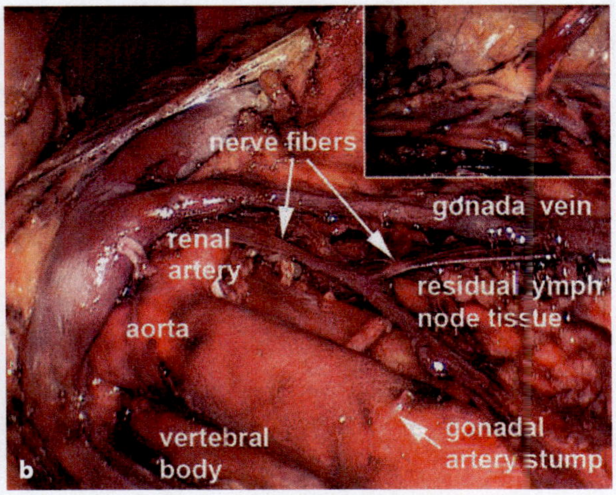

Further dissection of the para-aortic lymph nodes with preservation of the postganglionic nerve fibres is shown in Step 6a. Clips are applied on major lymph vessels underneath the renal artery. Care must be taken for the thoracic duct, which can be damaged during this manoeuvre, causing significant chylous ascites. Lumbar arteries and veins must be carefully identified and preserved to prevent troublesome bleeding. In Step 6b, most of the left template lymph nodes are removed. There are some residual para-aortic lymph nodes along the distal aorta and common iliac artery, which can now be resected. Dissection and removal of gonadal vessels from the renal hilum all the way to the internal inguinal ring is necessary (inset).

Step 7: Final inspection

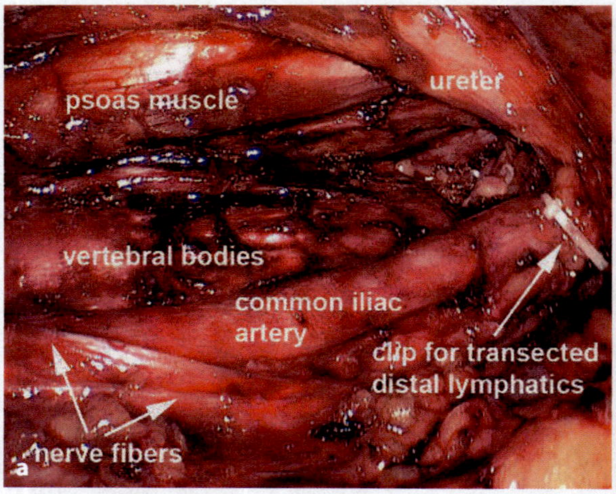

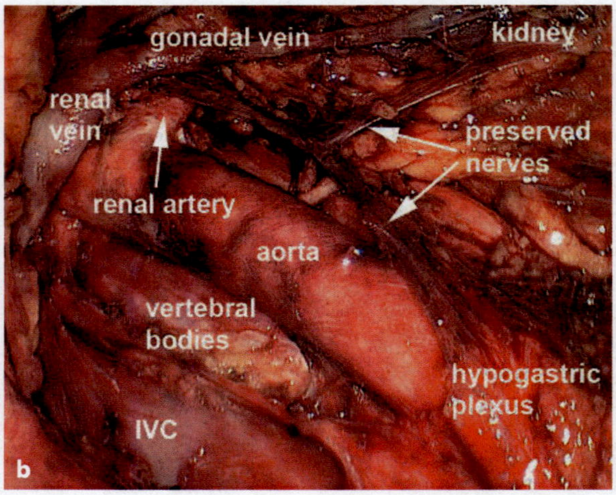

The final view in Step 7a demonstrates complete removal of the para-aortic lymph nodes all the way to the crossing of the left ureter over the iliac common artery. Large clips have been applied at the cranial and caudal end of the resection. A final inspection is made for bleeding or open lymphatic channels. The descending colon is placed back in its normal anatomic position and sutured in place. Step 7b demonstrates the anatomical location of the large number of nerves preserved following careful dissection of the lymphatic nodal package. Drain insertion is optional.

Postoperative Management

- Low-molecular-weight heparin until ambulatory
- Low-fat diet with middle-chain triglycerides for 3 weeks
- Light diet when bowel sounds return
- Large volume fluid replacement as per third space losses

References

1. Stephenson AJ, Klein EA (2009) Surgical management of low-stage nonseminomatous germ cell testicular cancer. BJU Int 104:1362–1368
2. Steiner H, Peschel R, Janetschek G, Höltl L, Berger AP, Bartsch G, Hobisch A (2004) Long-term results of laparoscopic retroperitoneal lymph node dissection: a single-center 10-year experience. Urology 63:550–555
3. Rassweiler JJ, Scheitlin W, Heidenreich A, Laguna MP, Janetschek G (2008) Laparoscopic retroperitoneal lymph node dissection: does it still have a role in the management of clinical stage 1 nonseminomatous testis cancer? A European perspective. Eur Urol 54:1004–1015
4. Neyer M, Peschel R, Akkad T, Springer-Stohr B, Berger A, Bartsch G, Steiner H (2007) Long-term results of laparoscopic retroperitoneal lymph-node dissection for clinical stage 1 nonseminomatous germ-cell testicular cancer. J Endourol 21:180–183

2.2 Transperitoneal Pelvic Lymph Node Dissection

Jens-Uwe Stolzenburg, Rowan Casey, Panagiotis Kallidonis, Minh Do, Anja Dietel, Matthias Winkler, Miguel Backhaus, Evangelos Liatsikos

Introduction

Currently, three variations of pelvic lymphadenectomy (PLA) exist: the limited (only obturator lymph nodes), the standard and the extended PLA. There is no consensus regarding the exact lymph node groups excised in each of the above PLA approaches. The standard PLA, which can be performed either trans- or extraperitoneally, should include the lymph nodes from the external iliac artery and vein extending up to level of iliac vessel bifurcation, the internal iliac artery and vein, and the obturator fossa [1].

There are several controversies that surround PLA. Firstly, examination of large series of patients with varied risk of lymph node metastasis has failed to prove that PLA has a significant impact in the biochemical relapse-free survival of the disease. Secondly, the extent of lymph node excision that should be performed is not known. It is generally accepted that the incidence of involved lymph nodes are detected more frequently when the extent of PLA increases and removal of greater that ten lymph nodes has been associated with more than double the incidence of metastasis compared to more limited lymphadenectomy (10.3% versus 4.6%). Extended PLA can result in retrieval of three times more lymph nodes compared to limited PLA [2].

Thirdly, recent evidence suggests that not all patients with prostate cancer should undergo an extensive PLA. Patients with PSA lower than 10 ng/dl, biopsy Gleason sum less than 7 and clinical stage T1c or T2 have a very limited (1–1.5% approximately) risk of harbouring nonobturator lymph node metastases [3].

For high-risk patients, a transperitoneal PLA is the most appropriate procedure as it allows extended lymph node dissection.

Indications

- High-risk prostate cancer
- Nomogram-based selection of patients

Contra-indications

- Uncorrectable coagulopathy
- Previous mesh placement for inguinal hernia repair limits the PLA. Lymph node groups covered by the mesh cannot be resected because of adhesions

Preoperative Preparation

- Similar to transperitoneal laparoscopic radical prostatectomy (see Sect. 3.10)

Step 1: Patient position and trocar placement

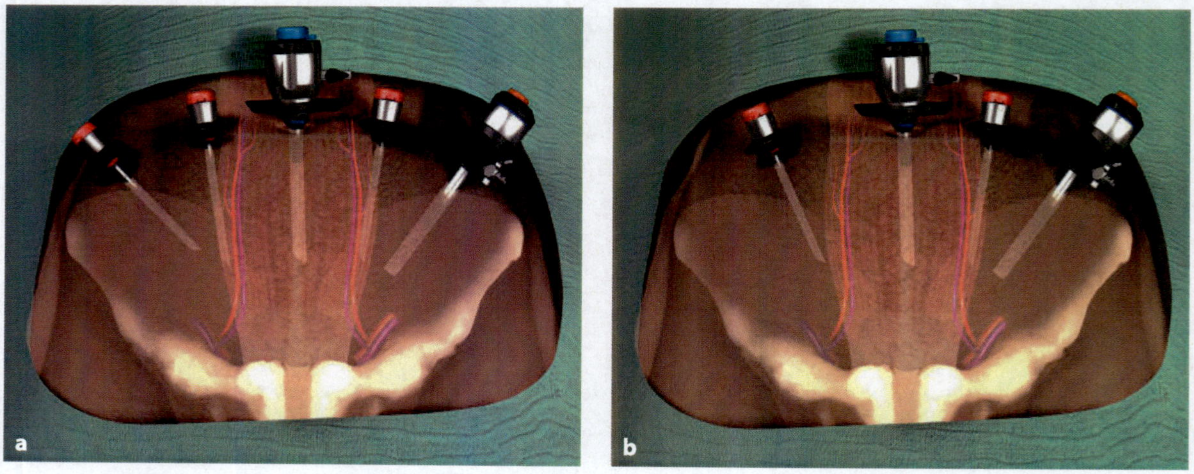

The patient is positioned as described in Sect. 3.1. In most cases, the PLA will be performed during laparoscopic RPE and for this reason five trocars are used. Step 1a illustrates this five-trocar set up. A 12-mm optical trocar is placed in the umbilicus. The other trocars are inserted under direct vision. Compared to the extraperitoneal access, the patient is more a head-down position and all the trocars are placed 2–4 cm more cranially to allow more proximal nodal dissection. Alternatively, when second assistant (camera holder) is not available, a four-trocar technique can be used (Step 1b). The first assistant holds the camera with his left hand and assists with his right hand through the 5-mm trocar in the right iliac fossa.

Step 2: Peritoneal incision and iliac vessel identification

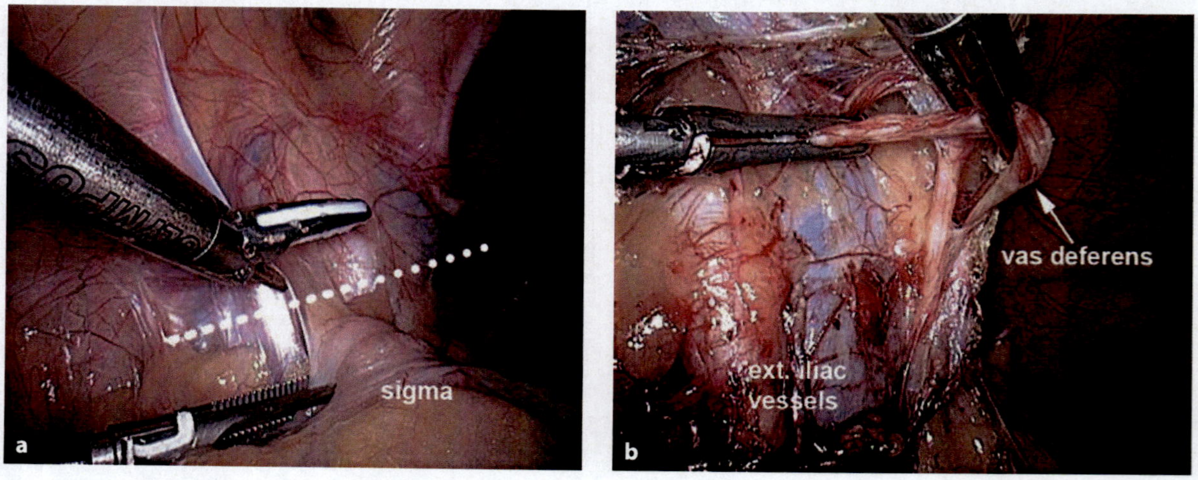

The 30° Trendelenburg position helps prevent the intestinal loops from covering the operative field. Mobilisation of the sigmoid colon or caecum and appendix should be performed as necessary for improved operative field exposure. The peritoneal fold covering the external iliac vessels is seen with the pulsations of the external iliac artery visible underneath. In thin patients, the ureter crossing the common iliac artery can usually be identified medially to the umbilical ligament. An incision in the peritoneum, over the iliac vessels, lateral to the sigmoid colon in a cephalad to caudal direction is performed (Step 2a). The vas deferens is identified and dissected (Step 2b).

Step 3: External iliac vein and artery lymph node dissection

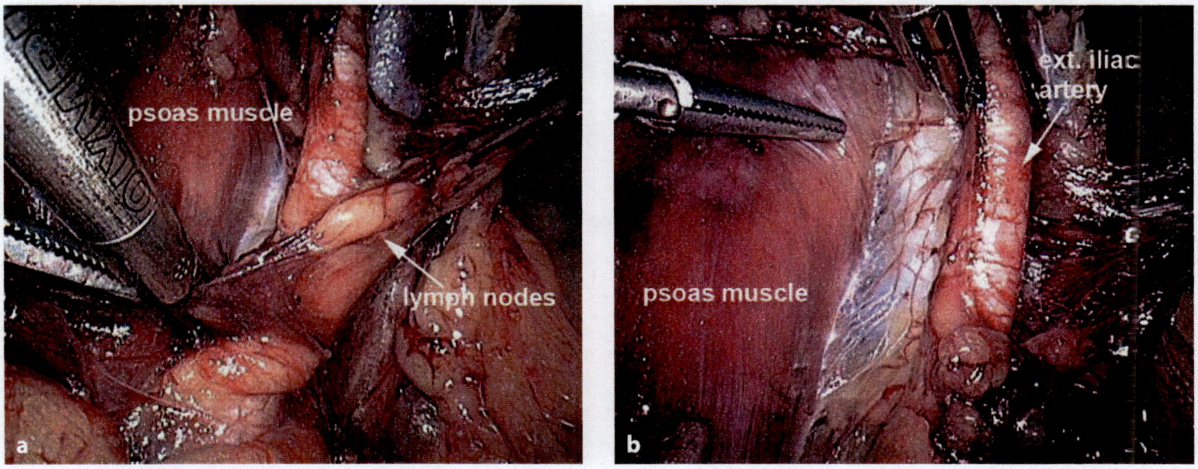

As shown in Step 3a and Step 3b, the external iliac vessels are visible after the dissection of the vas deferens and peritoneal covering. Careful en-bloc excision of the lymph node group located over the anterior and cranial aspect of the iliac artery and medially to the iliopsoas muscle takes place first. Retraction of the lymph node group to the contralateral side by the assistant using graspers facilitates the dissection. Dissection of lymph nodes requires a combination of clipping and coagulation. Larger lymphatic vessels should be clipped while smaller ones can be coagulated or cut with the SonoSurg device.

Step 4: Common iliac artery lymph node dissection

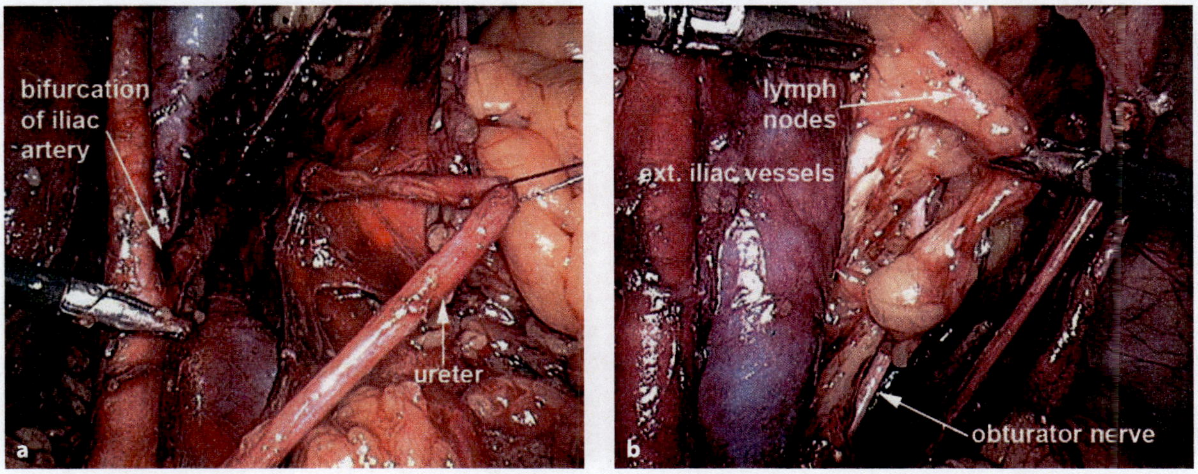

The dissection of the lymph node groups is continued up to the common iliac vessels. The common iliac artery and vein are completely cleared of lymph nodes. This may require further incision of the peritoneum and retraction of the large bowel. At this level, the ureter can be clearly mobilised and protected with a suture for retraction if necessary (Step 4a). Now attention is turned to the obturator fossa. The lymph nodes overlaying the pubic arc at the medial border of the external iliac vein are dissected (Step 4b). This is aided by medial retraction of the group of nodes by the assistant.

Step 5: Obturator fossa lymph node dissection

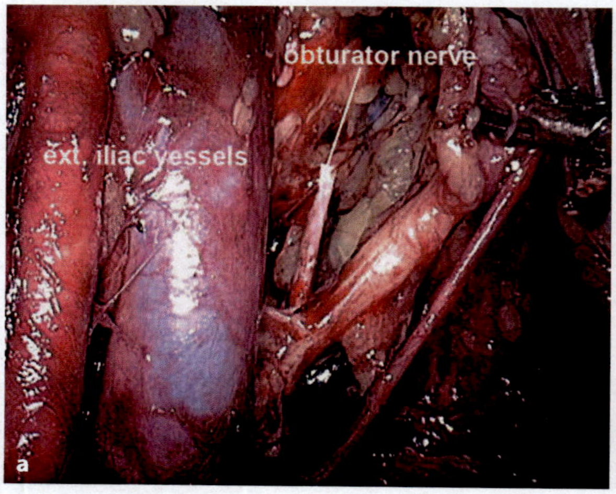

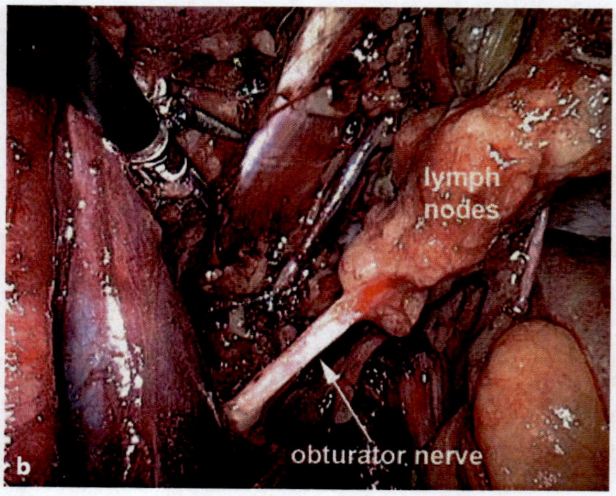

The dissection is continued deep in the obturator fossa and results in complete excision of the lymph node groups lying at the site. The external iliac vein and obturator nerve can be retracted gently with either the surgeon's or the assistant's instruments in order to allow complete dissection of the obturator packet (Step 5b). Careful diathermy at the base of the obturator fossa and behind the external iliac vein is necessary to ensure haemostasis. In case of bleeding, it is possible to clip the obturator artery and/or vein. The nodes ideally should be removed en-bloc. This requires the use of an EndoCatch bag.

Step 6: Internal iliac vessels lymph node dissection

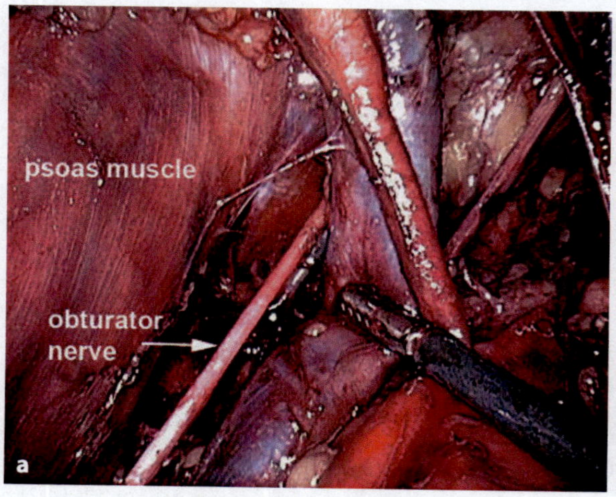

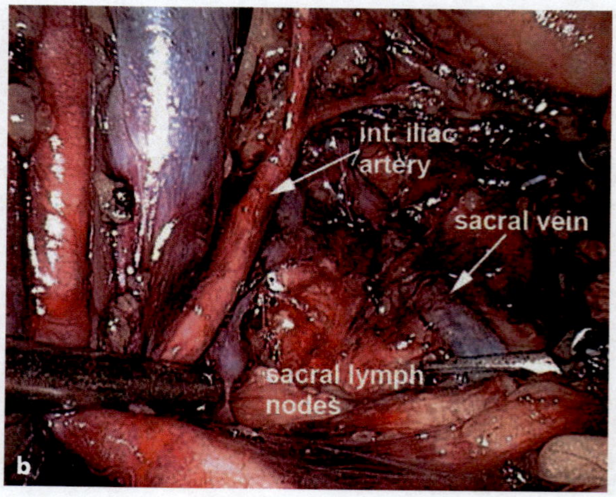

In Step 6a, the external iliac artery and vein are mobilised medially and this allows the obturator nerve to be fully skeletonised. This always should be done to check the completeness of obturator node dissection. The node excision now follows from the iliac artery bifurcation along the internal iliac artery and its branches in an antegrade direction. To make this possible, the assistant has to retract the bladder medially to obtain access. The dissection should also include presacral lymph nodes located between the internal iliac artery and the sacral vein. In this case, a large sacral vein is visible (Step 6b).

Step 7: Internal iliac vessels lymph node dissection

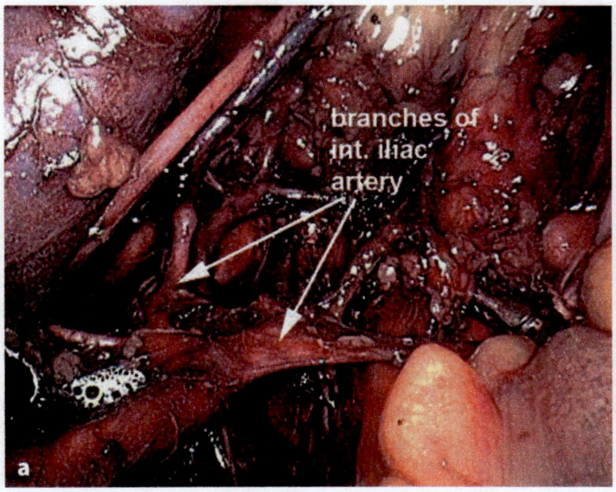

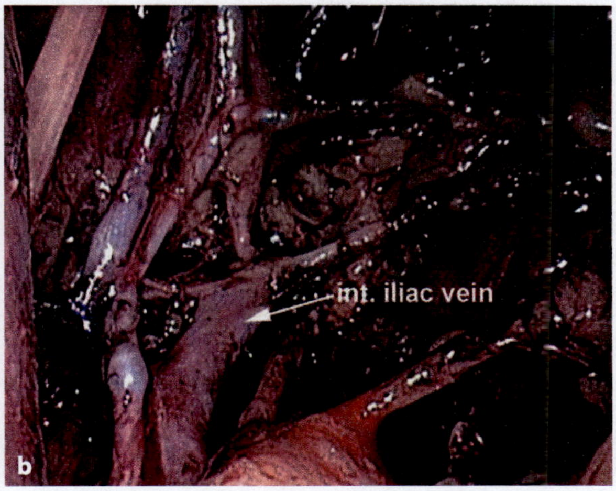

In PLA in patients with high-risk prostate cancer, it is important to perform a complete lymph node dissection, especially including all the branches of the internal iliac vessels. As shown in the figures, the branches can be thoroughly skeletonised laparoscopically. Venous bleeding can present a significant problem if encountered. For this reason, we prefer to use bipolar forceps in one of the surgeon's hands during the dissection to be able to control any bleeding immediately.

Step 8: Aortic bifurcation lymph node dissection

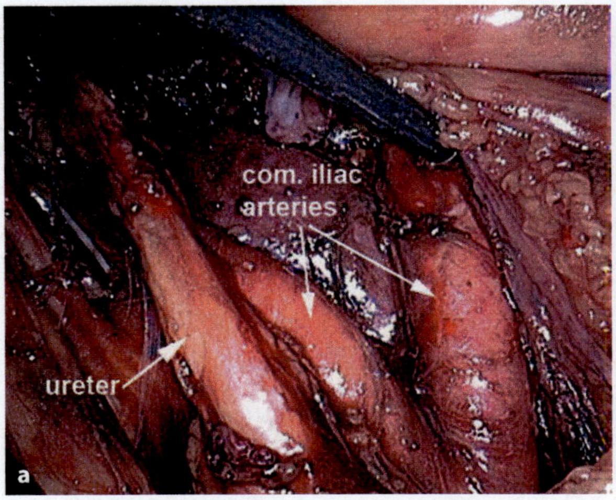

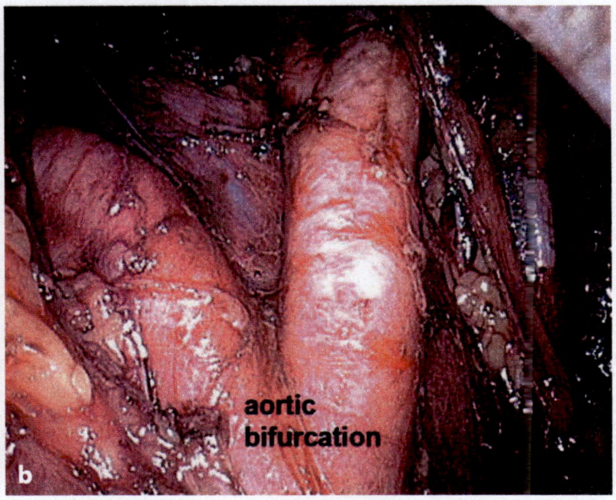

The confluence between the external iliac and the internal iliac artery represents the limit of excision for standard lymphadenectomy. In cases of extended pelvic lymphadenectomy, the dissection continuous in a cephalad direction towards the bifurcation of the aorta (Step 8b). Care should be taken to avoid injuring adjacent structures, especially the ureter. With the help of a stay suture from outside the abdomen, it can be placed either medially or laterally (Step 8a) to the iliac arteries. A further check is made for any bleeding or obvious open lymphatic channels or leaks and these are handled using a combination of clipping and coagulation. Finally a Robinson drain is placed in the iliac fossa.

Postoperative Management

- Clamp the drain on day 1 postoperatively
- Ultrasonic examination for detection of lymphocoele the following day
- If negative remove drain
- Final ultrasound on day before discharge

References

1. Sivalingam S, Oxley J, Probert JL, Stolzenburg JU, Schwaibold H (2007) Role of pelvic lymphadenectomy in prostate cancer management. Urology 69:203–209
2. Briganti A, Blute ML, Eastham JH, Graefen M, Heidenreich A, Karnes JR, Montorsi F, Studer UE (2009) Pelvic lymph node dissection in prostate cancer. Eur Urol 55:1251–1265
3. Studer UE, Collette L (2006) Morbidity from pelvic lymphadenectomy in men undergoing radical prostatectomy. Eur Urol 50:887–892

2.3 Extraperitoneal Pelvic Lymph Node Dissection

Jens-Uwe Stolzenburg, Panagiotis Kallidonis, Minh Do, Rowan Casey, Anja Dietel, Phuc Ho Thi, Alan Mc Neill, Matthias Winkler, Evangelos Liatsikos

Introduction

The extraperitoneal approach for performing pelvic lymphadenectomy (PLA) is an alternative to the transperitoneal method. The main advantages of the extraperitoneal approach are (1) lack of interference from intraperitoneal organs, thus minimising the risk of bowel injury and (2) ease of performing PLA in the case of intraperitoneal adhesions. However, the extraperitoneal approach only allows lymphadenectomy to be performed up to the level of the common iliac artery bifurcation, due to protrusion of the peritoneum and its contents, and not to the level of the aortic bifurcation. The extended PLA (including common iliac artery and presacral nodes) is technically very difficult, apart from in thin patients, by the extraperitoneal approach.

The benefits of the extended PLA beyond the level of the common iliac vessels remain questionable in terms of morbidity and cure rates [1]. A further disadvantage or the extraperitoneal technique is the higher rate of symptomatic lymphocoele formation. Various techniques to try to diminish lymphocoele formation have been attempted [2, 3], but bilateral fenestration of the peritoneum at the end of the procedure significantly reduces the incidence of lymphocoele formation [4)]

Indications

- Prostate cancer with PSA more than 10 ng/ml and the Gleason biopsy score is 7 or higher with or without the presence of palpable tumour
- Nomogram-based selection of patients
- Enlargement of pelvic lymph nodes as seen by imaging techniques or intraoperatively (relative indication)

Contra-indications

- Uncorrectable coagulopathy
- Previous extraperitoneal or transperitoneal mesh placement for inguinal hernia repair (because of adhesions technically impossible; the mesh covers the region of the nodes)

Preoperative Preparation

- Preoperative preparation of patients undergoing extraperitoneal PLA is similar to extraperitoneal laparoscopic radical prostatectomy

Step 1: Patient position and trocar placement

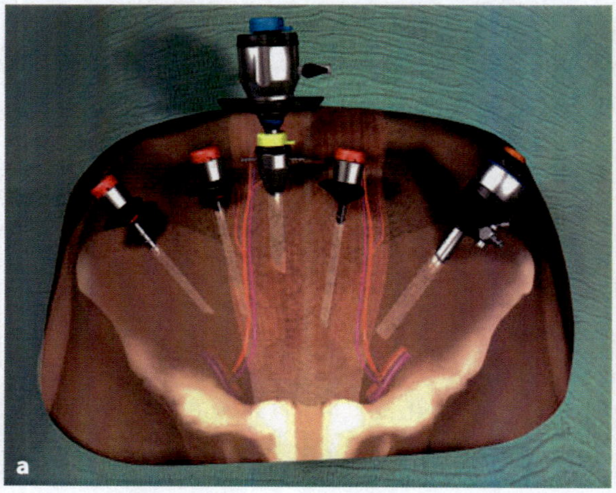

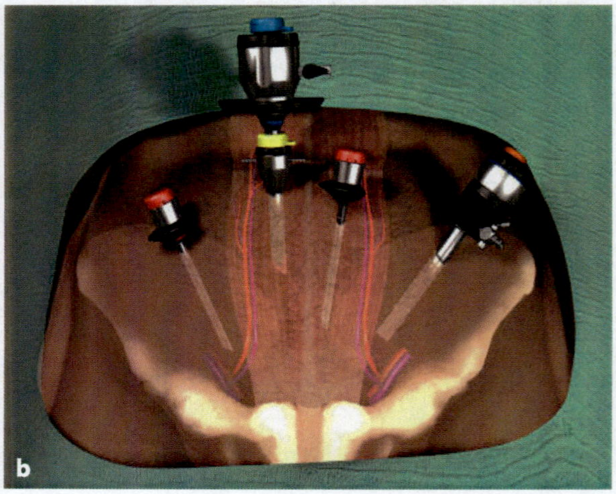

The patient is positioned the same way as for endoscopic extraperitoneal radical prostatectomy (EERPE). In most cases, the PLA will be performed during EERPE and for this reason the same five trocars are used (see Step 1a). The trocar placement is fully described in Sect. 3.4. If PLA is performed as a staging procedure (e.g. prior to radiotherapy) it is possible to use only four trocars. The difference to the five-trocar setup is that the assistant is holding the camera with his left hand and is assisting with his right hand. Therefore, a 5-mm trocar is placed in the right iliac fossa, as shown in Step 1b.

Step 2: External iliac vein and artery lymph node dissection

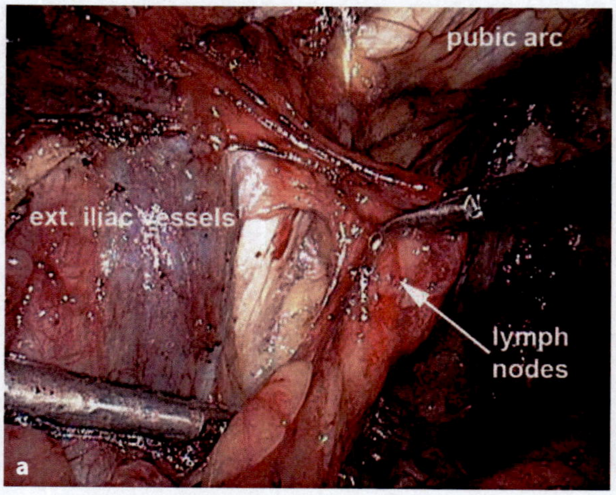

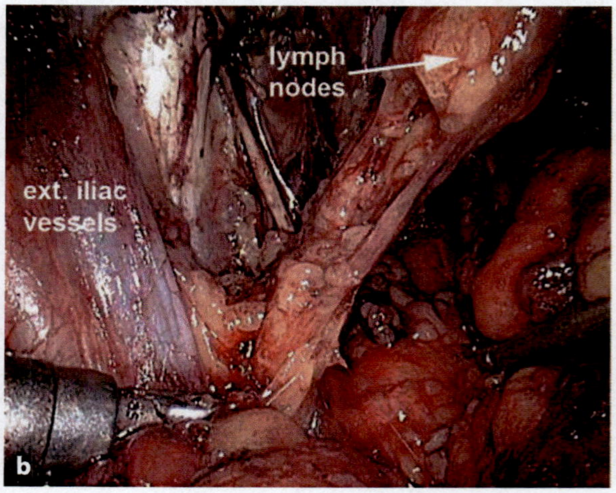

The extraperitoneal approach does not require any dissection of the peritoneum, mobilisation of the colon or division of vas deferens. The access provides direct visualisation of the external iliac vessels. Lymph node groups located medially to the external iliac vein, extending into the obturator fossa, are retracted medially by the assistant and carefully dissected. The dissection technique requires careful clipping and dissection of the lymphatic vessels, especially superior to the pubic bone. The dissection follows by removing any lymph node groups overlying the external iliac artery. The location of the external iliac vein must be noted when dissecting the artery as it lies in close proximity and must be correctly separated from the node group.

Step 3: Obturator fossa lymph node dissection

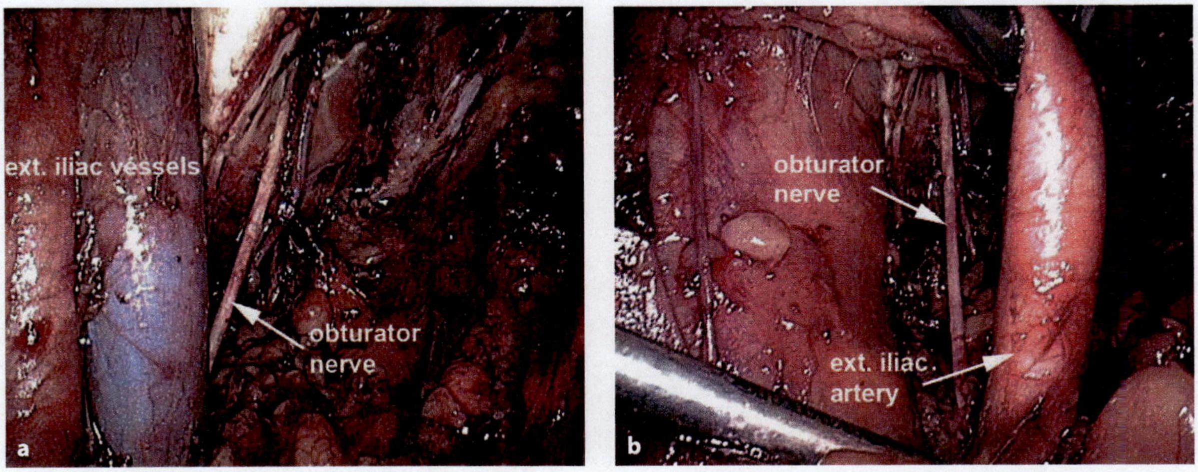

The dissection is continued into the obturator fossa. The obturator nerve should be kept in view at all times to prevent injury to the nerve. This dissection is continued deep in the obturator fossa on both sides of the obturator nerve. The assistant uses a sucker and grasping forceps in order to pull the node packet medially and retract the bladder to allow dissection. The surgeon uses a bipolar forceps and the SonoSurg device. The combination of clips + SonoSurg and bipolar coagulation helps to reduce the incidence of lymphocoele formation. In Step 3b, the external iliac artery is mobilised medially and this allows the obturator nerve to be fully skeletonised.

Step 4: Node dissection at the iliac bifurcation

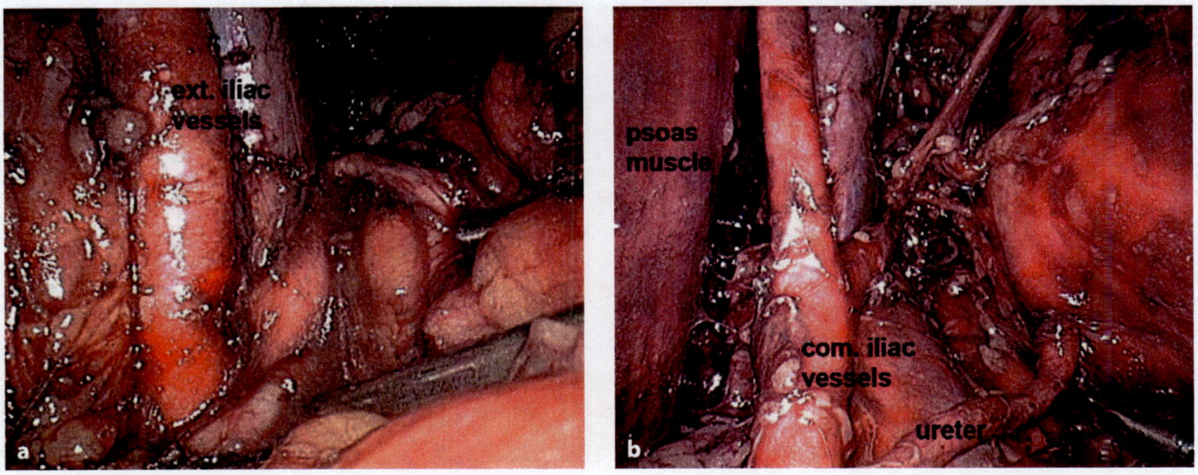

The dissection continues in a cephalad direction along the external iliac artery up to the level of the common iliac artery bifurcation. The assistant must provide sufficient retraction of the peritoneum with graspers and the bladder with the sucker in order to facilitate this. Step 4a shows the standard anatomical appearance in extraperitoneal PLA. The extraperitoneal approach allows lymphadenectomy to be performed up to the level of the common iliac artery bifurcation. In thin patients, it is possible to extend the level of PLA further up the common iliac artery. Beware of the ureter crossing the common iliac bifurcation.

Step 5: Internal iliac vessel node dissection

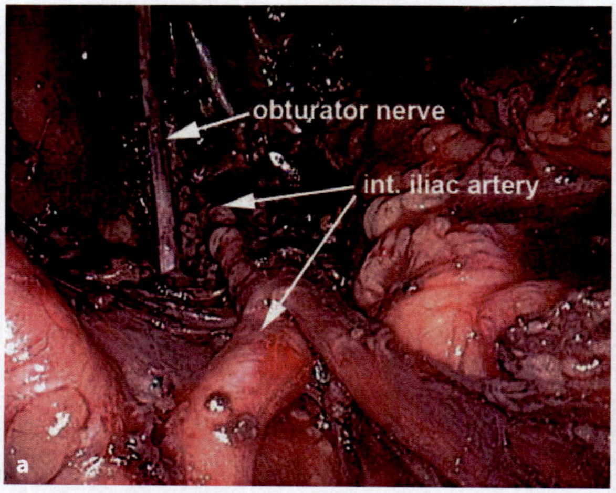

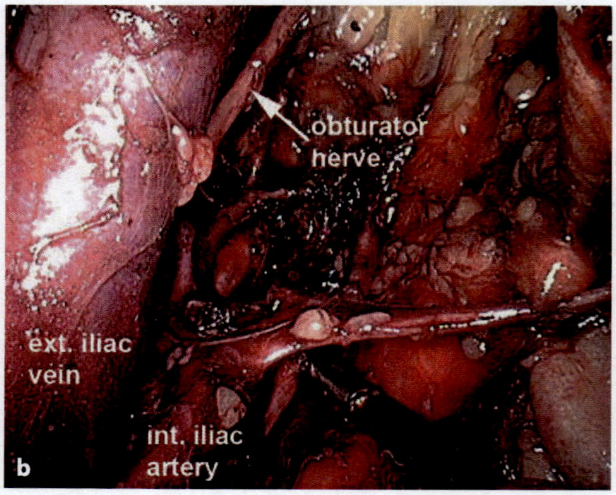

The dissection is now continued along the internal iliac artery. The branches of the internal iliac artery should be cleared of lymphatic tissue, as shown in Step 5a and Step 5b. The same procedure is now used on the lymph node groups on the contralateral side. This requires a slightly different technique as the main surgeon is on the left side of the patient. In this situation, the main surgeon retracts the lymph node packet medially and the assistant provides more assistance in retracting the external iliac artery and vein and surrounding tissue. Alternatively, the main surgeon may change sides. The 12-mm trocar is usually adequate for lymph node extraction, although it may require some dissection of nodal packages prior to removal.

Step 6: Fenestration of the peritoneum (right side)

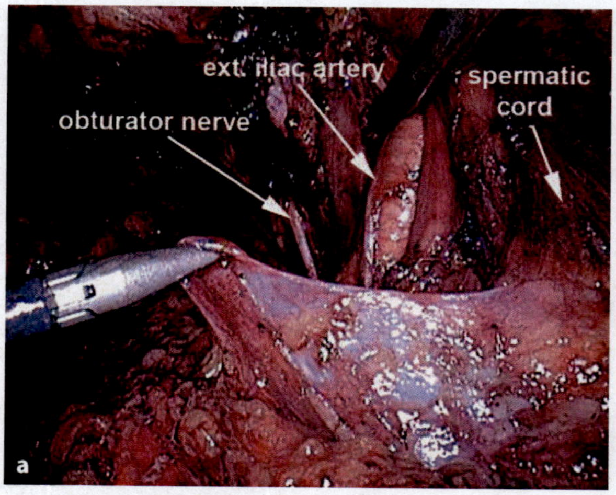

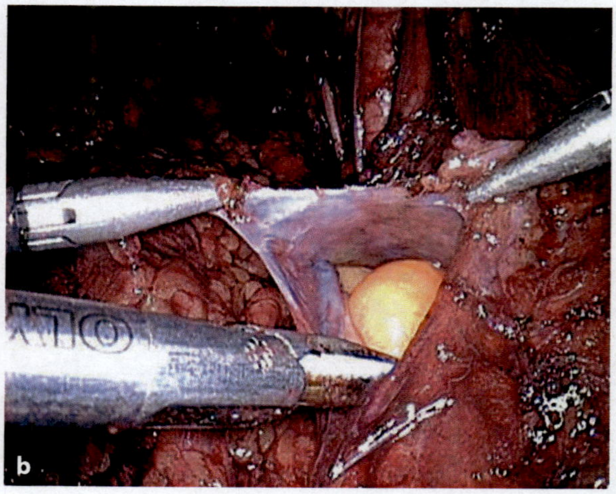

Fenestration of the peritoneum provides sufficient drainage into the peritoneal cavity to help prevent significant symptomatic lymphocoele formation (keep in mind this is an optional step). The surgeon and assistant grasp peritoneal fold proximally to the external iliac artery at the level of the spermatic cord (Step 6a). It is elevated to avoid bowel injury and incised using the SonoSurg device. The bowel within it is visualised (Step 6b) and the opening is developed towards the pelvis to enlarge it, as is shown in Step 7 for the left side, which must be carried out next.

Step 7: Fenestration of the peritoneum (left side)

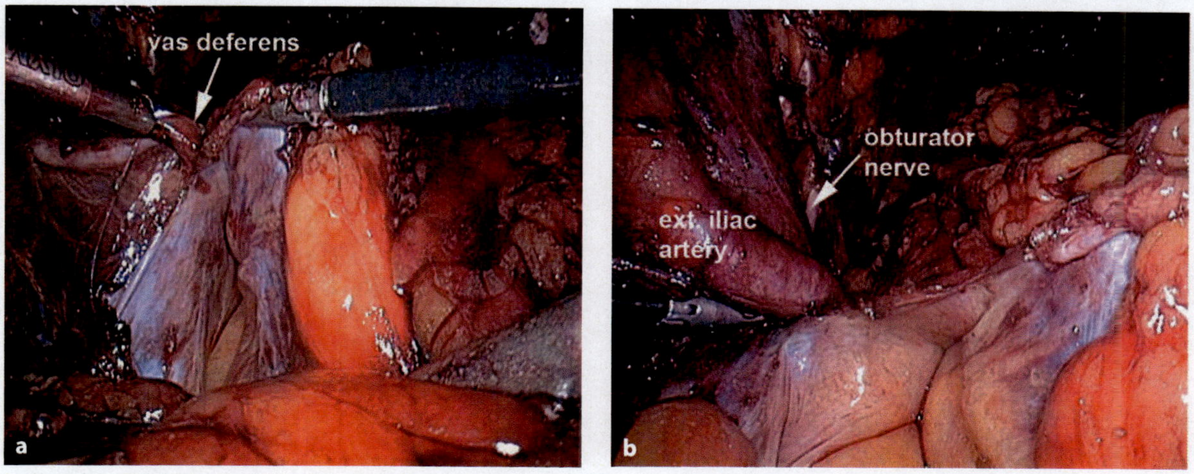

Following the initial peritoneal incision, the spermatic cord and vas are identified as the dissection proceeds distally. The vas can be divided at this point (Step 7a). The opening is now developed slightly further towards the obturator fossa (Step 7b). These openings should now be sufficient to provide drainage. If bowel adhesions from previous surgery are a possibility or other risk factors exist, we recommend fenestration only on one side. A nonsuction drain is inserted into the left iliac fossa through a 5-mm port site.

Postoperative Management

- Clamp the drain on day 1 postoperatively
- Ultrasonic examination for detection of lymphocoele the following day
- If negative remove drain
- Final ultrasound on day before discharge

References

1. Inderbir S Gill (2006) Textbook of laparoscopic urology. Informa Healthcare, New York
2. Simonato A, Varca V, Esposito M, Venzano F, Carmignani G (2009) The use of a surgical patch in the prevention of lymphoceles after extraperitoneal pelvic lymphadenectomy for prostate cancer: a randomized prospective pilot study. J Urol 182:2285–2290
3. Albala DM, Kevwitch MK, Waters WB (1993) Treatment of persistent lymphatic drainage after laparoscopic pelvic lymph node dissection and radical retropubic prostatectomy. J Endourol 7:337–340
4. Stolzenburg JU, Wasserscheid J, Rabenalt R, Do M, Schwalenberg T, McNeill A, Constantinides C, Kallidonis P, Ganzer R, Liatsikos E (2008) Reduction in incidence of lymphocele following extraperitoneal radical prostatectomy and pelvic lymph node dissection by bilateral peritoneal fenestration. World J Urol 26:581–586

Chapter 3

Urinary Bladder and Prostate

CONTENTS

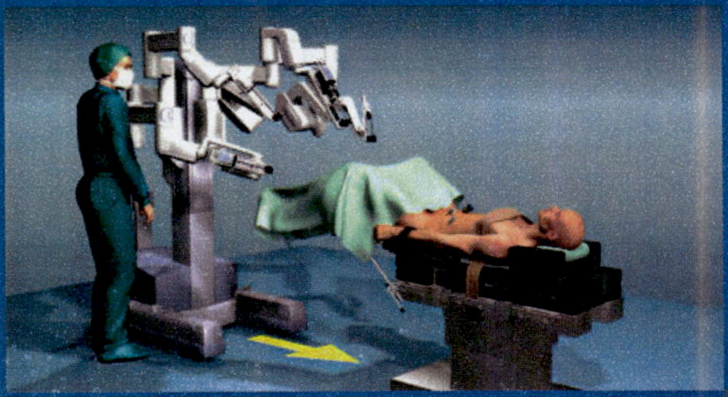

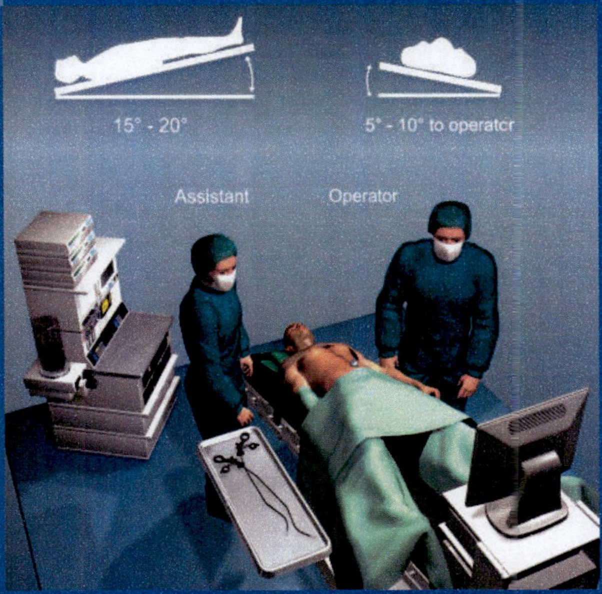

J.-U. Stolzenburg, I. Türk, E. Liatsikos: *Laparoscopic and Robot-Assisted Surgery in Urology*
DOI: 10.1007/978-3-642-00891-7_3, © Springer-Verlag Berlin Heidelberg 2011

3.1 Anatomical Considerations for Nerve-Sparing Pelvic Surgery

Thilo Schwalenberg, Jochen Neuhaus, Panagiotis Kallidonis, Evangelos N. Liatsikos, Jens-Uwe Stolzenburg

New operating procedures that spare the important neural structures of the urogenital tract have led to improved functional results in terms of bladder function, urinary continence and erectile potency. Well-described examples are nerve-sparing radical prostatectomy [1–3] and cystectomy (continence, potency) [3, 4], ureteric antireflux surgery (bladder function) [5], extended radical hysterectomy with total mesometrial resection (bladder function) [6] and rectal resection (continence, bladder function, potency) [7].

In general, the sympathetic innervation is responsible for secretory functions of prostate and seminal vesicles as well as ejaculation. Hence, injury to the pelvic sympathetic fibres during the concomitant extended lymphadenectomy of a radical cystectomy or retroperitoneal lymph node dissection for testicular cancer may cause retrograde ejaculation. Stimulation of parasympathetic nerves leads to dilatation of smooth-muscle-lined cavernosal sinuses, which effects influx of blood with subsequent tumescence. As a result, the parasympathetic system is the main neural component for erectile function.

The following table shows historically important publications which have profoundly influenced the understanding and surgical methodology in the quest for preservation of autonomic pelvic nerves.

Author	Findings
Müller (1835) F. Dummler, Berlin 1836	Detailed anatomic drawings of autonomic fibres within the pelvis; distinction of sympathetic and parasympathetic portions as well as fibres supplying the penis and, as a result of their proximity to the lateral surface of the prostate, the description of a plexus prostaticus; demarcation of the pudendal nerve
Budge (1858) Virchows Archive 15	First experimental investigations with electrical stimulation of the hypogastric nerve in animals and measurement of response at the ejaculatory duct and seminal vesicles
Eckard (1863) Anat Physiol 3:123–166	Experimental investigations and description of the relationship between pelvic plexus and erection in animals; definition of nervi erigentes as the main parasympathetic nerves for erection
Calabrisi (1955) George Washington University School of Medicine	Survey of the origin of cavernosal nerves and description of their anatomic pathway in the foetal and embryonic state
Davis and Jelenko (1975) South Med J 68:422–426	Reflections on sexual changes in patients after abdominoperineal resection; discussion of the protection of the pelvic plexus to preserve postoperative sexual function
Walsh and Donker (1982) J Urol 128:492–497	Description of the neurovascular bundle, coinage of the term "anatomical radical prostatectomy" with protection of the dorsolaterally localised neurovascular bundle; the first definition of a valid operational standard
Lue et al. (1984) J Urol 131:273–280	Comparative nerve topography of erection by means of cadaveric dissection in animal and man
Lepor et al. (1985) J Urol 133:207–212	Detailed nerve topography and precise relationship of cavernosal nerves of the pelvis plexus to urethra, lateral pelvic fascia, prostatica capsula and Denonvilliers fascia
Schlegel and Walsh (1987) J Urol 138:1402–1406	The importance of neurovascular bundle preservation in radical cystectomy
Jünemann et al. (1988) J Urol 139:74–80	Sacral and pudendal plexus, differentiated investigations of the sacral roots S2–S4
Fritsch (1989) Anat Embryol (Berl) 180:57–64	Topography of the pelvic plexus in the foetal state (21–29 weeks); Definition of pelvic connective tissues, study of fibre direction along the urethral sphincter
Stelzner et al. (1989) Chirurg 60:228–234	Experience from potency-preserving rectal surgery; investigation of embryos and newborns; relationship between nervi erigentes, anterior rectal wall, pelvic floor and the diaphragmatic part of the urethra before entering the two cavernosal bodies of the penis, exact determination of nerve density at the anterior rectal wall, preservation of sexual function using own patient population
Breza et al. (1989) J Urol 141:437–443	Cadaveric study on the description of vascular anatomy, in particular at the entrance to the cavernosal bodies; proof of connections between dorsal nerve and cavernosal nerve of penis at the crura penis
Stief et al. (1991) J Urol 146:771–776	Role of the sympathetic nervous system during erection

Author	Findings
Paick et al. (1993) Urology 42:145–149	Study on adult cadavers with detailed description of the autonomous nerve fibre direction distal to the prostate up to the entrance into the cavernosal bodies; description of medial urethral branches of the cavernosal nerve, interaction between cavernosal nerve and dorsal nerve of penis
Zvara et al. (1994) Br J Urol 74:182–187	Detailed neuroanatomy of the urethral sphincter, innervation of intrinsic and extrinsic segments of the urethral sphincter by sacral segments S2–4 of the pudendal nerve
Strasser et Bartsch (1996) Prostate 28:24–3125	Innervation of urethral sphincter (described as striated sphincter, "rhabdosphincter", by authors) by pudendal nerve, no role of cavernosal nerve and pelvic plexus; autonomous fibres of the pelvic plexus run to the membranous urethra
Höckel et al. (1998) Am J Obstet Gynecol 178:971–976	Development of the liposuction-assisted nerve-sparing extended radical hysterectomy to improve conventional gynaecological pelvic surgery and avoid urinary bladder dysfunction
Höer et al. (2000) Chirurg 71:1222–1229	Cadaveric study; detailed description of the topography of autonomic nerves and their lesions in pelvic surgery; the importance of a sympathetic lesion during high ligation of the inferior mesenteric artery; discussion of differences in terminology of the pelvic fascia and anatomical landmarks in pelvic surgery
Leißner et al. (2001) J Urol 165:1652–1655	Accurate topography of the pelvic plexus and related fibres on human cadavers fixed with Thiel solution; staining of the nerves with methylene blue; description of lesions of the pelvic plexus; clinical importance during antireflux surgery and trigonal reconstruction in prostate surgery; the article also refers to the possible intraoperative use of methylene blue to identify autonomic nerves
Akita et al. (2003) Surg Radiol Anat 25:387–392	Detailed cadaveric study on the origin and anatomical pathway of nerves supplying the urethral sphincter; innervation of the urethral sphincter by pudendal nerve and pelvic plexus
Kiyoshima et al. (2004) Jpn J Clin Oncol 34:463–468	Detailed investigations of the periprostatic fibromuscular stroma regarding the existence and course of fascial structures (Denonvilliers fascia, lateral pelvic fascia) and nerve structures, preparations after non-nerve-sparing radical prostatectomy; a dorsolateral-located neurovascular bundle (NVB) was found in only 48%, the NVB was separated by adipose tissue in 52% and neural structures were spread over the lateral surface of the prostate without classic bundling
Costello et al. (2004) BJU Int 94:1071–1076	Detailed topography of the NVB in cadavers; classification of the NVB into three functional compartments (posterior/posterolateral [rectum, lateral], levator ani, anterior, prostate/cavernosal nerves); clinical importance of sural nerve graft interposition after sacrifice of the cavernosal nerves during radical prostatectomy
Takenaka et al. (2005) Eur Urol 48:46–52	Interindividual variation in distribution of the extramural ganglion cells in the male pelvis; immunohistochemical differentiation into sympathetic and parasympathetic ganglia; description of autonomic cells not only in nerve components but also along viscera in coexistence with both cell types in a ganglion

Figure1: Sympathetic and parasympathetic system

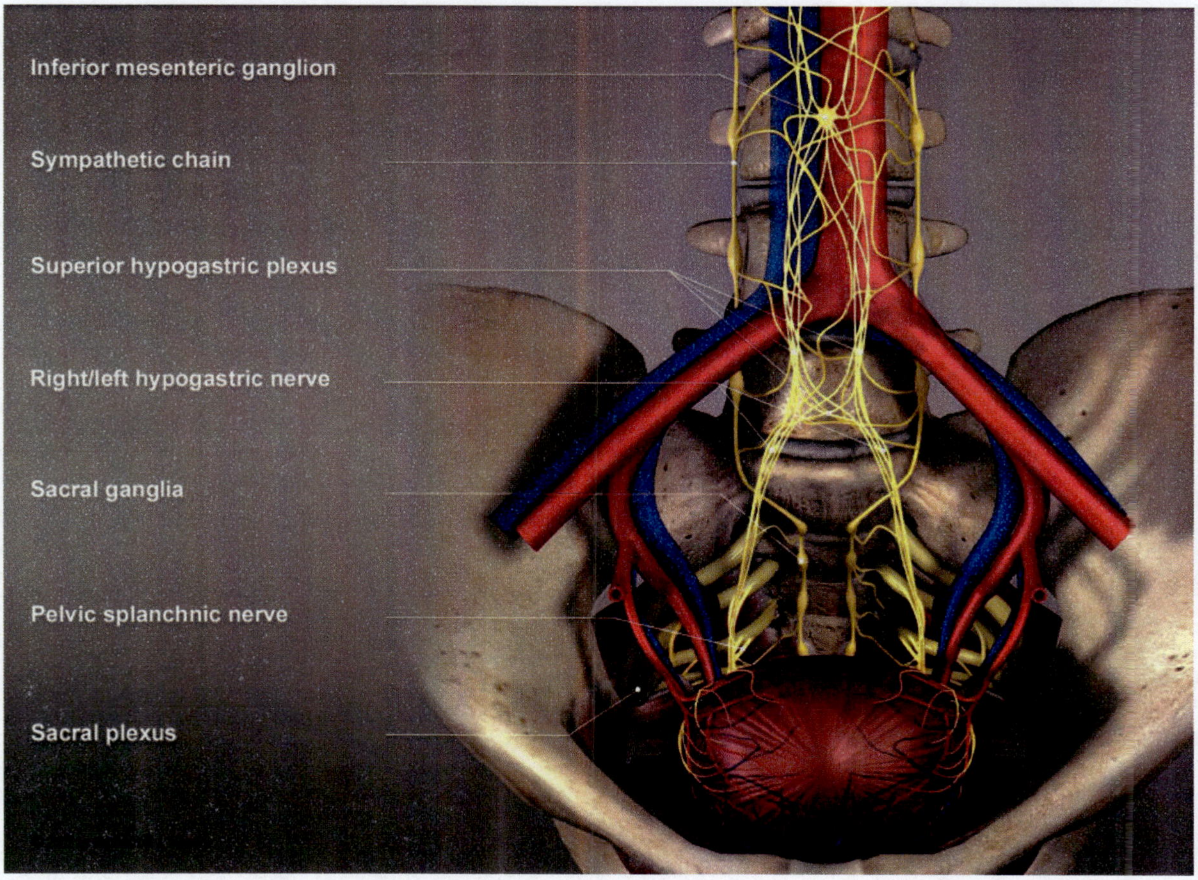

Sympathetic fibres responsible for the innervation of the lower urinary tract and male genital organs arise from thoracolumbar segments T10–12 and L1–2. They leave the spinal column via the anterior rami of the spinal nerves and finally reach the sympathetic chain via communicating rami albi. The main sympathetic effect at the end organ is vasoconstriction. The sacral component of the parasympathetic system originates from spinal segments S2–4. Sacral fibres run in the spinal nerves of the pudendal plexus but emerge shortly after exit from the sacral foramina as pelvic splanchnic nerves (see Fig. 2). Their further presynaptic course follows the rectum and the dorsolateral boundaries of the prostate.

Figure 2: Pelvic plexus (inferior hypogastric plexus, pelvic ganglion)

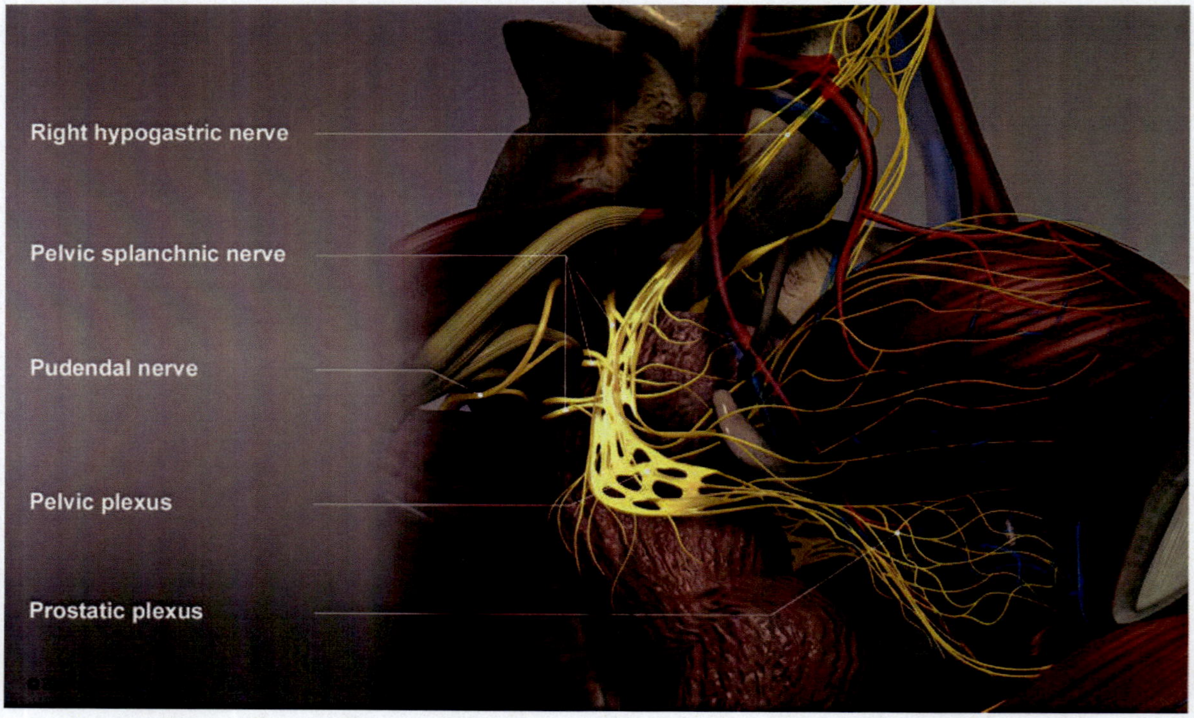

The sacral component of the parasympathetic system originates from spinal segments S2–4. Sacral fibres run in the spinal nerves of the pudendal plexus but emerge shortly after exit from the sacral foramina as pelvic splanchnic nerves. The pelvic plexus is a collection of ganglia which is located lateral to pelvic organs. It has a rhombic shape with a longitudinal diameter of approximately 5 cm and is located at the apex of the seminal vesicles. In the male, the plexus is situated laterally to the rectum, seminal vesicle, prostate and the posterior part of the bladder. These structures may be injured during radical cystectomy, rectal resection, ureteric antireflux surgery or extended radical hysterectomy (Wertheim operation).

Figure 3: Neurovascular bundle and prostatic plexus

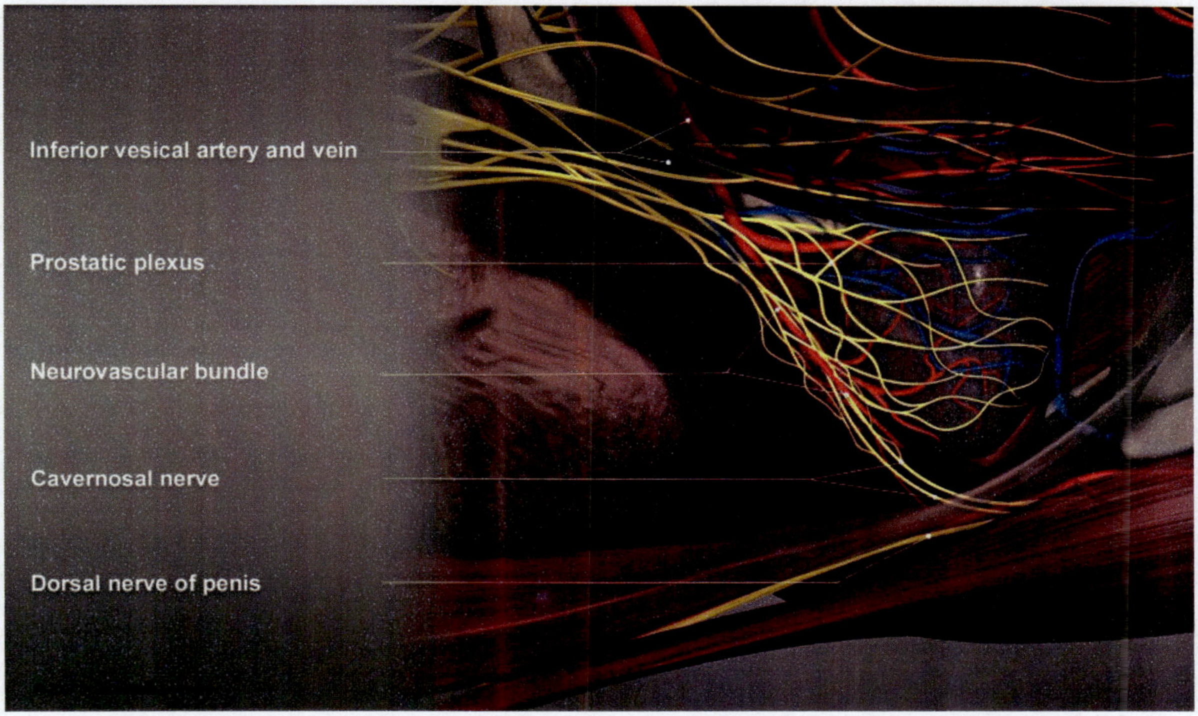

The nerve-sparing radical prostatectomy was developed to protect the pelvic plexus and the cavernosal nerves of the penis arising from the NVB. The nerve fibres of the NVB are of microscopic calibre and can only be recognised by the accompanying vascular structures. Accompanying arterial vessels arise from the prostatic arteries. Venous vessels channel into the prostatic venous plexus. In most patients, a nerve distribution on the whole lateral and partly on the posterior surface of the prostate can be found (prostatic plexus). The neurovascular bundle emerges from the pelvic plexus and continues distally as cavernosal nerves of the penis. The prostatic plexus supplies the prostate. The pudendal nerve continues as the dorsal nerve of the penis and lies externally to the levator hammock.

Figure 4: The cavernosal nerve

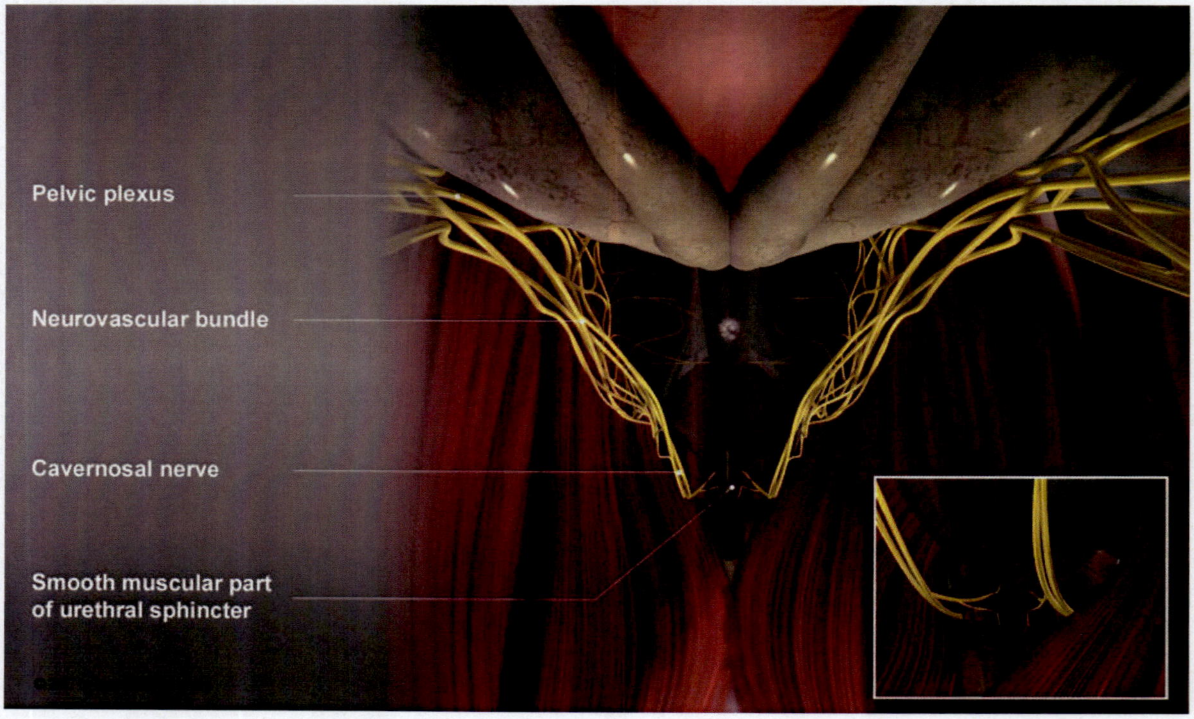

Figure 4 shows that the cavernosal nerves of the penis traverse the apex of the prostate at a distance of only a few millimetres from the prostatic capsule at the 5 and 7 o'clock positions. It divides into medial and lateral branches after penetration of the muscular pelvis. Medial branches innervate the smooth muscle component of the external urethral sphincter; lateral branches continue to enter the cavernosal bodies. Together with the deep artery and vein of the penis, the cavernosal nerves of the penis enter the crura after exiting from the muscular pelvis. Stimulation of parasympathetic nerves leads to dilatation of smooth-muscle-lined cavernosal sinuses, which effects influx of blood with subsequent tumescence. Hence, the parasympathetic system is the main neural component for erectile function.

Figure 5: Pudendal nerve

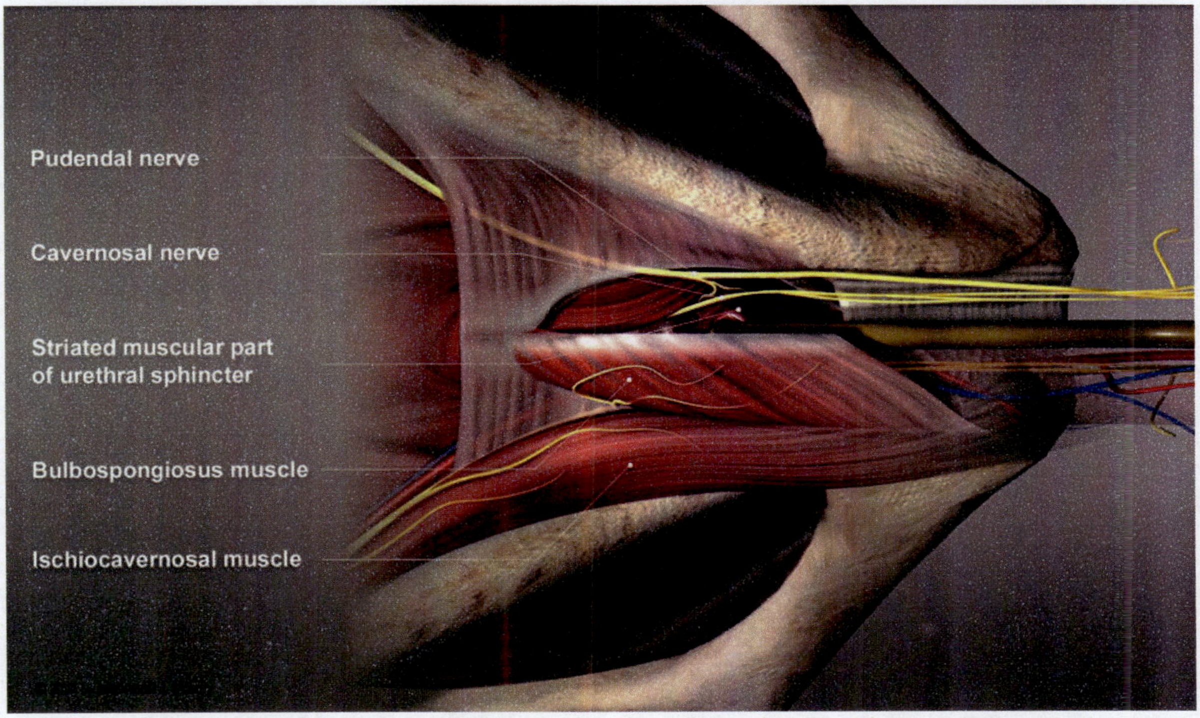

The pudendal nerve emerges from the pudendal plexus as essentially the cutaneous nerve and exits the small pelvis together with internal pudendal artery and vein. It runs in the direction of the ischiac spine and emerges from the ischioanal fossa in a fascial sheath of the internal obturator muscle (Alcock canal). The pudendal nerve is a somatosensory nerve with clear topographical separation from the cavernosal nerves of the penis, as shown in this figure. The pudendal nerve gives off motor branches to the bulbospongiosus muscle, ischiocavernosus muscle and the striated component of the external urethral sphincter. Contrary to pelvic bone injuries and injuries related to vaginal delivery, operations inside the pelvis have negligible risk of injuring the pudendal nerve.

Figure 6: Principles of intrafascial nerve-sparing radical prostatectomy

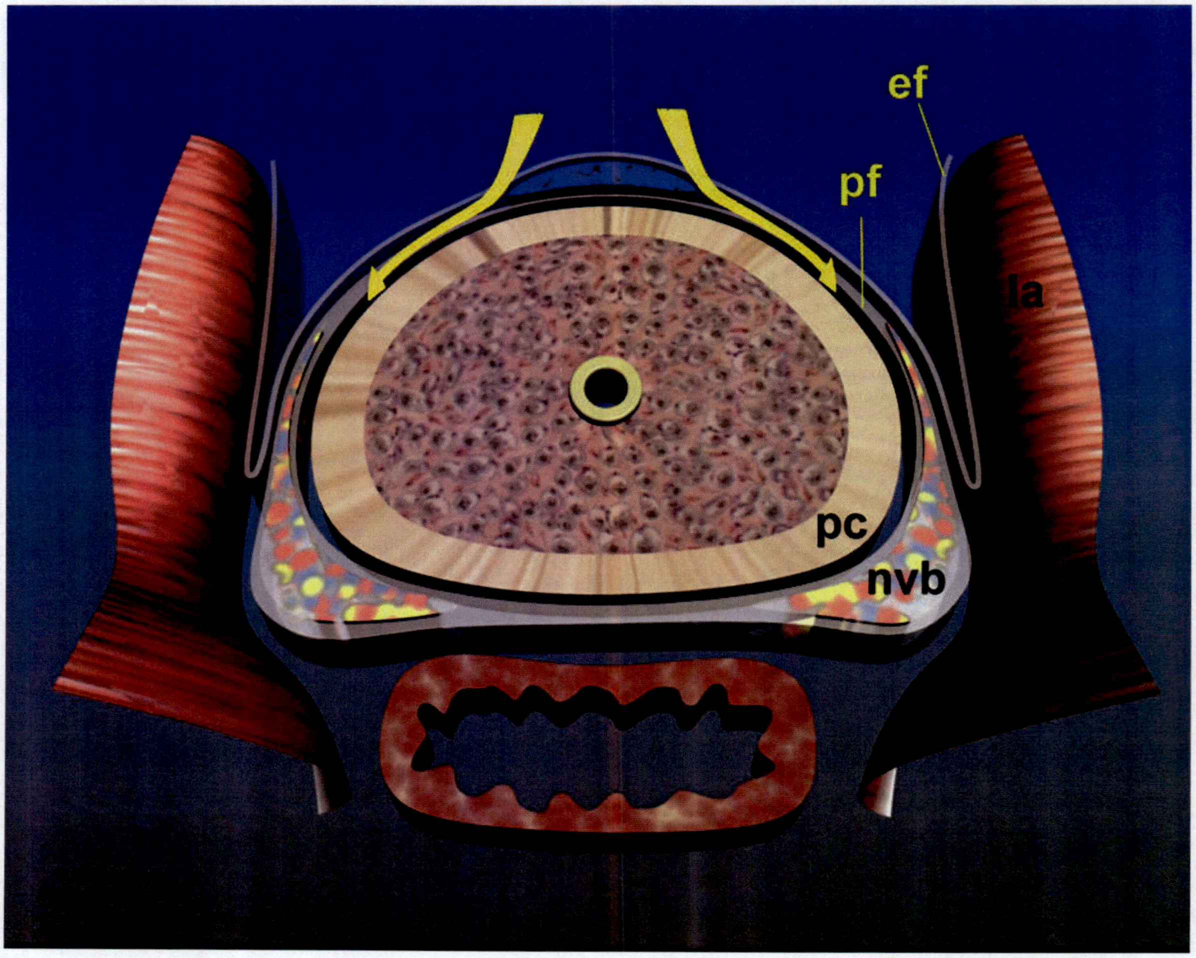

During the intrafascial nerve-sparing endoscopic extraperitoneal prostatectomy, the endopelvic fascia (ef) is incised only medially to the puboprostatic ligaments, while its portion overlying the levator ani (la) remains intact. The dissection is performed on the prostatic capsule, freeing the prostate laterally from its thin surrounding fascia (periprostatic fascia, pf) which contains small vessels and nerves. The dorsal dissection plane is between Denonvilliers fascia and prostatic capsula.

Figure 7: Interfascial and intrafascial nerve-sparing radical prostatectomy

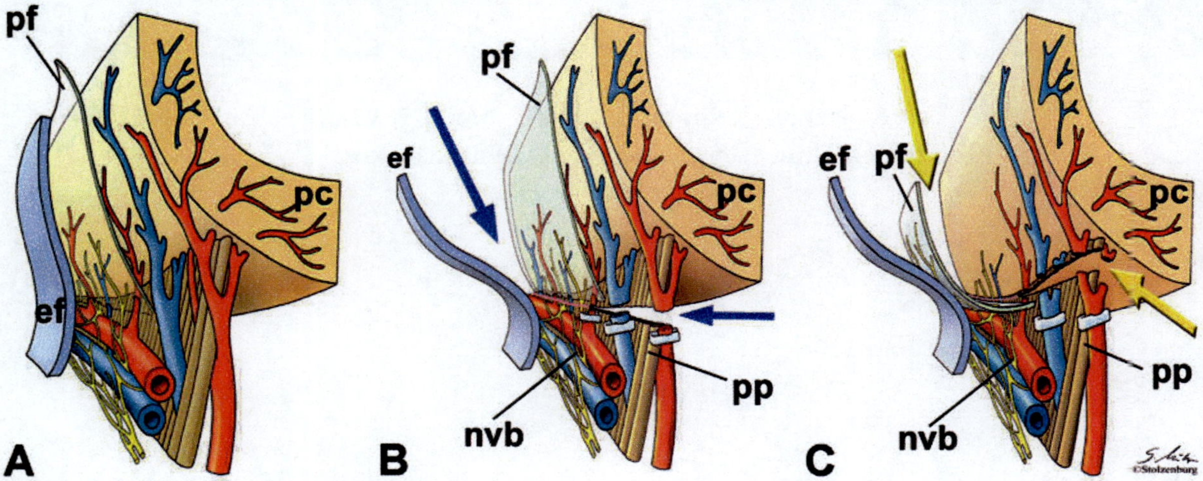

The prostate is covered by endopelvic and periprostatic fascia (Fig. 7a). The endopelvic fascia (ef) is incised and the neurovascular bundles (nvb) and prostatic pedicles (pp) are spared posterolaterally in the interfascial technique (Fig. 7b). In the intrafascial technique (Fig. 7c) the endopelvic fascia, the periprostatic fascia (pf) and the Denonvilliers fascia are not a part of the specimen because the dissection plane is directly on the prostatic capsula (pc).

References

1. Schwalenberg T, Neuhaus J, Liatsikos E, Winkler M, Loffler S, Stolzenburg JU (2010) Neuroanatomy of the male pelvis in respect to radical prostatectomy including three-dimensional visualization. BJU Int 105:21–27
2. Stolzenburg JU, Rabenalt R, Tannapfel A, Liatsikos EN (2006) Intrafascial nerve-sparing endoscopic extraperitoneal radical prostatectomy. Urology 67:17–21
3. Walsh PC, Schlegel PN (1988) Radical pelvic surgery with preservation of sexual function. Ann Surg 208:391–400
4. Schlegel PN, Walsh PC (1987) Neuroanatomical approach to radical cystoprostatectomy with preservation of sexual function. J Urol 138:1402–1406
5. Leissner J, Allhoff EP, Wolff W et al. The pelvic plexus and antireflux surgery: topographical findings and clinical consequences. J Urol. 2001;165:1652-1655
6. Hockel M, Horn LC, Hentschel B, Hockel S, Naumann G (2003) Total mesometrial resection: high resolution nerve-sparing radical hysterectomy based on developmentally defined surgical anatomy. Int J Gynecol Cancer 13:791–803
7. Stelzner F, Fritsch H, Fleischhauer K (1989) [The surgical anatomy of the genital nerves of the male and their preservation in excision of the rectum]. Chirurg 60:228–234

3.2 Patient Position for Pelvic Surgery

Jens-Uwe Stolzenburg, Rowan Casey, Jens Mondry, Minh Do, Anja Dietel, Tim Haefner, Thilo Schwalenberg, Evangelos Liatsikos

Step 1: Supine position

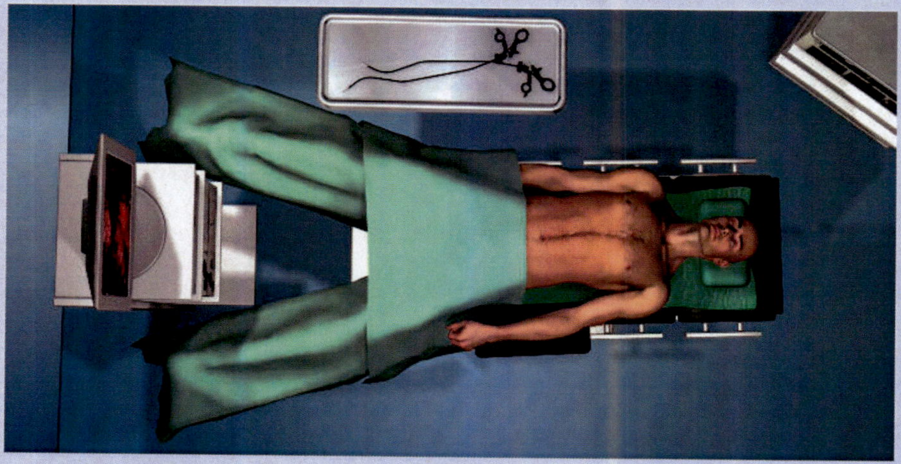

The steps described in this section will show the details of our preferred position in pure laparoscopic and robot-assisted pelvic surgery. The patient is positioned in a supine position. This can be done with the legs together or with abducted legs (as shown in Step 1) on movable leg-boards for three reasons. Firstly, it allows the monitor and laparoscopic stack to be positioned closer to the surgeon and assistant to optimise the ergonomic advantage for both. Secondly, it allows a cystoscopy prior to pelvic procedures such as prostatectomy. Thirdly, it allows access to the perineum intraoperatively. Furthermore, a roll of padding is placed in both popliteal fossae to prevent knee hyperextension.

Step 2: Position of the arms

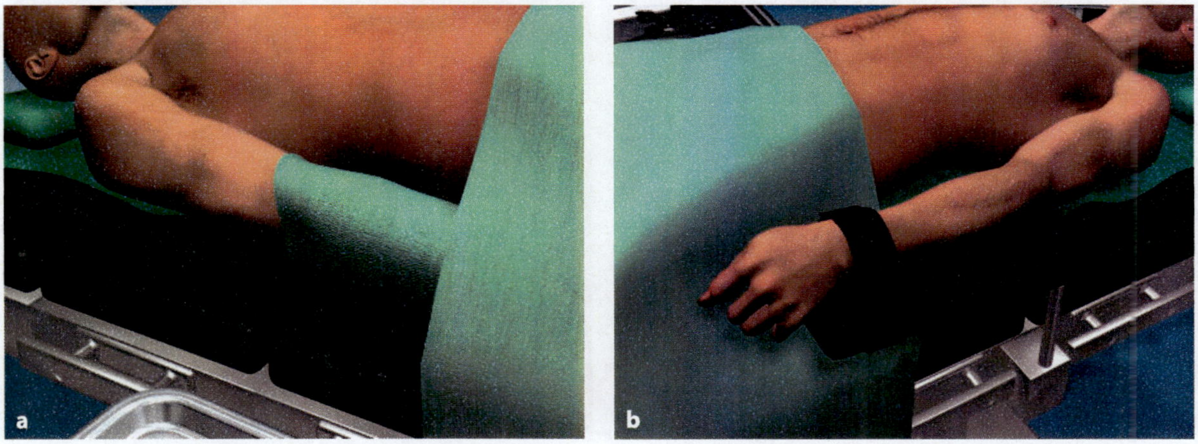

Both arms should be placed by the patient's side. The right arm is draped adherent to the patient's body and the drape is tucked underneath the patient's back to secure it. The elbow and wrist must be within the drape (Step 2a). This arm is used for the blood pressure cuff placement only. The left arm is positioned on an armboard and is secured with a Velcro strap (Step 2b). Two intravenous peripheral lines are placed in the left arm for use by the anaesthesiologists. Intravenous extension tubing should be placed by the anaesthesiologists so access can be ascertained after covering the patient's head.

Step 3: Fixation of the patient

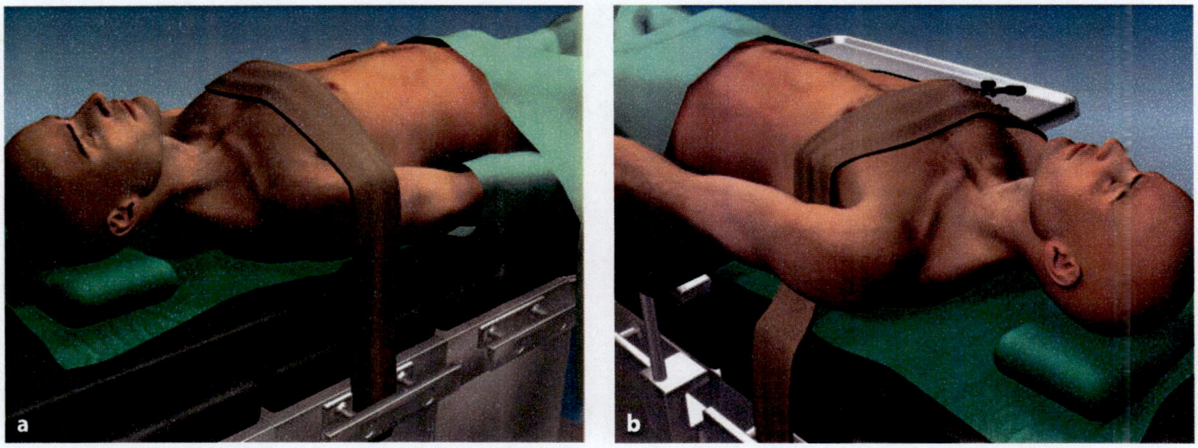

At this stage, the patient has to be secured on the table to avoid any movement when the table is placed in the Trendelenburg position during the actual procedure. It needs to be ensured that the patient is secure, as it will be difficult to access the patient once draped. Step 3a and Step 3b demonstrate the positioning of the chest belt in relation to the right and left shoulder. Caution should be made not to exert too much tension on the chest. We do not use shoulder harnesses due to the potential injury to the brachial plexus. Even in a 25° head-down position, the chest belt provides sufficient security.

Step 4: Trendelenburg position during extra- or transperitoneal surgery

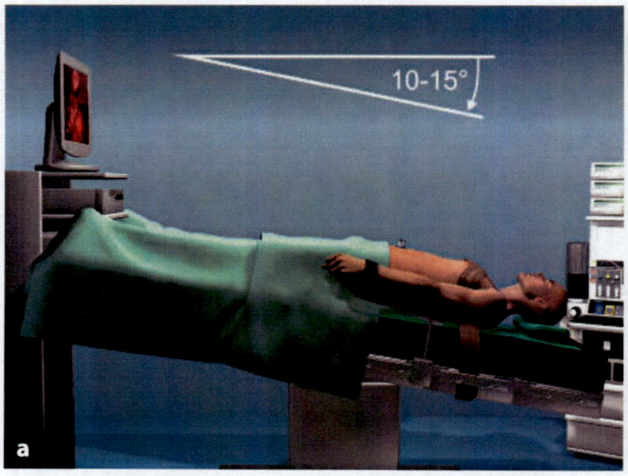

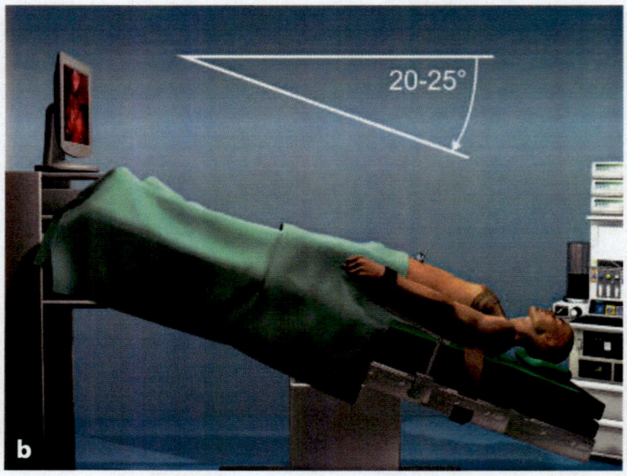

For extraperitoneal access to the pelvis, the ideal position of the patient is a 10–15° head-down position (Step 4a). In extraperitoneal pelvic surgery, there is no need for an extreme Trendelenburg position. The bowel does not interfere with the procedure. Step 4b demonstrates the extreme Trendelenburg position (20–25°) required for most transperitoneal procedures in order to allow sufficient access to the pelvis organs without bowel interposition. This extreme head-down position can be an anaesthetic contra-indication for laparoscopic intra- or transperitoneal surgery in patients with cardiorespiratory co-morbidities or intracranial pathology.

Step 5: Overview of the whole operative theatre setup

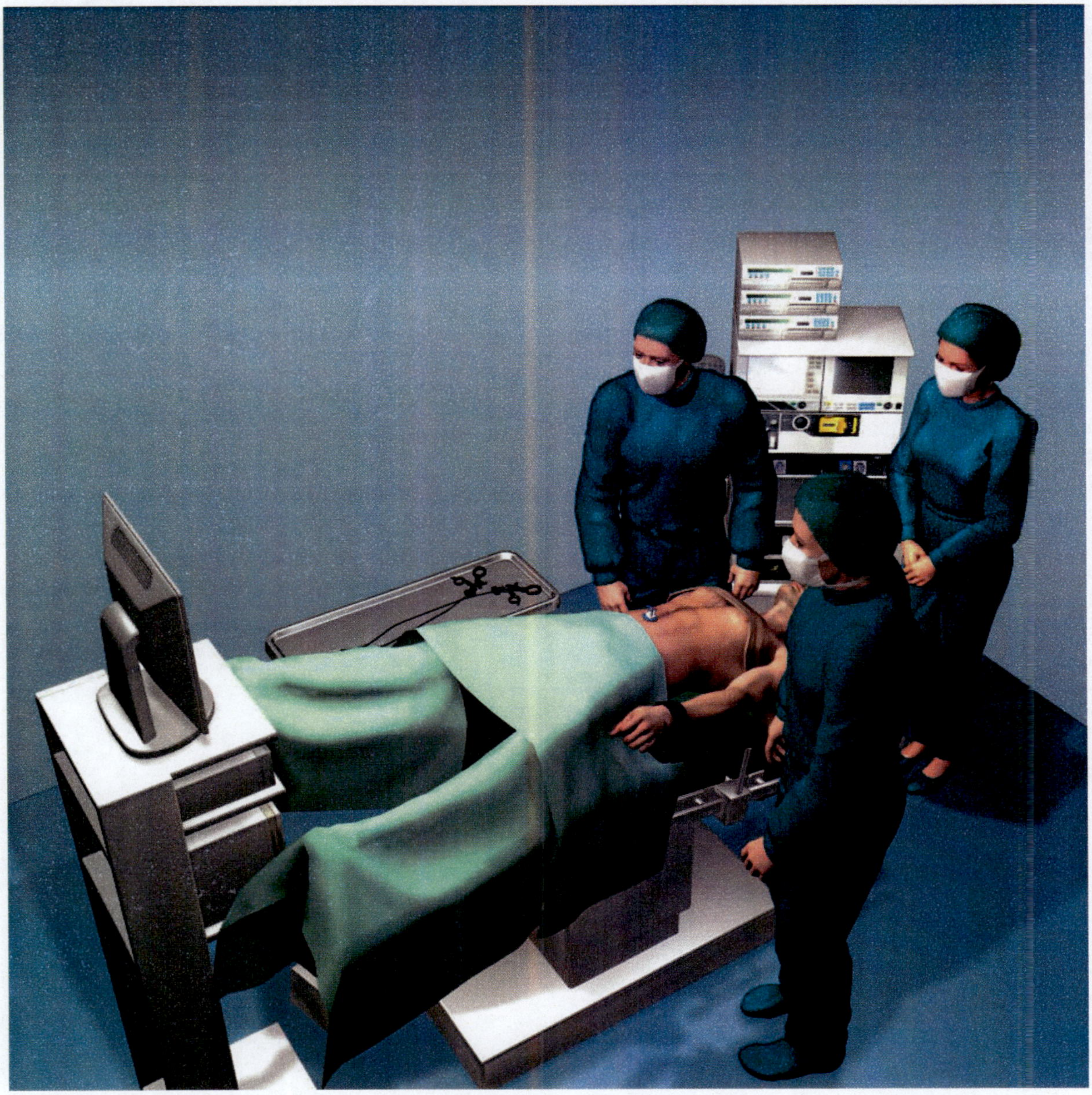

Step 5 gives an overview of the whole operative theatre setup. The patient is covered with Bair Hugger or blanket in order to assist maintenance of body temperature. It must also be noted that sequential compression stockings should be fitted to all patients prior to surgery. For most of the major pelvic surgery, the surgeon stands to the left of the patient with an assistant opposite. The camera-holder stands behind the patient's head. The scrub nurse can also act as camera holder because the procedure requires only a few instruments. Alternatively, the Freehand robotic camera holder or any other camera holder system can be employed as well.

Step 6: Landmarks for trocar placement

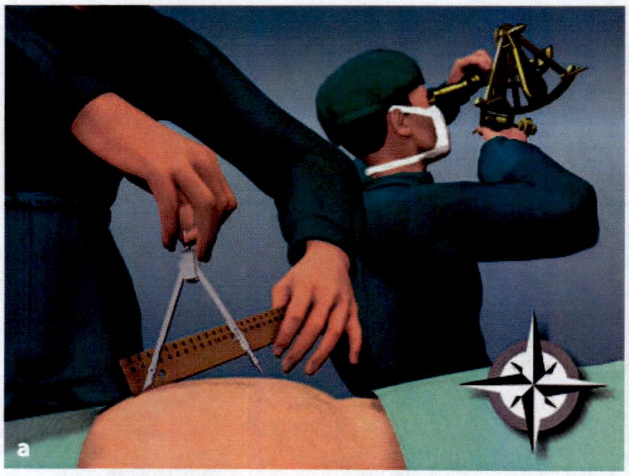

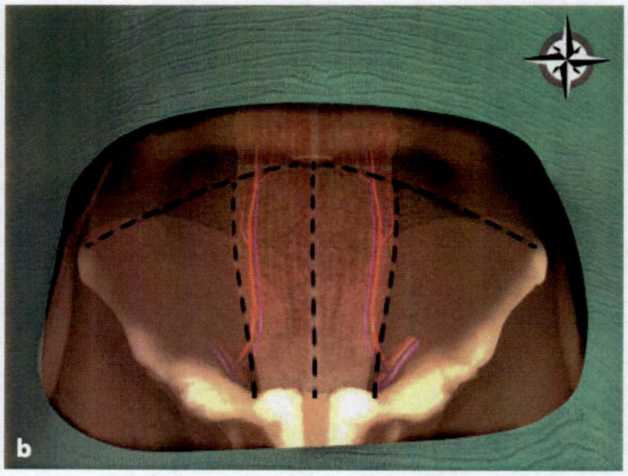

In the following sections, we represent trocar placement along a number of imaginary lines guided by anatomical landmarks on the patient (Step 6b). An imaginary line is drawn from the umbilicus to the anterior superior iliac spine on both sides. A line from the umbilicus to the symphysis pubis is drawn vertically along the linea alba. Lateral to this on both sides, the pararectal line can be identified. It is always important to be aware that the epigastric vessels course just medial to the pararectal lines. Trocar positions can slightly vary from patient to patient depending on body habitus, especially prior surgery, and cannot always be precisely measured as in Step 6a.

3.3 Setup of da Vinci Robot for Pelvic Surgery

Jens-Uwe Stolzenburg, Ingolf Tuerk, Panagiotis Kallidonis, Christopher Anderson, Harry Beerlage, Evangelos Liatsikos

Introduction

Robot-assisted laparoscopic radical prostatectomy (RALP) currently is a standard method for the management of localised prostate cancer [1, 2], while robot-assisted laparoscopic radical cystectomy (RALC) is an alternative to open and laparoscopic radical cystectomy [3–5]. The use of the robotic system requires preparation before every procedure. In the current section, the preparation of the robotic system for the performance of RALP will be described in detail. The robotic setup for RALC is similar and any differences will be discussed.

Step 1: Draping of the robot system and placement for surgical docking

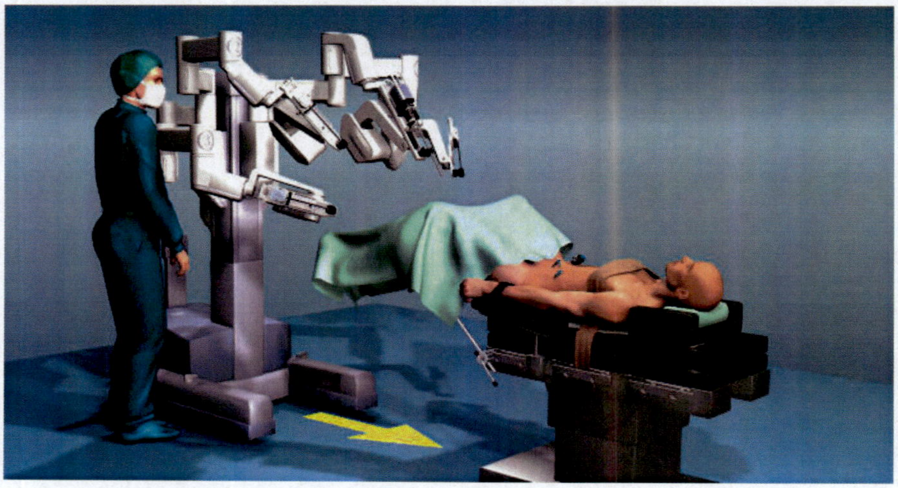

The console of the robotic system is started and allowed to go through the self-testing, component recognising process and camera and lens calibration. Adjustments for surgeon comfort (height and vision) are made. The movement of the robotic arms and camera are tested and the device is set to standby mode. Then, the da Vinci robotic system is draped with sterile sleeves away from the surgical table. All robotic arms as well as parts of the device that will come in contact with the patient or the surgical team are covered by sterile sleeves. The robotic arms are raised and brought together before docking to the patient. Step 1 shows the device being moved on the caudal side of the patient between his split legs.

Step 2: Patient position for robotic docking

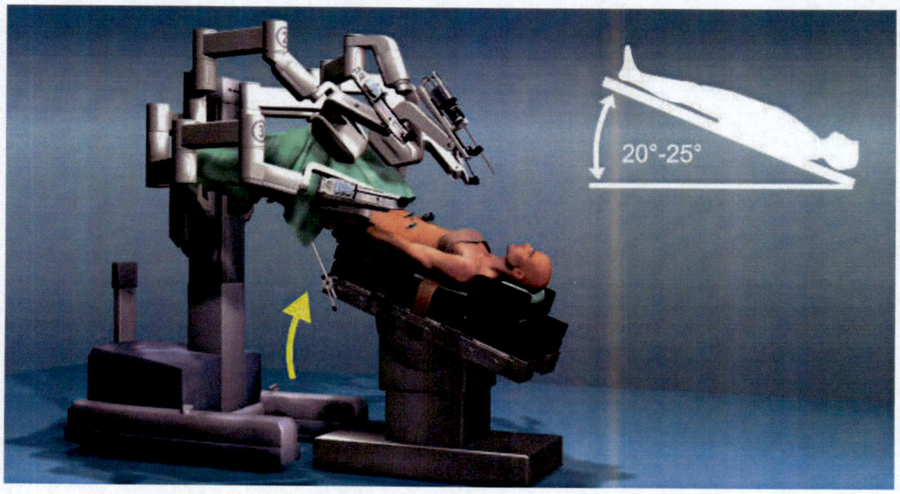

The patient is placed in the supine position with abducted legs and the ports are inserted. For the insertion of the appropriate ports, a Veress needle is used for the transperitoneal approach or balloon dilation of the extraperitoneal space is performed. The camera trocar is then inserted and the remaining trocars are inserted under vision. The transperitoneal and extraperitoneal approach for RALP can be performed by either a three-arm (five-port) or a four-arm (five- to six-port) robotic system. We present the trocar placement for a four-arm system. When the robotic system is placed on the patient's caudal side, the patient is positioned in the steep Trendelenburg position (20–25°), as shown in Step 2.

3

Step 3: Docking of the camera and medial left robot arm

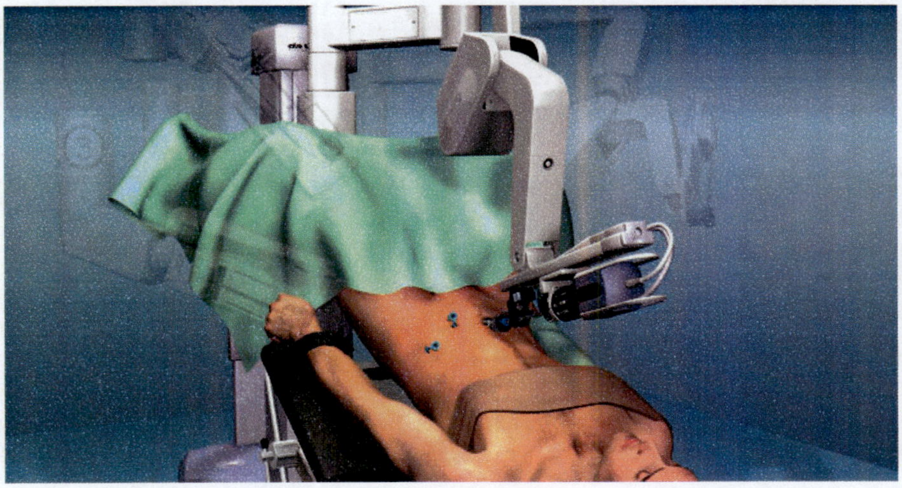

When the patient is positioned in the Trendelenburg position, care should be taken to avoid contact of the robotic system with the patient's body. The robotic arms are then docked. The image presents the docking of the camera arm to the trocar located in an umbilical site. The camera trocar is 10 mm in diameter and the camera arm possesses optics capable of providing three-dimensional stereoscopic vision. The working trocars are placed in the next step. It should be noted that the robotic camera is placed in a more caudal direction in obese patients, while a more cephalad direction is selected for RALC.

Step 4: Docking of the right working robotic arm

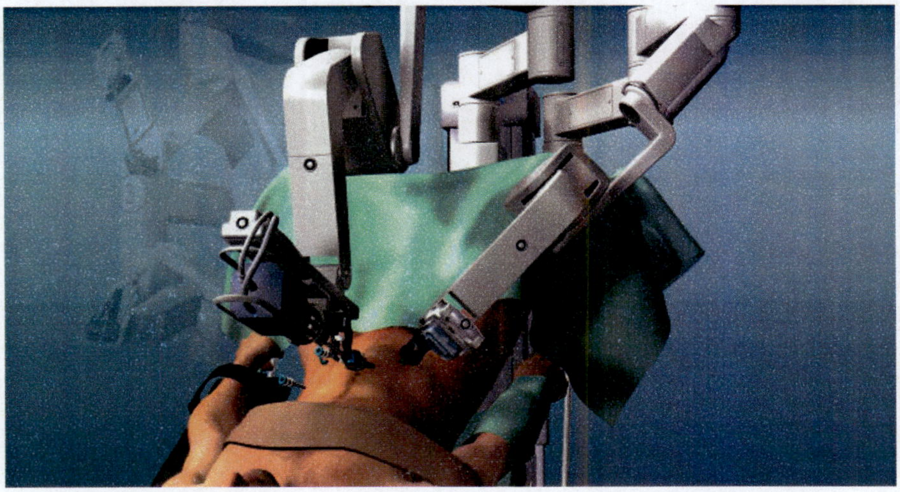

The remaining robotic arms are docked in sequence to the appropriate trocars. The first arm to the right medial robotic trocar (8 mm) is then docked. Step 4 shows the camera and right robotic arm in place. The high degree of movement of the instrument facilitates surgical tasks in dissection and suturing. It is important to note that after docking the robotic arm to the trocar, traction can be exerted on the abdominal wall, broadening the operative field and gaining space among the trocars. When placing the arms in their final position, a final check should be made to ensure that there is no compression of any body parts.

Step 5: Docking of the left working robotic arm

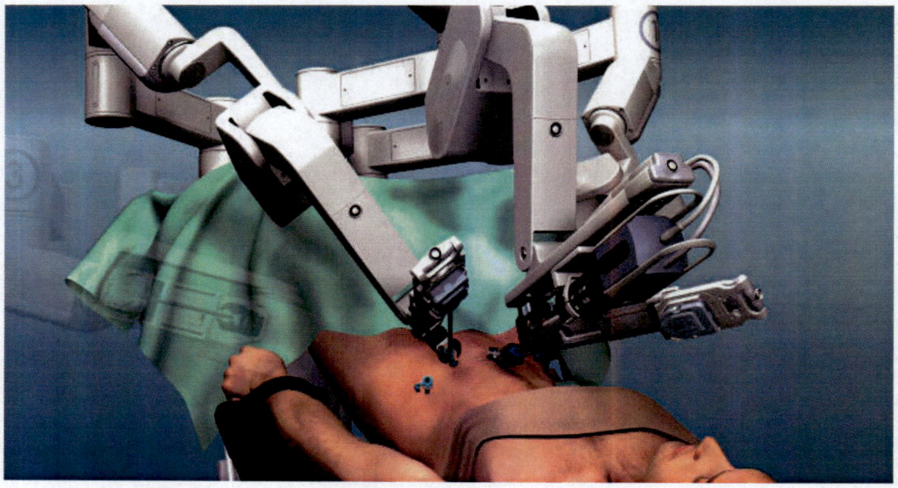

The left working robotic arm is then docked next in the appropriate 8-mm port. The two medial working arms are responsible for the performance of the procedure. All surgical tasks could be performed by these arms. The positioning of the working trocars and respective ports varies between the extraperitoneal and transperitoneal approach for prostatectomy. During the extraperitoneal prostatectomy, the medial working trocars are placed in a more caudal position in comparison to the transperitoneal prostatectomy. Both working trocars are positioned in a more caudal position in obese patients and more laterally in the RALC procedure.

Step 6: Docking of the fourth robotic arm

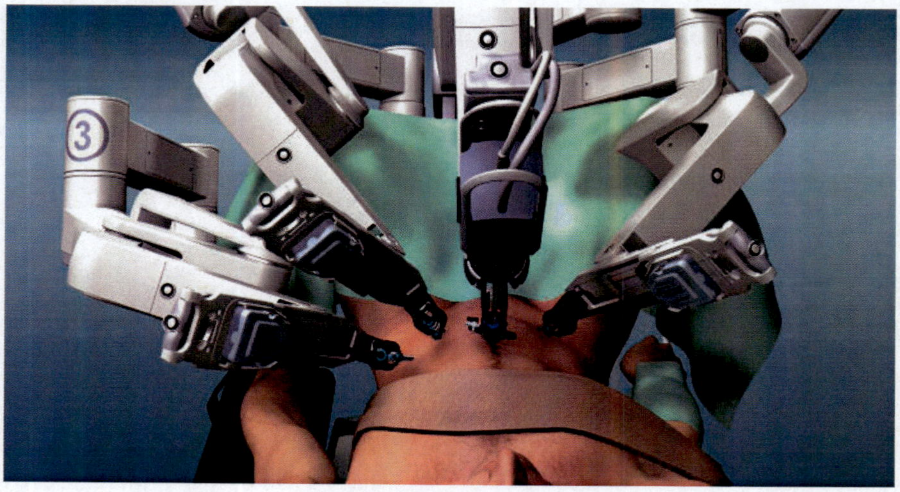

Final arrangement is made of all robotic arms after docking the fourth arm to the lateral trocar. Careful placement of all robotic arms avoids collision of the instruments intraoperatively. It should be noted that the insertion of a fourth robotic arm in the transperitoneal approach facilitates dissection as the fourth arm provides retraction. Nevertheless, the insertion of a fourth arm in the extraperitoneal approach is cumbersome since the caudal positioning of the trocars limits the space for robotic arm movements. Thus, the use of a fourth robotic arm in extraperitoneal prostatectomy should be considered according to the individual patient's anatomy.

Step 7: Activation of the robotic system

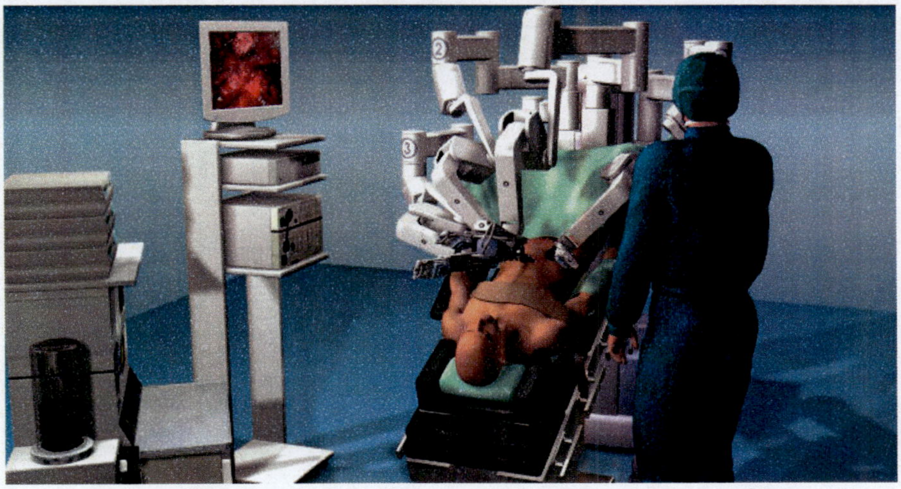

When all robotic arms have been docked, the robotic system is ready to perform the procedure. The intra-operative configuration of the robotic system is presented in Step 7. It is important to avoid any injury to the abdominal skin or the patient's legs from compression by any of the robotic arms. Thus, all arms should be carefully docked and the range of movement should be checked. In the operating room, a laparoscopic screen is placed near the assistant who does not have access to the robotic console as the surgeon does. Next to the robotic system, an appropriate cart containing the light-source device for the robotic camera is installed.

References

1. Ficarra V, Novara G, Artibani W, Cestari A, Galfano A et al (2009) Retropubic, laparoscopic, and robot-assisted radical prostatectomy: a systematic review and cumulative analysis of comparative studies. Eur Urol 55:1037–1363
2. Xylinas E, Ploussard G, Salomon L, Paul A, Gillion N, Laet KD et al (2010) Intrafascial nerve-sparing radical prostatectomy with a laparoscopic robot-assisted extraperitoneal approach: early oncological and functional results. J Endourol 24:577–582
3. Kasraeian A, Barret E, Cathelineau X, Rozet F, Galiano M, Sanchez-Salas R, Vallancien G (2010) Robot-assisted laparoscopic cystoprostatectomy with extended pelvic lymphadenectomy, extracorporeal enterocystoplasty, and intracorporeal enterourethral anastomosis: initial Montsouris experience. J Endourol 24:409–413
4. Pruthi RS, Nix J, McRackan D, Hickerson A, Nielsen ME, Raynor M, Wallen EM (2010) Robotic-assisted laparoscopic intracorporeal urinary diversion. Eur Urol 57:1013–1021
5. Manoharan M, Katkoori D, Kishore TA, Antebie E (2011) Robotic-assisted radical cystectomy and orthotopic ileal neobladder using a modified pfannenstiel incision. Urology 77:491–494

3.4 Extraperitoneal Access and Trocar Placement for Pelvic Surgery

Jens-Uwe Stolzenburg, Minh Do, Anja Dietel, Alan McNeill, Roman Ganzer, Matthias Winkler, Evangelos Liatsikos

Step 1: Patient position

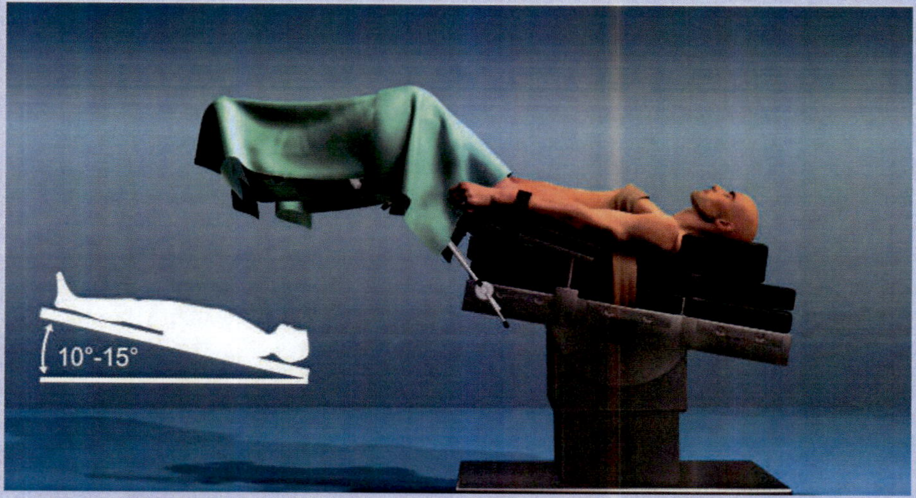

The patient is placed in a dorsal supine position with legs slightly apart, as described in Sect. 3.2. The laparoscopic tower is placed at the bottom of the operating table and the patient in a Trendelenburg position with the head tilted down at a 10° (maximum, 15°) angle. With increasing experience, we realised that there was no need for an extreme Trendelenburg position during extraperitoneal surgery since the bowel does not interfere with the procedure.

Step 2: Skin incision and incision of anterior rectus sheath

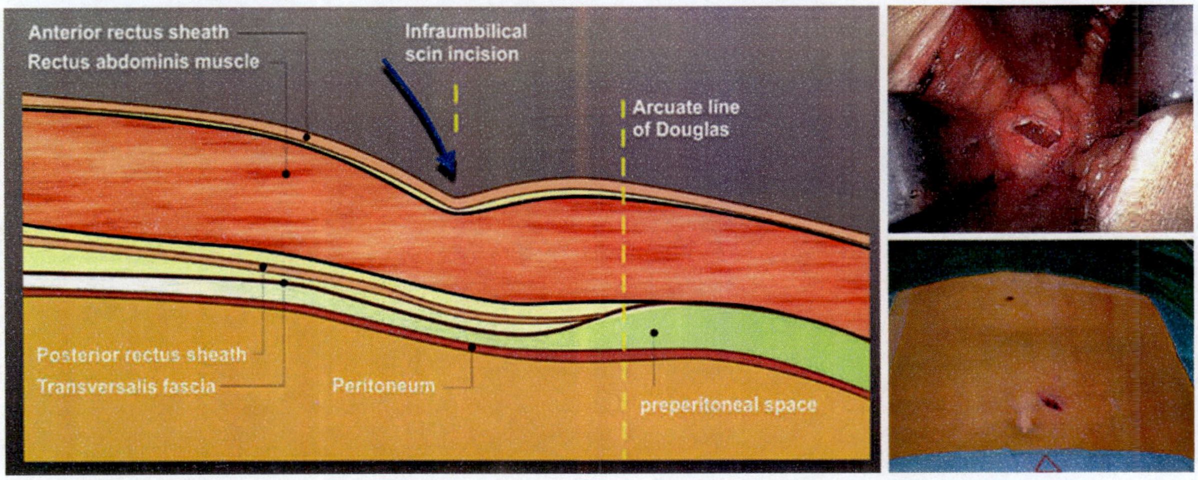

A 12- to 15-mm incision is made 1 cm below and lateral to the umbilicus (right infraumbilical incision) (Step 2, lower right). We prefer not to go in the midline, avoiding the linea alba adhesions. Step 2 (left) shows the layers of the abdominal wall. After the right infraumbilical incision, a blunt dissection is performed down to the anterior rectus sheath. The anterior rectus sheath is incised slightly horizontally (Step 2 upper right) and this opening is enlarged by blunt dissection (to prevent bleeding) using scissors. Hooks used by the assistant are very helpful. As soon as the horizontal fascial incision is made, the longitudinal muscle fibres of the rectus muscle become visible.

Step 3: Blunt dissection of rectus muscle and finger dissection of the preperitoneal space

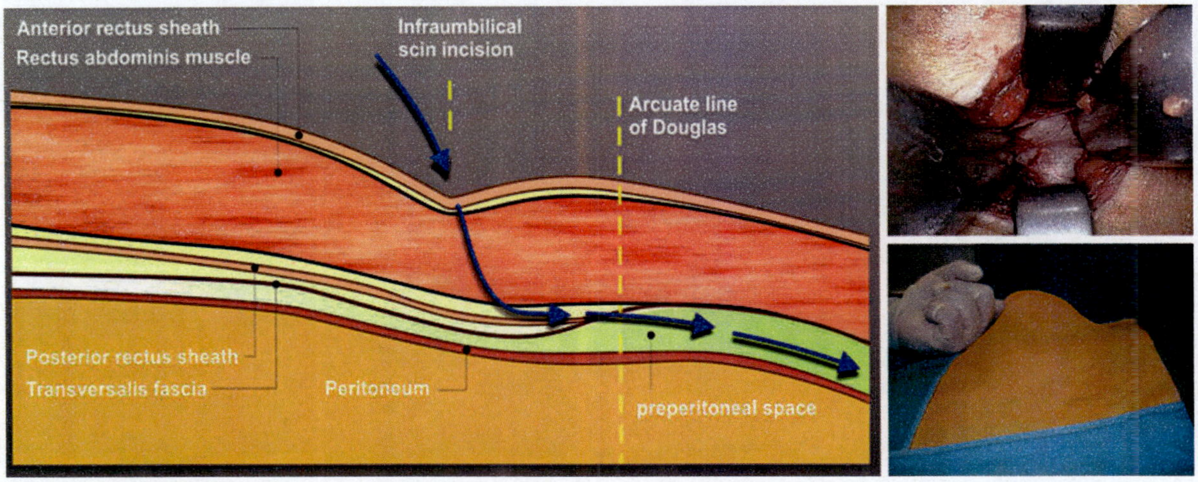

Only blunt dissection is used to separate the muscle fibres of the rectus muscle (rm). Again the specially designed hooks are very helpful. The assistant has to change the direction of the hook retraction from a horizontal to a vertical direction. The posterior rectus fascia is then exposed (Step 3, upper right). Be aware that the thickness of the muscle differs from patient to patient. In very obese patients, deeper hooks are needed. The space between the rectus muscle and the posterior rectus sheath is bluntly developed by finger dissection in the direction of the preperitoneal space (Step 3, lower right). Be careful with epigastric vessels on the right side: vigorous dissection could injure them. Extensive blunt finger dissection is not needed.

Step 4: Balloon dissection of preperitoneal space

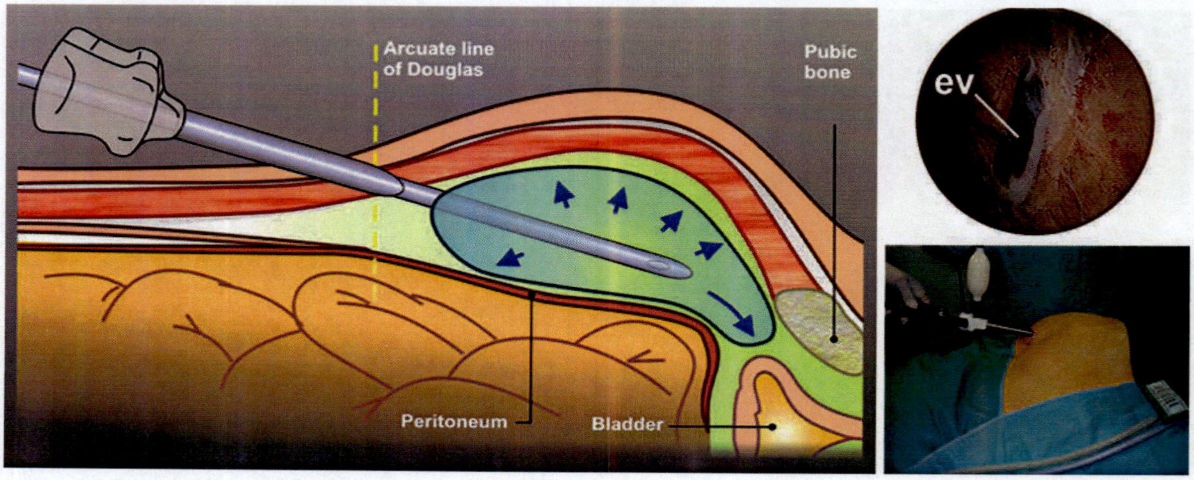

A balloon trocar is introduced superior to the posterior rectus sheath and insufflated under direct visual control. The posterior rectus sheath is absent inferior to the arcuate line. That is why the balloon dilation creates the preperitoneal space. The epigastric vessels (ev) are first seen ventrally compressed through the balloon (Step 4, upper right). The epigastric vessels (ev) and the pubic arch are the main landmarks during balloon dilation. The pubic arch becomes visible towards the end of the dissection.

Step 5: Optical trocar and first 5-mm trocar placement

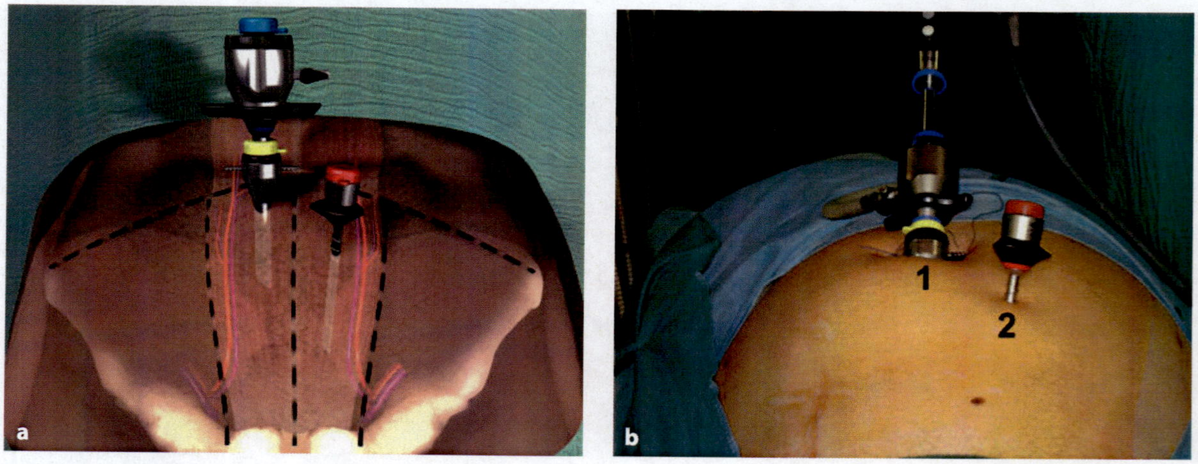

The balloon trocar is removed and stay sutures are then placed on either end of the anterior rectus sheath incision. An optical trocar (Hasson type) is inserted and fixed (trocar number 1). After insufflation with CO_2 (12 mmHg pressure), a 5-mm trocar (trocar number 2) is positioned two finger widths left, lateral to the midline (at a one-third to two-thirds ratio from the umbilicus to the pubic arch).

Step 6: Trocar placement into the right iliac fossa

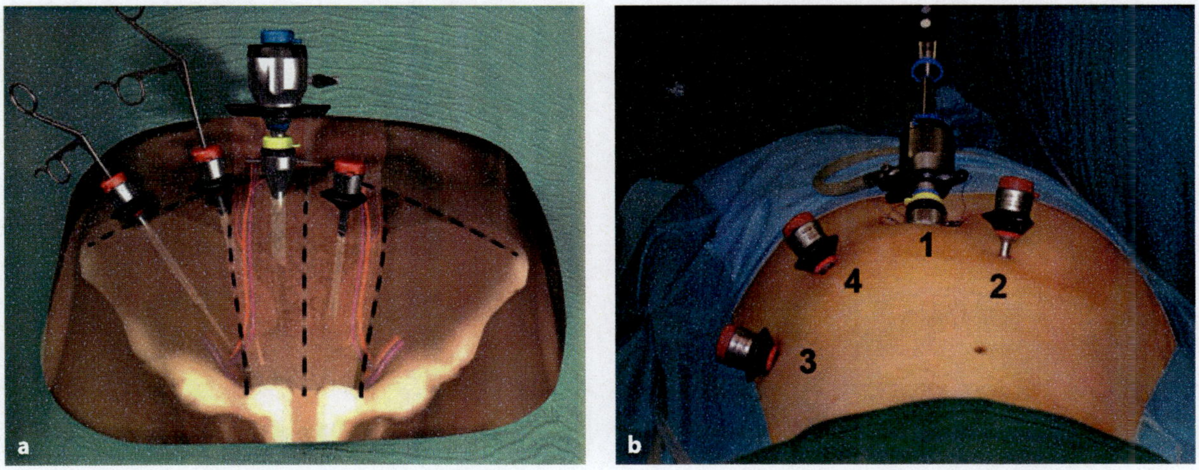

A 5-mm trocar (trocar number 3) is then positioned two finger widths medial to the right anterior superior iliac spine (in the line from the spine to the umbilicus). Another 5-mm trocar (trocar number 4) is placed in the right pararectal line (on the same theoretical line from the spine to the umbilicus), taking care to avoid injury to the epigastric vessels.

Step 7: Beware of the risk of injury to epigastric vessels

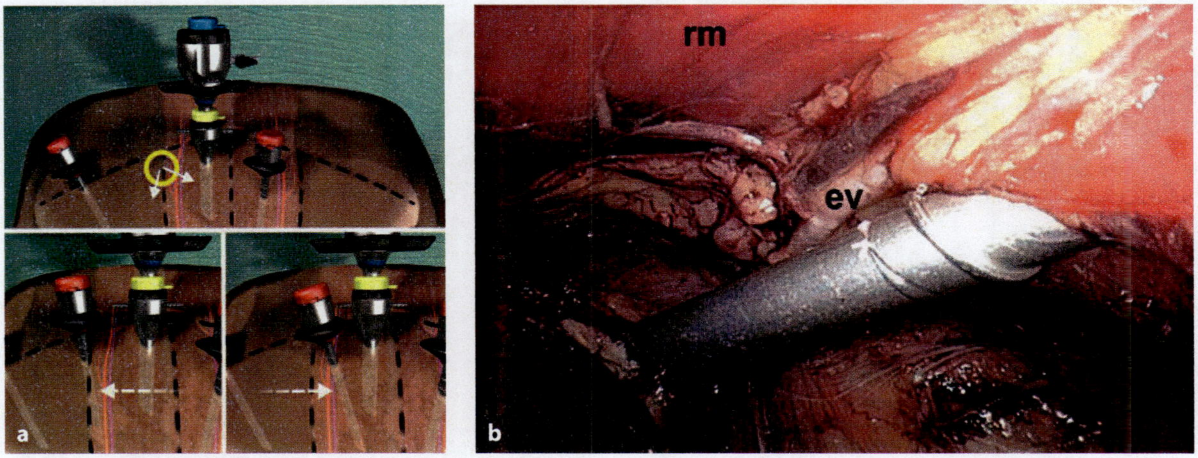

The epigastric vessels (ev) can be injured during insertion of the fourth trocar (pararectal line, right iliac fossa). For this reason, this is the most dangerous trocar for bleeding. Injury to the epigastric vessels can be avoided by careful inspection of the abdominal wall via the laparoscope before trocar insertion. The fourth trocar position has to be varied medially or laterally (see arrows) aiming to avoid epigastric vessel injury. Another way to reduce the risk of injury is to use a VersaStep trocar.

Step 8: Dissection of the left preperitoneal space

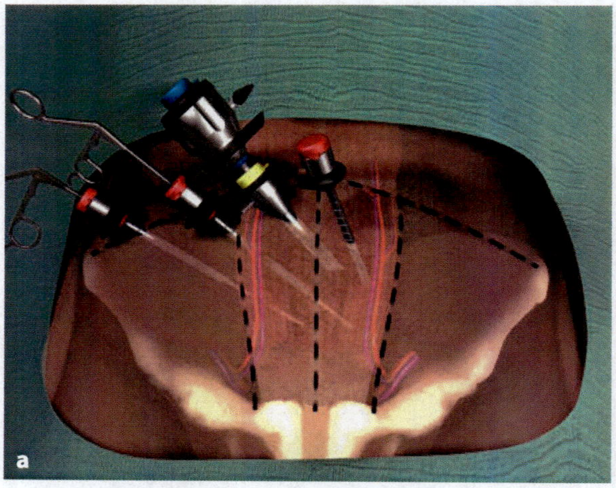

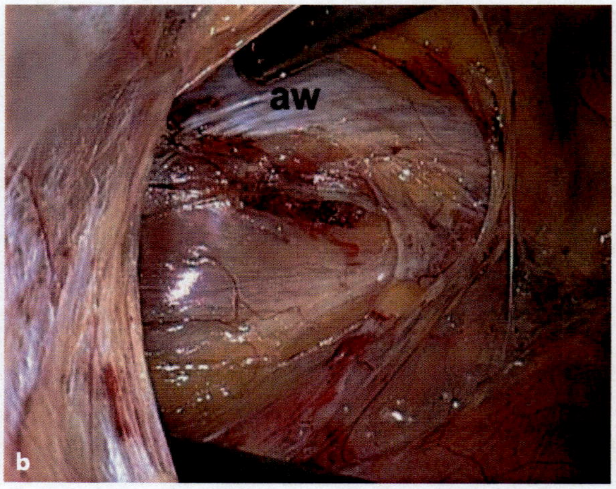

Operating bimanually through trocars number 3 and 4, dissection is continued bluntly to the left preperitoneal space. Follow the pubic arch from right to left and then identify the iliac vessels and spermatic cord. Go ventrally and dissect underneath the epigastric vessels to the left side. Most dissections can be performed bluntly. If the assistant is not experienced, the surgeon should then change his position and move to the right side of the patient for this step (abdominal wall, aw).

Step 9: Placement of 12-mm trocar in left iliac fossa

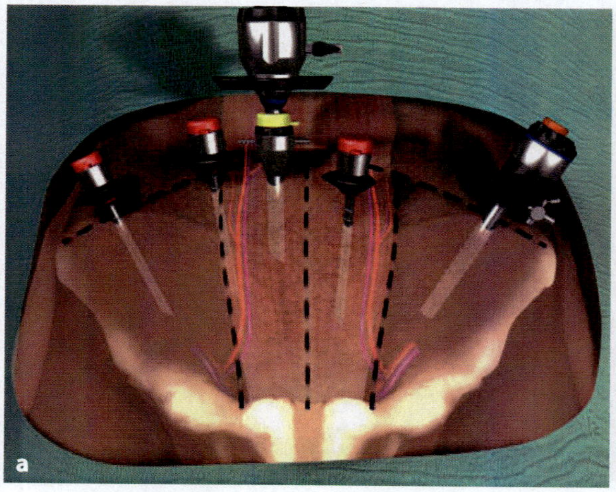

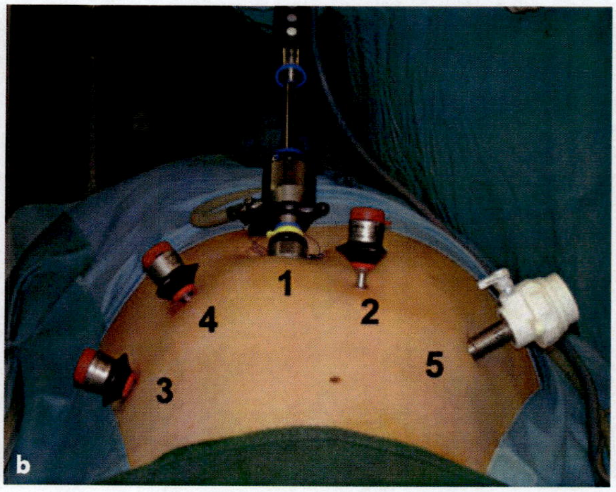

The final 12-mm trocar is placed approximately three finger widths medial to the left anterior superior iliac spine (on a hypothetical line from the spine to the umbilicus). Avoid placement too distally or too close to the iliac spine, because this can cause problems during apical dissection and anastomosis. This is the trocar through which all the lymph nodes are extracted. Furthermore, the needles are inserted and extracted through this trocar.

Step 10: Summery of all trocars for major pelvic surgery

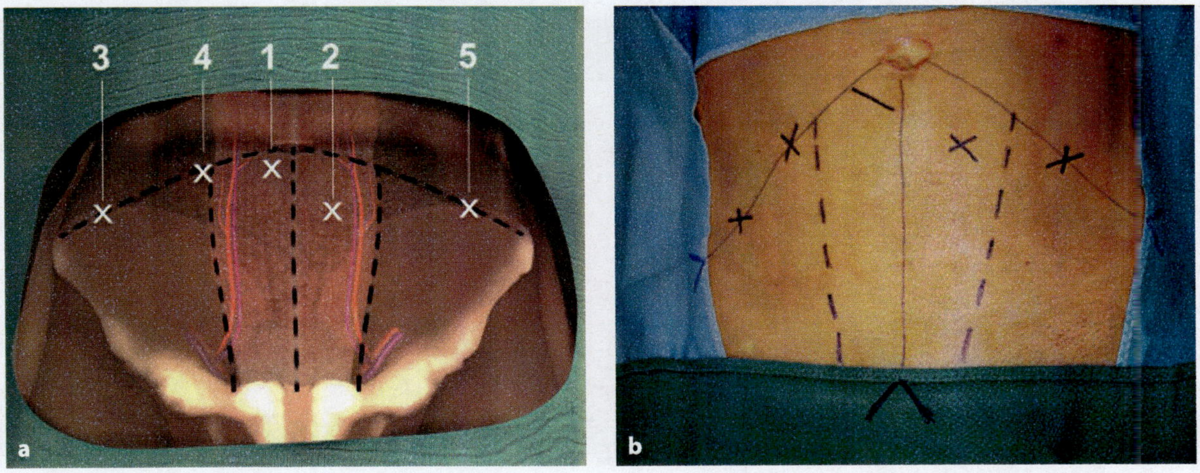

The position off all trocars is summarised in Step 10. The imaginary lines drawn in Step 10a and Step 10b are helpful for orientation (from umbilicus to anterior superior iliac spine, continuous lines; pararectal line, dashed lines). The numbers give the sequence of trocar placement.

Step 11: Trocar placement in obese or very tall patients

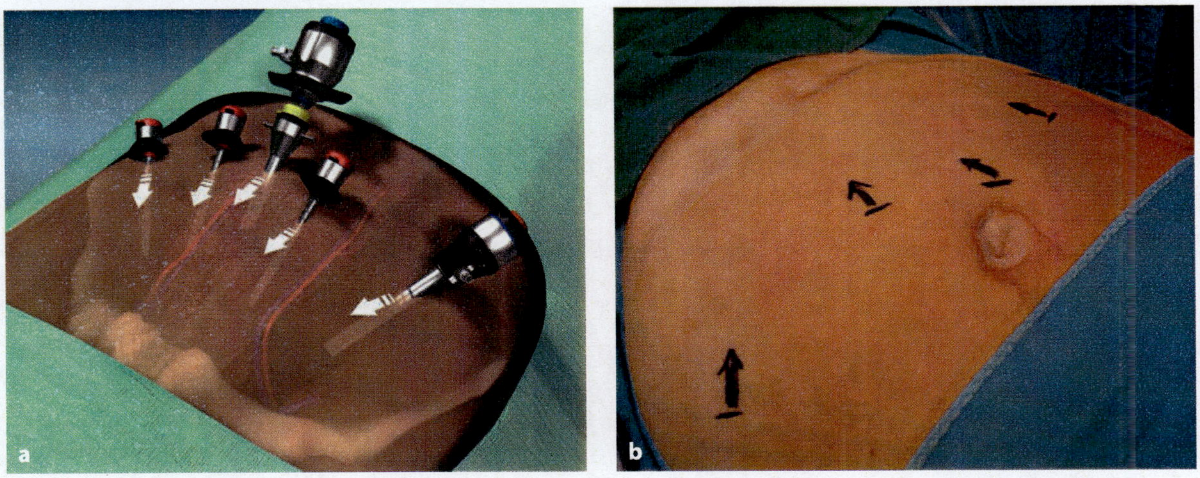

In extremely obese or very tall patients, all trocars should be placed 1–3 cm caudally, depending on the size of the patients, for optimal access to the retropubic space. The principles of trocar placement are the same. In extremely obese patients, a 10 + 5° head-down position is recommended.

3.5 Bladder Diverticulectomy (Laparoscopic and LESS)

Jens-Uwe Stolzenburg, Minh Do, Rob Mills, Holger Till, Rowan Casey, Anja Dietel, Panagiotis Kallidonis, Evangelos Liatsikos

Introduction

A bladder diverticulum is a thin-walled, urothelium-lined outpouching from the bladder lumen. Congenital diverticula are rare and usually solitary [1]. Acquired diverticula are much more common, often multiple and usually secondary to bladder outflow obstruction. Small diverticula are usually asymptomatic and do not require treatment. Larger diverticula may present with symptoms related to poor bladder emptying as the diverticulum may accommodate a large proportion of the bladder volume during attempted voiding, may not empty fully and therefore more frequently require surgical intervention [2]. If surgical treatment is required a number of approaches are possible: endoscopic fulguration (only if small) or resection by an open, transvesical, endoscopic extraperitoneal, laparoscopic or the laparoendoscopic single-site surgery (LESS) approach [3, 4]. Prior to surgical removal, it is helpful to perform a cystoscopy in order to identify the ureteric orifices and stent them if necessary to reduce the risk of injury during the dissection at the diverticular neck. On occasion, the ureteric orifice may become incorporated into a diverticulum as it develops, necessitating ureteric reimplantation at the time of surgical resection [5]. Voiding cystourethrography is also usually performed to examine the functional effect the diverticulum has on bladder emptying. Here we illustrate both the laparoscopic and the LESS approaches.

Indications

- Voiding dysfunction with large residual urine caused by the diverticulum
- Pain or recurrent urinary tract infection

Contra-indications

- Active urinary infection

Preoperative Preparation

- Midstream urine should be sterile
- Single-shot broad-spectrum antibiotic preoperatively

Step 1: Cystoscopy and placement of balloon catheter into the diverticulum

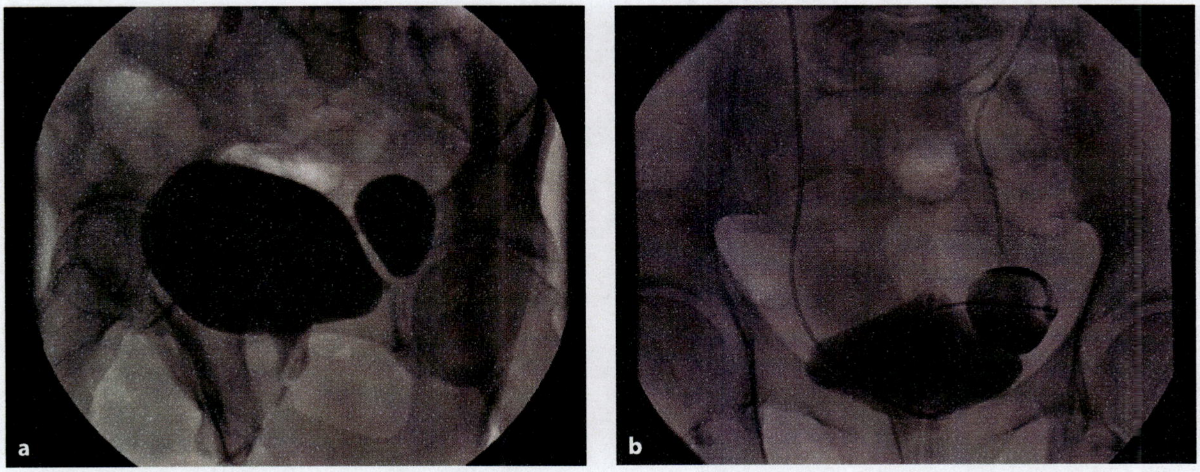

Cystoscopy and fluoroscopy are performed on table to delineate the diverticulum. In Step 1a, the diverticulum can be seen on the left side of the bladder. A double-J catheter is placed in one or both ureters depending on the location of the diverticulum. Bilateral stents have been inserted in this case. A guidewire is then passed transurethrally and guided into the diverticulum fluoroscopically. A balloon catheter with an open-ended tip is then passed over the guidewire into the diverticulum. The balloon is inflated to greatly facilitate laparoscopic identification of the distended diverticulum (Step 1b).

Step 2: Patient position and operative setup

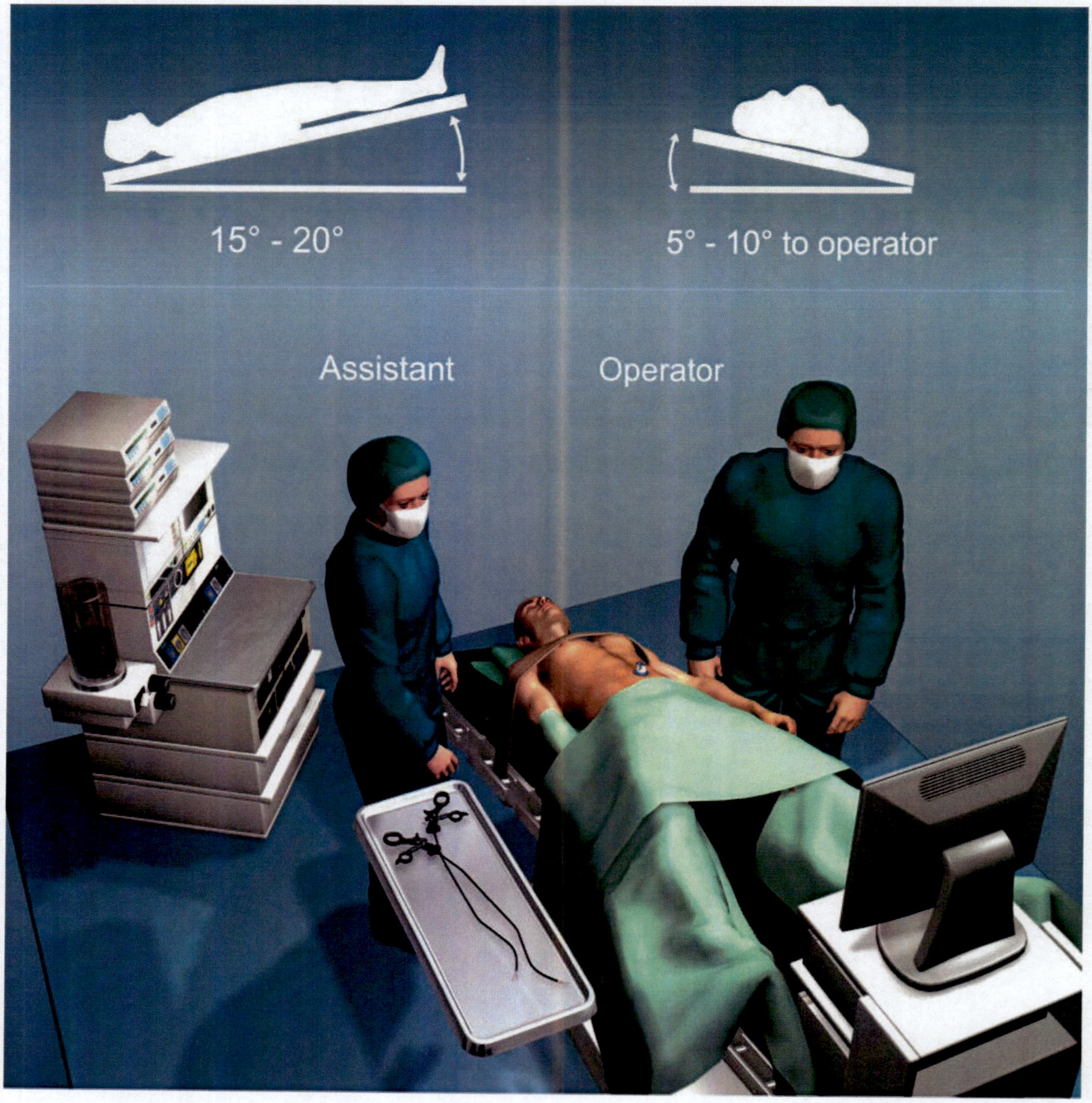

The patient is placed supine in a 15–20° head-down position. When performing LESS, the table is also tilted towards the operator in order to make initial Triport or Quadport access at the umbilicus easier and more ergonomic, as shown in Step 2. The main surgeon stands on the patient's left side with an assistant on the opposite side. The assistant can also be positioned at the head of the table.

Step 3: Trocar placement

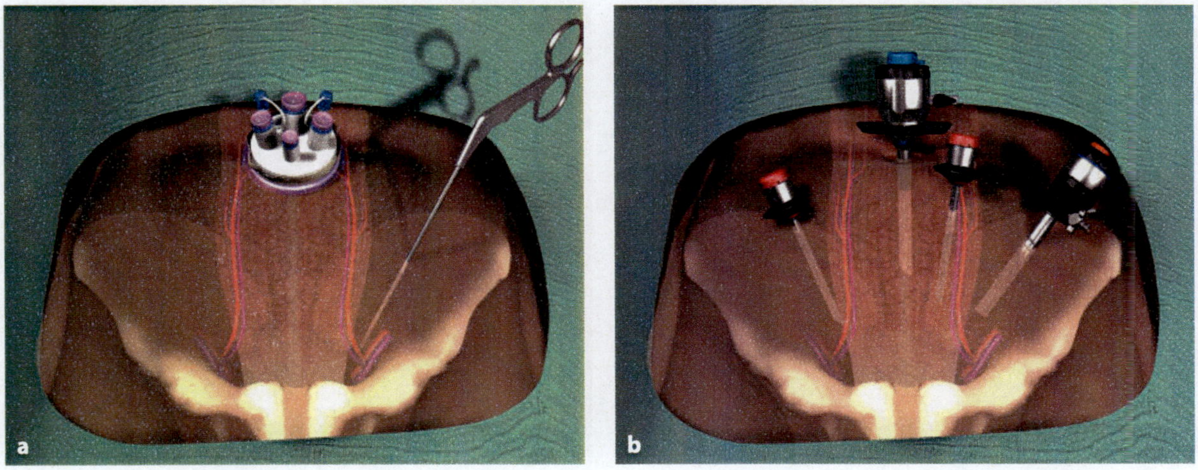

Step 3a shows the placement of the Quadport for the LESS procedure. It is also possible to use a Triport for this procedure as it is not one of the more technically demanding procedures. The bladder reconstruction is aided by the addition of a 3-mm instrument (forceps or needle holder) placed laterally to the Quadport, especially if no prebent needle holder is available. Step 3b demonstrates port placement for conventional laparoscopic diverticulectomy (optic trocar at the umbilicus, 10- to 12-mm trocar three fingerbreadths medial to the left anterior superior iliac spine on a line towards the umbilicus, a 5-mm trocar two fingerbreadths left of the midline and a 5-mm trocar into the right iliac fossa, as shown.

Step 4: Incision of the peritoneum (LESS)

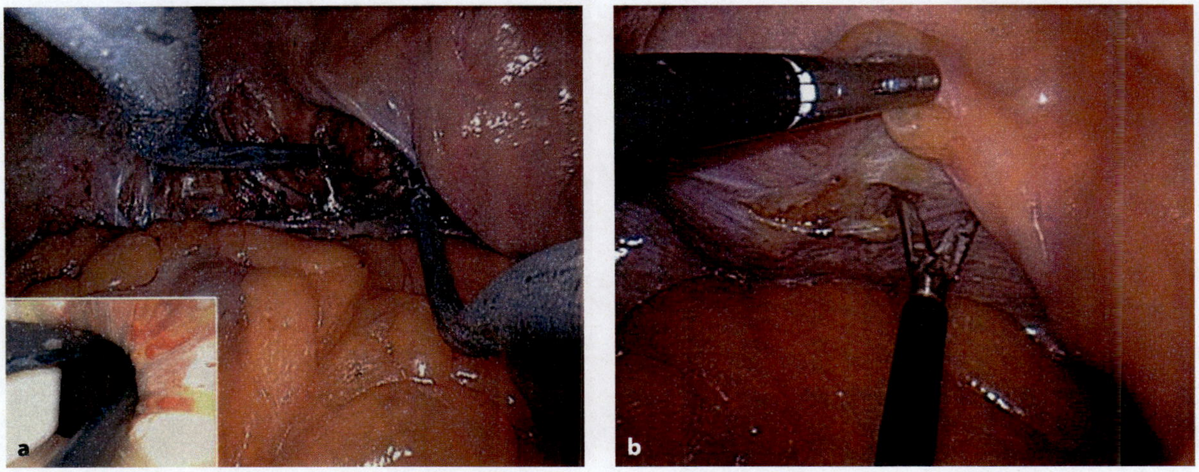

During the LESS procedure, all instruments are inserted via the Quadport or TriPort. Two prebent instruments can be seen (forceps and scissors) in both images. With the aid of the head-down tilt, the bowel is retracted out of the pelvis to reveal the bladder. If the position of the diverticulum is not readily discernible the balloon catheter may be manipulated to aid identification. The peritoneum over the diverticulum is then incised. Note that one instrument is being used to retract superiorly to provide vision and counter-traction, while the scissors are used to incise the peritoneum over the diverticulum. The scissors can be either a prebent or a straight instrument.

Step 5: Ventral and lateral dissection of the diverticulum (LESS)

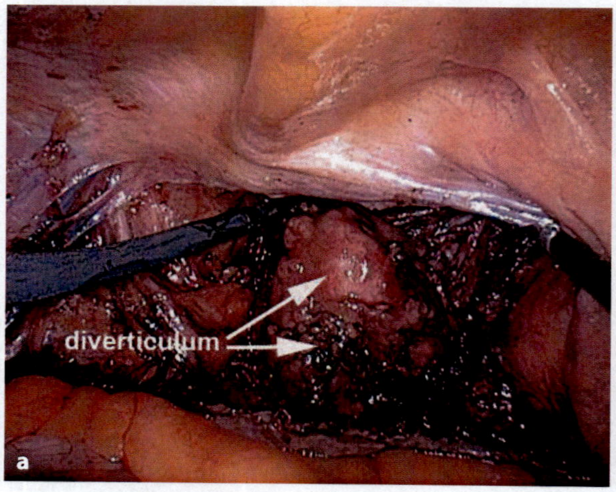

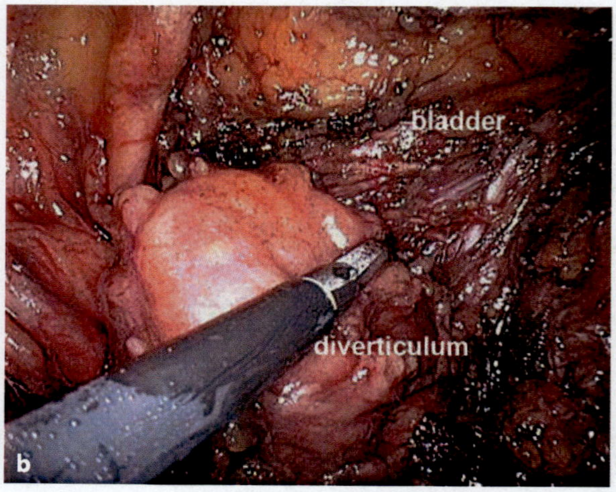

Identification of the diverticular margin is facilitated by palpation of the catheter balloon with the instruments. One prebent instrument is used for tissue retraction, enabling the other instrument to dissect the perivesical tissue, thus exposing the diverticulum. In this case, the dissection was started ventrally and then followed circumferentially around the neck of the diverticulum.

Ensure that the horizontal incision of the peritoneum is large enough to expose the whole diverticulum. If the diverticulum is located close to the ureter, the ureter should be identified and isolated prior to dissection of the diverticulum. It may be helpful to elevate the ureter laterally with a suture, which is brought in through the anterior abdominal wall.

Step 6: Dissection of the neck of the diverticulum (LESS)

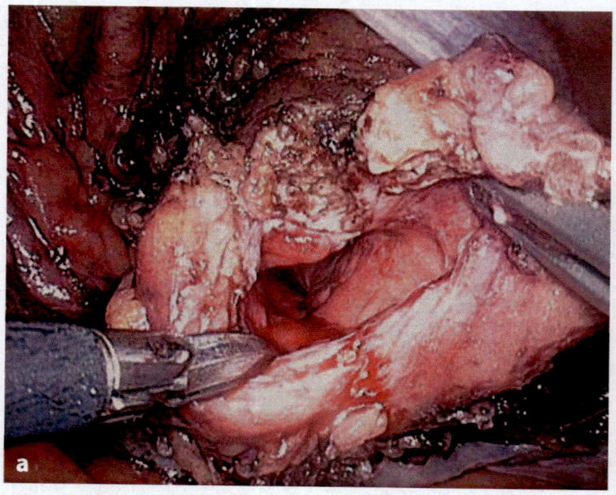

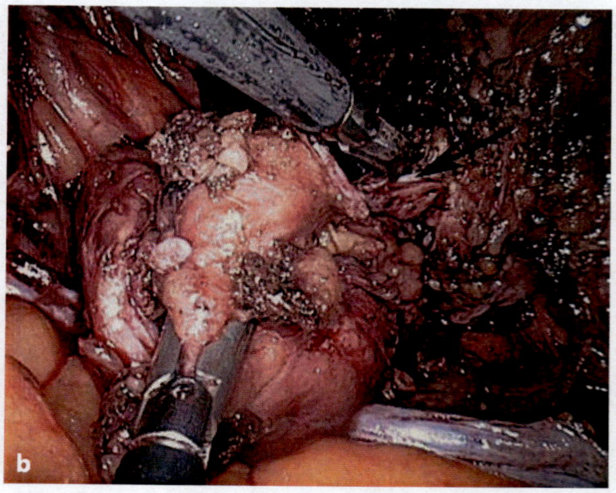

If it is difficult to dissect out and circumscribe the diverticular neck satisfactorily at this stage, then the diverticulum may be opened to aid orientation. In Step 6a, we see the urothelium of the normal bladder and the diverticulum, thus making it easier to appreciate the junction between diverticulum and normal bladder wall. Step 6b demonstrates that the subsequent ventral approach to the neck of the diverticulum is now more straightforward, since the internal aspect of the diverticulum has been inspected. By the end of this stage of the procedure, the neck of the diverticulum should be clearly demarcated at its junction with the normal bladder wall.

Step 7: Dissection and incision of the diverticulum (conventional laparoscopy)

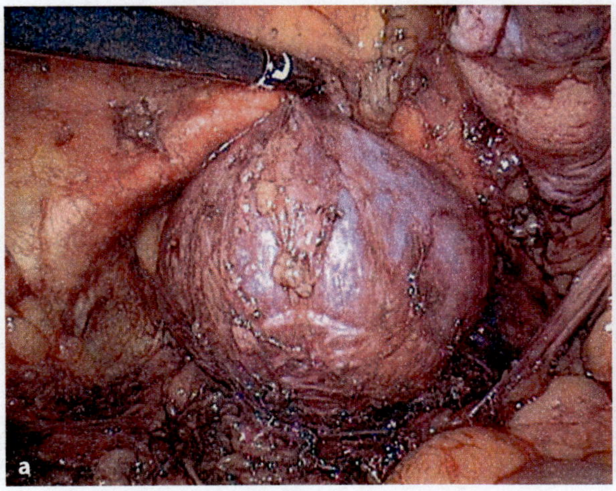

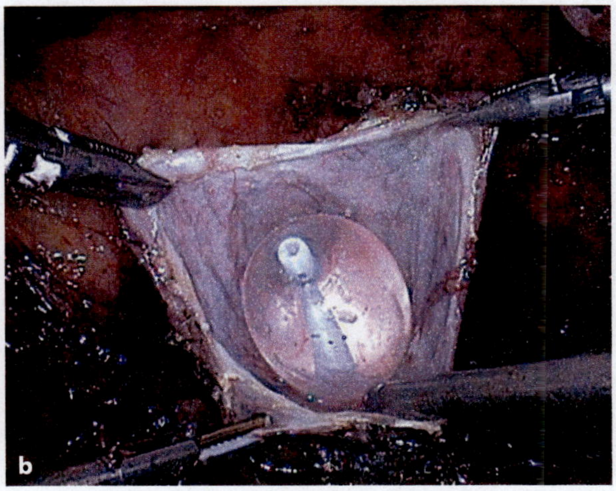

The Step 7 images were taken from a conventional laparoscopic approach to a large diverticulum. In this case, dissecting out the diverticulum was possible without opening it. Distension of the diverticulum with the balloon catheter made identification of landmarks possible. Once the diverticular wall has been incised, the balloon of the open-ended catheter is visible. In conventional laparoscopy, most of the dissection is performed using the SonoSurg device and a bipolar forceps used by the surgeons. In difficult cases, an additional 5-mm trocar can be placed to allow assisting with suction and forceps, as shown in Step 7b.

Step 8: Identification of the neck of the diverticulum (conventional laparoscopy)

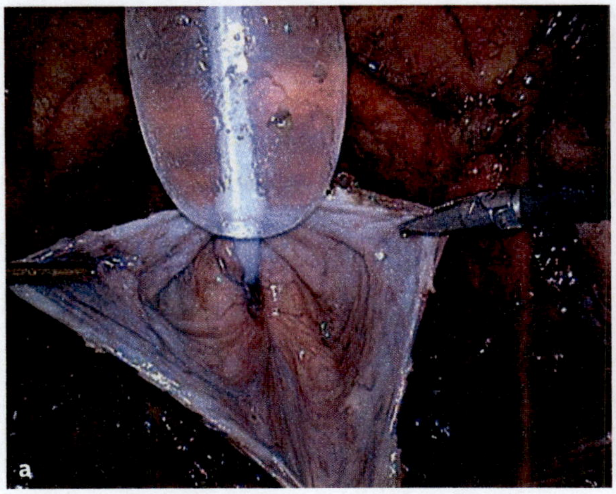

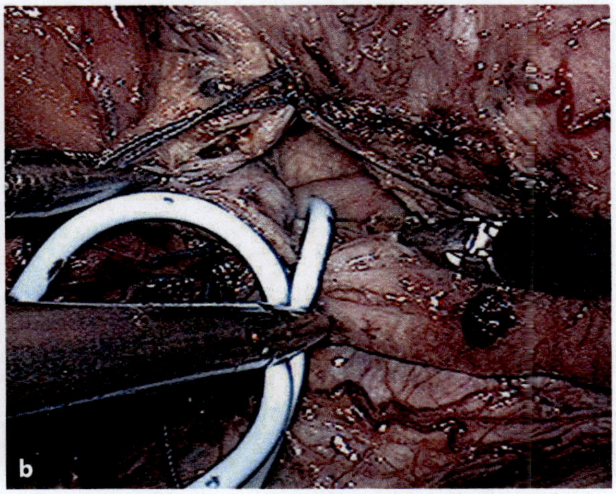

Elevation of the catheter and retraction of the walls of the diverticulum reveals the junction of the neck of the diverticulum and the bladder (Step 8a). The balloon catheter has been removed, providing a view into the bladder. The diverticulum is completely dissected from the bladder at the neck. Identification of the ureteric orifices is aided by the presence of double-J stents (Step 8b), thus reducing the risk of injury. As seen in this case, double-J stents may be removed during the procedure or alternatively at the time of catheter removal postoperatively.

Step 9: Dissection of the posterior side of the neck of the diverticulum (LESS)

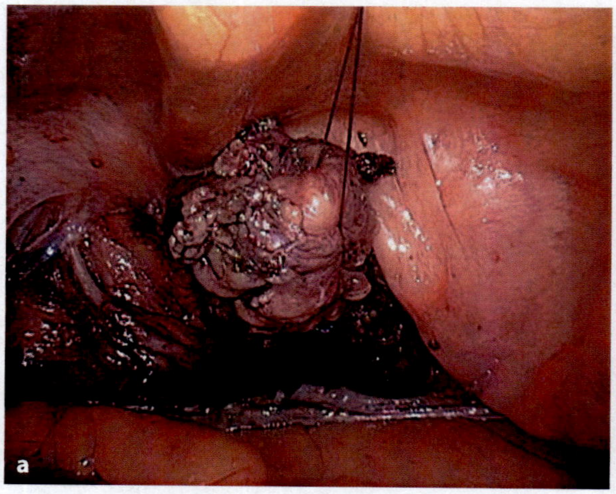

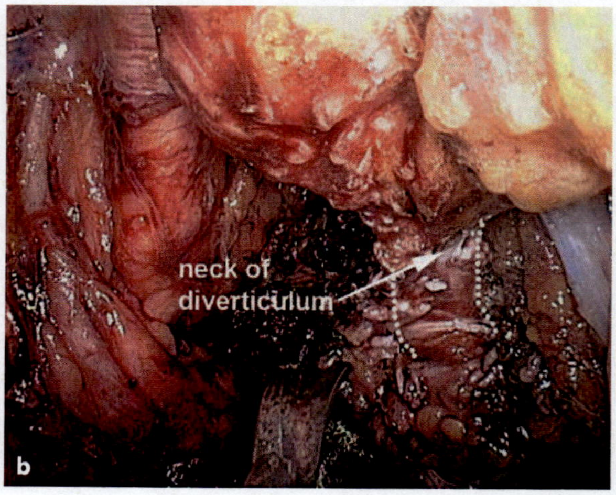

The dissection of the posterior aspect of the diverticulum may be more difficult and this process can be facilitated by fixing the diverticulum to the ventral abdominal wall using a suture in the LESS procedure. Under direct vision, a long straight needle is passed through the abdominal wall, through the diverticulum and back out through the abdominal wall. A clip is then placed at the skin surface to tent up the cyst, allowing easier access to the posterior diverticular neck, as in Step 9a. The posterior diverticula neck dissection is now completed safely using prebent scissors.

Step 10: Complete diverticulum dissection and bladder wall suturing (LESS)

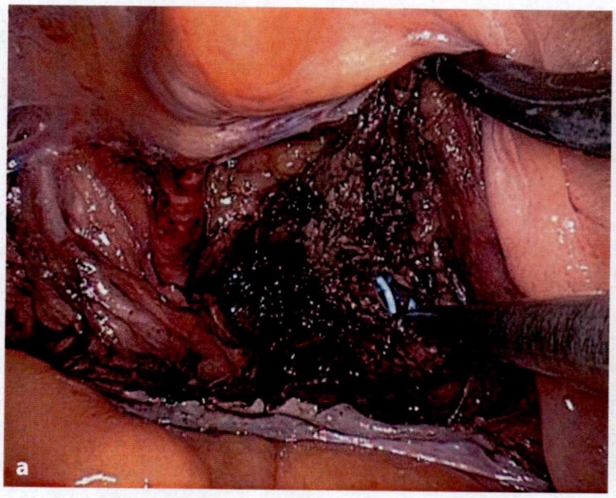

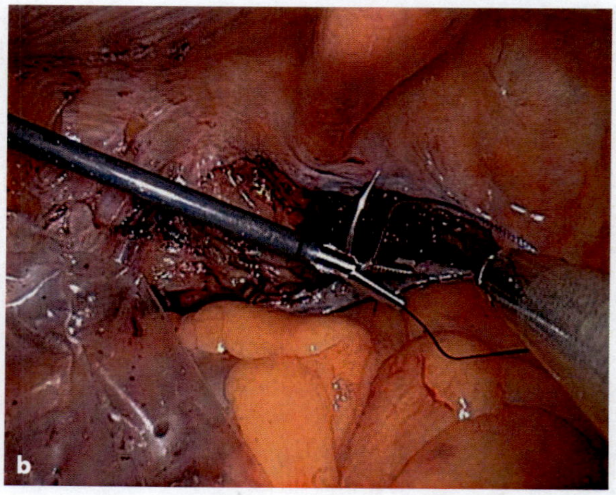

Step 10a demonstrates the bladder wall defect with the bottom end of the double-J stent visible in the bladder during the LESS procedure in which the diverticulum was removed. The resected diverticulum is placed in an EndoCatch bag (bottom left, Step 10b) and will be removed with the Quadport at the end of the procedure. In LESS procedures, the defect in the bladder is sutured using a straight needle holder and prebent forceps (Step 10a). If this is technically difficult a 3-mm needlescopic instrument can be inserted via a 3-mm trocar or directly through the skin as additional forceps providing triangulation for suturing. Step 10b shows these needlescopic forceps together with a 5-mm straight needle holder being used.

Step 11: Suturing the bladder wall (LESS)

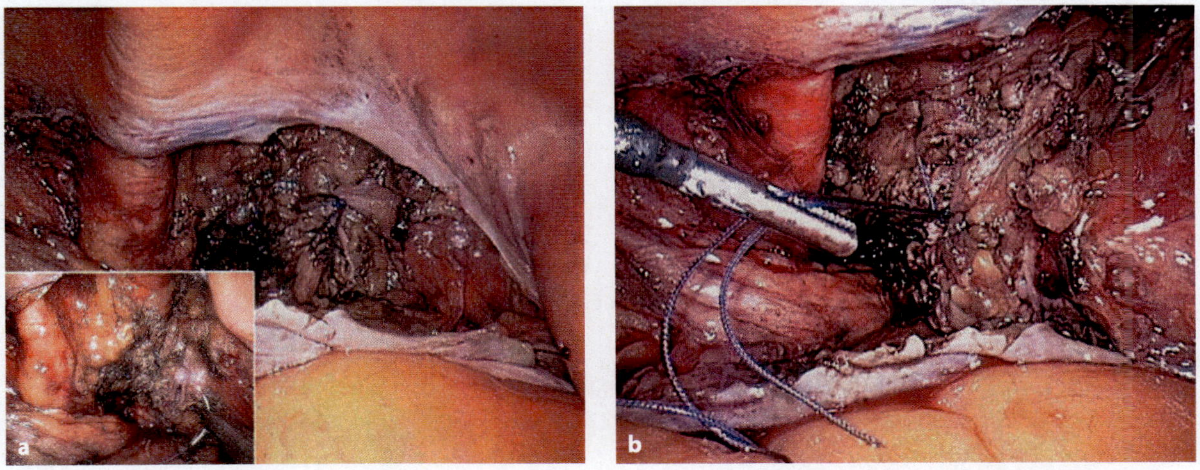

The defect in the bladder from the diverticulum neck is closed using interrupted or continuous sutures (2/0 Polysorb on a GU-46 needle or 2/0 Vicryl on a UR-6 needle), as in Step 10a. The inset in Step 11a demonstrates this detail. Following bladder closure, saline (200–300 ml) is infused via the urethral catheter in order to check that the repair is watertight (Step 11b). Additional sutures may be placed as necessary. Ensure that there is no inadvertent fixation of the double-J stent or closure of the ureter if it is located close to the resected neck of the diverticulum.

Step 12: Closure of the peritoneum and drain placement (LESS)

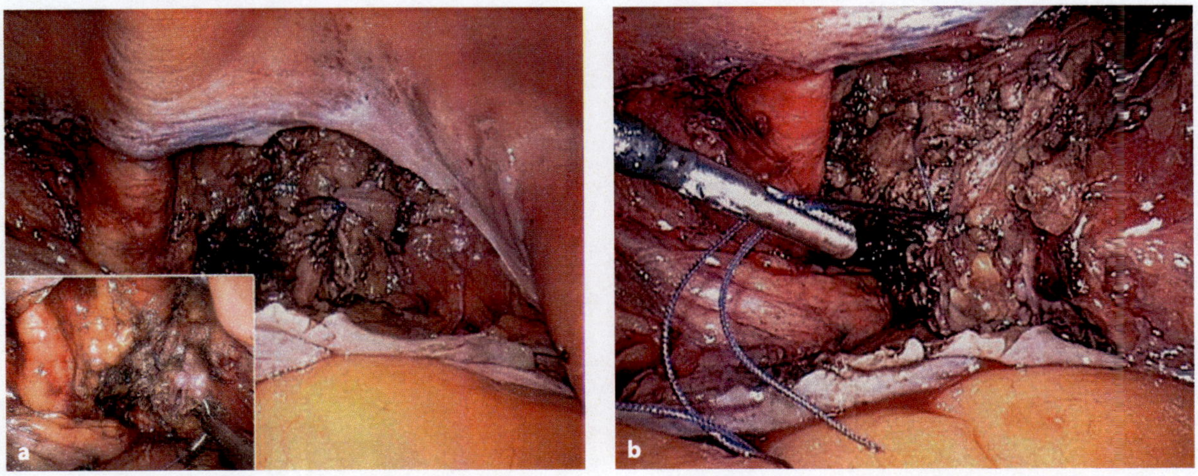

Once it has been confirmed that the bladder is watertight, the peritoneum is closed with running or interrupted sutures (Step 12a). Ideally the whole peritoneal incision is closed. This may occasionally be difficult to achieve because of tension due to previous colon mobilisation. In Step 12, the entire peritoneal opening is not closed, thus allowing a small drain to be placed through the 3-mm skin incision or through the Quadport into the extraperitoneal space. The endoscopic bag containing the diverticulum is retracted into the Quadport, which is then removed and the umbilical incision is closed. In conventional laparoscopy, the endobag is removed through one of the trocar sites.

Postoperative Management

- A catheter should be left in place for 8–10 days
- A cystogram should be performed prior to catheter removal
- Antibiotic cover until catheter removal is recommended

References

1. Blane CE, Zeron JM, Bloom DA (1994) Bladder diverticula in children. Radiology 190:695–697
2. Wilson B, Klufio G (1985) The radiological and urodynamic significance of large bladder diverticula. Clin Radiol 36:521–524
3. Faramarzi-Roques R, Calvet C, Gateau T, Ballanger PH (2004) Surgical treatment of bladder diverticula: laparoscopic approach. J Endourol 18:69–72
4. Thawini A, McLeod A, Nambirajan T (2008) Laparoscopic bladder diverticulectomy. J Laparoendosc Adv Surg Tech A 18:849–851
5. Shukla AR, Bellah RA, Canning DA et al (2004) Giant bladder diverticula causing bladder outlet obstruction in children. J Urol 172:1977–1979

3.6 Ureteral Reimplantation (Ureteroneocystostomy)

3.6.1 Robot-Assisted Psoas Hitch

Alexandre M. Mottrie, Vincenzo Ficarra, Nazareno Suardi, Geert Denaeyer

Introduction

The management of distal ureteric strictures is a potentially challenging task. When ureteral length is insufficient for direct reimplantation, additional length can be gained by a psoas hitch, necessitating mobilisation of the bladder to perform a tension-free anastomosis. Reimplantation with a psoas hitch was first described by Zimmerman et al. in 1960 [1]. Harrow [2] modified this technique with the addition of the submucosal tunnel to prevent reflux. The psoas hitch has the advantage of maintaining urothelial continuity, and it avoids compromising the function of the normal contra-lateral ureter. It also avoids the risk of chronic urinary tract infections and electrolyte abnormalities, which are advantages over transureteroureterostomy and ileal substitution, respectively [3].

The optimal benefit of robotic technology appears to be in procedures in which extensive reconstruction is required in small confined regions of the body. Robotic prostatectomy and pyeloplasty have shown the benefits to both the patient and the surgeon. Now these benefits appear to be extending further to other reconstructive procedures. We describe our technique for robot-assisted laparoscopic distal ureterectomy and ureteral reimplantation with psoas hitch [4].

Indications

- Lower ureteric lesions (strictures, fistulae, tumours)
- Failed primary ureteral reimplantation

Contra-indications

- Active urinary tract infection
- Neurogenic bladder dysfunction
- Contracted bladder, low-capacity bladder
- Bladder malignancy

Preoperative Preparation

- Cystogram to determine bladder capacity
- Imaging of the kidneys, ureters and bladder in malignant cases
- Imaging to determine the upper and lower borders of the ureteric pathology
- Clear fluids and bowel preparation the day before surgery

Step 1: Patient position and trocar placement

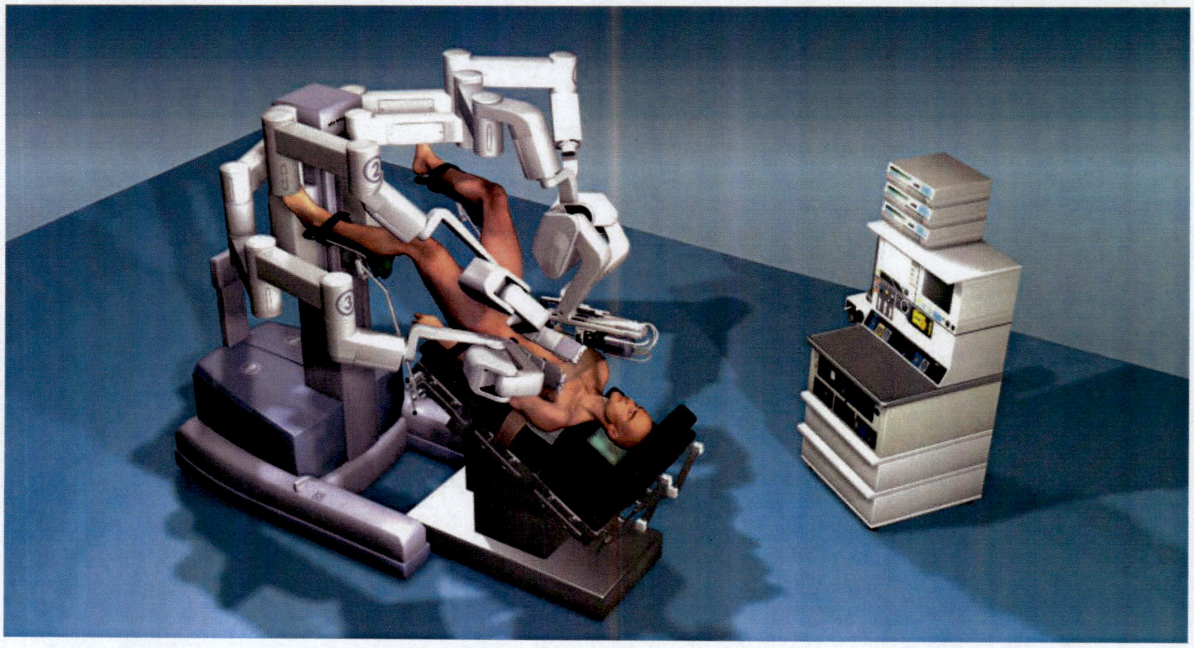

The patient is placed supine and in a 20° head-down position with a slight tilt to the contra-lateral side. The patient is then prepped and draped. Care should be taken to ensure that all pressure points are adequately protected. After this, the patient is catheterised on table using a standard urethral catheterisation technique. On-table catheterisation allows intraoperative filling and emptying of the bladder during the different stages of the operation, which is performed using the transperitoneal approach.

Step 2: Patient position and trocar placement

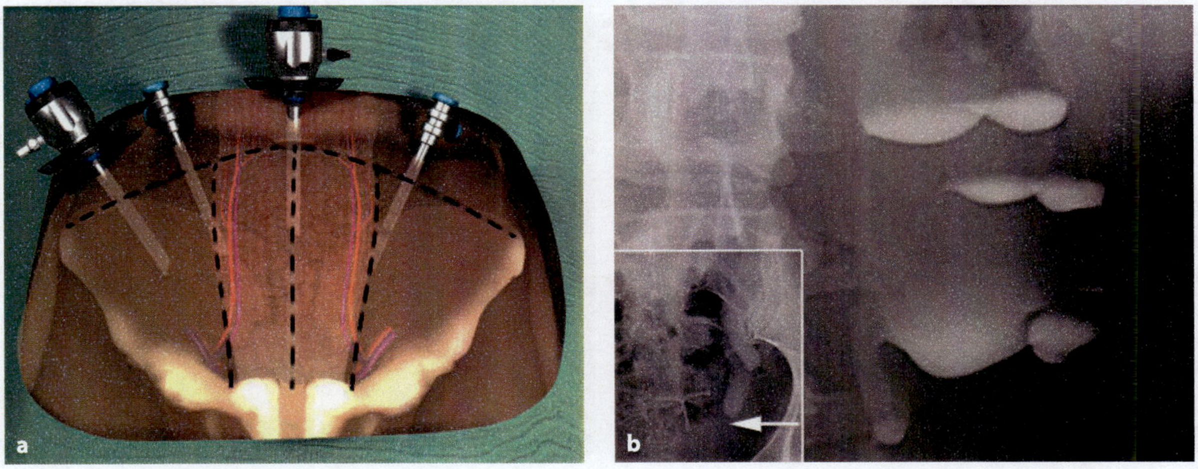

The trocar position is similar to robot-assisted radical prostatectomy, but only three robotic arms are used (Step 2a). A 12-mm camera trocar is placed at the level of the umbilicus. About 8 cm lateral to the umbilicus, an 8-mm robotic trocar is placed bilaterally and a 12-mm assistant trocar is placed laterally, as shown in the Step 2a and opposite to the side of planned reconstruction. Step 2b shows the intravenous urogram of a patient with obstructed ureter (inset, arrow), who is a candidate for stricture resection and ureteral reimplantation.

Step 3: Dissection of ureter and bladder dome

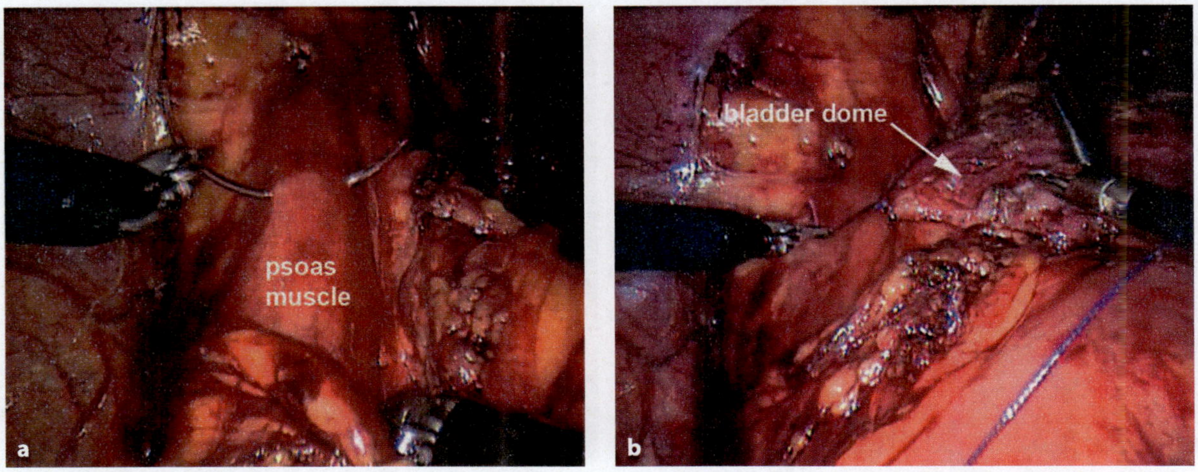

The ureter is first identified as it crosses the iliac vessels and then mobilised with its periureteral blood supply intact. Just cranial to the site of the ureteric obstruction, the ureter is clipped distally and transected. The ureter is now carefully freed cranially to allow tension-free alignment at the psoas muscle. The bladder is filled with approximately 200 ml of normal saline and mobilised until the psoas muscle can be reached. In cases of inadequate mobilisation, the contra-lateral vesical vascularisation (superior vesical artery) can be transected, which will offer greater mobility to the bladder dome. In contrast to open surgery, the psoas hitch is performed now, as it will align the posterior bladder wall in the direction of the ipsilateral robotic trocar and facilitate access to the submucosa for tunnelling.

Step 4: Psoas hitch and opening of the bladder

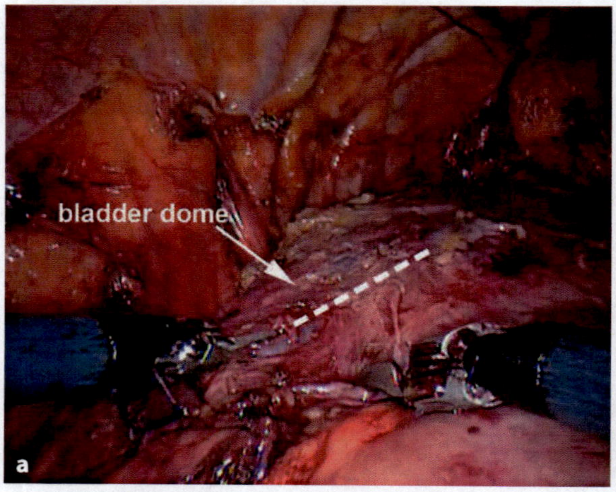

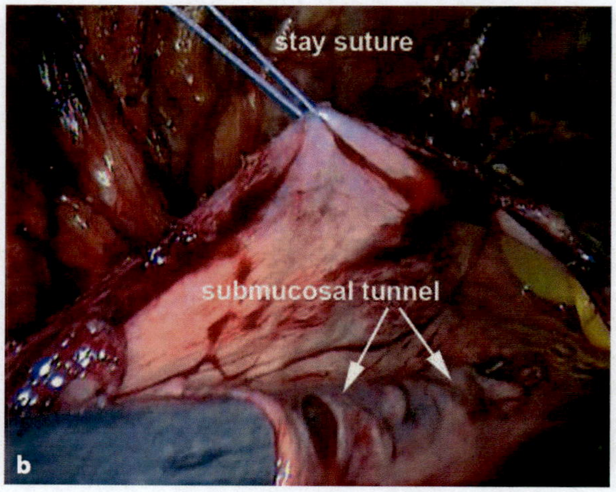

The bladder dome is fixed to the psoas muscle with two Vicryl 1 stitches approximately 1.5 cm apart. Care is taken to place the stitches through the detrusor muscle superficial to its mucosa. The bladder dome is opened from the psoas hitch downwards in the direction of the bladder neck over 6–7 cm (Step 4a). With a straight needle, two stitches are placed through the abdominal wall and used to keep the bladder incision open, which allows easy access to the posterior bladder mucosa and facilitates submucosal tunnelling (Step 4b). The submucosa is entered at the psoas hitch between the two stitches. An avascular plane is entered with the Hot Shears via the ipsilateral trocar that is in the same orientation as the planned tunnel. Once a tunnel of about 4 cm has been reached, the mucosa is perforated.

Step 5: Formation of antireflux tunnel and formation of ureteroneocystostomy

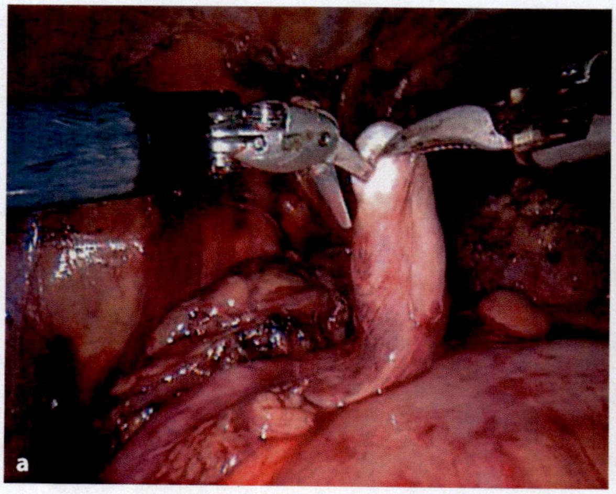

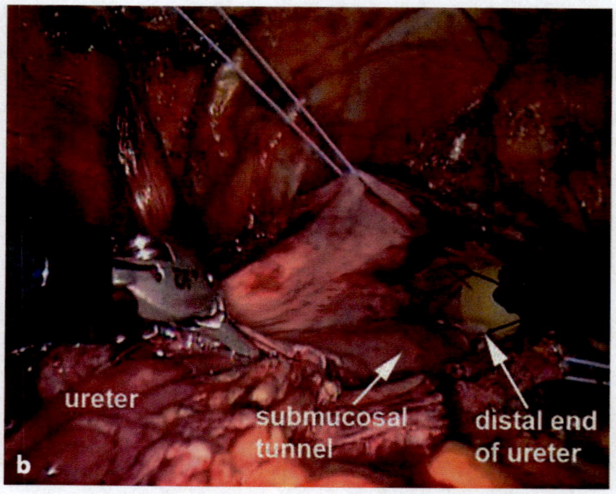

The ureter is now spatulated anteriorly over 1–1.5 cm (Step 5a). It is important that the ventral aspect of the ureter (not the posterior part) is spatulated. A suture of approximately 5 cm is placed at the distal end of the ureter. ProGrasp forceps are exchanged for the Hot Shears and the suture at the distal end of the ureter is grasped and brought through the submucosal tunnel. Using this procedure, the ureter can be carefully pulled through the tunnel without tension (Step 5b).

Step 6: Creation of ureteroneocystostomy

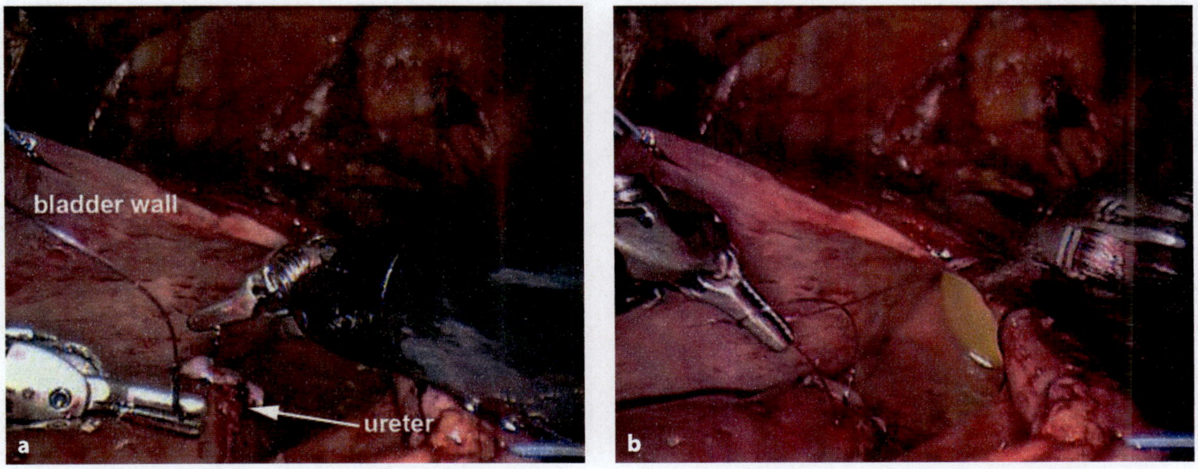

The ureteroneocystostomy is started with two anchoring Monocryl 4/0 stitches passed through the distal ureter and the full thickness of the bladder. The ureteroneocystostomy is finished with three more interrupted Monocryl 4/0 stitches of the spatulated ureter to the mucosa of the bladder only. A guidewire is inserted into the spatulated ureter through the 12-mm assistant trocar by the assistant surgeon. The surgeon then manipulates the guidewire with graspers through the ureteroneocystostomy, up the ureter and into the renal pelvis (not shown).

Step 7: Double-J stent insertion and bladder closure

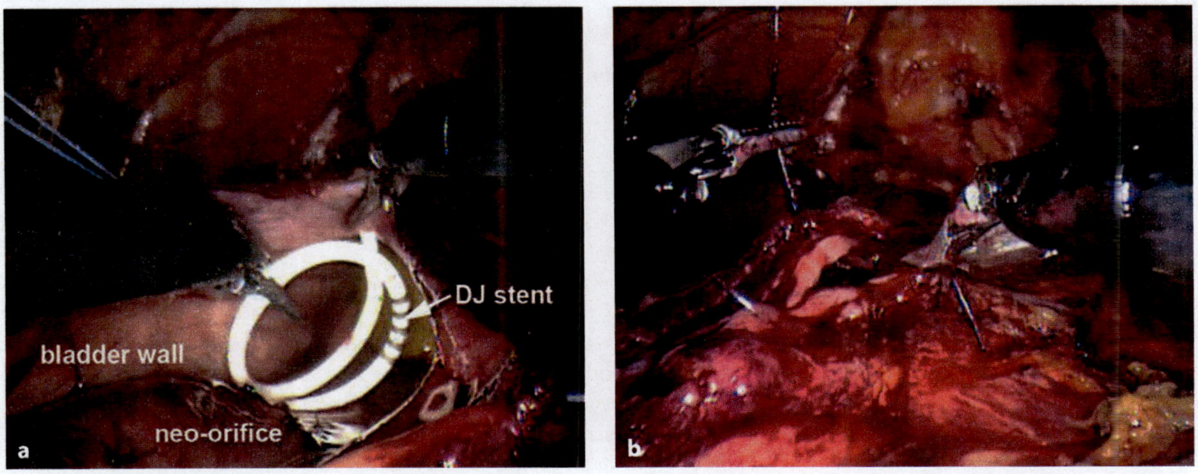

With the guidewire in place, a double-J stent is passed carefully over it, initially by the assistant from the 12-mm lateral port and then by the surgeon, until it is placed in the correct position. The guidewire is now removed. Step 7a shows the caudal end of the double-J stent in the bladder. The bladder is now closed in two layers starting from the psoas hitch (Step 7b). The mucosa of the bladder is closed with a running Monocryl 4/0 suture and the detrusor muscle is closed with a running Vicryl 2/0 suture. Care is taken not to close the muscularis too tightly over the ureter at the psoas hitch.

Step 8: Final bladder closure and postoperative cystogram

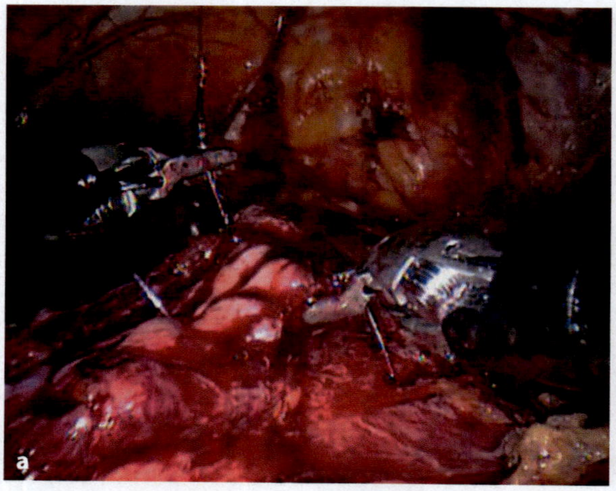

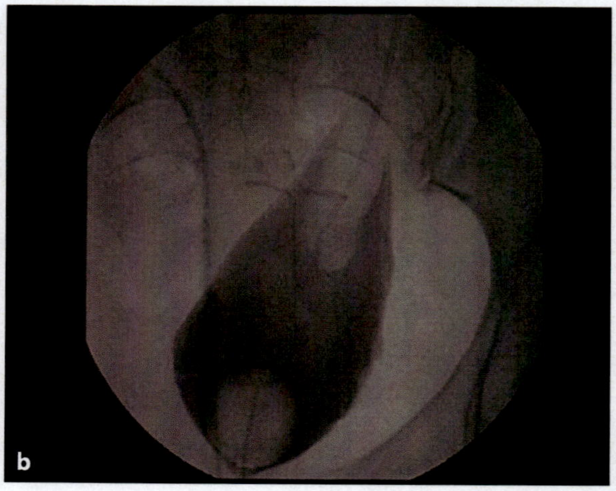

The two-layer bladder closure is completed in Step 8a. A drain is placed through the lateral robotic port site. The Foley catheter is left in situ for approximately 7–10 days. Step 8b shows a cystogram done on the 7th postoperative day demonstrating the left-sided double-J stent, psoas hitch and indwelling Foley catheter through which the cystogram was performed. There is no leak and therefore the catheter can be safely removed.

Postoperative Management

- Remove bladder catheter after cystogram on day 7
- Remove double-J stent at 3–4 weeks
- Intravenous urogram or renal ultrasound at 3 months

References

1. Zimmerman IJ, Precourt WE, Thompson CC (1960) Direct ureterocysto-neostomy with the short ureter in the cure of ureterovaginal fistula. J Urol 83:113–115
2. Harrow BR (1968) A neglected maneuver for ureterovesical reimplantation following injury at gynaecologic operations. J Urol 100:280–284
3. Ahn M, Loughlin KR (2001) Psoas hitch ureteral reimplantation in adults – analysis of a modified technique and timing of repair. Urology 58:184–187
4. Patil NN, Mottrie A, Sundaram B, Patel VR (2008) Robotic-assisted laparoscopic ureteral reimplantation with psoas hitch: a multi-institutional, multinational evaluation. Urology 72:47–50

3.6.2 Robot-Assisted Boari Flap

Ingolf A. Tuerk, Rowan Casey, Evangelos Liatsikos, Jens-Uwe Stolzenburg

Introduction

In 1894, Casati and Boari first described the flap reimplantation procedure in a canine model [1]. In 1947, it was first attempted in humans [2]. Various other groups further described the minimally invasive (laparoscopic and robot-assisted) Boari flap procedure in a variety of clinical settings [3, 4]. It is the ideal procedure for mid- to distal ureteric defects and may allow bridging a 10- to 15-cm ureteric defect in a tension-free manner. It may need to be combined with a psoas hitch procedure for further length. Robot-assisted laparoscopic surgery has been successfully applied to patients requiring distal ureteral surgery and displays similar benefits that laparoscopy has proven over open surgery in terms of improved vision, analgesia requirements and shorter hospital stays. However, maintaining sound open surgical principles in this operation is of paramount importance.

Indications

- Mid- and lower ureteric lesions (strictures, fistulae, tumours)
- Failed primary ureteral reimplantation

Contra-indications

- Active urinary tract infection
- Neurogenic bladder dysfunction
- Contracted bladder, low-capacity bladder
- Bladder malignancy

Preoperative Preparation

- Cystogram to determine bladder capacity
- Imaging of the kidneys, ureters and bladder in malignancy cases
- Imaging to determine the upper and lower borders of the ureteric pathology
- Clear fluids and bowel preparation the day before surgery

Step 1: Patient position

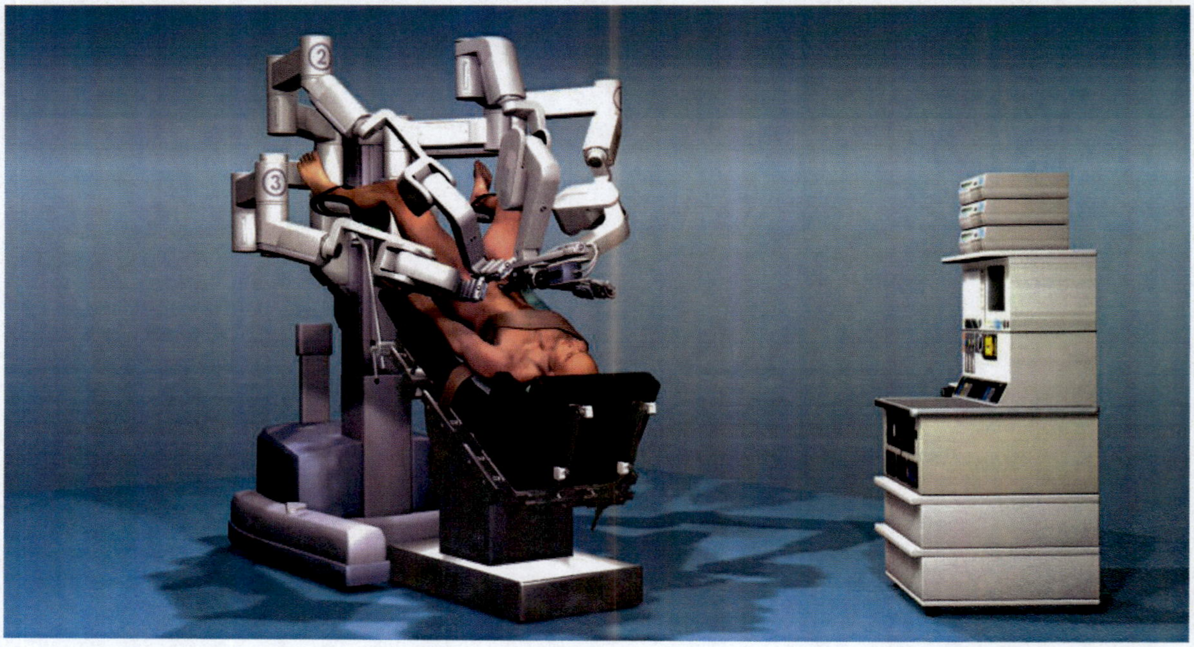

The procedure is performed transperitoneally. The patient is placed in the supine position in a 20° head-down position. The patient is catheterised on table to allow filling of the bladder during the procedure as described in the previous section. Normally, the patient's head is fully draped (not shown in the figure). For this reason, the anaesthetist chooses to use longer infusion lines to facilitate safe access. The surgical assistant sits at the left side of the patient and uses the 12- and 5-mm ports, as shown in Step 2. The surgeon sits at the robotic console throughout the entire procedure.

Step 2: Trocar placement

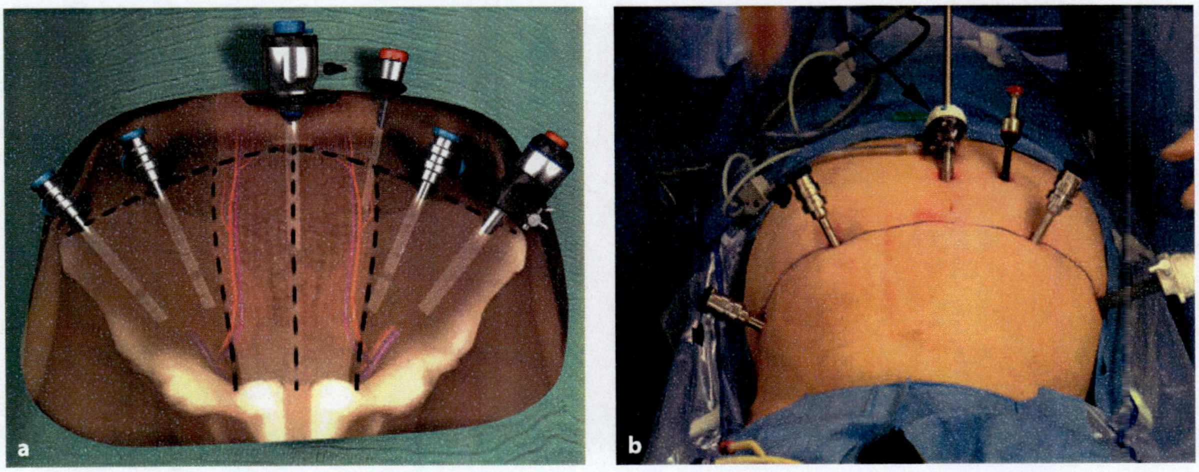

The trocar position is similar to robot-assisted radical prostatectomy. A 12-mm camera trocar is placed 3–4 cm above the umbilicus. Three fingerbreadths lateral to this on the left side, a 5-mm suction trocar is placed. Three 8-mm and one 12-mm assistant ports are placed along a line at the level of the umbilicus, as shown in Step 2a and Step 2b.

Step 3: Distal ureteric dissection

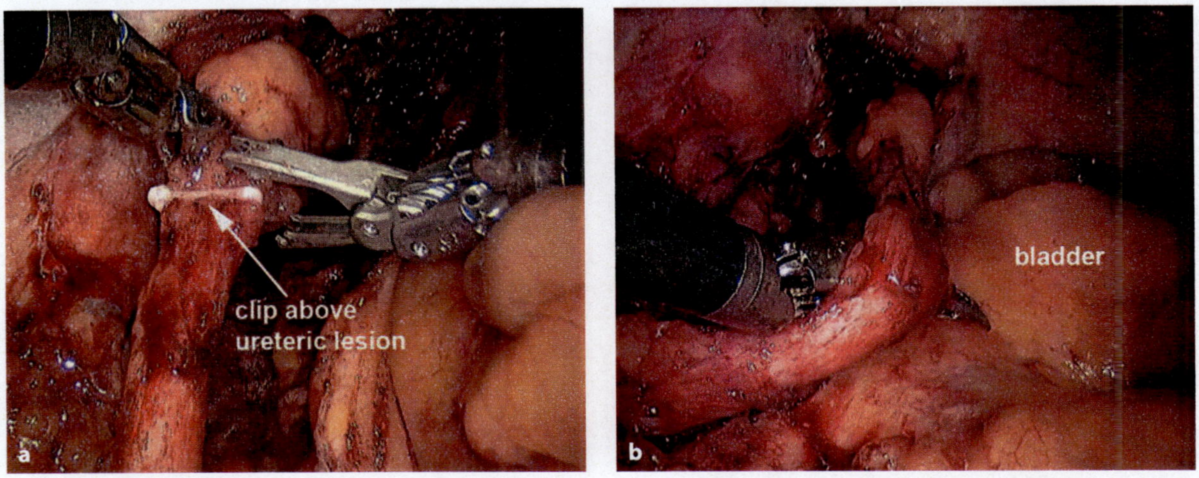

In this case, a distal left ureteric tumour is obstructing. The distal left ureter is identified and mobilised, making sure to protect the periureteral blood supply. The site of ureteric obstruction and the length of defect is confirmed intraoperatively. At this stage, the surgeon assesses whether the Boari flap will bridge the defect, although this is not perfectly accurate. The dissection of the distal left ureter is commenced (Step 3a). Robotically delivered clips are placed proximally and distally to the tumour to avoid urine spillage and potential tumour seeding during resection (Step 3b).

Step 4: Resection of the bladder cuff

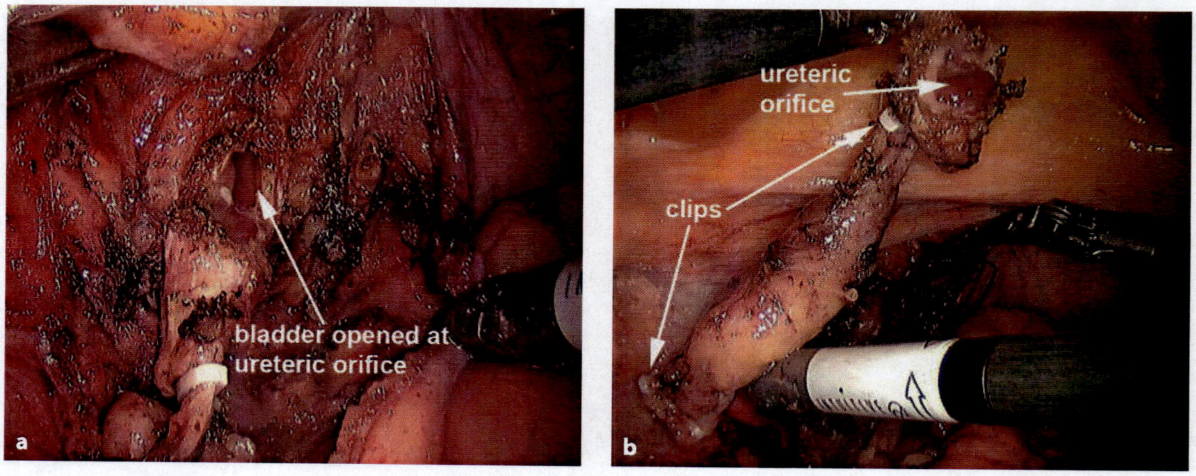

The ureter distal to the tumour is mobilised to the intramural portion of the bladder. The bladder is now opened around the ureteric orifice along the line of the ureter. The specimen, with the ureteric orifice and bladder cuff intact, is resected under direct vision whilst the bladder is open (Step 4a). Step 4b shows the resected specimen of the distal ureter with clips proximally and distally to the tumour and bladder cuff to prevent tumour spillage.

Step 5: Bladder closure and mobilisation

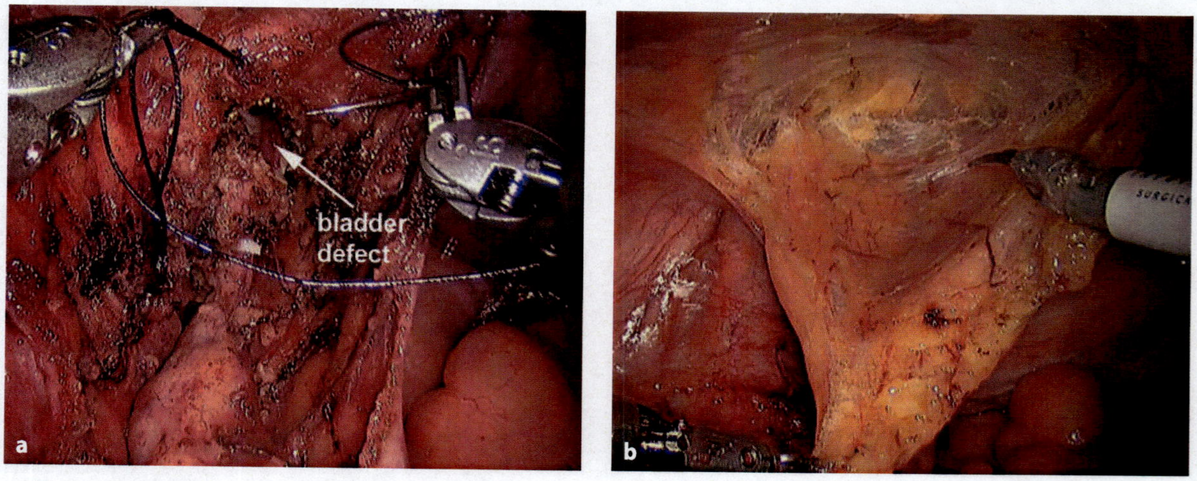

The bladder defect is now closed in two layers using 2/0 Vicryl on an SH needle in a continuous fashion for the inner mucosal and muscular layer (Step 5a). Interrupted sutures can be used for the outer serosal and fat layers. The bladder now needs to be fully mobilised to allow adequate length for a tension-free anastomosis. It is mobilised from the anterior abdominal wall, Retzius space (Step 5b) and on the contra-lateral side to the anastomosis. Posteriorly, further mobilisation may be useful. It must not be mobilised on the ipsilateral side of the Boari flap because the flap depends on its vascularity from this side.

Step 6: Boari flap formation

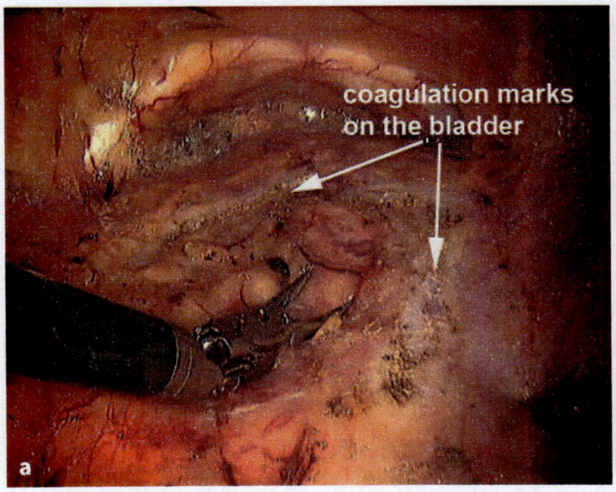

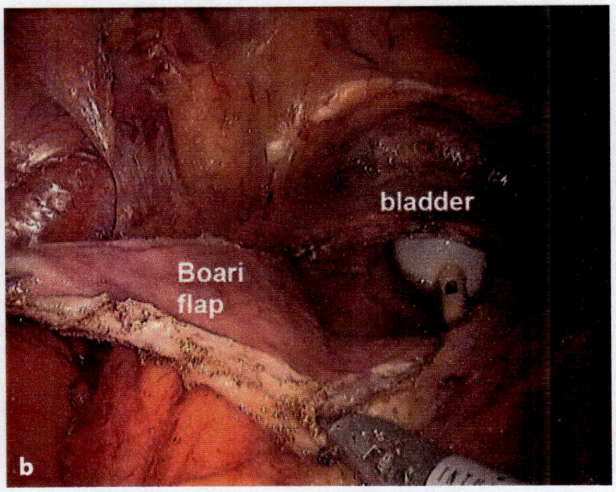

The mobilised bladder is filled with 300 cc saline in order to aid identification of dissection planes. To aid orientation, the margins of the Boari flap are marked on the perivesical fat with coagulation, as in Step 6a. The flap should be positioned obliquely across the bladder towards the contralateral side and the base should be wider than the neck to ensure good vascularity. Step 6b demonstrates the development of the Boari flap as the base is dissected from the contra-lateral side of the bladder (towards the bladder neck) and brought out of the pelvis on its pedicle towards the ureter.

Step 7: Anastomosis of ureter and Boari flap

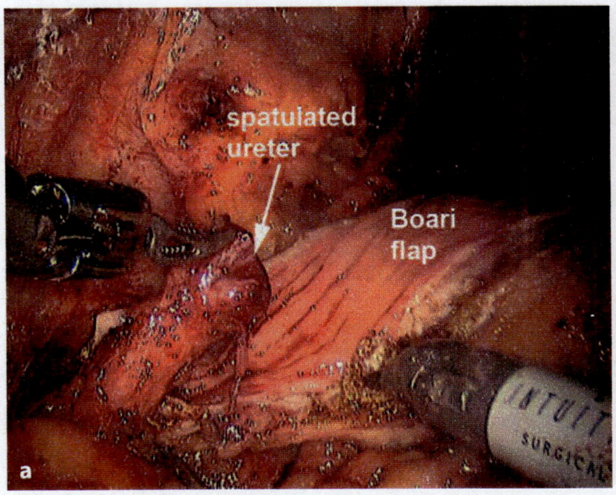

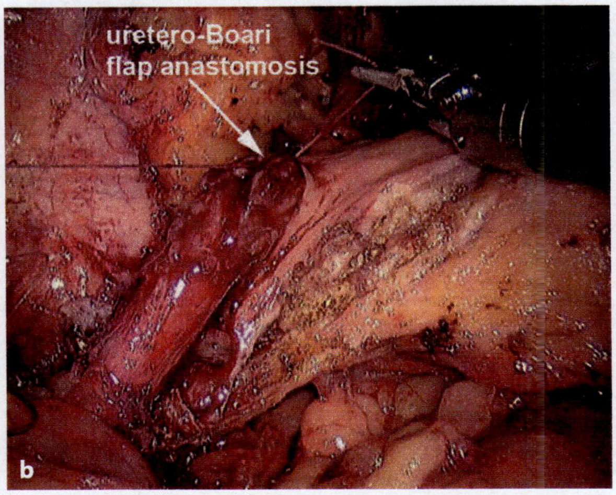

The left ureter is spatulated anteriorly, and both the ureter and Boari flap are approximated at this point to determine if there is sufficient length for a tension-free anastomosis. The ureter often is dilated and allows the scissors to be inserted easily for spatulation. Step 7b shows the ureter being fixed within the Boari flap with 4/0 Vicryl interrupted sutures on an RB-1 needle for later ureteric tunnelling. The ureter is anchored to the Boari flap with three stitches.

Step 8: Insertion of ureteric stent

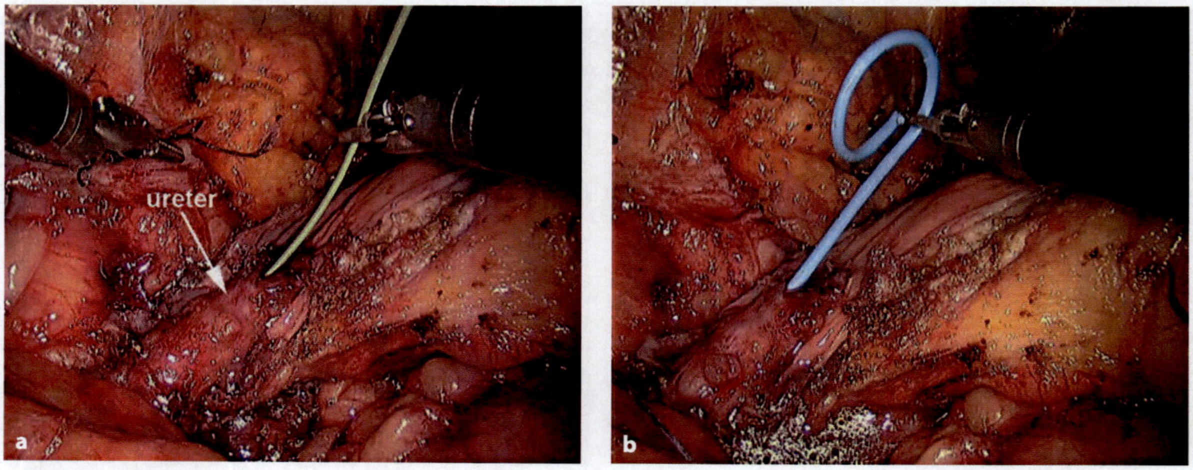

A guidewire is inserted into the spatulated ureter through the 5-mm suction trocar by the side surgeon. This is manipulated into the ureter and threaded up the ureter with graspers and into the renal pelvis, as in Step 8a. Over this guidewire, a double-J stent is passed through the 5-mm suction trocar. The guidewire is now removed. Leave enough length on the double-J stent to allow the pigtail to be positioned in the bladder rather than the Boari flap.

Step 9: Boari flap closure

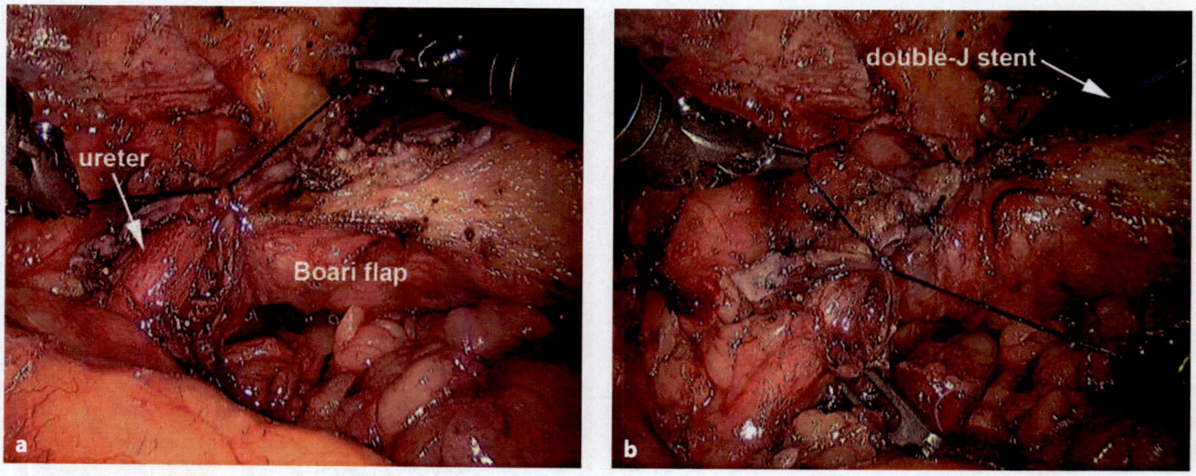

The submucosal tunnel can now be created to form a nonrefluxing anastomosis. We use a nontunnelled uretero-Boari flap anastomosis in situations where free reflux of urine is not a concern. To perform this, the ureter is not tunneled but rather there is an incision of the mucosa underneath the ureter and closure of the mucosa over the ureter. The Boari flap is now rolled and closed over the ureter with interrupted 2/0 Vicryl sutures on an SH needle. Continued closure of the Boari flap over the ureter is now carried out towards the bladder.

Step 10: Bladder closure and psoas hitch

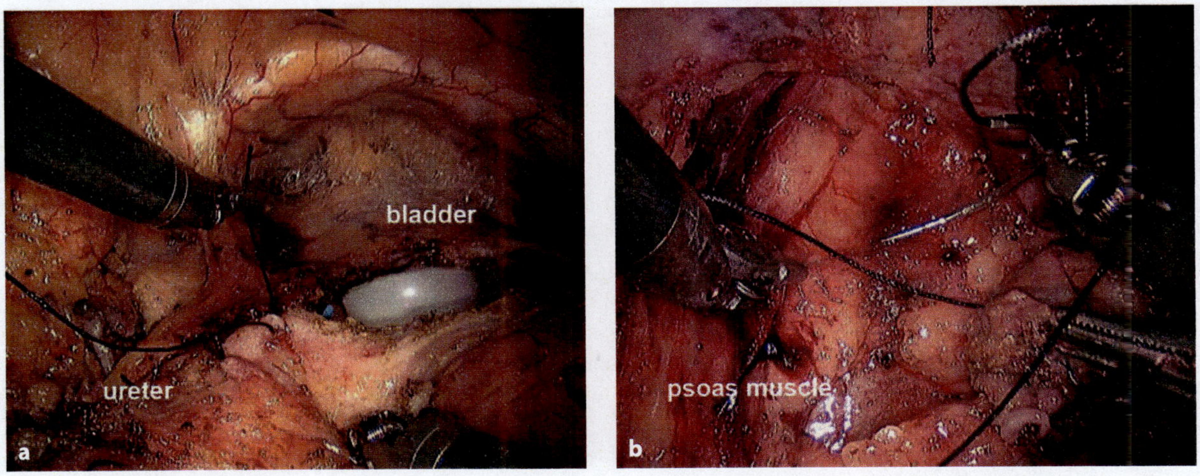

Anteriorly, the bladder had been opened to create the Boari flap. It is now closed in one or two layers from the Boari flap to the base of the bladder incision. We perform a psoas hitch stitch next using three 0 Vicryl sutures on a CT-1 needle from the psoas muscle to the Boari flap in order to provide further stability to the anastomosis. This is easily performed with the excellent vision provided with robotic surgery.

Step 11: Finished result

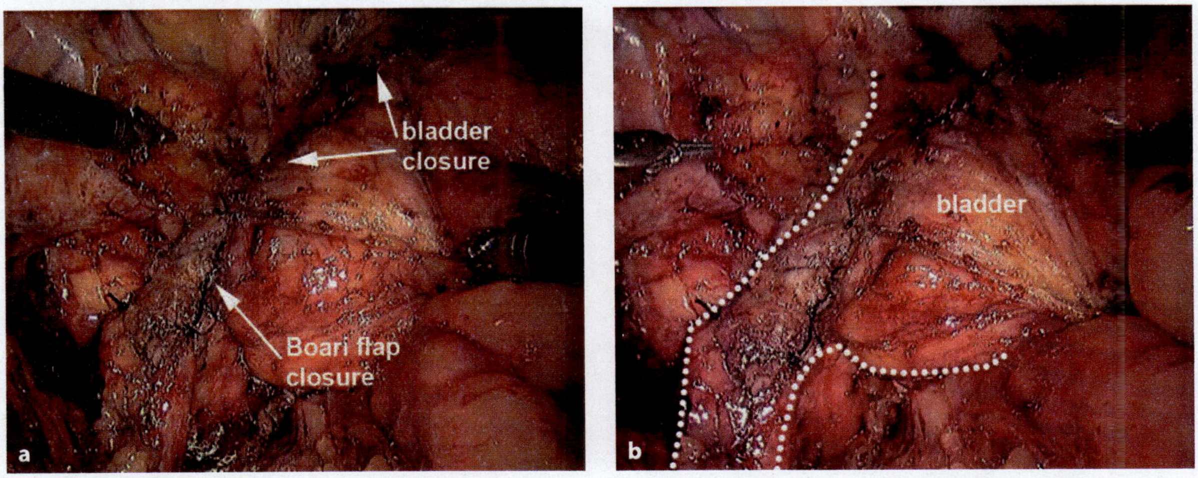

The finished result is shown in Step 11a and Step 11b. The insertion of a suprapubic catheter is not necessary prior to bladder closure. The bladder can be filled with 200 ml of water of dilute methylene blue to check that there are no leaks. A nonsuction drain is placed in the left iliac fossa. A final check is made for bleeding and to ensure that there is no tension on the ureter or bladder.

Postoperative Management

- Remove urethral catheter after cystogram on day 10
- Remove double-J stent at 4–6 weeks
- Intravenous urogram or renal ultrasound at 3 months to check uretero-Boari flap anastomosis

References

1. Casati E, Boari A (1894) Contributo sperimentale alla plastic dell'uretere. Communicazione preventive. Atti Acad Sci Med Nat 14:149
2. Ockerblad NF (1947) Reimplantation of the ureter into the bladder by a flap method. J Urol 57:845
3. Gözen AS, Cresswell J, Canda AE, Ganta S, Rassweiler J, Teber D (2010) Laparoscopic ureteral reimplantation: prospective evaluation of medium-term results and current developments. World J Urol 28:221–226
4. Symons S, Kurien A, Desai M (2009) Laparoscopic ureteral reimplantation: a single center experience and literature review. J Endourol 23:269–274
5. Schimpf MO, Wagner JR (2009) Robot-assisted laparoscopic distal ureteral surgery. JSLS 13:44–49

3.7 Radical Cystoprostatectomy

3.7.1 Laparoscopic Radical Cystoprostatectomy

Jens-Uwe Stolzenburg, Tony Riddick, Thilo Schwalenberg, Anja Dietel, Minh Do, Rowan Casey, Evangelos Liatsikos

Introduction

Open radical cystectomy with extended pelvic lymphadenectomy (PLA) remains the gold standard and most effective treatment of patients with organ-confined muscle-invasive or high-risk bladder cancer [1]. However, radical cystectomy remains an aggressive procedure with significant morbidity and mortality, especially given that bladder cancer is usually diagnosed in older persons who most often have medical co-morbidities.

Laparoscopic approaches to radical cystectomy have been introduced in order to maintain high-quality outcomes but with less morbidity associated with the laparoscopic approach.

Current techniques allow for the performance of cystectomy in selected patients with improvements in estimated blood loss. Early results also show that the technique adheres to the oncologic principles required for cancer control, including obtaining negative margins and performing an adequate extended lymph node dissection [2]. While completely intracorporal approaches are technically feasible, currently they are associated with significant increases in operative times and perioperative complications. With the current techniques available, the best results seem to be with cystectomy and extended lymph node dissection being performed laparoscopically and the urinary reconstruction performed in a limited open fashion. While laparoscopic cystectomy remains investigational, intermediate cancer control outcomes are favourable compared to open surgery. Since publication of the first reports by Sánchez de Badajoz [3] and Puppo [4] and after a decade of progress, laparoscopic radical cystectomy continues to be a pioneering technique that is only performed in centres with extensive experience in laparoscopy [5, 6]. However, long-term outcome data are currently being accrued and this may allow a shift in the standard of care to minimally invasive approaches for select patients.

Indications (EAU guidelines 2009/2010)

- Non-muscle-invasive bladder cancer (high risk of progression)
  - Multiple recurrent high-grade tumours (despite resection and intravesical chemotherapy)
  - High-grade T1 tumours (grade 3 poorly differentiated tumours (according to the 1973 WHO grading) are equivalent to high-grade papillary urothelial carcinoma (according to the updated WHO/ISUP [International Society of Urological pathology] 2004 grading system)
  - High-grade tumours with concomitant carcinoma-in-situ
  - T1 tumours with high risk of progression (multifocality, large size [>3 cm])
  - Bacillus Calmette-Guerin (BCG) failures
- Muscle-invasive bladder cancer
  - Recommended in T2–4a, N0–Nx, M0 bladder cancer

Contra-indications

- Bulky or locally advanced bladder malignancy (relative)
- Prior pelvic radiation or prostate surgery (relative)
- Extensive abdominal surgery (relative)
- Cardiovascular co-morbidities

Preoperative Preparation

- Optimal site of (contingency) stoma marked on skin
- Sorbitol 100 ml two days before surgery, clear liquid diet
- Two sachets MoviPrep 1 day before surgery, clear liquid diet
- Enema bowel preparation the day before
- Broad-spectrum antibiotic coverage
- DVT thromboprophylaxis (compression stockings and low-molecular-weight heparin) until the patient is ambulatory
- Nasogastric tube and urinary catheter inserted on table

Step 1: Patient position and trocar placement

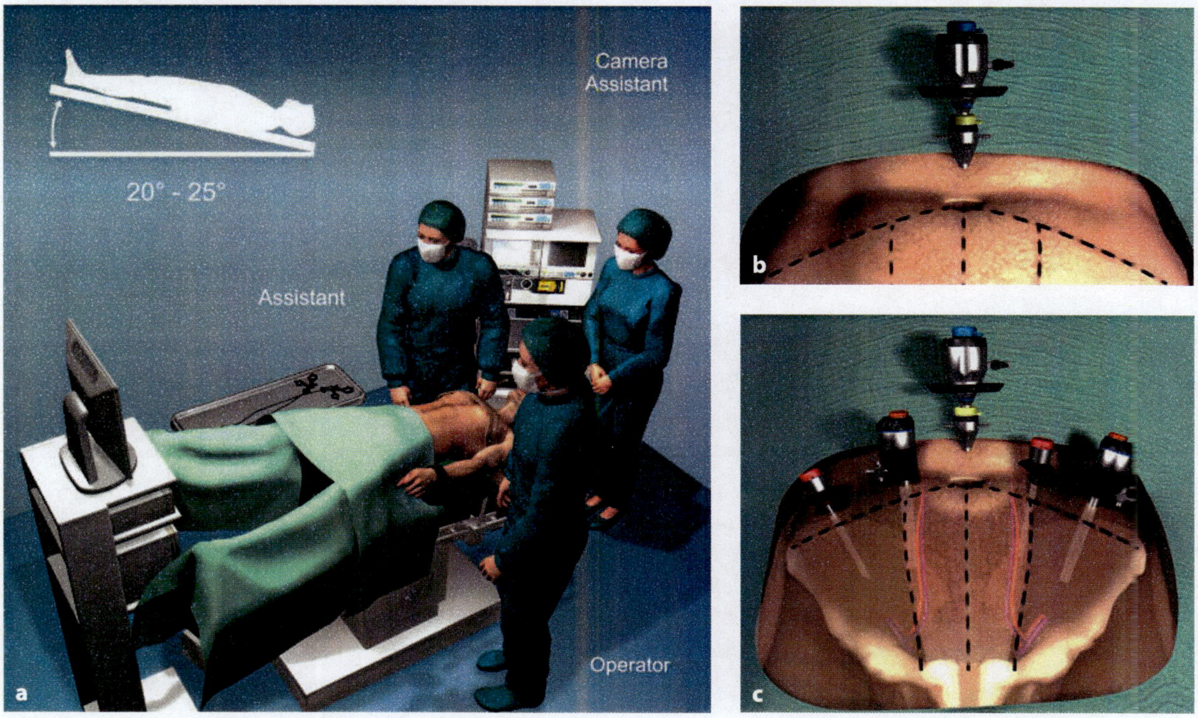

The patient is placed in a dorsal supine position with a 20–25° Trendelenburg position. The operating surgeon stands on the left side of the patient, the assistant on the opposite side, the camera holder behind the head of the patient. A 15-mm incision is made 3–4 cm cranial to the umbilicus for placement of the camera laparoscopic port (Step 1b). Two 12-mm and two 5-mm ports are placed at the level of the umbilicus on the left and on the right as shown in Step 1c. These five port positions enable the extended lymphadenectomy described below. If a Bricker stoma is planned the position of the right 12-mm port is variable and depends on where preoperatively it has been decided to site the Bricker stoma.

Step 2: Anatomical landmarks

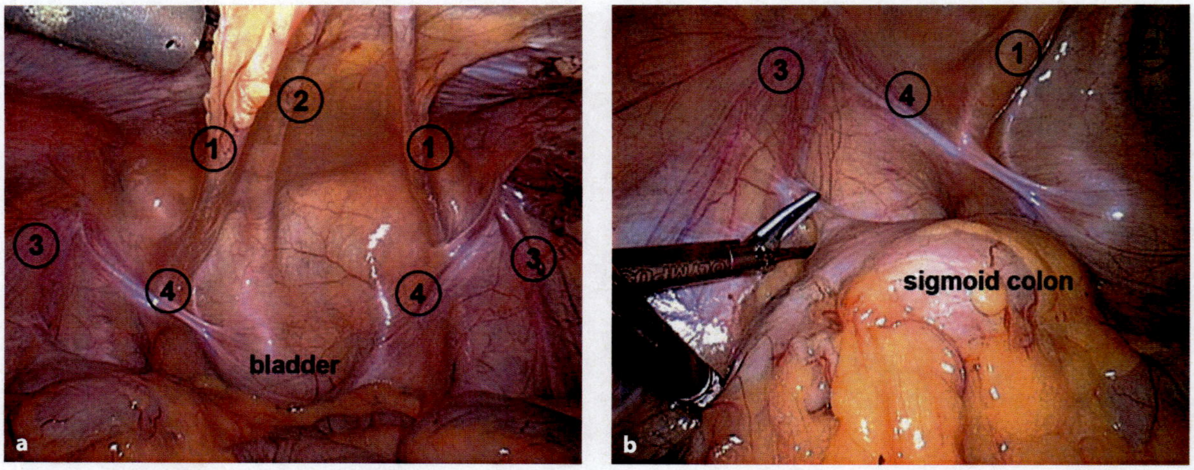

Initial inspection of the pelvis should clearly reveal the abdominal wall with the right and left obliterated umbilical arteries (1) and the obliterated urachus in the midline (2). The spermatic cord (3) and vas deferens (4) can be identified bilaterally. Any adhesions will need to be divided before peritoneal incision. The next step is the mobilisation of the descending colon and sigmoid colon. On the right side, the caecum has to be mobilised. The full mobilisation of the colon along the line of Toldt on both sides is a requirement for extended lymphadenectomy.

Step 3: Dissection of the vas and seminal vesicle mobilisation

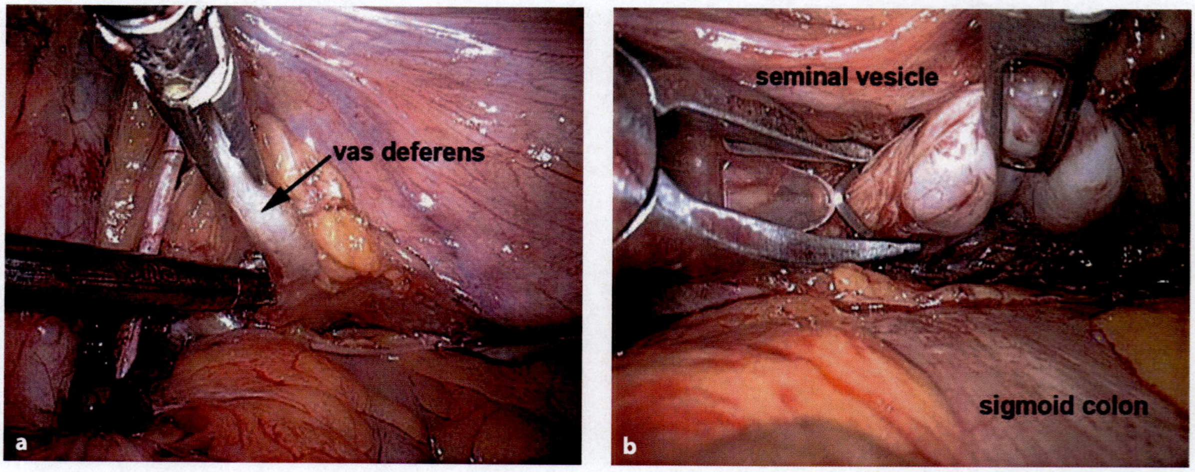

The peritoneal incision on each side is continued towards the pelvis along the course of the vas deferens. Both vas deferens are completely mobilised, revealing the ampullary portions of the vas deferens, which are then dissected. The seminal vesicles are easily identified slightly lateral to the vas deferens and completely dissected. Dissection in the region of the tips of the seminal vesicles is performed with clips and cold scissors in order to avoid injury to the pelvic plexus in a nerve-sparing procedure. In a non-nerve-sparing procedure, the whole dissection can be performed with the SonoSurg device.

Step 4: Incision of Denonvilliers fascia

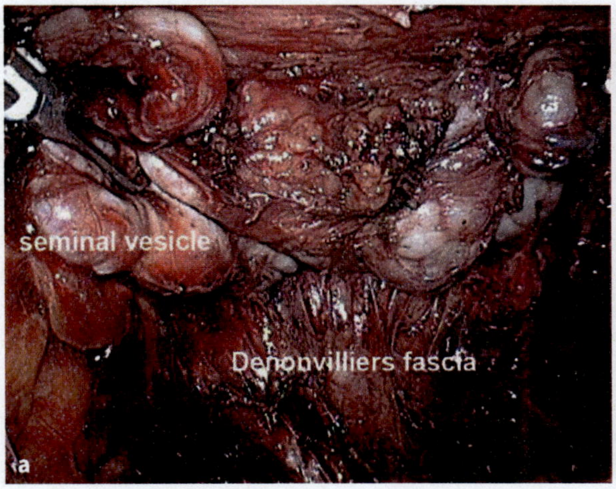

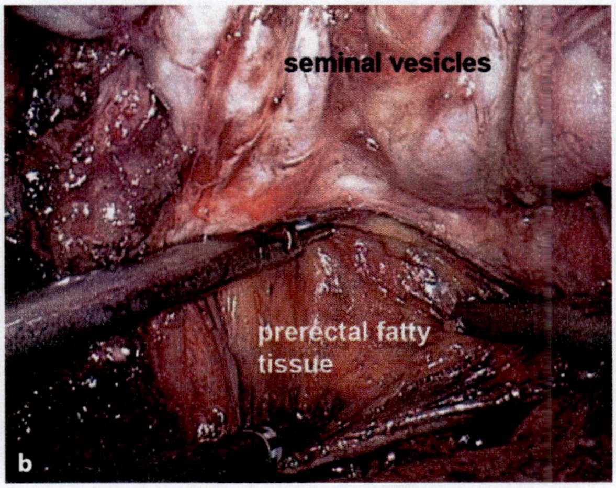

After dissection of the seminal vesicles, the assistant holds the right ampulla and the right seminal vesicle and the operating surgeon the left ampulla and the left seminal vesicle in a craniolateral direction. With this manoeuvre, a window is developed encompassing the dorsal aspect of the prostate and the prostatic pedicles. The Denonvilliers fascia is clearly seen between these structures. The posterior layer of the Denonvilliers fascia is then incised and the prerectal fatty tissue (yellow) is visualised. The dissection is continued in a blunt and sharp fashion as far as possible towards the apex of the prostate and strictly in the midline in order to avoid injury to the neurovascular bundles. Visualisation of the posterior plane of the prostate helps determine a safe plane of dissection.

Step 5: Pelvic lymphadenectomy

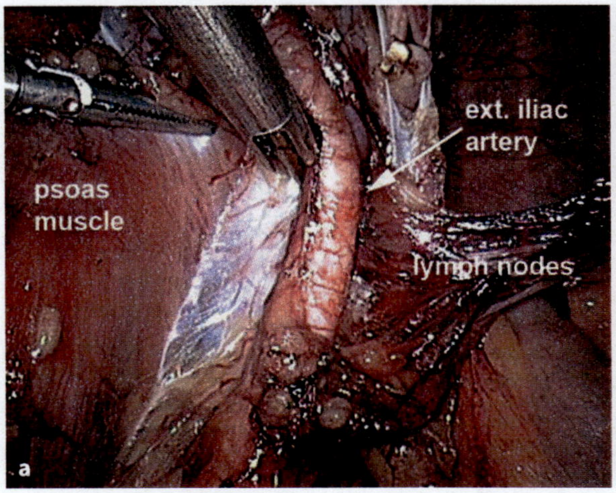

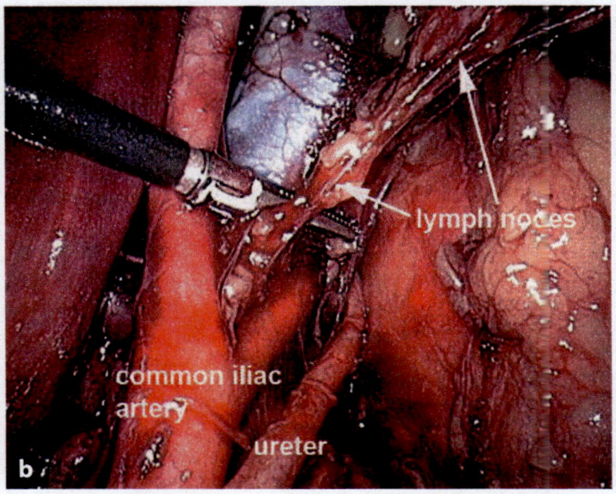

It is essential to perform an extended pelvic lymphadenectomy in patients with transitional cell carcinoma nodal metastases, rather than a limited PLA, because of the benefits in cancer-specific survival. The technique is described in detail in Sect. 2.2. The lymph node packages around the external iliac artery and vein need to be carefully cleared from these vessels (Step 5a, Step 5b). The lymphadenectomy must include the common iliac artery (Step 5b). The dissection should be continued in a cranial direction up to the bifurcation of the aorta. Some authors recommend dissection up to the inferior mesenteric artery. Performing this laparoscopically is technically very challenging.

Step 6: Pelvic lymphadenectomy

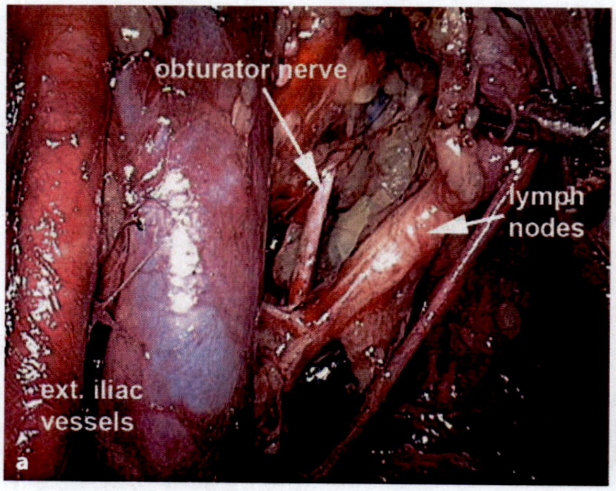

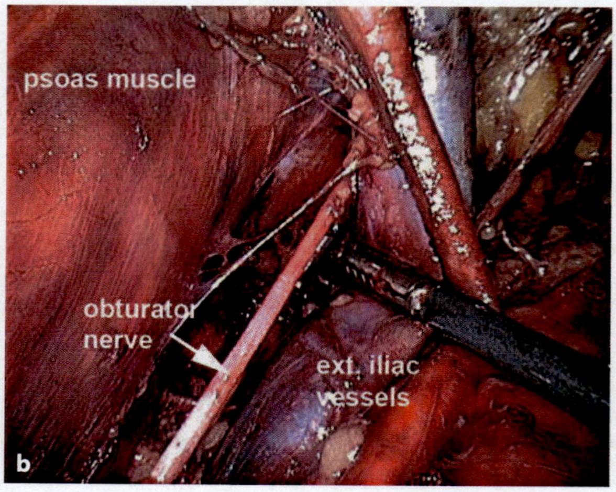

The assistant grasps and retracts the lymph node package to the contralateral side (Step 6a) while the surgeon performs the PLA. The obturator fossa must be completely dissected free of lymph nodes. This can be confirmed by retracting the external iliac artery and vein medially. The window between the psoas muscle and the external iliac vessels, as shown in Step 6b, allows further access to the obturator fossa to complete the nodal dissection. Where bleeding occurs, the vessels should be clipped and extensive coagulation should be avoided. This thermal injury to the obturator nerve caused by excess coagulation may result in neurapraxia that can take months to recover.

Step 7: Pelvic lymphadenectomy

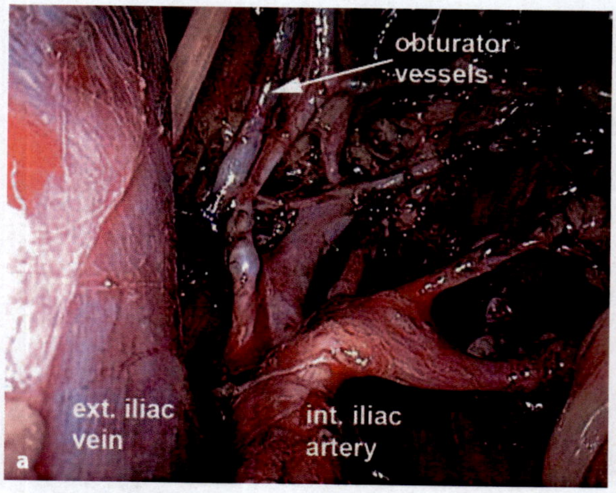

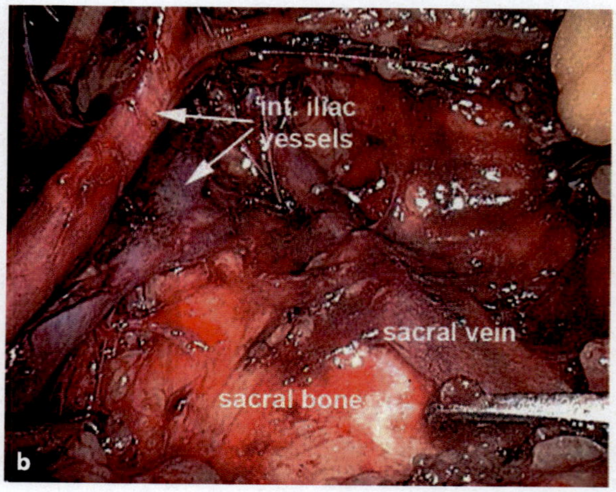

In an extended PLA, all the branches of the internal iliac artery and vein are freed from lymph nodes, as shown in Step 7a. The lymphadenectomy must also include the presacral nodes. Finally, the sacral bone and sacral vein should be visible on complete dissection, as shown in Step 7b. All the lymph nodes should be placed in an EndoCatch bag intact and en bloc if possible. For proper clinical staging, it is recommended to use different bags for each level of dissection on each side. Dissecting the node packages in pieces to remove them via the 12-mm trocar can potentially lead to tumour spillage or port site metastasis and therefore should not be performed.

Step 8: Dissection of the ureter

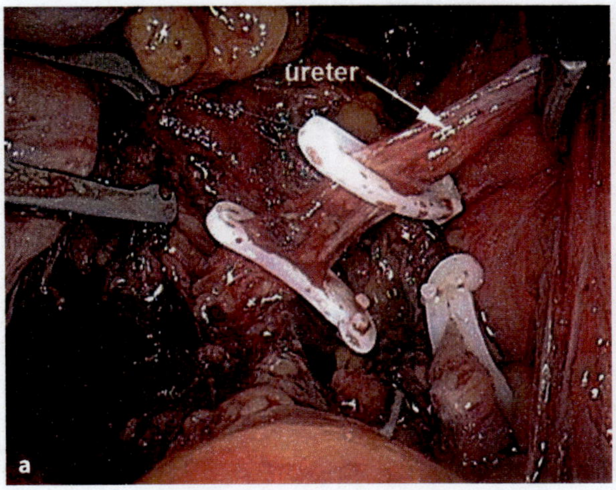

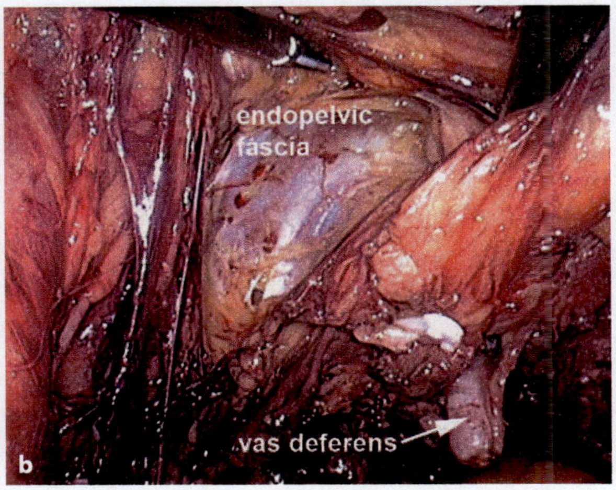

The next step is the identification and mobilisation of the ureter. The ureter is normally clearly identifiable during the lymphadenectomy. It is mobilised to the point of insertion into the bladder. Care must be taken not to skeletonise the ureter. This can be prevented if the tissue bridge (blood supply to the ureter) between the ureter and gonadal vessels is protected. On the left side, the ureter must be divided as close to the bladder as possible in order to provide sufficient length to perform the ureteroileal anastomosis, especially in the case of a Bricker stoma. It is divided between two clips (Step 8a) and a frozen section taken from the caudal end of the divided ureter. Then prior to the bladder pedicle dissection, all the fatty and areolar tissue on top of the endopelvic fascia is cleared using the bipolar forceps (Step 8b).

Step 9: Bladder pedicle dissection

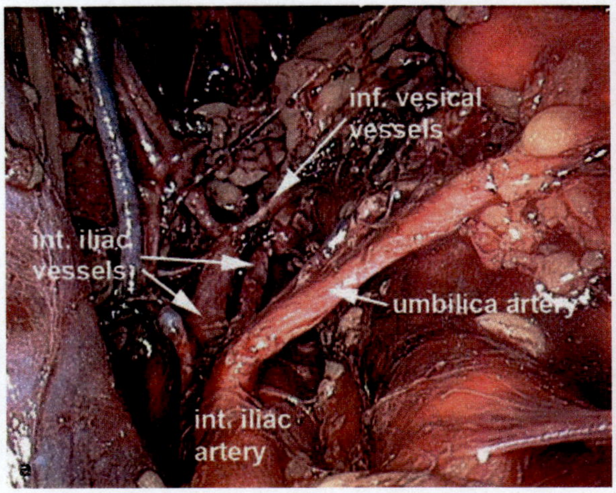

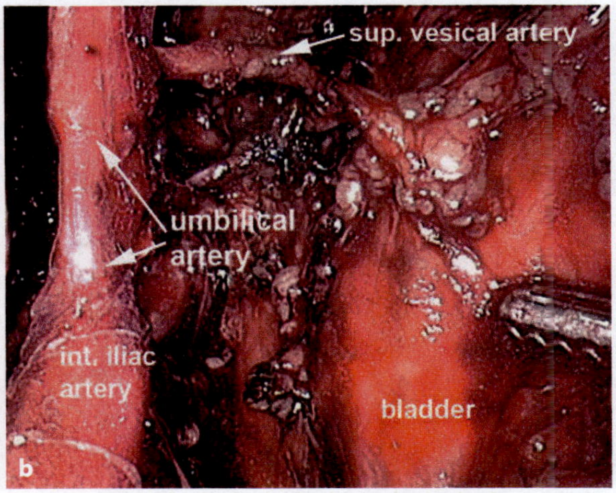

Anatomically, the superior vesical artery is the first branch of the umbilical artery, which originates from the internal iliac artery in the majority of patients, as shown in Step 9. Step 9b shows the detail of this topographic anatomy. There are a number of anatomical variations which will be shown in Step 10. Despite some authors preferring to perform PLA after cystectomy, performing the PLA first provides excellent visualisation of the bladder pedicle vessels, allowing selective clipping of individual vessels.

Step 10: Anatomical variants of bladder pedicle

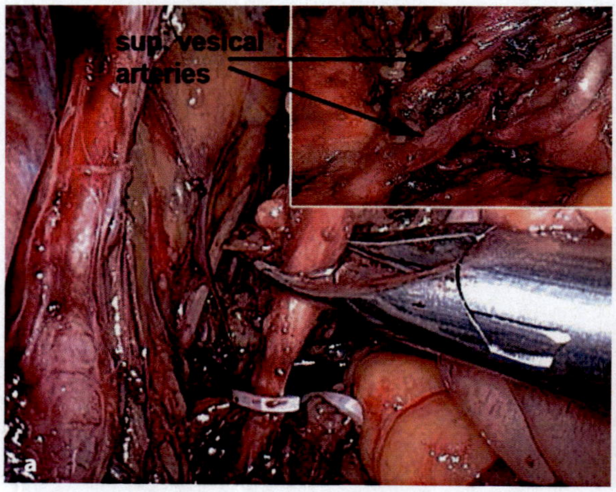

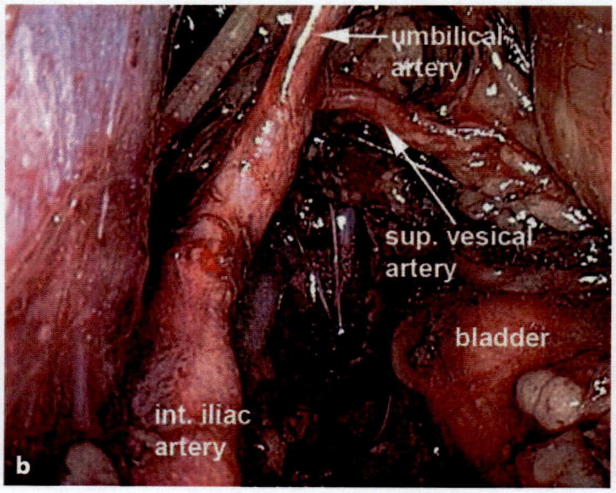

To secure the bladder pedicle, the umbilical artery is dissected and divided between Hem-o-lok clips (two clips on the proximal internal iliac artery side). Ligaclips can be used on the distal bladder side. Alternatively, the superior vesical artery can be selectively clipped and divided. The inset in Step 10a demonstrates an anatomical variant with two superior vesical arteries originating directly from the internal iliac artery. Step 10b shows another anatomical variant where the umbilical artery and superior vesical artery arise directly from internal iliac artery. In case of severe bleeding from the bladder pedicle or branches from the internal iliac artery, the whole internal iliac artery should be clipped. This must be done caudal to the origin of the superior gluteal artery.

Step 11: Access to the Retzius space

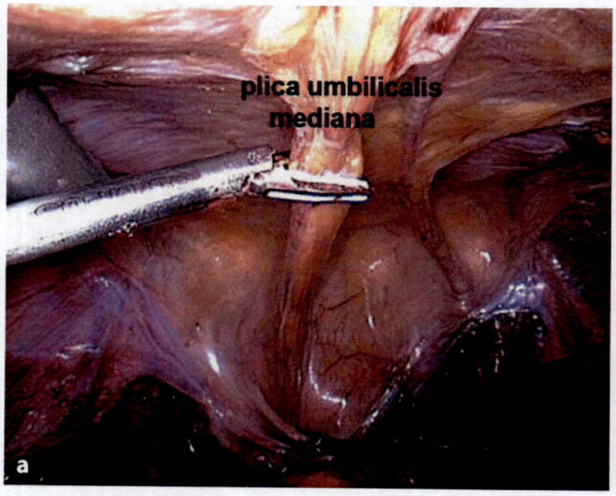

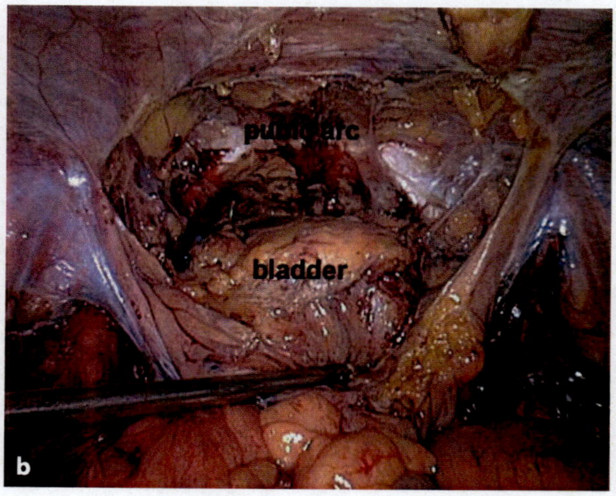

The operation continues with the dissection of the Retzius space. The parietal peritoneum is incised between the two medial umbilical folds, and the two medial umbilical ligaments (obliterated umbilical arteries) are divided using the SonoSurg device. If bleeding occurs (when the umbilical artery is not clipped or obliterated) bipolar forceps can be used to gain control. The dissection is continued in the lateral direction towards the inguinal ring. The gas insufflation helps to dissect the Retzius space. The pubic arch and the symphysis are widely exposed and the incision of the peritoneum is continued in the lateral direction up to the external iliac vessels and the endopelvic fascia.

Step 12: Endopelvic fascia incision and Santorini plexus ligation

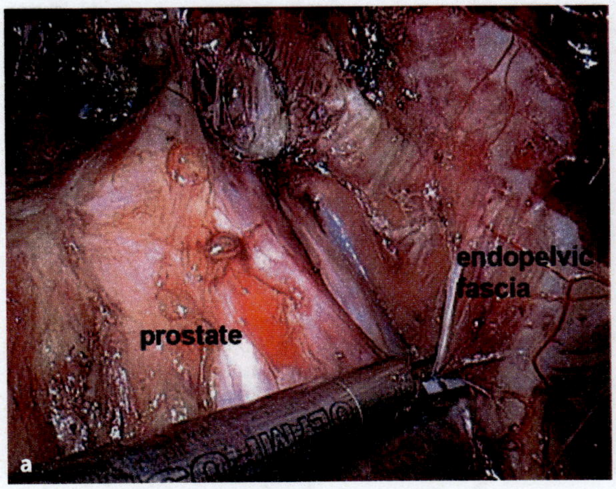

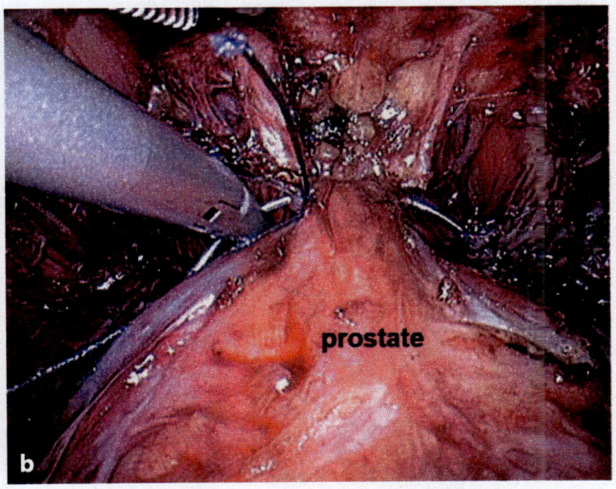

The endopelvic fascia is incised on both sides, as demonstrated in Step 12a. At this level, the distinction between the lateral side of the prostate and the endopelvic fascia covering the levator ani muscle becomes clear. Then both puboprostatic ligaments are fully dissected with cold scissors. The Santorini venous plexus is situated directly under the ligaments and care should be taken not to cut too deeply when dividing these ligaments. The Santorini plexus is ligated with 2/0 Polysorb (GS-22 needle, slightly straightened) by passage of the needle underneath the plexus from left to right. For safe ligation, we recommend a second ligation with the same suture, as shown in Step 12b. Even if the first suture is not perfectly placed the second stitch always allows accurate placement of the suture.

Step 13: Preservation of neurovascular bundle and urethral dissection

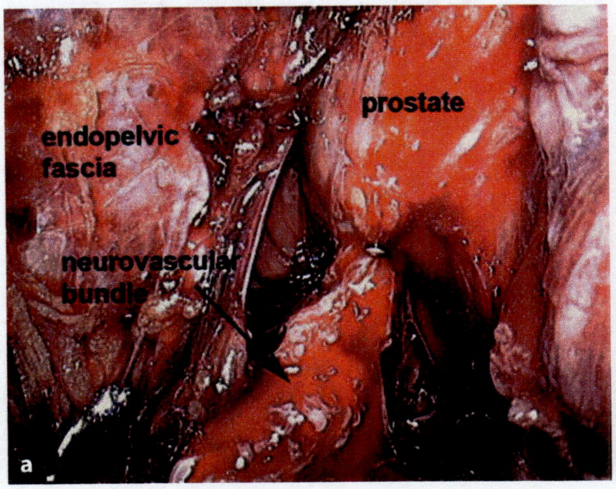

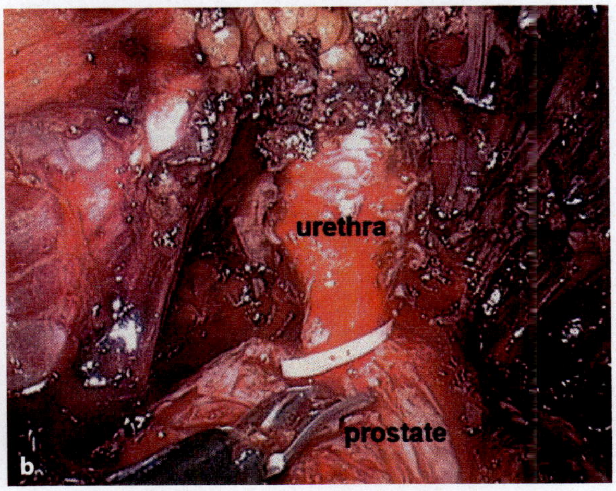

The seminal vesicles are now lifted by the assistant up towards the symphysis pubis. This allows clear identification of the prostatic pedicles. The prostatic pedicles must be clipped and cut with cold scissors step by step. In nerve-sparing procedures, it is not recommended to use the SonoSurg or bipolar diathermy. When the main prostatic pedicles have been fully dissected, the remaining neurovascular bundles can be detached from the prostatic capsule (Step 13a). Now the urethra can be developed and clipped before cutting to avoid any urine leakage into the abdominal cavity (remember to remove the catheter immediately before clipping).

Step 14: Final inspection and haemostasis

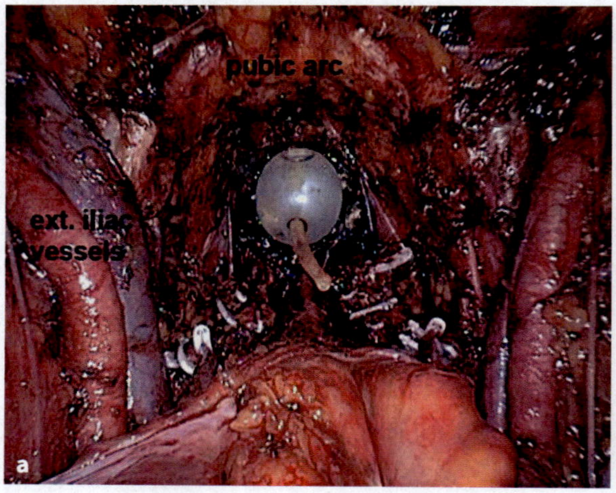

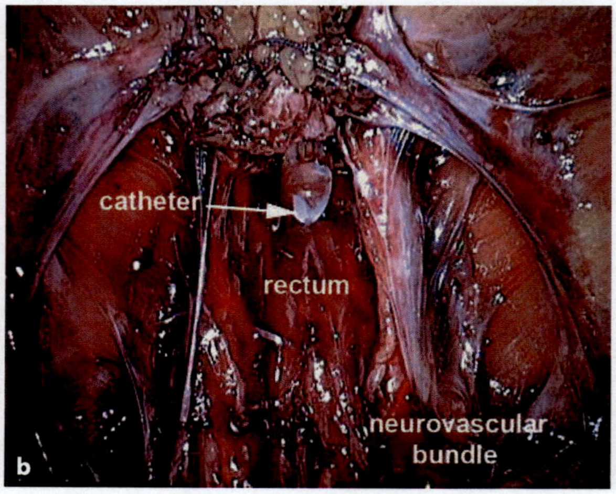

Step 14a demonstrates the view of the pelvis after radical cystoprostatectomy. At this point, it is essential to check for bleeding. Minor urethral bleeding can be controlled by traction on the balloon catheter (Step 14a). Surgicel is placed under the inflated balloon of the catheter.

Step 14b demonstrates a view of the pelvis following a nerve-sparing laparoscopic radical cystoprostatectomy with the neurovascular bundles clearly identifiable. Coagulation should be avoided in nerve-sparing procedures. When arterial bleeding occurs, we recommend the accurate placement of a haemostatic suture (e.g. 4/0 Vicryl). For venous oozing, Tachosil or FloSeal can be used. If a rectal injury is suspected the pelvis is filled with water and air is insufflated via a rectal catheter (no bubbles, no leak).

Step 15: Bagging the specimen

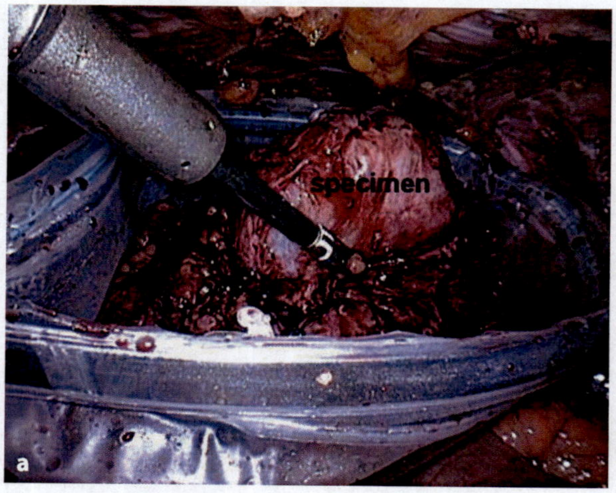

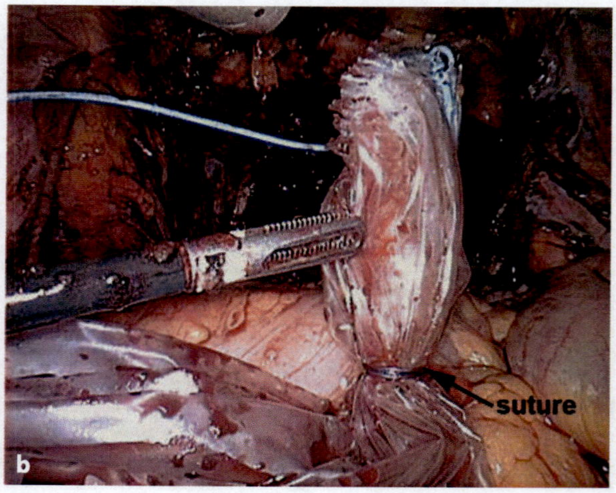

The cystoprostatectomy specimen is placed into an EndoCatch bag, which is partly removed through the 12-mm trocar in the left iliac fossa. This allows a suture to be tied around the neck of the bag before being placed back into the abdominal cavity. This suture safely seals the bag and prevents any inadvertent tumour spillage. The bag is removed via a midline laparotomy created from the optical trocar to the umbilicus prior to construction of a neobladder or an ileal conduit. The bags containing the lymph node packages are removed separately at the same time.

Step 16: Urethroneovesical anastomosis

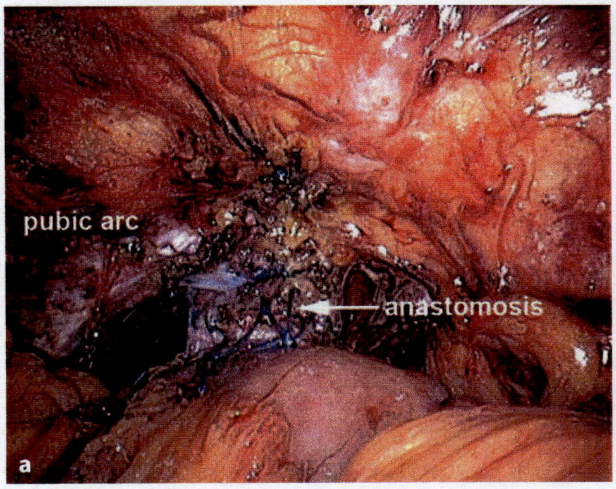

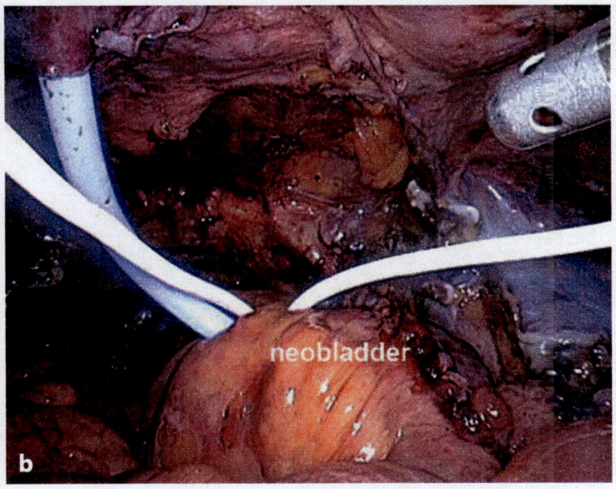

If the patient is a candidate for a neobladder it is fashioned extracorporally, via a small midline laparotomy (incisions 3–4 cm cranially and 3–4 cm caudally to the umbilicus). See Sect. 3.9.2.1. The completely sutured neobladder including two ureteral stents and a suprapubic catheter is placed in the pelvis and the laparotomy wound closed. Pneumoperitoneum is re-established as before and the anastomosis (interrupted sutures, six to eight stitches) is performed laparoscopically. The technique is comparable to the urethrovesical anastomosis during endoscopic extraperitoneal radical prostatectomy (EERPE) (clockwise, starting from 8 o'clock with posterior wall first). Step 16b demonstrates the view into the pelvis at the end of the procedure with the neobladder in place. Finally, one or two 20-F Robinson drains are placed and the wounds are closed.

Postoperative Management

- Mobilise early
- Continue deep vein thrombosis (DVT) prophylaxis
- Nasogastric tube removal on day 1
- Oral antibiotic cover for 5 days
- Drain removal if minimal output and no urine leak on day 3–5
- If Bricker anastomosis, ureteric stent removal on days 14 and 15 (each stent should be removed on different days)
- If neobladder, cystogram and catheter removal at day 18–21 (after mono-J stent removal) if no leak in cystogram

References

1. Dalbagni G, Genega E, Hashibe M, Zhang ZF, Russo P, Herr H, Reuter V (2001) Cystectomy for bladder cancer: a contemporary series. J Urol 165:1111–1116
2. Irwin BH, Gill IS, Haber GP, Campbell SC (2009) Laparoscopic radical cystectomy: current status, outcomes, and patient selection. Curr Treat Options Oncol 10:243–255
3. Sánchez de Badajoz E, Gallego Perales JL, Reche Rosado A, Gutiérrez de la Cruz JM, Jiménez Carrido A (1995) Laparoscopic cystectomy and ileal conduit: a case report. J Endourol 9:59–62
4. Puppo P, Perachino M, Ricciotti G, Bozzo W, Gallucci M, Carmignani G (1995) Laparoscopically assisted transvaginal radical cystectomy. Eur Urol 27:80–84
5. Puppo P, Naselli A (2005) Laparoscopic radical cystectomy. Curr Urol Rep 6:106–108
6. Simonato A, Gregori A, Lissiani A, Bozzola A, Galli S, Gaboardi F (2003) Laparoscopic radical cystoprostatectomy: a technique illustrated step by step. Eur Urol 44:132–138

3.7.2 Robot-Assisted Radical Cystoprostatectomy

Stefan Siemer, Jörn Kamradt, Michael Stöckle

Introduction

Radical cystectomy is the standard treatment in cases of muscle-invasive bladder cancer. Although mortality is low (1–3%), the morbidity of the open procedure is still quite high (25–60%). Minimally invasive procedures such as the robot-assisted cystectomy (RAC) offer a significant reduction of perioperative morbidity and complications. A reduction in blood loss, lower transfusion rates, quicker resumption of oral intake and a shorter hospitalisation time after RAC seem to outweigh the longer operation time [1]. Using a small laparotomy incision not only for removing the bladder, but also for performing an extracorporal urinary diversion can reduce operative time as well. Alternatively, the urinary diversion can be performed intracorporally [2, 3]. Compared to the conventional laparoscopic procedure, the RAC procedure seems to be an improvement due to the additional options only the RAC procedure offers: 3D view, EndoWrist instruments and intuitive movement [4].

Indications

- Non-muscle-invasive bladder carcinoma (high risk of progression)
- Muscle-invasive bladder carcinoma suitable for a cystectomy

Contra-indications (see Sect. 3.7.1)

- Cardiovascular co-morbidities

Preoperative Preparation

- Bladder catheter
- Nasogastric tube
- Single-shot antibiosis
- Thrombosis prophylaxis

Step 1: Patient position and trocar placement

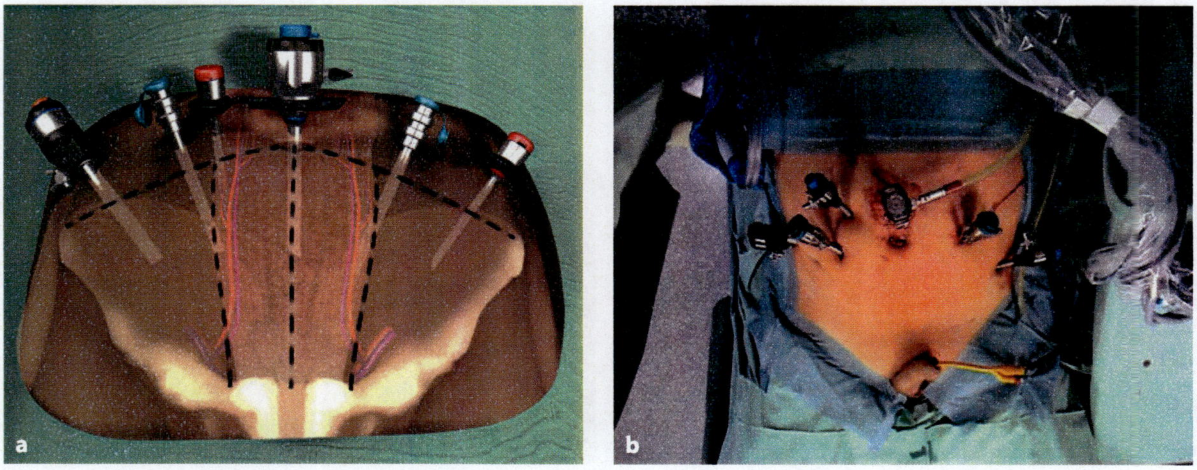

A 3-cm supraumbilical incision for a Hasson access (alternatively a puncture using the Veress needle) is used to place the 12-mm camera port. Two da Vinci trocars (8 mm) are placed 8 cm lateral of the umbilicus under visual control. Using a four-armed da Vinci system, the fourth robot port is placed above the anterior superior iliac spine (ASIS) on the left side. Alternatively, a single port (5 mm) can be placed here for the assistant's instruments. Another port (5 mm) is placed between the right da Vinci port and the camera, and another port (12 mm) above the ASIS on the right side. The patient is now placed to the modified Trendelenburg position (supine situation, approximately 40–45°, lowered head) and the legs are bedded in conventional leg support systems.

Step 2: Colon mobilisation and ureteric dissection

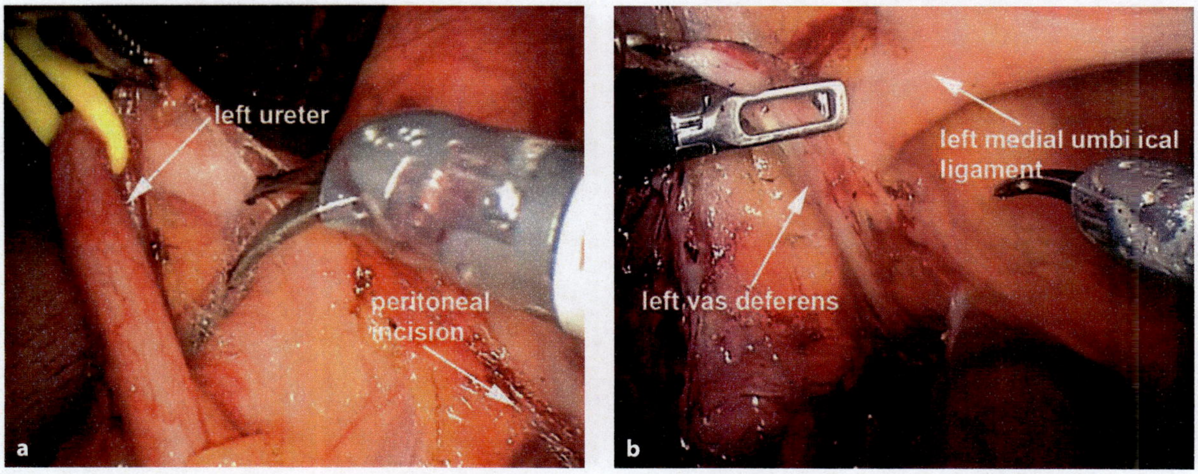

The peritoneum is incised and the sigmoid colon is mobilised to identify the left ureter (Step 2a). Mark the left ureter using a rubber sling (secured with a clip). The same steps are carried out on the right side and the ureters must be mobilised down to the bladder without injuring the periureteral vessels. Furthermore, mobilisation of the ureters is performed in the cranial direction to gain enough length for the appropriate urinary diversion later on. The vas deferens must be located and cut on both sides (Step 2b).

Step 3: Mobilisation of bladder from rectum

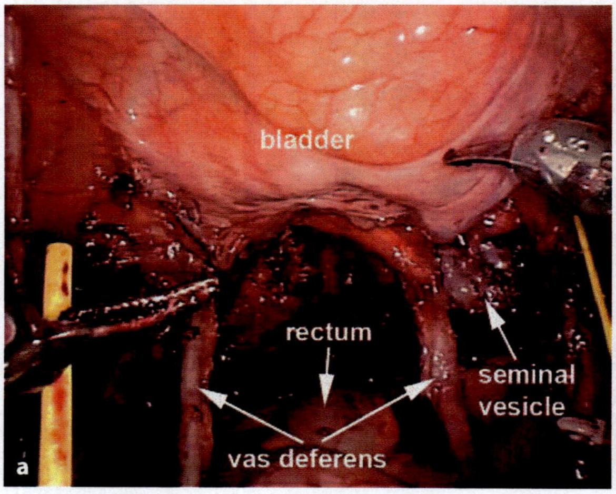

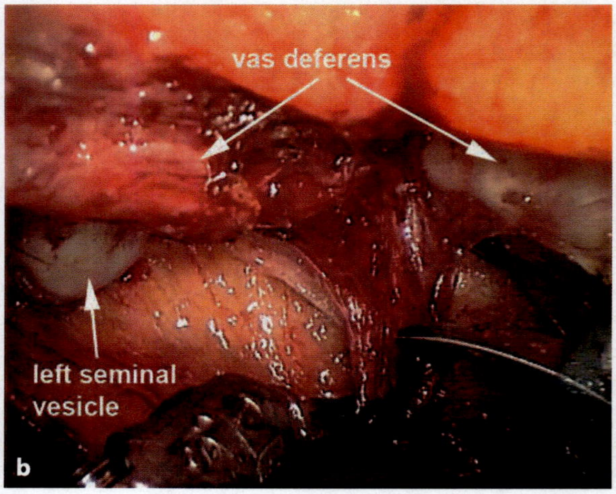

The peritoneum is incised along the vas deferens in the direction of the pouch of Douglas. In this procedure, the incisions are joined with each other in the midline behind the bladder. The rectum and peritoneum must now be detached from the posterior bladder wall in the avascular layer (Step 3a). In case of suspected tumour infiltration, the peritoneum is left attached to the bladder. Now both seminal vesicles are dissected laterally on each side up to the peritoneal fold of the Denonvilliers fascia.

Step 4: Incision of Denonvilliers fascia

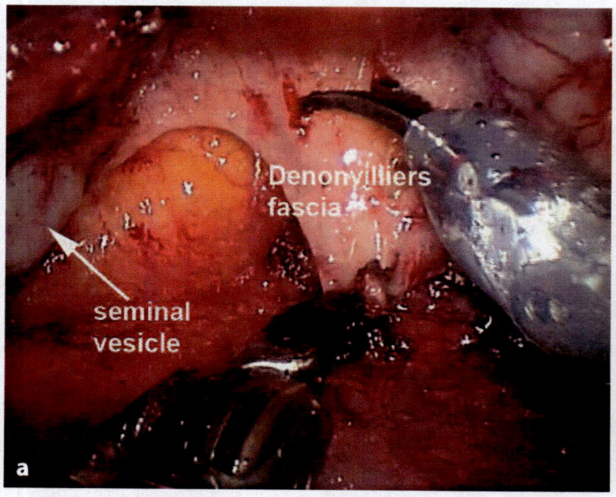

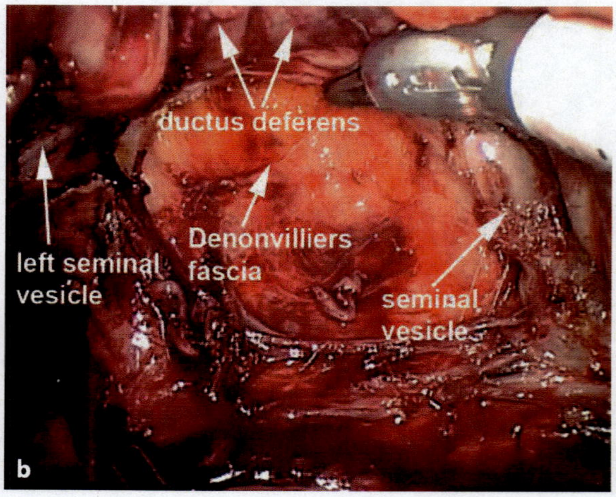

Incise Denonvilliers fascia and detach the rectum off the dorsal prostate gland surface. If a nerve-sparing procedure is intended an intrafascial preparation can be performed, similar to intrafascial radical prostatectomy (see Sect. 3.12.1.2), but it must be established first that the patient does not have co-existing prostate cancer. The dissection of this layer should go as far as possible in the direction of the urethra and towards the lateral direction, making it easier to separate the prostate pedicle later. This should be done without thermal energy if possible.

Step 5: Dissection in preparation for lymphadenectomy

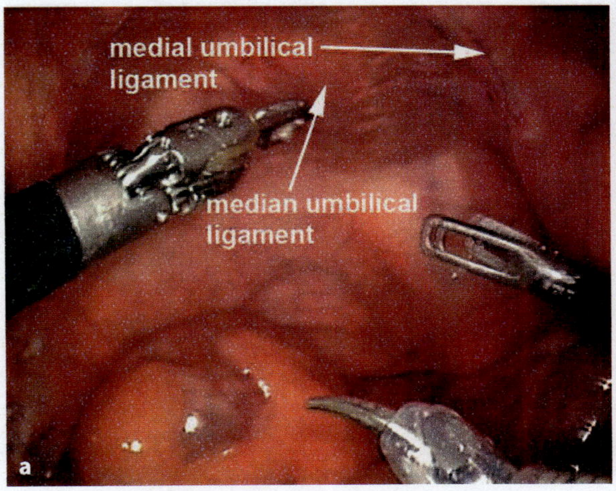

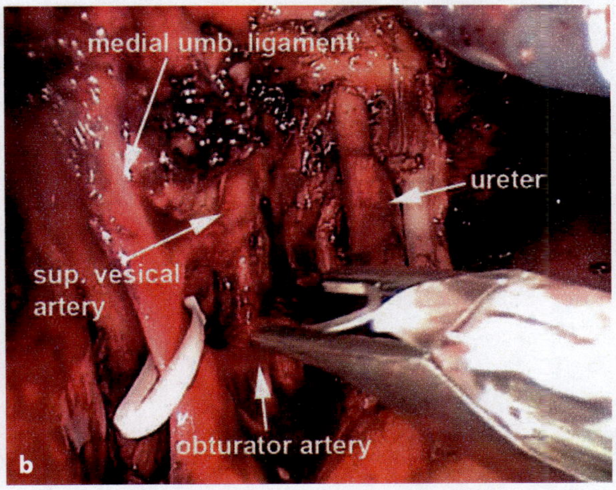

For lymphadenectomy, the first incision is placed lateral to the medial umbilical ligament (preferably up to the umbilicus) and followed by the preparation of the Retzius space down to the endopelvic fascia. Now we recommend the incision of the endopelvic fascia and preparation up to the urethra as far as possible. Later, the prostate pedicle can easily be resected. We recommend following the medial umbilical ligament up to the insertion at the internal iliac artery and to clip it at this particular point (Step 5b).

Step 6: Lymphadenectomy (limited and extended)

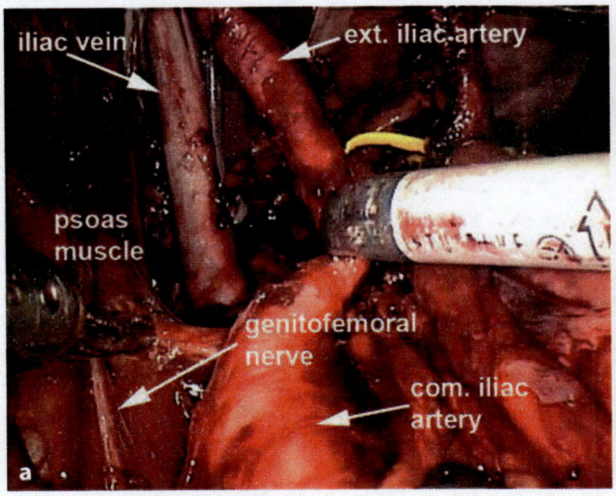

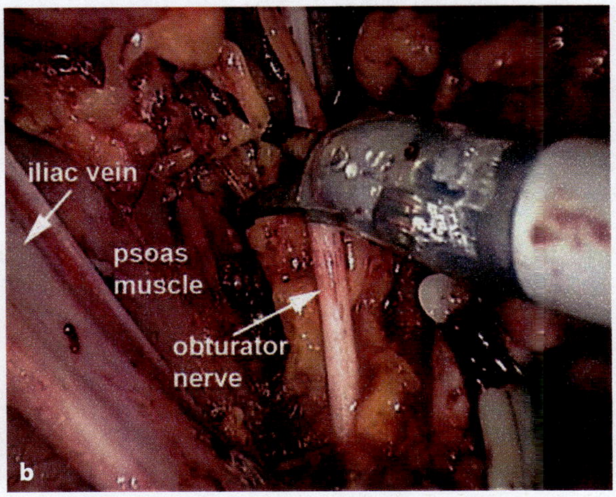

Depending on the indication, a standard or extended lymphadenectomy is performed. The spermatic vessel is the lateral border and the obturator nerve the caudal border for the standard procedure. All lymph nodes, even between the psoas muscle and the external iliac artery and vein, are removed. On this occasion, dissection between the psoas muscle and the external iliac vessels make the entire lymphatic package easier to remove (Step 6b). During the standard lymphadenectomy, the common iliac artery is exposed and forms the cranial limit of lymph node removal (Step 6a). The lymphadenectomy is performed bilaterally. The lymph nodes are stored separately in a recovery bag and are not extracted directly through the port due to the potential risk of tumour cell scattering.

Step 7: Ureteric preparation

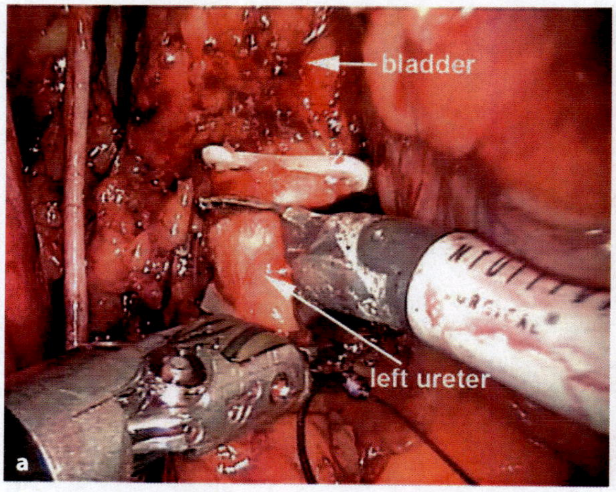

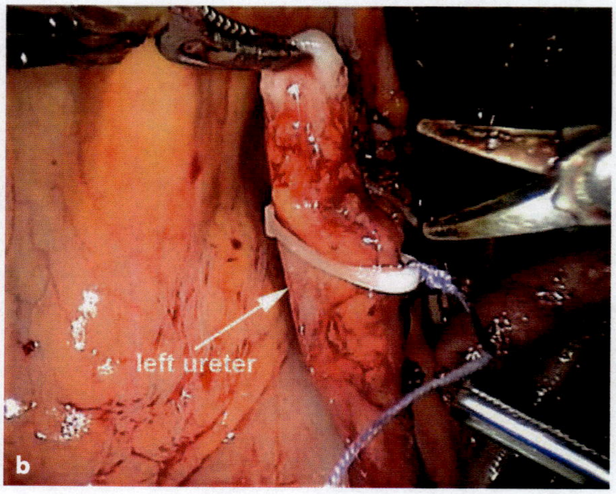

A Hem-o-lok clip is placed distally on each ureter as close to the bladder as possible. A second Hem-o-lok clip is prepared outside the abdomen first, by tying a approximately 10-cm-long Vicryl suture to it. The clip is then introduced with the suture attached and clipped about 1 cm above the previous clip on each side. This suture allows the ureter to be located more easily and moved under the colonic mesentery later. Both ureters are divided just above the bladder between the two Hem-o-lok clips (Step 7a). A segment of each ureter, approximately 1 cm long, is excised and sent for frozen section (Step 7b).

Step 8: Bladder and prostatic pedicle division

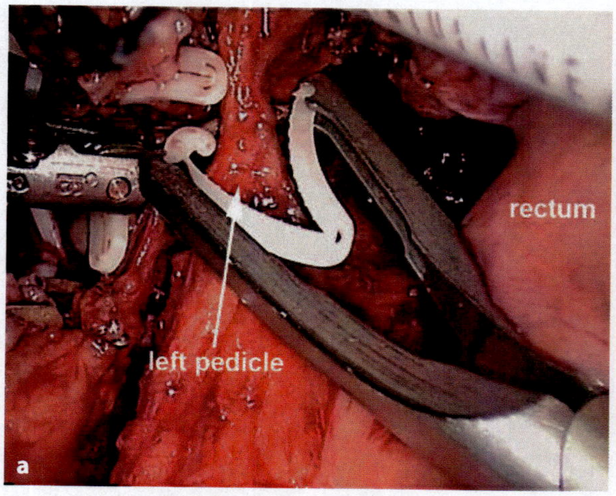

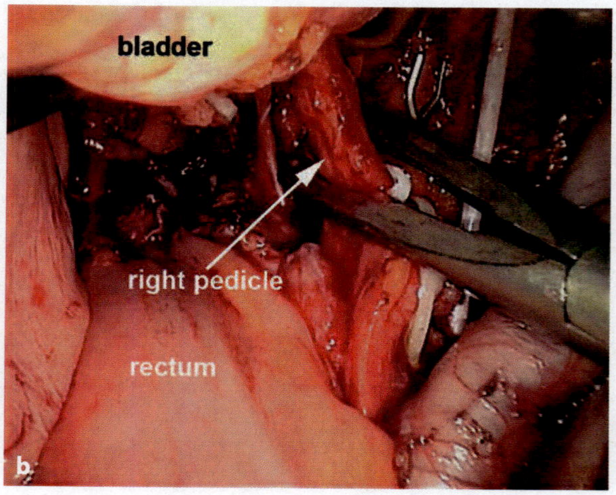

Using the fourth da Vinci arm (alternatively, the assistant uses alligator forceps), the bladder pedicle is stretched by pulling the vas deferens up and out of the pelvis (alternatively, the medial umbilical ligament). Afterwards, the bladder pedicle vessels are located separately and divided between Hem-o-lok clips. In case of larger blood vessels, two clips should be used to minimise the risk of bleeding. During a nerve-sparing operation, no more thermal energy should be used. The pedicles are prepared as far as possible in the direction of the urethra.

Step 9: Ventral mobilisation and further dissection of bladder and prostatic pedicle

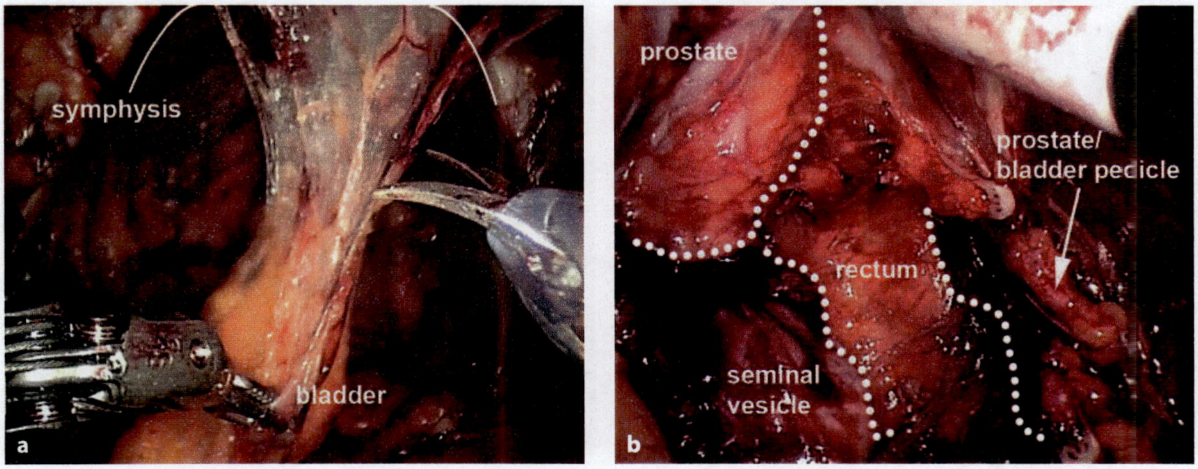

At this point of the procedure, the ventral attachments of the bladder are completely dissected (Step 9a). This facilitates the separation of the bladder from the rectum and the bladder pedicle dissection. Now we recommend dividing the median and the medial umbilical ligaments as close as possible to the umbilicus. This approach offers an almost avascular layer for preparation to dissect the bladder from the abdominal wall. Using the fourth da Vinci arm or the assistant's port, the bladder is turned to the left in order to keep tension on the bladder to expose the prostate gland pedicle (Step 9b).

Step 10: Apical and urethral dissection

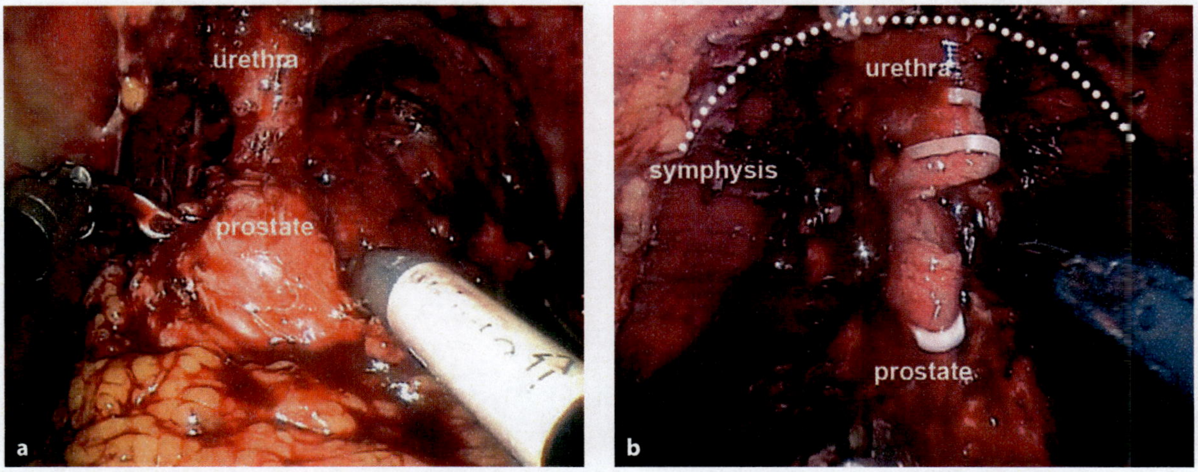

Analogue to the radical or nerve-sparing prostatectomy procedure, the neurovascular plexus is either dissected radically or preserved. In order to improve continence, the puboprostatic ligaments are spared. After dissecting the Santorini plexus (if nerve-sparing is intended), a complete circular mobilisation of the urethra is necessary. Attention must be paid to possible lesions of the urethra (tumour spreading). The urethral catheter is removed and the urethra sealed using a clip as near as possible to the prostate gland (Step 10b). If a neobladder is planned the urethra is left open. If a conduit is constructed the urethra is sealed by another clip and then detached. Ligation in the area of the Santorini plexus is not necessary in most cases. If there is persistent bleeding, we recommend a sequential 4/0 Vicryl ligation.

Step 11: Specimen removal

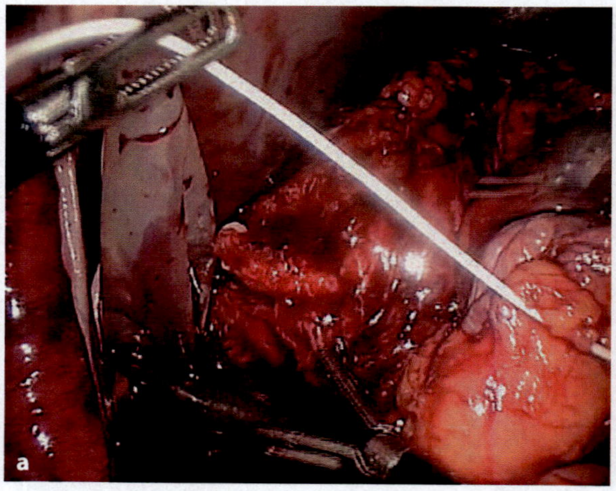
a

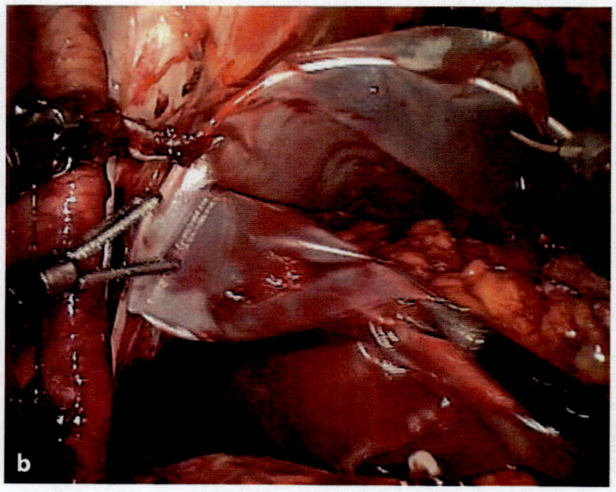
b

The bladder and attached prostate gland are recovered using a recovery bag followed by a detailed inspection for haemostasis. To check for any rectal injury, air is insufflated via a rectal tube inserted now or at the start of the operation. In uncertain cases, the pelvis can be filled with water and air is insufflated via the rectal tube. Bubbles should not be seen in the water in the pelvis if the rectum is intact.

Step 12: Ureteroileal anastomosis

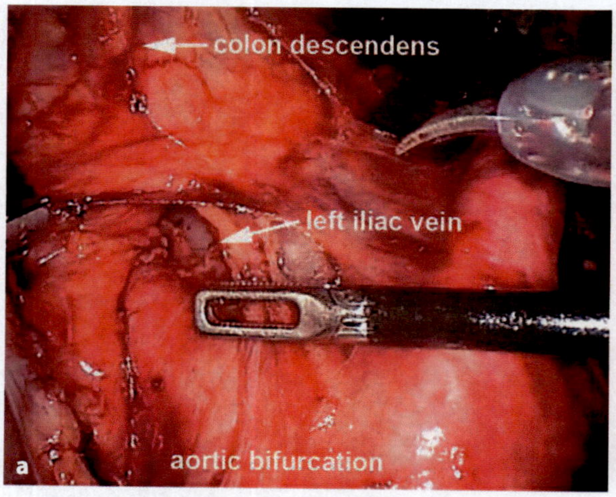

a

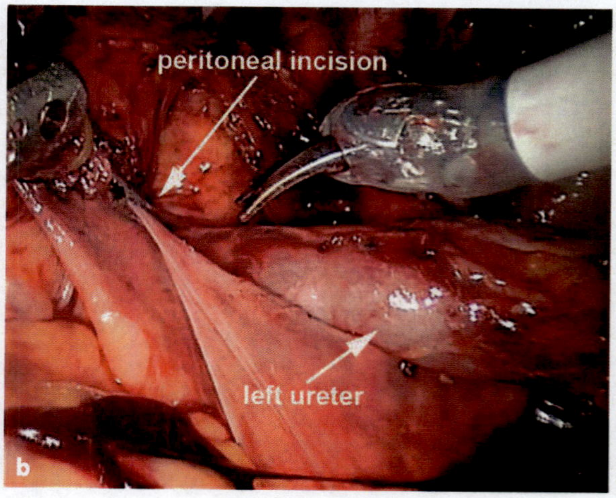

b

For constructing the ureteroileal anastomosis, we prefer the Wallace procedure for all different types of urinary diversion. The left ureter is brought beneath the sigmoid mesocolon to the right side. Further mobilisation of the peritoneum and the mesocolon (Step 12a, Step 12b) is probably necessary to ensure that the (1) the pathway through the mesocolon is large enough to afford a tension-free anastomosis and (2) the mobilised ureter is long enough to reach the left abdominal wall. After the pathway through the mesocolon is formed, the assistant is able to conduct the left ureter carefully using alligator forceps to the right abdominal wall. At the end, a careful check is made for haemostasis with the intra-abdominal pressure at 4–5 mmHg.

Postoperative Management

- Fast-track procedure
  - Quick return to solid food
  - Early mobilisation after surgery (usually 6 h)
- Sab Simplex if required to reduce intestinal flatulence

References

1. Wang GJ, Barocas DA, Raman JD, Scherr DS (2008) Robotic vs. open radical cystectomy: prospective comparison of perioperative outcomes and pathological measures of early oncological efficacy. BJU Int 101:89–93
2. Hemal AK (2009) Role of robot-assisted surgery for bladder cancer. Curr Opin Urol 19:69–75
3. Kaul SA, Menon M (2007) Da Vinci assisted cystoprostatectomy and urinary diversion: a paradigm shift in surgical management of bladder cancer. Minerva Urol Nefrol 59:149–157
4. Dasgupta P, Rimington P, Murphy D, Challacombe B, Hemal A, Elhage O, Khan MS (2008) Robotic assisted radical cystectomy: short to medium-term oncologic and functional outcomes. Int J Clin Pract 62:1709–1714

3.8 Robot-Assisted Radical Cystectomy in Female Patients

Stefan Siemer, Jörn Kamradt, Michael Stöckle

Introduction

Radical cystectomy is the standard treatment of muscle-invasive bladder cancer. In female patients, the removal of the uterus, fallopian tubes, ovaries and the anterior wall of the vagina along with the bladder is indicated. Nevertheless, fallopian tubes and ovaries could be preserved in younger, premenopausal women. The open procedure is related to low mortality rates (1–3%) but significant morbidity rates ranging between 25% and 60%. Minimally invasive procedures such as the robot-assisted radical cystectomy (RARC) offer a significant reduction of perioperative morbidity and complications. The reduction in blood loss, the lower transfusion rates, the quicker resumption of oral intake and the shorter hospitalisation time after RARC seem to outweigh the longer operative time [1]. The RARC procedure offers improvements over the conventional laparoscopic approach due to the 3D view provided by the robotic system, the use of EndoWrist instruments and their intuitive movement [2]. A small laparotomy incision is used not only for removal of the bladder, but also for the performance of the extracorporal urinary diversion and may result in reduced operative time. Alternatively, the urinary diversion can be performed intracorporally [3, 4]. The removal of the bladder through the vagina is also possible. In the current section, the technique for RARC in female patients is described.

Indications

Patient suitable for cystectomy with:

- Muscle-invasive bladder carcinoma
- High-risk, stroma-invasive bladder carcinoma (pT1G3)
- Nonresectable superficial bladder carcinoma (high risk carcinoma)
- Recurrent carcinoma in situ of the bladder after intravesical immuno- or chemotherapy

Contra-indications

- Acute thrombotic incident
- T4 bladder cancer

Preoperative Preparation

- Bladder catheter
- Nasogastric tube
- Single-shot antibiotic
- Deep venous thrombosis prophylaxis
- Enema (bowel preparation)

Step1: Patient and trocar positions

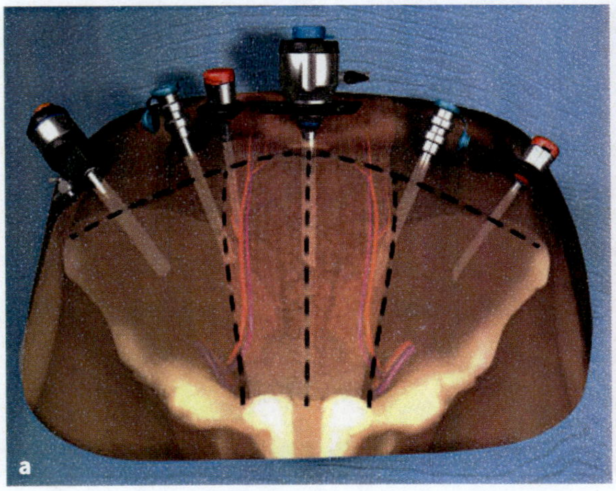

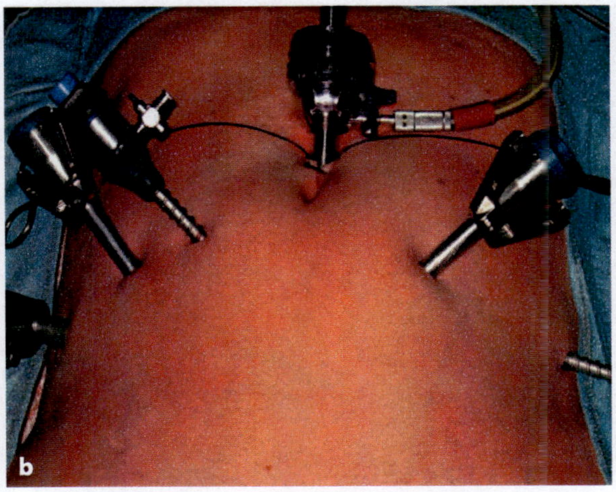

The patient is placed in the supine position with abducted legs. A 3-cm supraumbilical incision is made and a 12-mm camera trocar is inserted with the Hasson technique. Two da Vinci trocars (8 mm) are placed under visual control on the lateral margin of the rectus muscle approximately 2 cm caudally to the umbilicus. When a four-arm da Vinci system is used, the fourth robotic port is placed above the anterior superior iliac spine on the left side. Alternatively, a single port (5 mm) can be placed here for the assistant instruments. A 5-mm port is placed between the right robotic port and the camera trocar and a 12-mm port above the right anterior superior iliac spine (Step 1a). The patient is now placed in the modified Trendelenburg position (supine position, head down approximately 40–45°).

Step 2: Mobilisation of sigmoid colon and left ureteric dissection

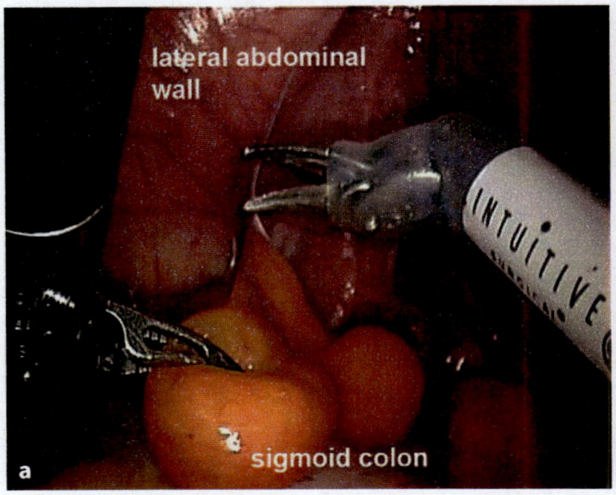

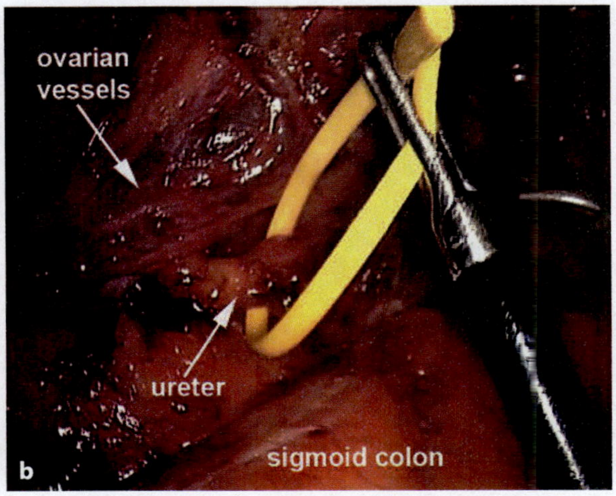

Step 2a shows the incision of the peritoneum (line of Toldt) starting at the level of the sigmoid colon. The left colon is mobilised away from the operative field. The left ureter is identified across the common iliac artery and mobilised from the psoas muscle. The ovarian vessels are also identified over the psoas muscle lateral to the ureter (Step 2b). The left ureter is marked by using a rubber sling secured with a clip. The ureter is mobilised to the level of the bladder and in its cranial direction without injuring the periureteral vessels. It is important to preserve adequate periureteral tissue over the mobilised ureter in order to preserve generous vascular supply. The mobilisation of the ovarian vessels from the pelvic wall is useful for gaining access to the iliac vessels and the obturator fossa.

Step 3: Preparation of the retropubic (Retzius) space

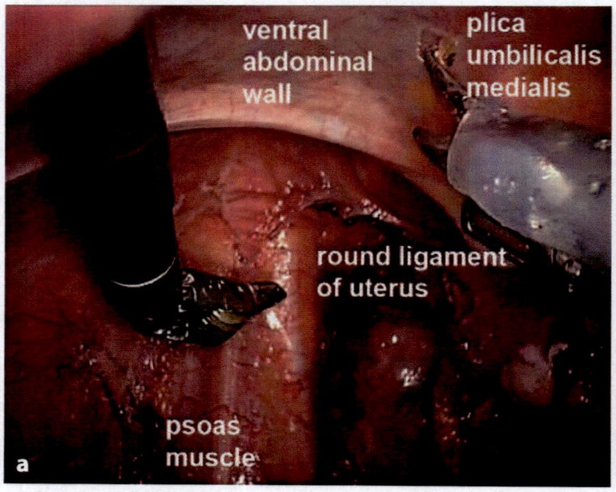

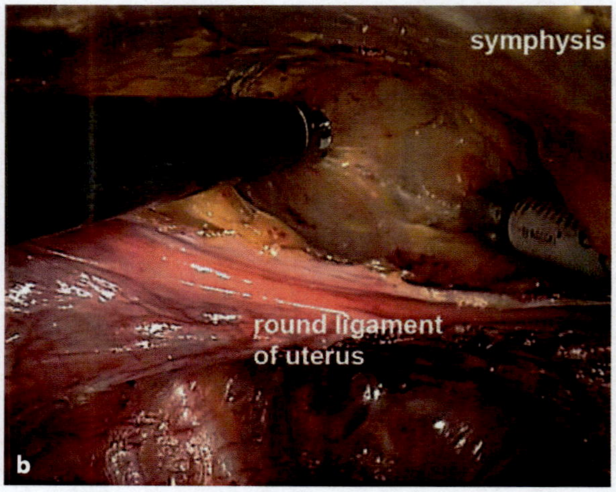

An incision of the peritoneum laterally to the medial umbilical ligament follows (Step 3a) and the avascular layer down to the endopelvic fascia is developed. The borders of the dissection are the umbilical ligament medially, the round ligament of uterus dorsally and the abdominal wall ventrally (Step 3b). A combination of blunt and sharp dissection is carried out. The continuous gas insufflation often helps define the avascular layer and minimises bleeding. The inferior epigastric vessels may interfere with the dissection field during the preparation of the preperitoneal space. Careful dissection is critical to prevent injury to these vessels.

Step 4: Transection of the round ligament of uterus

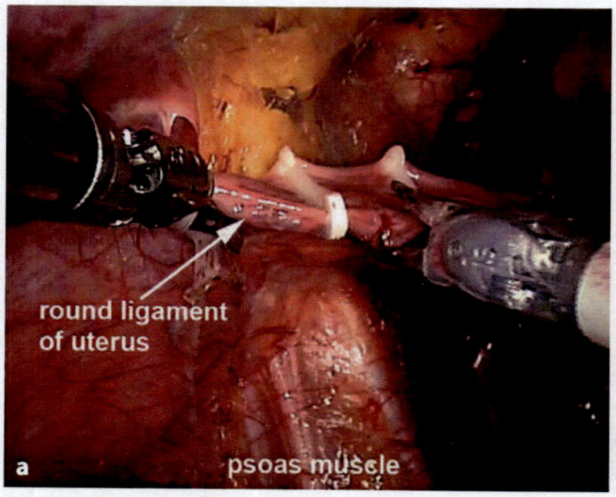

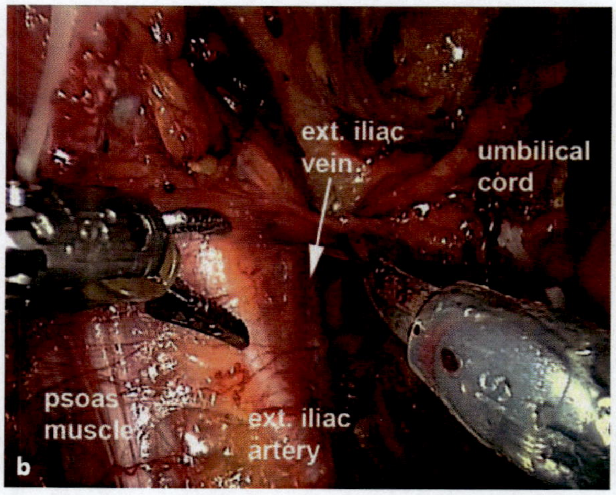

When the retropubic space is developed, the anterolateral bladder wall is mobilised from its attachments and the transection of the round ligament of the uterus will eventually fully mobilise the left side of the bladder wall and the uterus from the left anterolateral pelvic wall. Elevation of the uterus by the fourth arm is helpful. The round ligament of uterus is ligated by Hem-o-lok clips and transected between them (Step 4a). Metal clips could also be used for the ligation. The complete mobilisation of the bladder and uterus from the lateral pelvic wall provides access to the obturator fossa (Step 4b). The external iliac vessels and the obturator fossa (including vessels and nerve) are now accessible for the performance of lymph node dissection.

Step 5: Right ureteric dissection and preparation of Retzius space

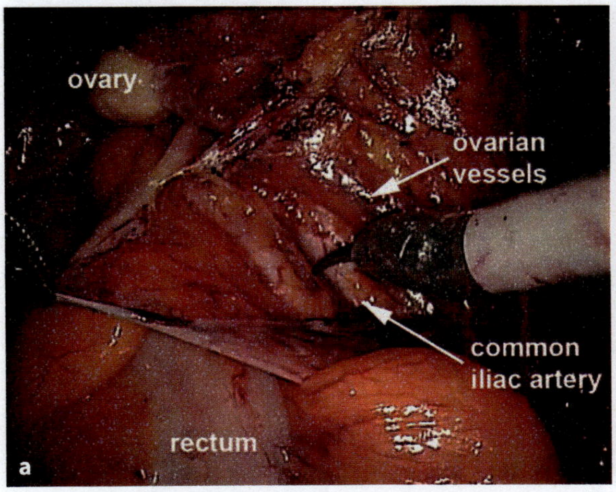

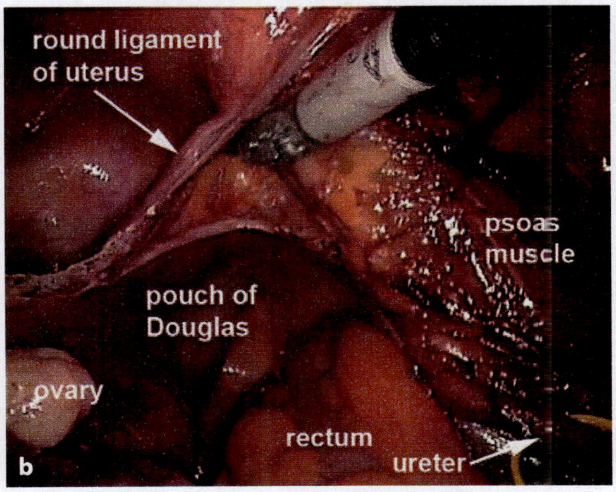

On the right side, the peritoneal fold over the right common iliac artery and the ureter is incised and the ovarian vessels are also identified (Step 5a). The ureter and ovarian vessels are mobilised from the psoas muscle and surrounding tissue, as described above. The gentle handling of the ureter and its surrounding tissue minimises traction and ureteral trauma and the risk of ureteral strictures is significantly reduced. The mobilisation of the caecum and terminal ileum is sometimes necessary for the identification of the ureter. The caecum is divided from its lower attachments and the dissection is extended towards the pouch of Douglas (Step 5b). The use of coagulation near the bowel should be avoided. Preparation of the preperitoneal space on the right side to the endopelvic fascia follows.

Step 6: Pelvic lymphadenectomy I

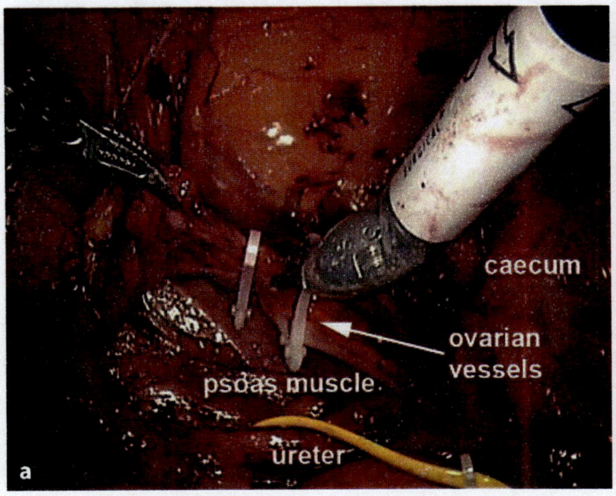

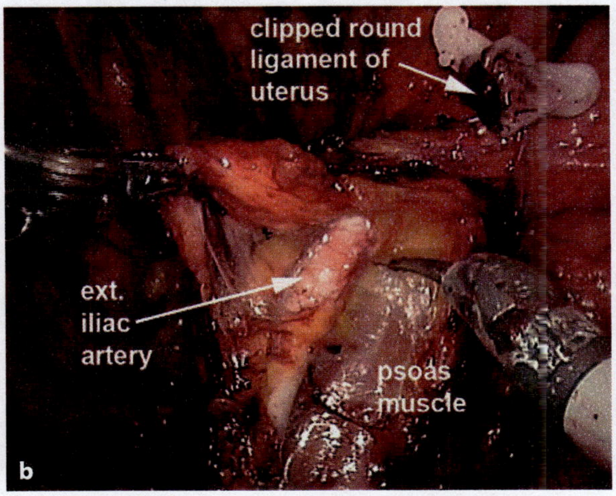

Hem-o-lok clips are placed on the right round ligament of the uterus and the structure between clips transected. Thus, the anterior bladder wall and uterus are mobilised and the right external iliac vessels and obturator fossa are accessible. The ovarian vessels are located at the lateral border of lymphadenectomy. The ovarian vessels can be transected after ligation with Hem-o-lok clips to facilitate lymph node dissection (Step 6a). Pelvic lymphadenectomy includes the lymphatic tissue surrounding the external and internal iliac vessels, the obturator fossa as well as the common iliac vessels. The dissection starts over the psoas muscle and is guided over the external iliac vessels towards the obturator fossa.

Step 7: Pelvic lymphadenectomy II

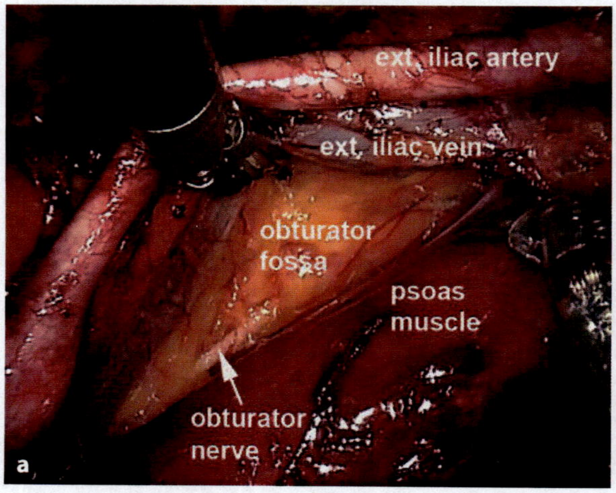

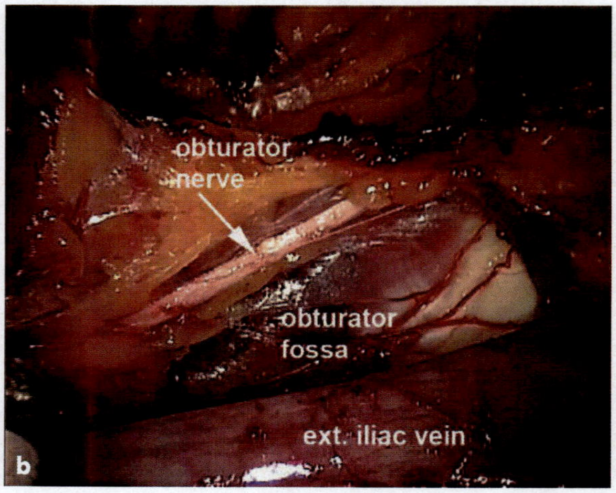

After the excision of the lymphatic tissue surrounding the external iliac vessels, these vessels could be mobilised from the psoas muscle easily, using the EndoWrist instruments. The latter manoeuvre facilitates the complete resection of lymphatic tissue at the obturator fossa (Step 7a). The resection is complete when the obturator nerve is fully freed from its surrounding lymphatic tissue (Step 7b). The anatomic limits of the lymph node dissection are the following: laterally, the internal surface of the external iliac vein and the iliopsoas muscle; medially, the umbilical ligament; caudally, the pectineal ligament and obturator nerve; anteriorly, the iliopubic branch of the pelvis; cephaladly, the confluence of the external iliac vein and the internal iliac vein. All lymph node groups should be excised en bloc.

Step 8: Pelvic lymphadenectomy III

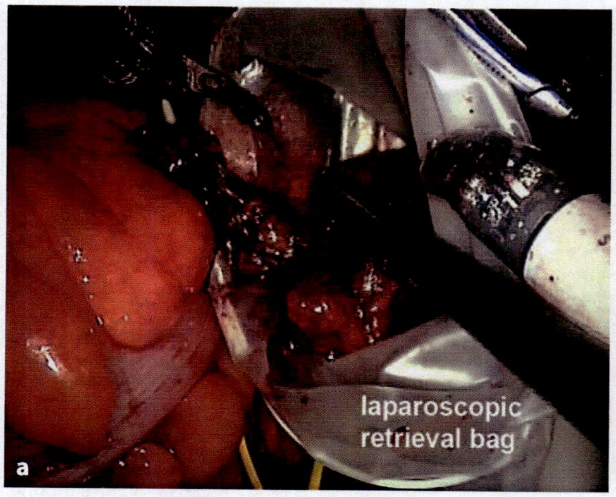

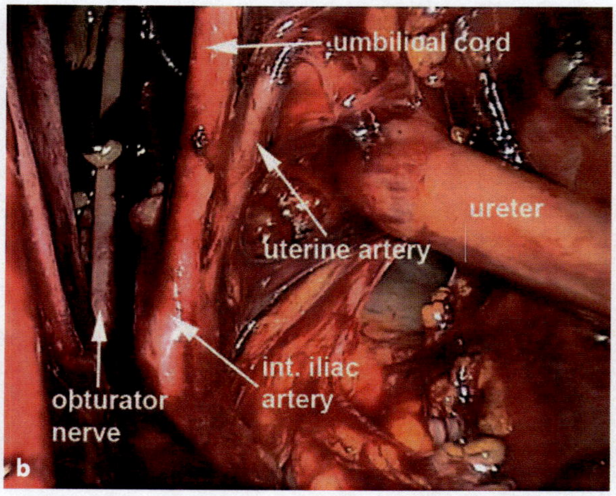

The removed lymphatic tissue excised from the obturator fossa and external iliac vessels should be placed a retrieval bag (Step 8a). Lymphatic tissue surrounding the common iliac vessels should be retrieved separately in a different bag in order to distinguish the sites of possible lymph node invasion and to accurately evaluate lymph node involvement. Pelvic lymphadenectomy can also be performed after cystectomy. Nevertheless, all major pelvic vessels are freed from their surrounding tissue up to the common iliac vessels during the lymphadenectomy and the cystectomy is facilitated by an excellent exposure of the bladder vessels as they derive from the internal iliac artery (Step 8b).

Step 9: Transection of branches from the internal iliac artery

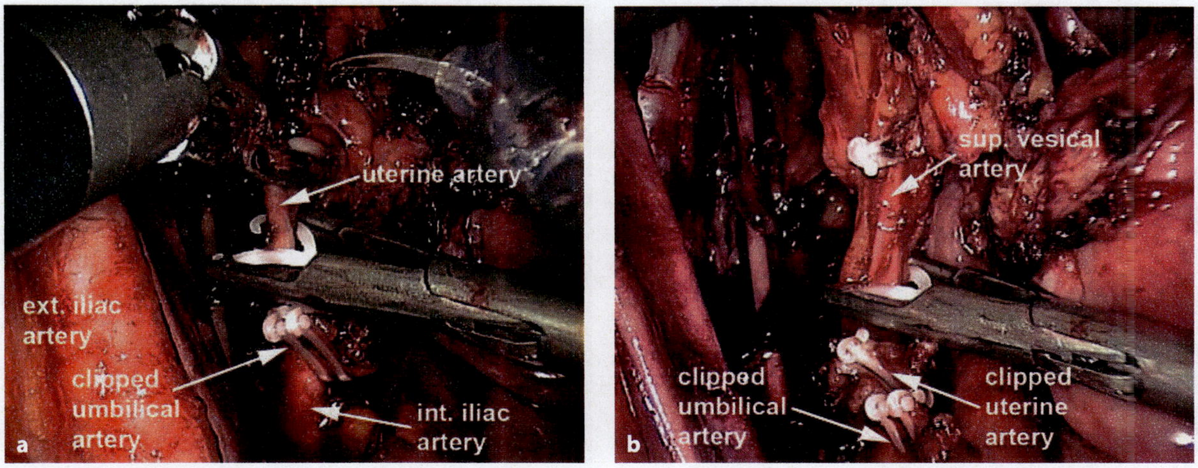

The internal iliac artery is the landmark for the identification of the vessels supplying the organs that are about to be excised. During its course, the internal iliac artery provides several arterial branches that should be ligated. The umbilical artery is the first to be identified and is ligated and transected between Hem-o-lok clips. Step 9a shows the transected umbilical artery and the uterine artery, which is ligated by clips and will be transected. Then the superior vesical artery is transected after secure ligation with clips (Step 9b). The application of two clips on the proximal side of the vessels and on the distal side provides adequate haemostasis.

Step 10: Dorsal incision of the peritoneum

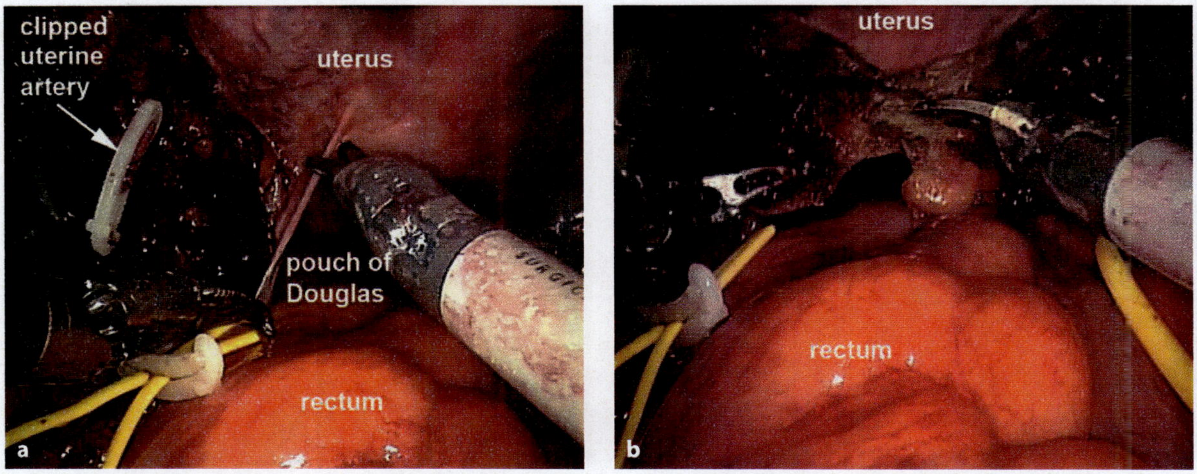

The next step is the dorsal incision of the peritoneum beginning lateral to the posterior fornix of the vagina starting from both sides and expanding the incision medially. A sponge stick or Hegar dilatator could be inserted in the vagina to facilitate the identification of the posterior fornix. The fourth arm is used to elevate the uterus. Step 10a shows the initiation of the dissection of the peritoneal fold on the left lateral posterior fornix. The pouch of Douglas is just posterior to the dissection site. Step 10b demonstrates the complete incision of the posterior fornix, which was started laterally and expanded to the middle position of the fornix. A combination of sharp dissection with coagulation provides efficient bloodless dissection.

Step 11: Transection of the ureters

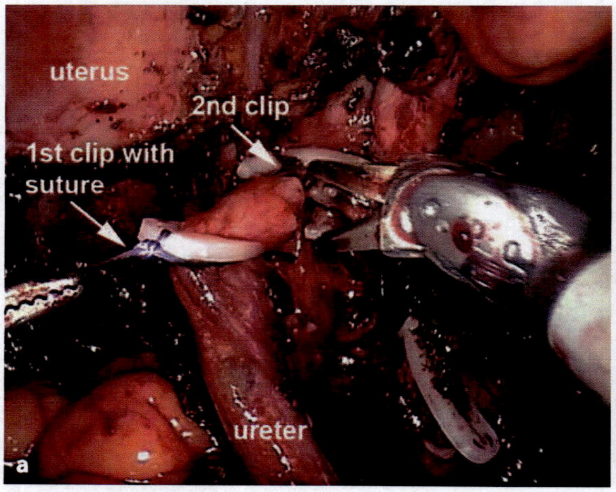

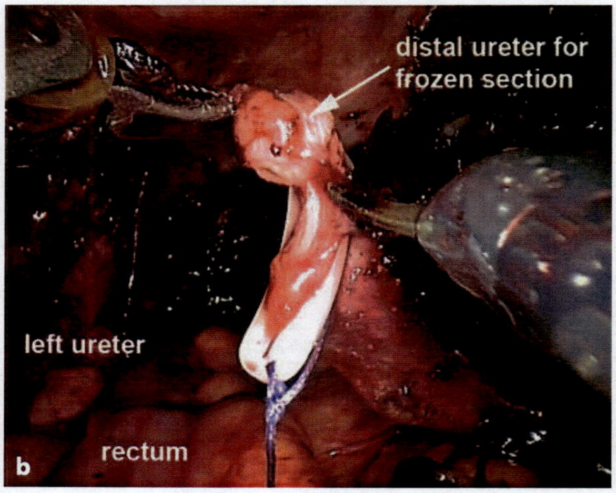

A Hem-o-lok clip is placed distally on each ureter as close to the bladder as possible. A second Hem-o-lok clip is prepared with an approximately 10-cm-long Vicryl suture to it. This clip is used to ligate the ureter about 1 cm proximal to the previous clip (Step 11a). The same manoeuvre is performed on the other side. After the placement of the clips, the ureteral segment of each ureter between the clips is excised and sent for frozen section (Step 11b). The suture placed on the clip is useful for the handling the ureter during the following steps of the cystectomy and the performance of the urinary diversion procedure.

Step 12: Incision of the posterior fornix of vagina

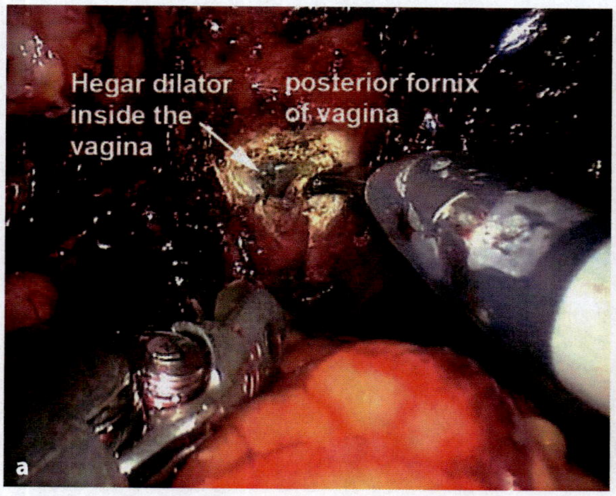

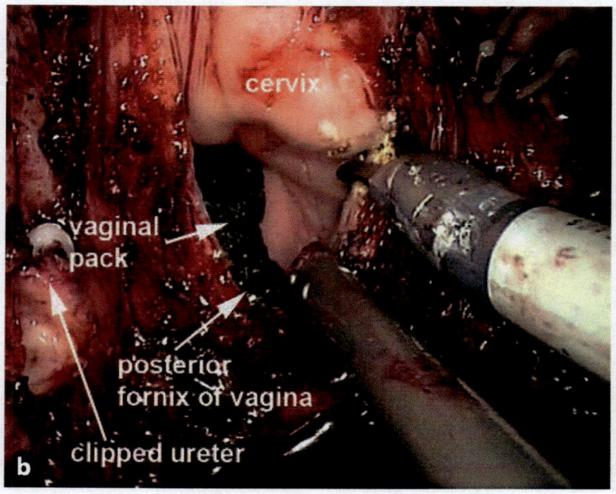

The incision of the posterior fornix is expanded and access to the vagina is gained. Scissors in combination with coagulation could be used. In Step 12a, the incision of the posterior fornix provided access to the vagina. The Hegar dilator located in the vagina is visible. The incision to the vagina is elongated laterally to both sides. The direction of the incision is guided from the posterior portion of the vagina to the anterior side where the urethra is located (Step 12b). Traction of the uterus in the ventral direction is provided by the one robotic arm while the assistant provides dorsal traction to the posterior vaginal wall.

Step 13: Transection of bladder pedicles and ventral mobilisation

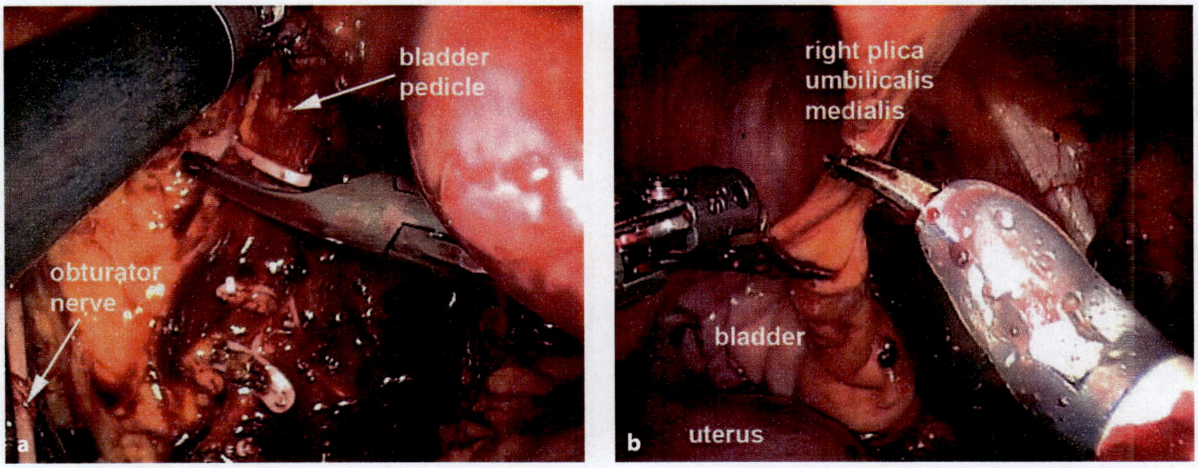

As the bladder is still attached to the anterior abdominal wall, the lateral vascular pedicles are easily identified. The bladder is gently retracted to the opposite side to the dissection using one of the robotic arms. Thus, the vascular pedicles are set in tension and the pedicles are ligated by Hem-o-lok clips. Step 13a demonstrates the placement of the clips on the vascular pedicle, which is under tension. The transection of the pedicle is about to follow. Once the vascular supply of the bladder is completely dissected, the medial umbilical ligaments and the urachus are transected close to the umbilicus with a combination of scissors and coagulation (Step 13b). Then the anterior bladder wall is mobilised in the avascular plane caudally to the level of the pubic symphysis.

Step 14: Urethral dissection and specimen removal

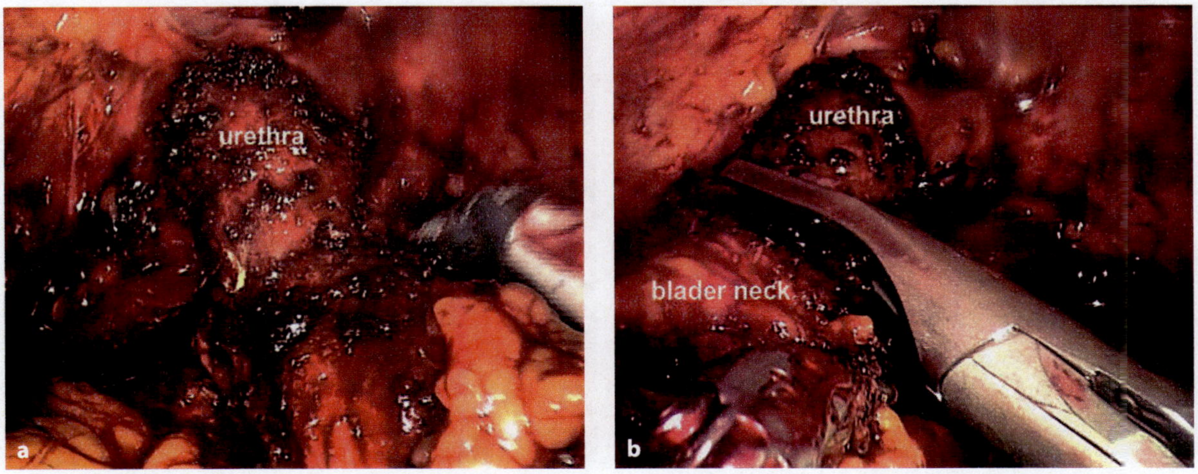

In case of a urinary diversion with the ileal conduit or heterotopic pouch, the urethral meatus can be excised along with the anterior wall of the vagina. An orthotopic pouch requires preservation of the urethra. Therefore, the urethra and bladder neck are divided in circumferential fashion (Step 14a). The urethral catheter is removed and the urethra is ligated with a clip at the bladder neck in an attempt to minimise the risk of tumour spilling when transecting the urethra (Step 14b). The specimen containing the bladder with the uterus, fallopian tubes, ovaries and anterior vaginal wall is placed in a large retrieval bag. Depending on the size of the specimen, the bag can be removed through the open vagina or through a small median laparotomy incision. The vagina is closed by a polydioxanone surgical (PDS) running suture.

Step 15: Transposition of the left ureter to the right side

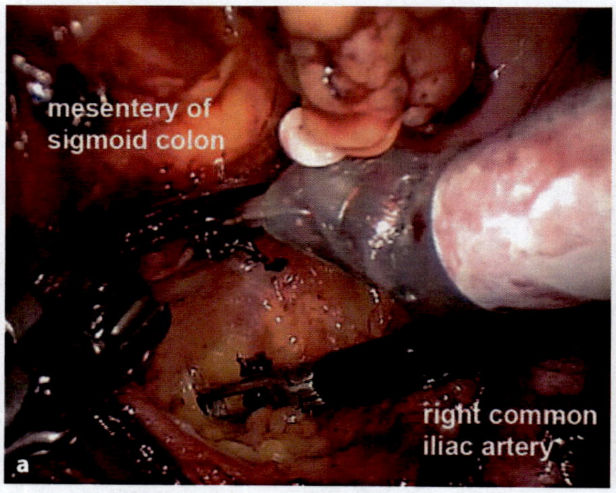

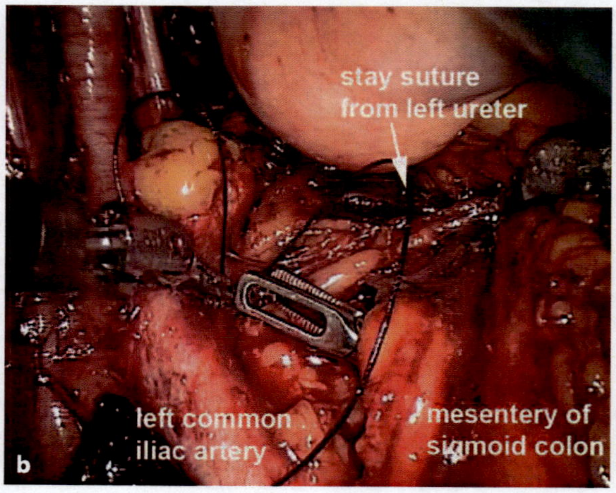

The tissue medial to the right common iliac artery is dissected as close to the aortic bifurcation as possible. It is important to keep the dissection plane near the aortic bifurcation and away from the mesenterium in order to prevent injuries to mesenteric vessels. A conventional laparoscopic grasper is placed at the site (Step 15a). Then the sigmoid colon is retracted to the right side and the left common iliac artery is exposed. The tip of the grasper is identified and the suture (on the clip) of the left ureter is grasped by the instrument (Step 15b). The left ureter crosses underneath the sigmoid mesenterium by carefully pulling out the grasper.

Step 16: Placing anastomotic sutures for the ileal neobladder

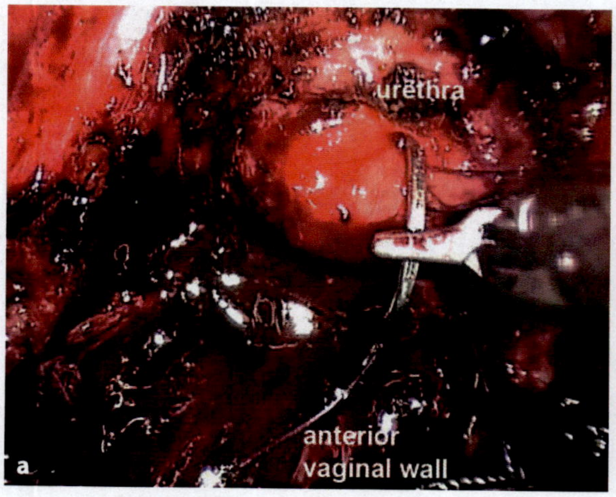

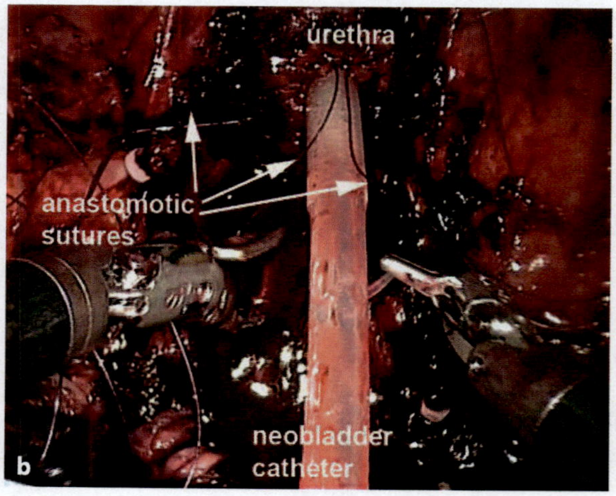

If an orthotopic neobladder is selected as the urinary diversion, the sutures for anastomosis between the urethra and the lower portion of the neobladder can be placed. These sutures are initially placed on the urethral stump and left in place until the neobladder has been formed and is ready for anastomosis. The sutures to the urethra are placed from inside to outside (Step 16a). Articulating robotic instruments provide additional manoeuvrability for the performance of the suturing tasks in comparison to conventional laparoscopic equipment. Several urethral sutures have been successfully placed in Step 16b.

Postoperative Management

The postoperative management is associated with the urinary diversion that is performed after the cystectomy. In general, the following should be considered:

- Continuous antibiotic treatment for 5 days after surgery is recommended
- Intravenous fluids until bowel function is regained
- Diet is gradually advanced when bowel function is regained
- Early mobilisation

References

1. Wang GJ, Barocas DA, Raman JD, Scherr DS (2008) Robotic vs. open radical cystectomy: prospective comparison of perioperative outcomes and pathological measures of early oncological efficacy. BJU Int 101:89–93
2. Dasgupta P, Rimington P, Murphy D, Challacombe B, Hemal A, Elhage O, Khan MS (2008) Robotic assisted radical cystectomy: short to medium-term oncologic and functional outcomes. Int J Clin Pract 62:1709–1714
3. Hemal AK (2009) Role of robot-assisted surgery for bladder cancer. Curr Opin Urol 19:69–75
4. Kaul SA, Menon M (2007) Da Vinci assisted cystoprostatectomy and urinary diversion: a paradigm shift in surgical management of bladder cancer. Minerva Urol Nefrol 59:149–157

3.9 Urinary Diversion

3.9.1 Extracorporeal Ileal Conduit

Stephan Siemer, Jörn Kamradt, Michael Stöckle

Introduction

Minimally invasive laparoscopic or da Vinci cystectomy (RAC) is a challenging procedure with high demands on a surgeon's skill and a long operative time. An incision is necessary to remove the bladder. This access can also be used to construct the urinary diversion. Therefore, the invasiveness of the procedure is not increased and the operative time can be reduced, similar to the time needed for open surgery [1, 2]. The incision can be made as a midline laparotomy below the umbilicus or as a pararectal incision over a length of about 4–6 cm [3]. We prefer the infraumbilical access, which offers good access to the terminal ileum as well as to both ureters positioned laparoscopically in the right lower abdomen.

Indications

- Cases not suitable for orthotopic urinary bladder substitute
- Infiltration of the urethra
- Existing urinary incontinence

Contra-indications

- Short-bowel syndrome
- Crohn disease

Preoperative Preparation

- Mark the conduit position at the abdominal wall using water-resistant markers
- Bladder catheter
- Nasogastric stomach tube (removed after operation)
- Single-shot antibiosis
- Thrombosis prophylaxis

Step 1: Ureteric spatulation and cannulation

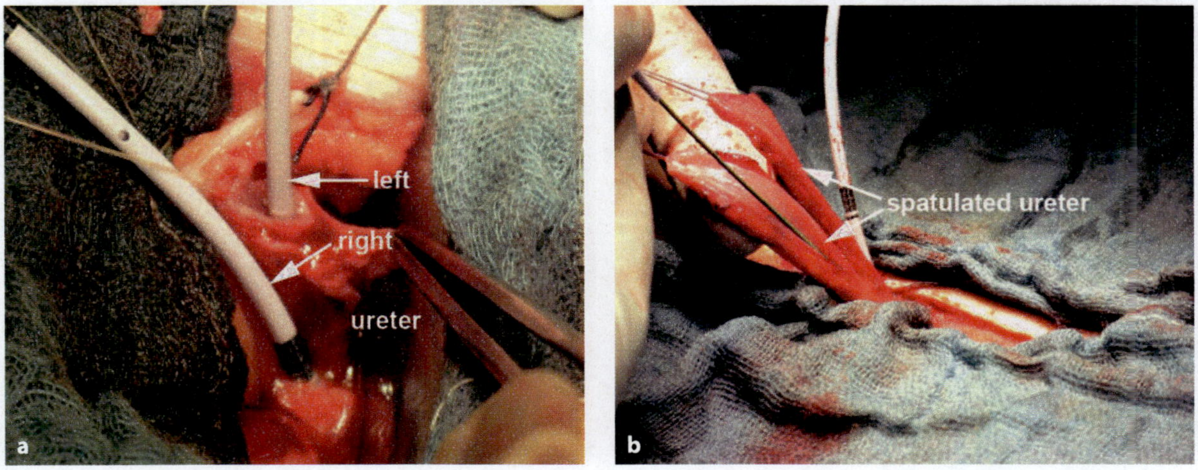

After disconnecting the da Vinci system, all ports are removed. A skin incision is made approximately 4–6 cm infraumbilically. After careful access to the intraperitoneal space is made, the previously mobilised ureters are brought out through the incision. They should have been clipped intraoperatively to avoid urinary contamination. The clips are now removed from the dilated ureters. Mono-J ureteric stents (6–8 Ch) are inserted in both ureters (Step 1a). The proper position, especially of the left stent, must be checked very carefully. For constructing the ureterointestinal anastomosis, we prefer the Wallace procedure. Therefore, both ureters are spatulated for approximately 3 cm, as shown in Step 1b.

Step 2: Wallace anastomosis

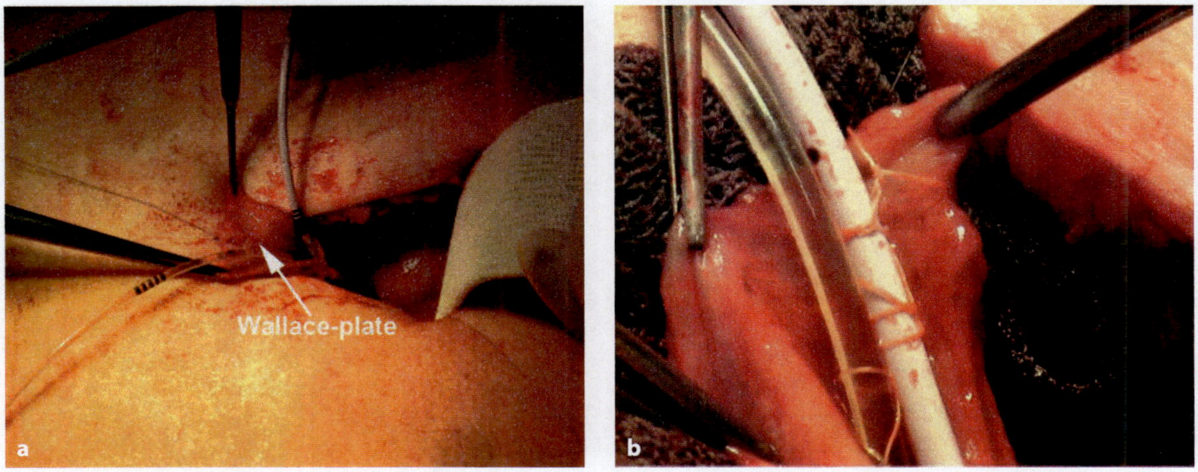

To perform the Wallace procedure, we recommend constructing the posterior wall using a 5/0 Monocryl suture as a continuous suture method to form the Wallace plate (Step 2a). The first suture must be placed precisely at the lowest point of the spatulated ureters. Afterwards, both ureteral stents are fixed onto the Wallace plate with a 5/0 Vicryl rapide suture (Step 2b). The front wall of the Wallace anastomosis is sutured at a distance of approximately 5–8 mm with single interrupted stitches to create a single-lumen ureter. Afterwards, the Wallace anastomosis is repositioned in the intraperitoneal area.

Step 3: Ileum mobilisation

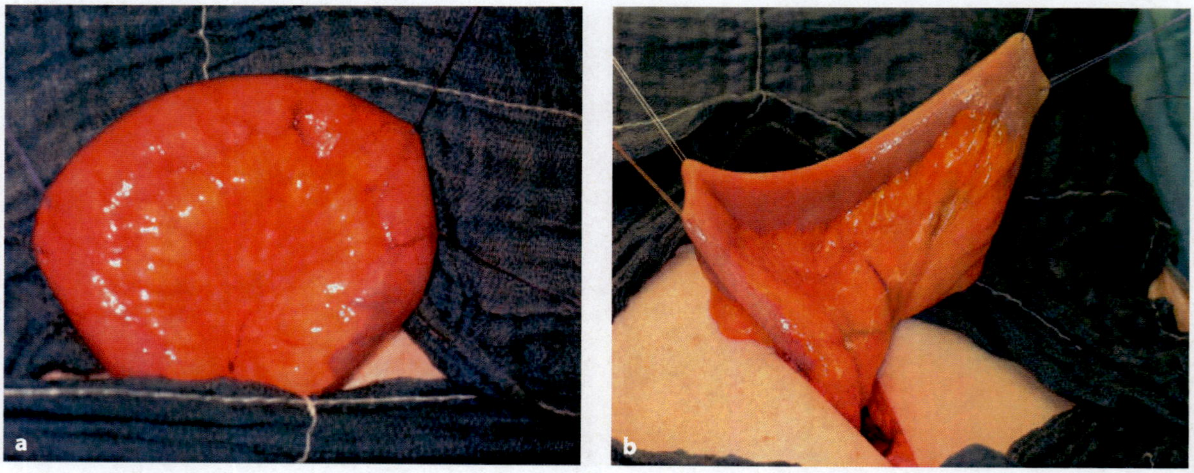

Even through the skin incision (approximately 4–6 cm), the terminal ileum (approximately 15 cm proximally from the ileocaecal (Bauhin valve) can be easily mobilised out of the incision (Step 3a). If there are intestinal adhesions, we recommend performing this beforehand using the da Vinci system, since an adhesiolysis through this small incision is generally difficult. As a rule, 10–12 cm of small intestine are required for an ileal conduit. Step 3b demonstrates this length held between two marking sutures and elevated. Only very obese patients require a longer intestinal segment.

Step 4: Ileum and mesenteric dissection

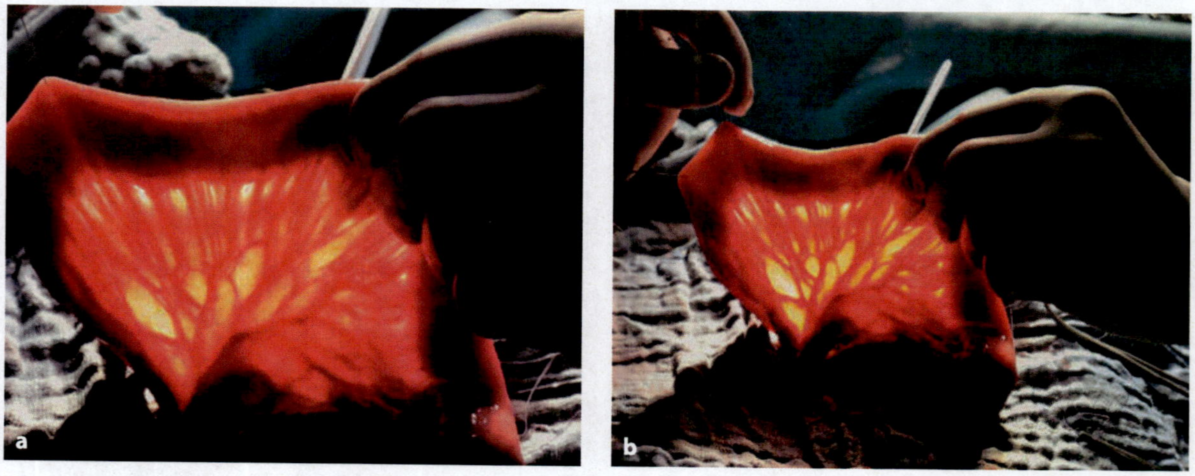

Shining the theatre light through the mesentery (diaphanoscopy) demonstrates the vascular arcades very well in most cases (Step 4a, Step 4b). Consideration is now given to the vascular arcades. The small bowel mesentery is now incised with cautery. Larger vessels are ligated. Haematoma in the mesentery should be avoided, since it can lead to serious complications. At least one large vascular arcade must be preserved for the maintenance of the conduit perfusion. The skin incision is covered with abdominal packs to avoid stool contamination of the abdomen. Now the small intestine is divided with the scissors. We flush the conduit with saline solution.

Step 5: Ileal re-anastomosis

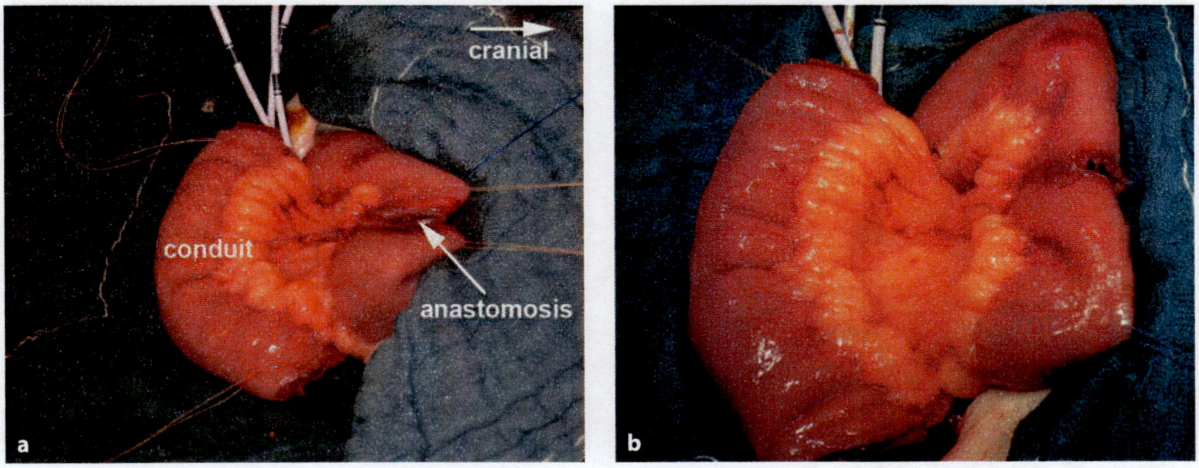

The mesenteric adipose tissue at the free ends of the cut small bowel should be removed to make the end-to-end anastomosis easier. The re-anastomosis of the small intestine limbs is performed, using a sequential, all-layer seromuscular suture (4/0 PDS). Alternatively, the small intestine can be restored in two layers. The small access used necessitates careful attention to avoid unnoticed rotation of the intestinal loops and intra-abdominal examination is usually not possible later. The re-anastomosis is performed cranially to the ileal conduit (Step 5a) and we use 3/0 or 4/0 Vicryl for the closure of the mesenteric defect to prevent internal hernia (Step 5b).

Step 6: Ureteroileal anastomosis

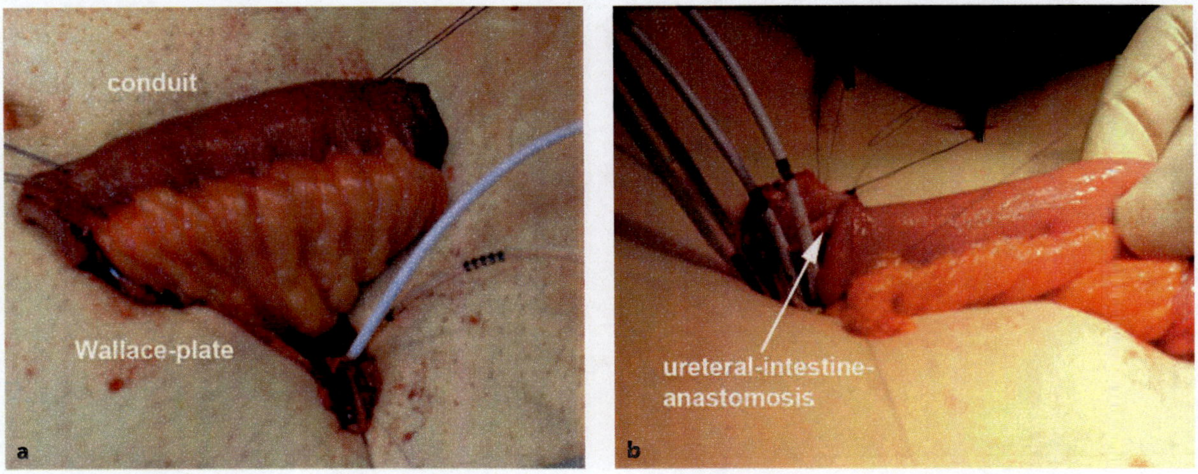

The Wallace plate is returned to the skin (Step 6a) and the ureterointestinal anastomosis is begun (Step 6b) with 4/0 Monocryl continuous sutures. For water-tight anastomosis, attention should be paid to the inversion of the bowel mucous membrane. Before tightening the front wall, the stents are diverted through the conduit using a long right-angled clamp. Finally, the anastomosis is checked for any leakage by filling the conduit with approximately 60 ml of saline solution. If the anastomosis is sufficient it can be replaced to an intraperitoneal position.

Step 7: Ileal conduit spout formation

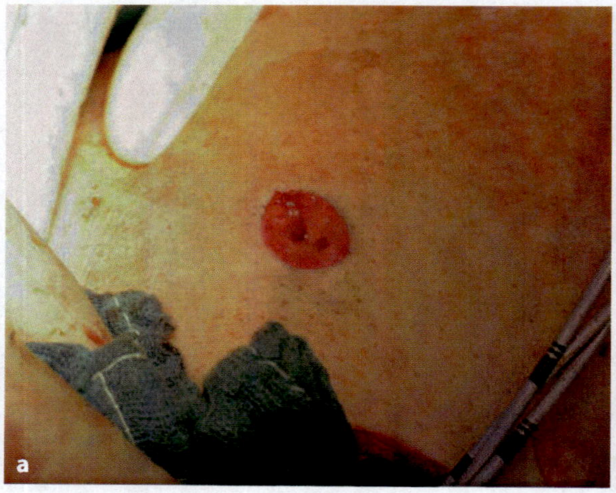

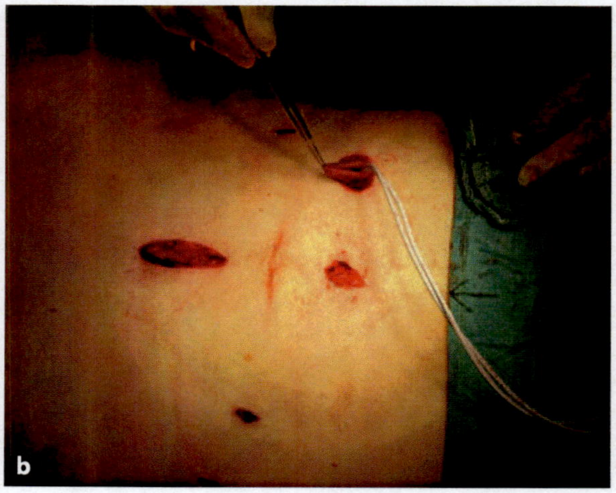

To construct the conduit, excise a circular disc of skin from the presurgically marked conduit exit point (Step 7a) (preferably a port position). We recommend a star-shaped incision of the fascia and exiting the conduit through the rectus muscle to avoid hernia formation. Fix the conduit wall in the fascia with Vicryl single interrupted stitches.

Use 3/0 Monocryl single interrupted stitches for fixation of the conduit to the skin (Step 7b). Attention should be paid to prevent a stretched or angled course of the conduit through the abdomen, as this can lead to problems during the following years.

Step 8: Final inspection and skin incisions

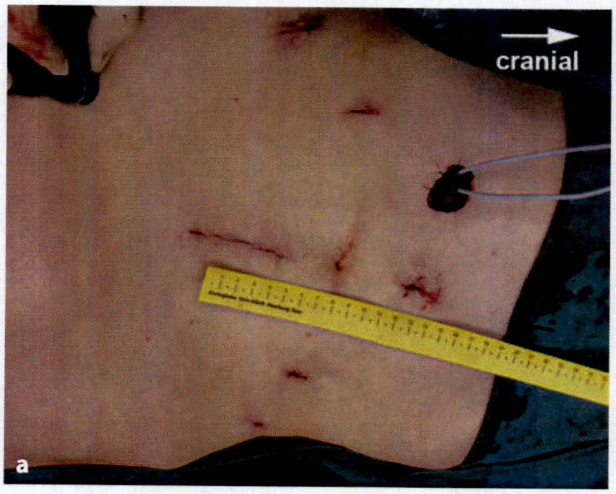

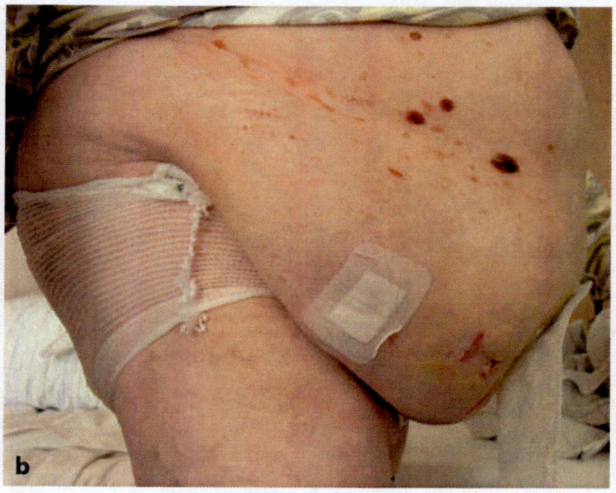

A final check for bleeding is performed through the incision. A drain is not necessary in all cases. For wound closure, we recommend fascial sutures for the median laparotomy and 10- or 12-mm ports. Skin incisions should be avoided in the area of the stoma bag. If this cannot be avoided the incision should be carefully closed to avoid later excessive scarring, for example.

In particular, very obese patients may benefit from this procedure where skin incisions are kept to a minimum (Step 8a, Step 8b).

Postoperative Management

- Fast-track concept
  - Quick return to solid food
  - Early mobilisation of the patient if possible 6 h postoperatively
- Remove the ureteric mono-J stents after 8–10 days

References

1. Hemal AK (2009) Role of robot-assisted surgery for bladder cancer. Curr Opin Urol 19:69–75
2. Kaul SA, Menon M (2007) Da Vinci assisted cystoprostatectomy and urinary diversion: a paradigm shift in surgical management of bladder cancer. Minerva Urol Nefrol 59:149–157
3. Dasgupta P, Rimington P, Murphy D, Challacombe B, Hemal A, Elhage O, Khan MS (2008) Robotic assisted radical cystectomy: short- to medium-term oncologic and functional outcomes. Int J Clin Pract 62:1709–1714

3.9.2 Neobladder

3.9.2.1 Extracorporal Neobladder

Thilo Schwalenberg, Evangelos Liatsikos, Jens-Uwe Stolzenburg

Introduction

Within the spectrum of continent diversion after cystectomy, orthotopic reconstruction using an ileal neobladder is currently the most popular choice for male and female patients alike. The main advantages of a neobladder over other forms of continent diversion are firstly that the native urinary sphincter can be utilised, and secondly that the patient is more likely to experience the normal pelvic sensation of bladder filling.

While the indications for neobladder creation have broadened over recent years, and the technique for ureteric implantation has evolved, the principles of neobladder formation are well established. In many centres, including our own, the Hautmann principles are employed to construct a low-pressure spherical reservoir. This is created by a W-shaped reconstruction of detubularised ileum. This technique, above others, allows for the closest approximation to a sphere, optimising capacity-to-surface area ratio, thus minimising metabolic complications. The lower pressure of this reservoir also reduces the incidence of reflux.

We recommend achieving an incremental increase in neobladder capacity, through timed voiding, until this functional capacity is reached. We have found that the functional neobladder capacity of 400–500 ml, in conjunction with a length of bowel not exceeding 60 cm, is the optimum for long-term satisfactory function.

The advantages of minimal access surgery are many. However, there must be no compromise in the high standard of urinary reconstruction already established in the open field. The debate over intra- versus extracorporal reconstruction is less important than the quality and reproducibility of the technique.

Indications

The procedure is indicated for all cancer patients who are candidates for curative cystectomy and those with refractory benign disease in the presence of an intact sphincter. In the former, the indications have widened in recent years to include those with more advanced bladder cancer, cancer in locations such as the bladder neck and the urethra, and women who would previously have undergone routine urethrectomy. The origins of these changing paradigms can be traced to a consensus conference in 2004 [1]. The point remains, though, that there should be no suspicion of residual disease at the time of orthotopic reconstruction.

Contra-indications

- Incomplete tumour resection
- Multifocal urethral CIS or prostatic stromal tumour infiltration
- Neurogenic pelvic floor dysfunction
- Posterior exenteration without omental interposition
- Chronic renal disease (serum creatinine > 150–200 μmol/l)
- Chronic hydroureteronephrosis
- Short bowel syndrome
- Chronic inflammatory bowel disease
- Radiation enteritis
- Recurrent urethral stricture disease
- Inability to perform Clean Intermittent Self-Catheterisation
- Significant physical and cognitive impairment (no absolute contra-indication based on age alone)

Preoperative Preparation

- We recommend a 2-day preoperative bowel preparation
- On preoperative day 2, the patient is restricted to liquids only, and takes 100 ml sorbitol
- On preoperative day 1, the patient takes MoviPrep (made up to 1 l), and 1 l more of clear fluid
- The site of a potential ileal conduit is marked
- Intravenous cefuroxime and metronidazole are administered at induction of anaesthesia

Step 1: Enlargement of skin incision for reconstruction

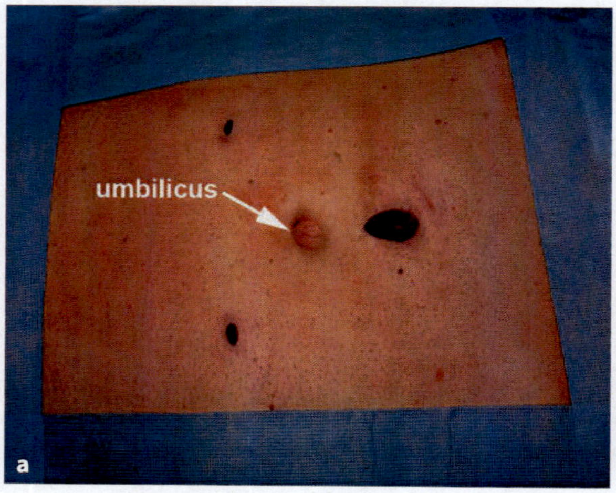

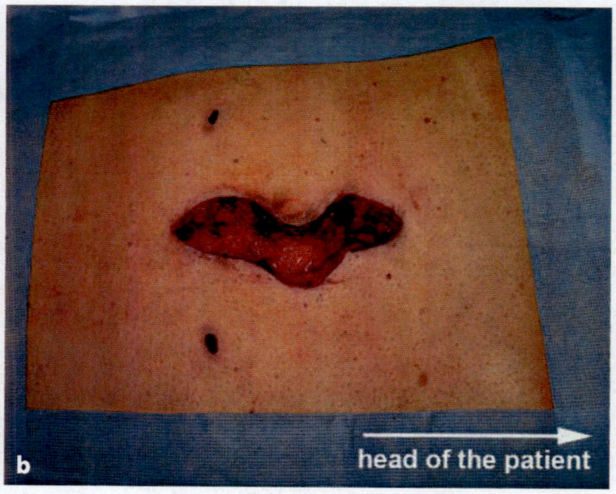

Step 1a demonstrates the abdomen after port removal after cystectomy. An 8- to 10-cm midline incision is made, skirting the umbilicus to the left. This incision incorporates the camera-port incision. An incision that is too cranial to the umbilicus can create problems during the mobilisation of the mesenteric root. We prefer an incision cranially and caudally to the umbilicus only because of the incorporation of the camera port shortening the final overall length of the incision. Alternatively, an infraumbilical median laparotomy can be performed.

Step 2: Entry to peritoneal cavity and bowel mobilisation

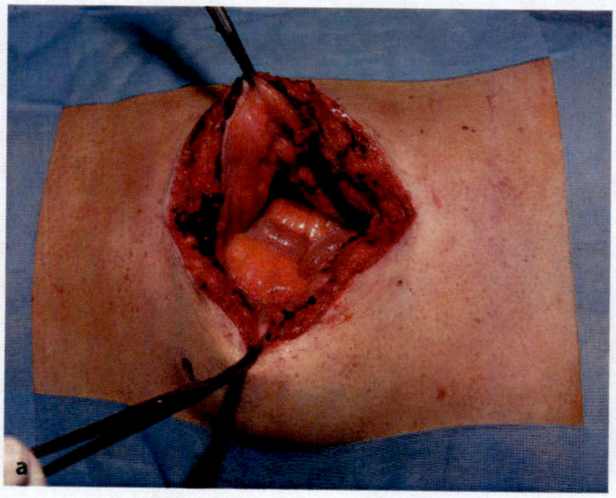

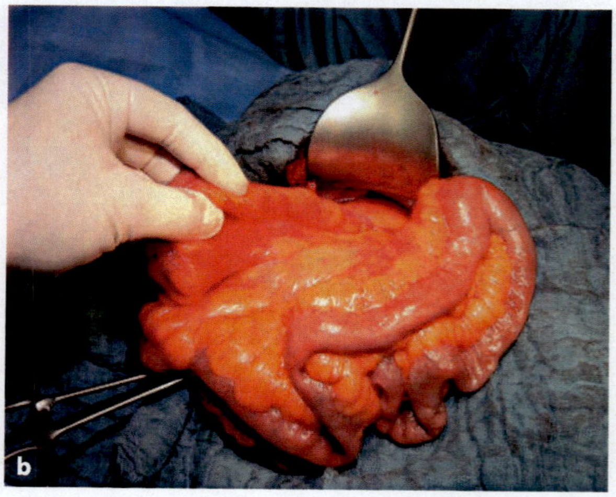

The margins of the wound are retracted (e.g. with Mikulicz clamps) to allow the operator's hand entry to the abdomen (Step 2a). Adequate access and exposure are required to allow mobilisation of the root of the mesentery, as well as the ureters. It must also be remembered that occult bleeding, previously tamponaded by the pneumoperitoneum, may now become apparent. Adequate access is required to manage this. The assistant retracts the wound edge to facilitate bowel mobilisation and exteriorisation (Step 2b). Care must be taken to maintain bowel orientation. While this is not normally a problem during open surgery, the potential to twist the small bowel on its mesentery is much greater in a mini-laparotomy procedure.

Step 3: Transillumination of the mesenteric vessels, ileal resection and ileoileal anastomosis

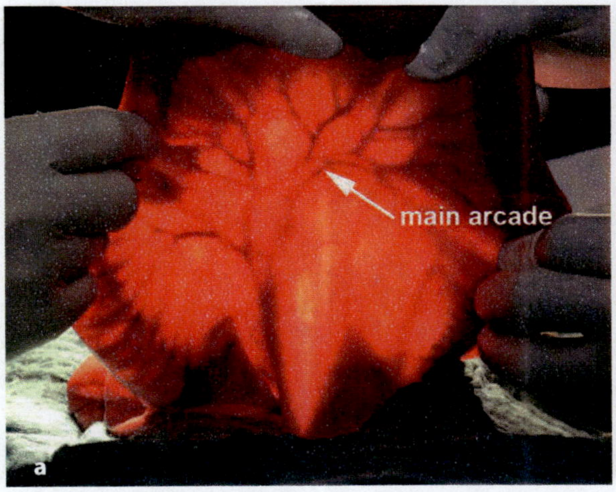

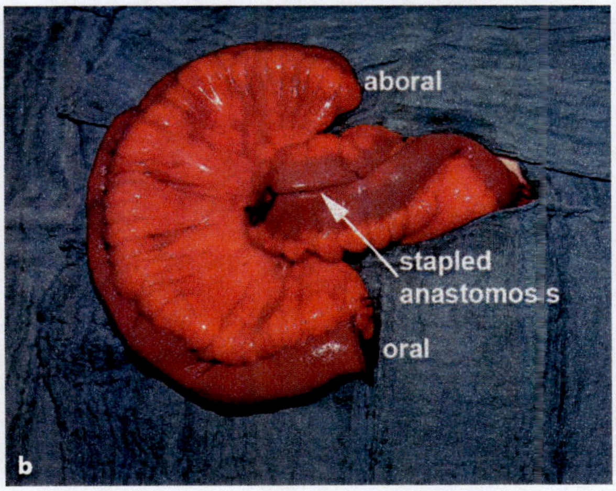

The technique of transillumination facilitates identification of the mesenteric vessels (Step 3a). The main arcade must be preserved. Approximately 50–60 cm of terminal ileum is required, sparing the distal 10 cm. For bowel anastomosis, we prefer the functional end-to-end stapled technique (Step 3b). The mesenteric window should be closed, and the isolated bowel segment must lie caudal to the anastomosis. Before incising the bowel to create the neobladder, an appreciation must be gained of the mobility required by the bowel segment to enable a tension-free urethral anastomosis within the pelvis. If necessary, further dissection of the mesentery must be performed to allow this. The temptation to overcome the problem of mobility by harvesting an excessive length of ileum (maximum, 60 cm) must be avoided.

Step 4: W-configuration of the neobladder and detubularisation

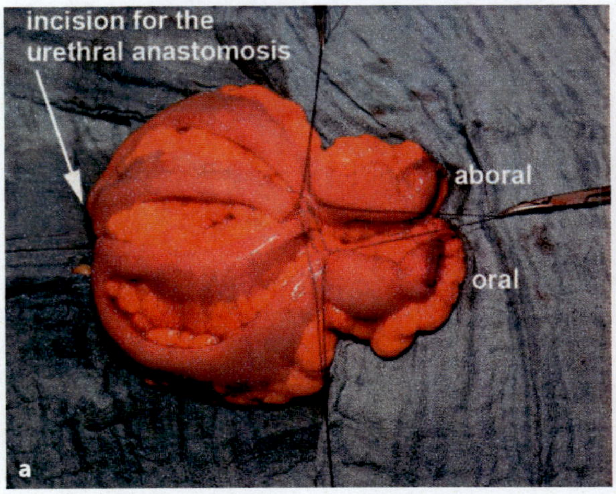

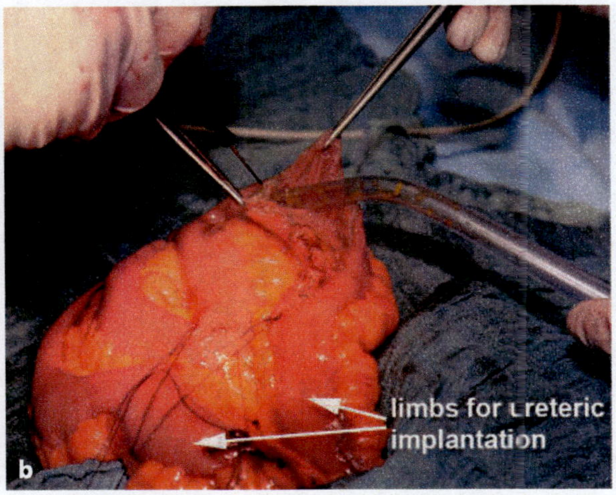

The ileum is configured in the W-formation, and stay sutures are inserted. For the ureteric implantation, each end of the ileal segment is left protruding from the pouch. Typically, 5 cm long, these limbs can be longer if necessary to allow for reduced proximal ureteric length, the goal being a tension-free anastomosis. Detubularisation of the bowel (Step 4b) is performed precisely on the antimesenteric border. This can be facilitated by the use of cutting diathermy over an instrument such as a plastic suction device, placed in the lumen. In some instances the bowel circumference may seem too small to allow safe and easy anastomosis of the urethra between the ileoileal suture line and the mesentery. In such a case, a detubularisation incision of the ileum in a sinusoidal fashion can help overcome this problem.

Step 5: Approximation of ileal wall margins and construction of posterior wall

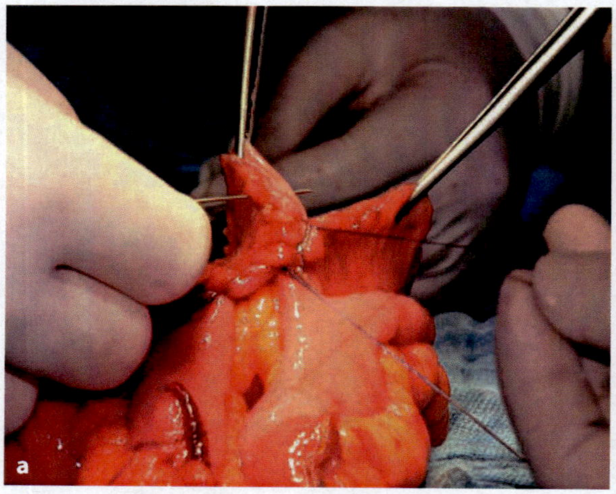

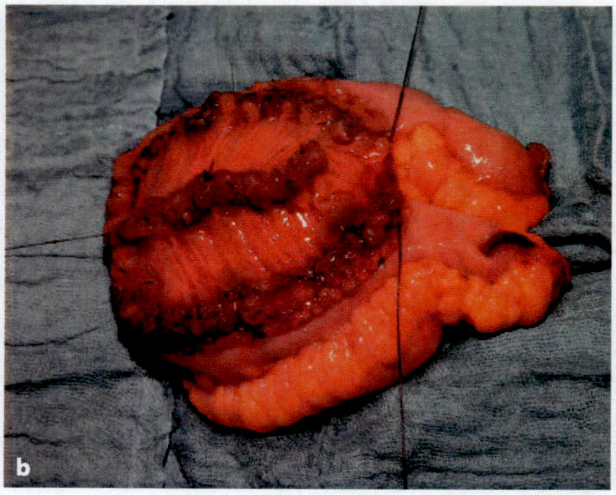

The free edges of ileum (all layers) are anastomosed with continuous 3/0 braided synthetic (e.g. Polyglactin) sutures. To enhance the integrity, we place a knot at regular intervals in the otherwise continuous anastomosis. The use of a straight needle may prove faster than a mounted curved needle for this part of the procedure.

The margins of the posterior wall are completely closed (Step 5b). The site of the urethral anastomosis is separate from the ileoileal suture line.

Step 6: Closure of the anterior wall and preparation of limbs for ureteric implantation

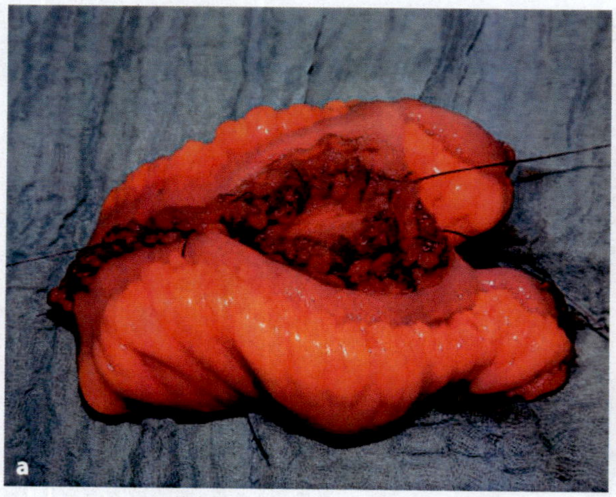

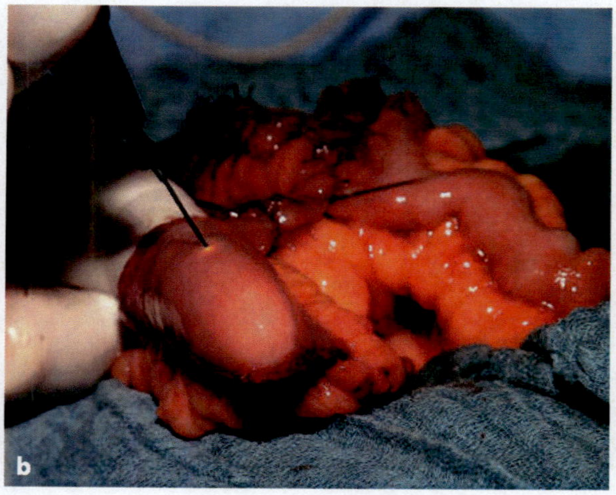

The anterior wall of the neobladder is now closed, though not completely at first (Step 6a). The correct placement of the urethral catheter (silicon Charrière 20) and ureteric implantation must be performed before the complete closure of the neobladder. A suprapubic catheter may also be placed, at the surgeon's discretion. A final check is made to confirm that the ureteric length is appropriate for the position of the proposed anastomosis. The limbs of the ileal segment are then incised antimesenterically in preparation for implantation (Step 6b).

Step 7: Refluxing ureteric implantation (button hole technique)

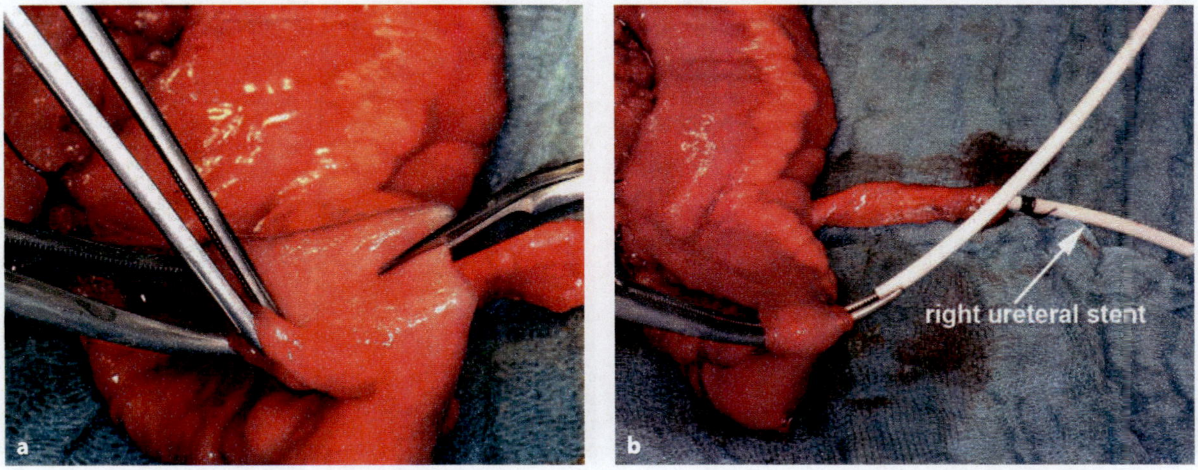

The bowel wall is incised over a curved dissector, as shown in Step 7a. The stented ureter (Mono-J stents, 7 or 8 F) is brought carefully into the limb (Step 7b). The ureter is brought directly into the ileum, without submucosal tunnelling. Only then is a ureter spatulation performed. The anastomosis is performed entirely intraluminally, which we believe to be more secure than one performed extraluminally. The stent is fixed with a rapidly dissolving suture after the ureteric anastomosis is complete.

Step 8: Ureteric implantation

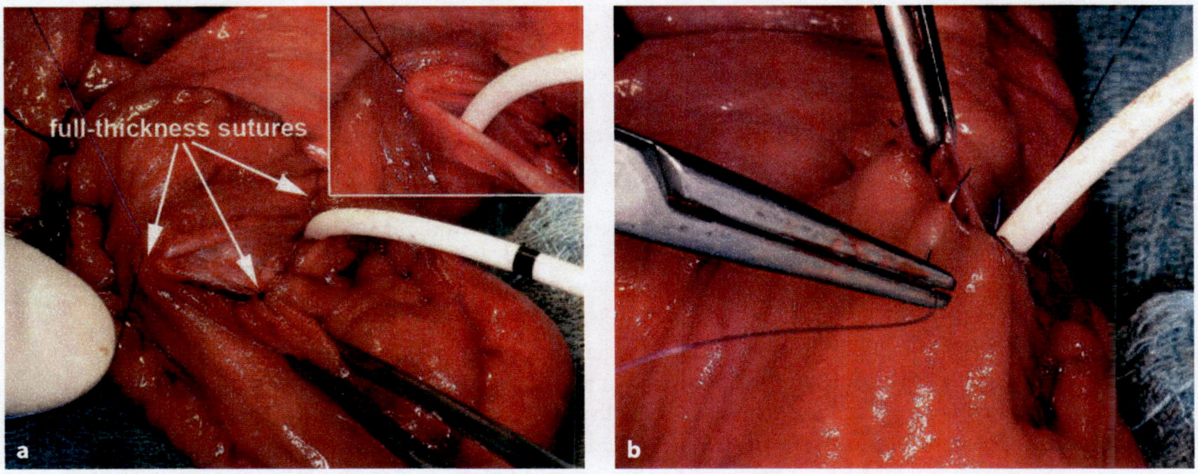

Full-thickness sutures are placed at all three corners, completed with mucosal sutures in between (Step 8a). The principles and technique of the button-hole refluxing technique are as follows: Firstly, there is no ureter tunnelling. Secondly, the ureter is spatulated. Thirdly, the ureter is fixed at three corners with 5/0 monofilament suture (e.g. Polydioxanone). Fourthly, the anastomosis is completed in between with interrupted 5/0 monofilament mucosal sutures. The purpose of the corner sutures is to secure the anastomosis.

Step 9: Completed ureteric anastomosis

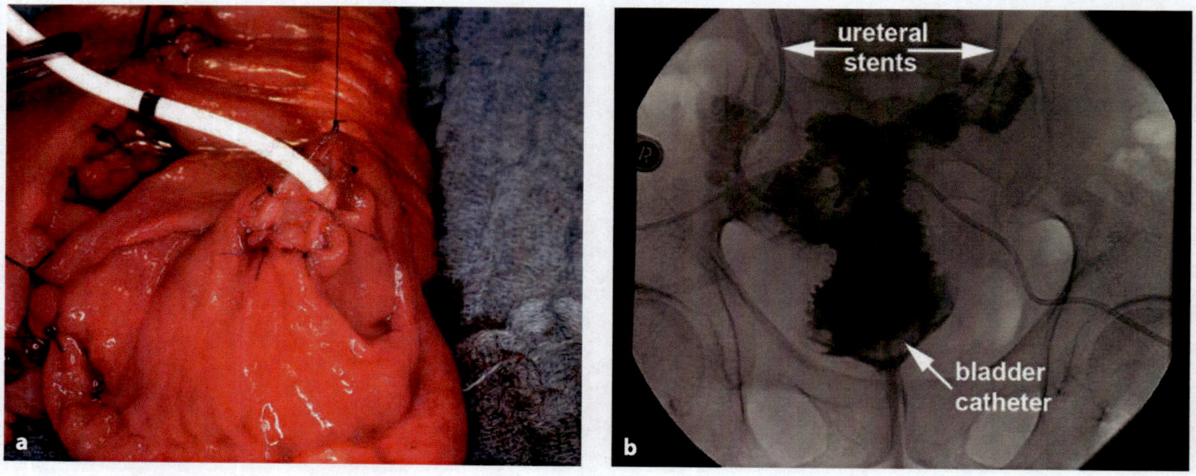

The ureteric anastomosis is now complete. Note that we have used the initial (proximal) corner suture as a retractor to facilitate the rest of the anastomosis (Step 9a). We now secure the stents with a rapidly dissolving suture to the bowel mucosa. The stents are exteriorised. This is accomplished by first crossing the stents over one another within the pouch and passing them through small incisions made in its anterior wall. The stents are passed through the anterior abdominal wall by the most direct route. Although it may be tempting to use an existing port site for this purpose, this should only be done if there is no risk of kinking or twisting the stent in the process. Step 9b shows a cystogram done on day 14 before removing the urethral catheter. The optimal (physiological) bladder capacity is 400–500 ml.

Postoperative Management

- Parenteral feeding is given until restoration of bowel peristalsis. Diet is introduced, if appropriate, from day 3 postoperatively
- Cefuroxime and (optional) metronidazole are given for 7 days postoperatively
- Bladder lavage on a daily basis is performed to evacuate mucous
- Stents are inspected on a daily basis to ensure patency and flushed with sterile saline if there is suspicion of occlusion
- Cystogram at 14 days postoperatively
  If there is no leak, the suprapubic catheter (if placed) and then the stents are removed sequentially 24 h apart
- The urethral catheter is removed at 21 days postoperatively, although it can be left in place longer at the discretion of the surgeon if there is any concern about the anastomosis
- When the catheter is removed, the patient should commence self-catheterisation to confirm complete bladder emptying and so that mucous can be evacuated
- Timed voiding is commenced, gradually increasing the interval between micturition until an optimal functional capacity of 400–500 ml is reached.
- Prior to discharge, we recommend close monitoring of acid-base status and renal function. Sonography is also performed to ensure complete voiding and to exclude upper tract dilation

References

1. Hautmann RE, Abol-Enein H, Hafez K, Haro I, Mansson W, Mills RD, Montie JD, Sagalowsky AI, Stein JP, Stenzl A, Studer UE, Volkmer BG (2007) Urinary diversion. World Health Organization (WHO) Consensus Conference on Bladder Cancer. Urology 69: 17–49

3.9.2.2 Intracorporal neobladder

N. Peter Wiklund, Abolfazl Hosseini, Martin C. Schumacher, Martin N. Jonsson

Introduction

The construction of the urinary diversion after robot-assisted radical cystectomy (RARC) is probably the most challenging part of the procedure, especially using a totally intracorporal approach. Currently available experience counts more than 200 RARCs worldwide [1, 2]. Robot-assisted intracorporal ileal conduit, orthotopic neobladder, and neobladder urethral anastomosis have been performed and described in the literature [3, 4]. The preferred method of performing the neobladder intracorporally or extracorporally is based on the surgeon's preference [5]. The operative time used for the reconstruction is one of the important factors in deciding whether to perform the diversion extra- or intracorporally. The completely intracorporal approach would certainly be advantageous in the female patient in whom transvaginal specimen extraction is the most elegant way to extract the specimen. At this point in time, intracorporally performed urinary diversion may be recommended in the hands of experienced surgeons at high-volume centres.

Indications

- Patients who are candidates for robot-assisted cystectomy

Contra-indications

- Reduced kidney function (serum creatinine more than 1.8 mg/dl or creatinine clearance less than 60 ml/min)
- Presence of tumour in prostatic urethra in men (relative contra-indication)
- Presence of tumour in the bladder neck in women (relative contra-indication)
- Decreased pulmonary compliance that would not tolerate the Trendelenburg position
- Patients with a history of previous extensive abdominal surgery (relative contra-indication)

Preoperative Preparation

- For intracorporal orthotopic neobladder: mechanical bowel preparation (osmotic laxative) should be used the day prior to surgery
- For an extracorporal urinary diversion: enema early in the morning
- A stoma site is also marked the day prior to surgery
- Anticoagulant treatment with low-molecular-weight heparin is started the day before the surgery
- Broad-spectrum intravenous antibiotics are administrated at the beginning of the procedure

Step 1: Patient position

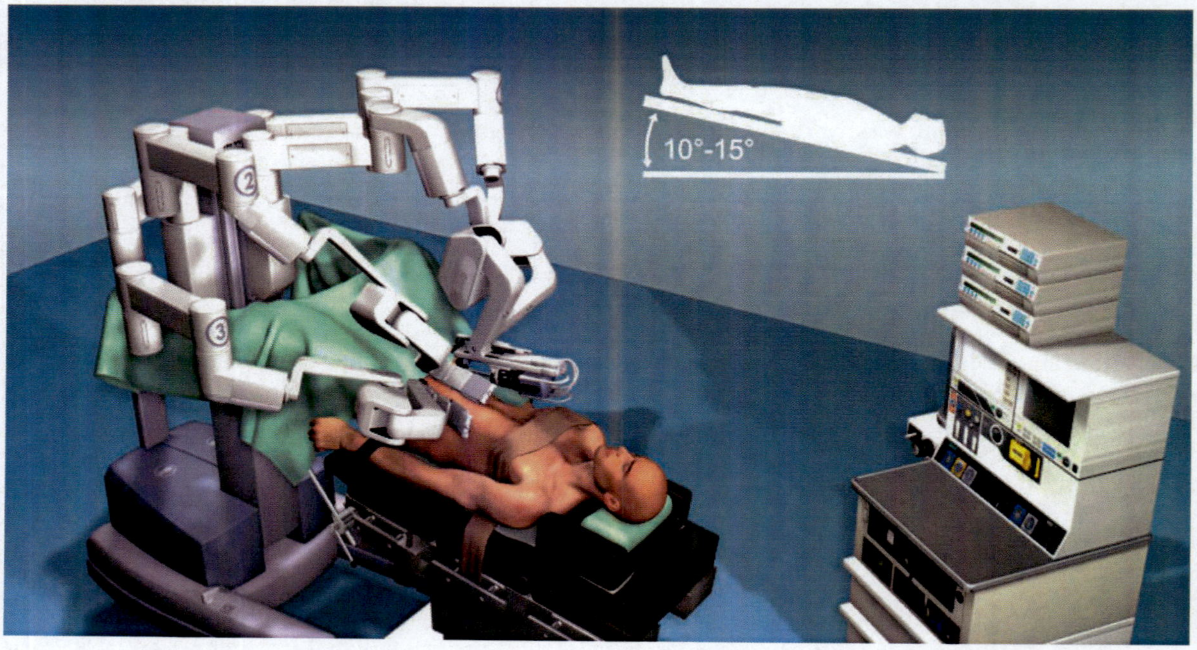

For robot-assisted radical cystoprostatectomy, the patient has to be placed in the extreme Trendelenburg position (20–25°) to allow sufficient access to the pelvis organs without bowel interposition. After the cystoprostatectomy and the extended pelvic lymph node dissection are finished, the urinary diversion is performed. For the urinary diversion, the extreme Trendelenburg position is not necessary or is not helpful. The Trendelenburg position is decreased to 10–15°, as shown in Step 1.

Step 2: Trocar placement

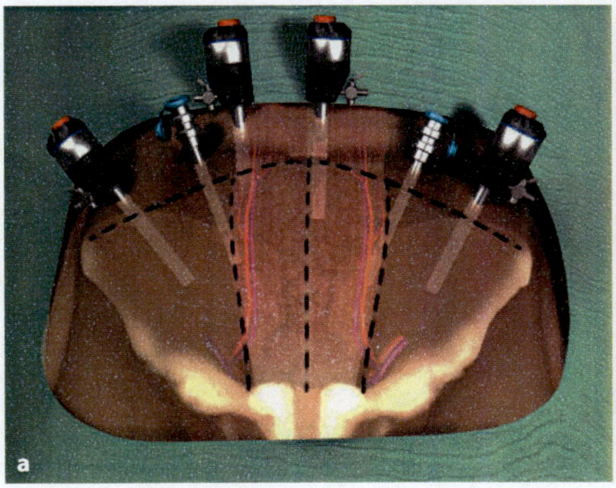

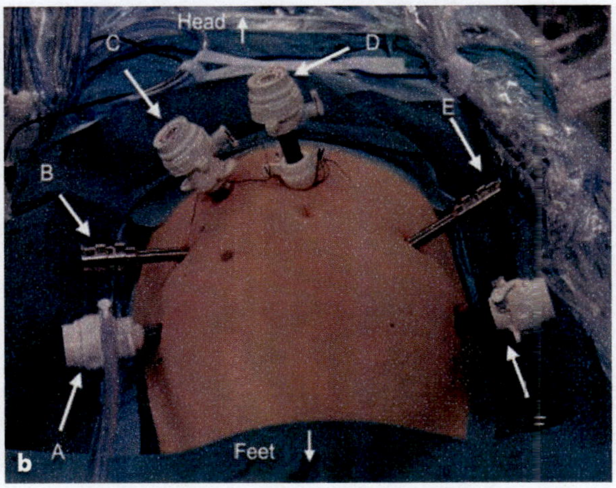

Trocar placement for the standard da Vinci system is presented in Step 2. If the Si daVinci system is used, all the ports may be placed 3 cm more cranially compared to the standard (non-Si) system. The possibility to place the ports more cranially is helpful during the lymph node dissection, since the area close to the aortic bifurcation is easier to reach. Furthermore, the mobilisation of the ileum is also helped by a more cranial placement of the trocars. Trocars designated as B and E in Step b are 8-mm robotic arm trocars, whereas the 15-mm F trocar is useful for the fourth arm (grasping and stapling). The camera trocar is designated as D.

Step 3: Anastomosis between the urethra and ileum

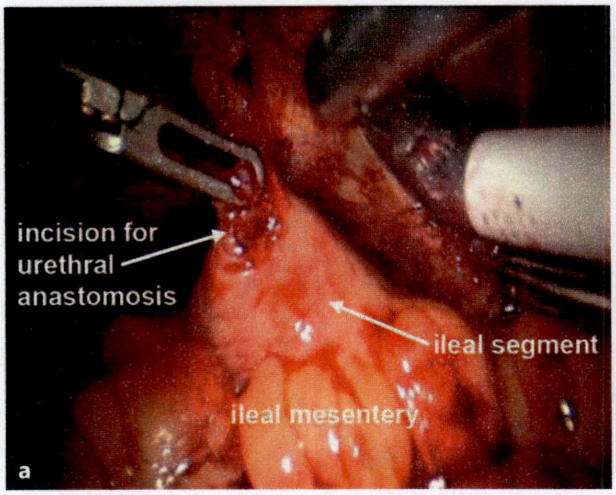

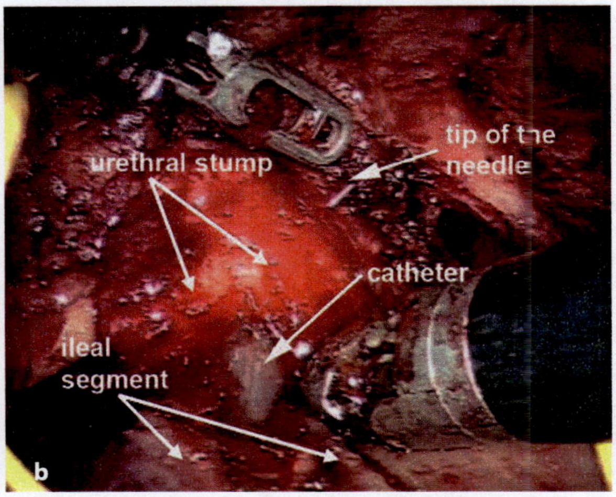

The 0° lens is used for this initial step. The ileum is sufficiently mobilised to reach down to the urethra in an attempt to provide a tension-free anastomosis between the neobladder and urethra, while the neobladder will be placed correctly in the small pelvis during the whole procedure. A 20-Ch opening is made using robotic scissors on the antimesenteric side of ileum (Step 3a). The anastomosis is performed according to the Van Velthoven running suture technique with two 18-cm 4/0 Biosyn® sutures allowing for 10–12 stitches (Step 3b). A needle driver and a grasper are used to establish the anastomosis. A 22-F urethral catheter is inserted.

Step 4: Isolation of 50 cm of ileum

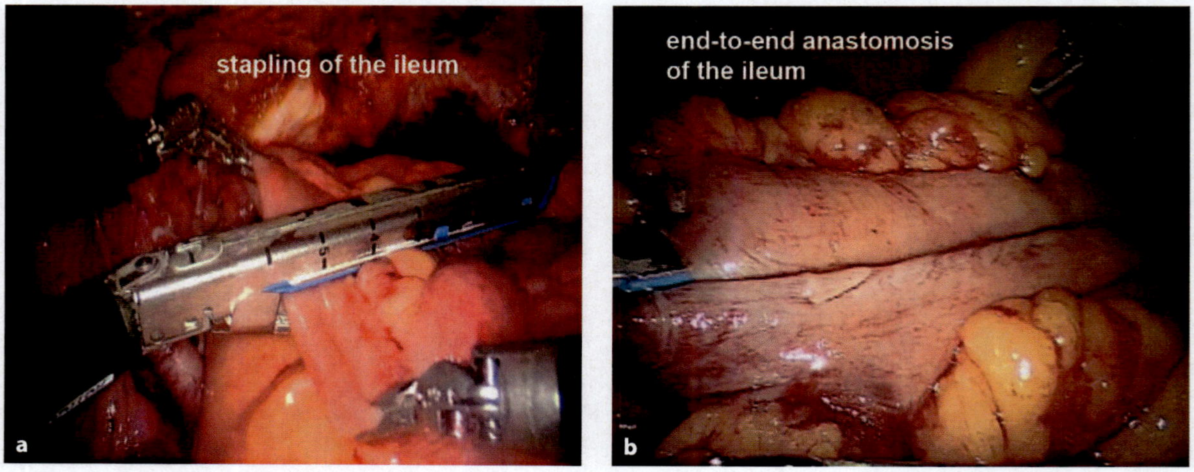

The orthotopic neobladder is fashioned from a 50-cm segment of terminal ileum. Sparing the 15- to 20-cm section from the ileocaecal junction of the terminal ileum is advisable. The intestine is isolated using laparoscopic the Endo-GIA with a 60-mm intestinal stapler by transecting proximally and distally (Step 4a). The stapler is inserted by the assisting surgeon, using the 15-mm port on the left side. The ileum is stapled 40 cm proximally to the urethroileal anastomosis. The continuity of the small bowel is restored by using the Endo-GIA with a 60-mm intestinal stapler, positioning the distal and proximal end of the ileum side to side with the antimesentery parts facing each other (Step 4b). While handling the bowel, it is important not to interfere with the major mesenteric vasculature.

Step 5: Detubularisation

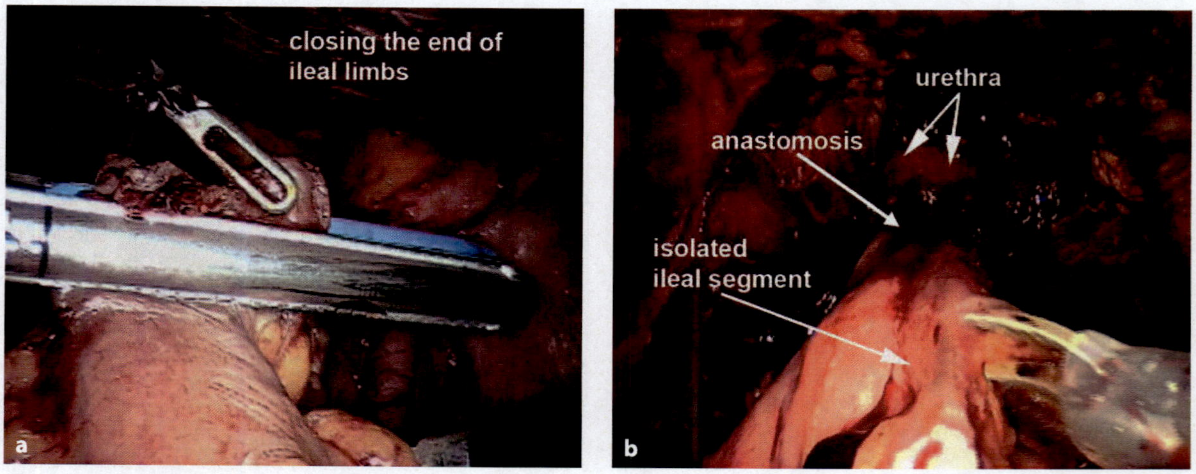

An additional transverse firing of the Endo-GIA stapler is used to close the open ends of the ileal limbs due to the aforementioned incisions (Step 5a). Stay sutures may be used to attach the intestinal segment before stapling them together. The distal 40 cm of the isolated ileal segment is detubularised along its antimesenteric border with cold scissors, leaving a 10-cm intact proximal isoperistaltic afferent limb while avoiding interfering with the sutures of the anastomosis to the urethra (Step 5b). When the detubularisation is complete, the posterior part of the Studer reservoir is closed using multiple running sutures (25 cm 3/0 Biosyn®) in a seromuscular fashion, avoiding suturing the mucosa. After the posterior part has been sutured, the distal half of the anterior part of the reservoir is sutured, using the 25 cm 3/0 Biosyn® suture. The proximal half of the anterior part of the reservoir is left open (approximately 3 cm).

Step 6: Preparation of ureters for ureteroneovesical anastomosis

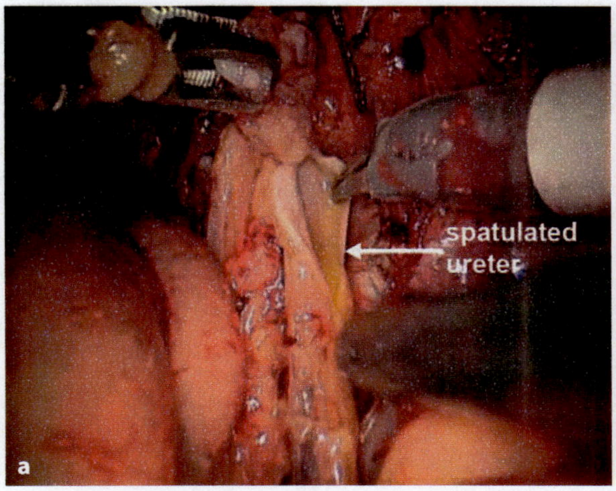

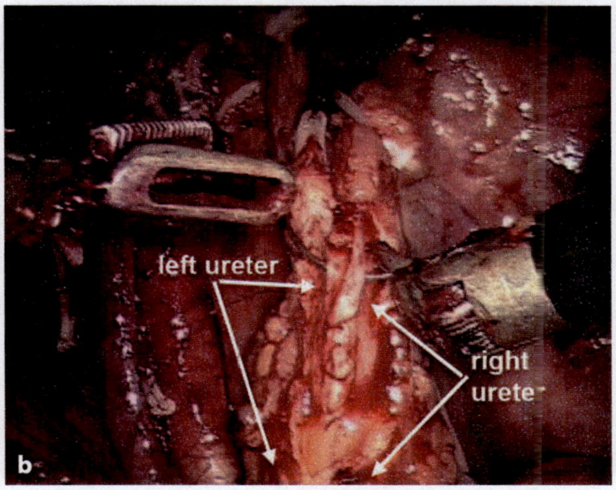

The opened anterior part of the reservoir is closed in the last part of the procedure by the anastomosis of the ureters to the neobladder. The anastomosis between the ureters and the afferent limb is performed according to the Wallace technique using a 0° lens camera. A 3/0 Biosyn® suture is placed at the distal end of each ureter for retraction purposes. The left ureter is tunnelled under the sigmoid mesentery to the right side. The distal segment of the ureters are then incised and spatulated for 2 cm (Step 6a). The posterior walls of the ureters are sutured side to side, using 15 cm running 4/0 Biosyn® suture (Step 6b). Before the anastomosis between the ureters and the isolated intestinal loop is performed, two single-J 40-cm ureteric stents are inserted using the Seldinger technique through two separate 4-mm ports at the lower part of abdominal wall.

Step 7: Ureteroneovesical anastomosis

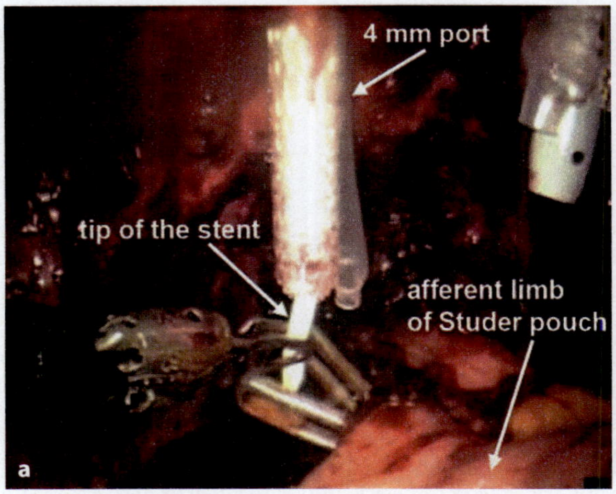

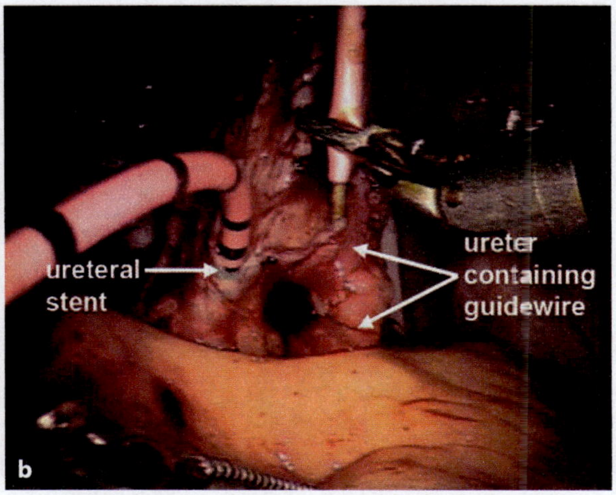

The stents are pulled through the trocars and inserted to the afferent limb (Step 7a). The ureters are gently pulled by their holding sutures and the stents are pushed in the ureters up to the renal pelvis on each side. The distal portion of the stents is passed through the neobladder wall. The ureters are then sutured to the afferent limb of the Studer pouch, using two 15-cm 4/0 Biosyn® suture (Step 7b). The standard method for the implantation of the ureters is used. After the ureterovesical anastomosis is completed, the distal segment is pulled through the lateral trocars and fixed to the skin.

Step 8: Closure of the Studer reservoir

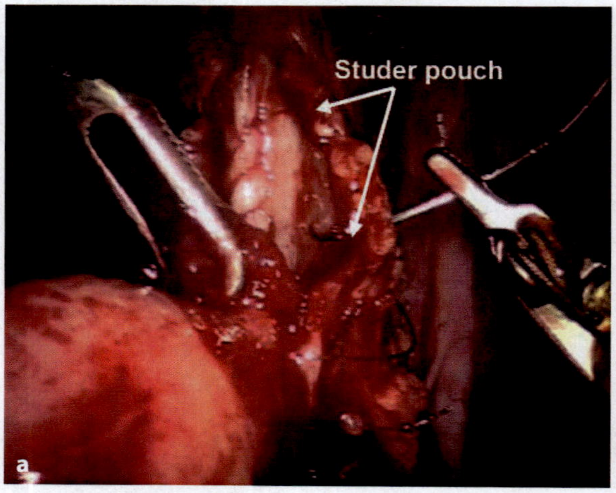

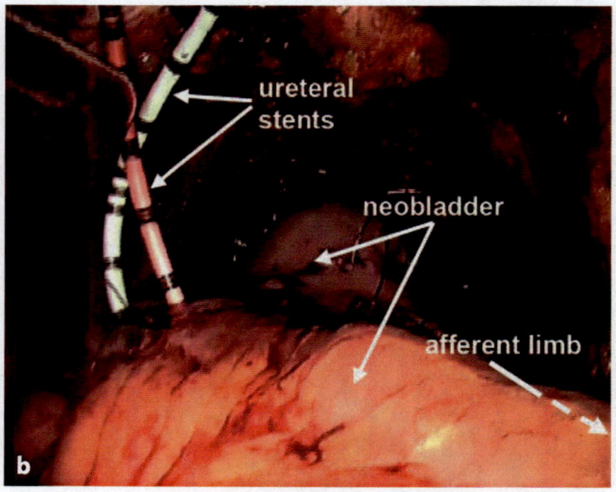

The remaining part of the reservoir is then closed with a running 3/0 Biosyn® suture, using a 0° lens laparoscopic camera (Step 8a). The balloon of the indwelling urethral catheter is filled with 10 cc saline. The neobladder is then filled with 50 cc of saline to check for leakage (Step 8b). If leakage is observed extra sutures should be considered. A 21-Ch passive drainage is introduced and placed in the small pelvis. The drainage should be placed carefully so as to not interfere with the anastomotic lines of the neobladder. In female patients, the specimen may be retracted through the vagina, whereas in males the specimen can be retracted through an enlarged infraumbilical incision (3–4 cm) in the midline of the abdominal wall.

Postoperative Management

- Continuous antibiotic treatment for 5 days after operation is recommended
- Remove the abdominal drain when the draining liquid is less than 200 cc/day
- Ureteral stent extraction 7 days after the surgery. A single shot of 240 mg Garamycin is administered 0.5 h before the removal of the stents
- Extraction of the catheter from the neobladder is performed 21 days after the surgery

References

1. Binder J, Kramer W (2001) Robotically-assisted laparoscopic radical prostatectomy. BJU Int 87:408–410
2. Guru KA, Kim HL, Piacente PM, Mohler JL (2007) Robot-assisted radical cystectomy and pelvic lymph node dissection: initial experience at Roswell Park Cancer Institute. Urology 69:469–474
3. Hemal AK, Abol-Enein H, Tewari A, Shrivastava A, Shoma AM, Ghoneim MA, Menon M (2004) Robotic radical cystectomy and urinary diversion in the management of bladder cancer. Urol Clin North Am 31:719–729
4. Menon M, Hemal AK, Tewari A, Shrivastava A, Shoma AM, Abol-Ein H, Ghoneim MA (2004) Robot-assisted radical cystectomy and urinary diversion in female patients: technique with preservation of the uterus and vagina. J Am Coll Surg 198:386–393
5. Guru KA, Jonsson MN, Wiklund NP (2008) Robot-assisted radical cystectomy. In: Jhona, Wiklund NP (eds) Robotic Urology Springer, Berlin Heidelberg New York, pp. 189–202

3.10 Prostatic Adenomectomy

3.10.1 Laparoscopic Adenomectomy

René Sotelo Noguera, Camilo Mejia Buendia

Introduction

Open surgery has been the gold standard for the treatment of benign, symptomatic, large-volume prostatic hyperplasia. Since 2002, many laparoscopic studies have been conducted that duplicate this technique. These investigators have achieved results comparable to open surgery, while maintaining the advantages of a minimally invasive approach.

Mariano et al. [1] first reported the use of a laparoscopic approach for simple prostatectomy that was performed in a patient with benign prostatic hyperplasia (BPH). In this case report, a longitudinal vesicocapsular incision was made to extract a 120-g prostate adenoma, with a total of four haemostatic sutures used for vascular control. Van Velthoven et al. [2] reported their initial experience with laparoscopic extraperitoneal Millin prostatectomy in 18 patients, duplicating the open technique. Sotelo et al. [3, 4] described a horizontal cystotomy incision proximal to the junction of the bladder and prostate. The technique was performed for laparoscopic simple prostatectomies in 17 patients with symptomatic significant prostatomegaly as well as robotically in seven patients. A French group [5] has described how to assist the enucleation with the finger. In this section, we will describe the developed technique in detail.

Indications

Preoperative evaluation includes history and physical examination, as well as digital rectal examination and routine laboratory tests. These include prostate-specific antigen, International Prostate Symptom Score (IPSS) and quality of life (QOL) questionnaires, uroflowmetry, and transrectal ultrasound (TRUS) evaluation with prostate volume measurement.

- Selection criteria are symptomatic BPH with a TRUS and an estimated gland weight of 60 g or more.

Contra-indications

- Prostate cancer
- Morbid obesity
- Anticoagulation therapy
- Anaesthetic contra-indications

Preoperative Preparation

- The patient should stop taking antiplatelet or any anticoagulant medication at least 8 days before surgery

Step 1: Port placement

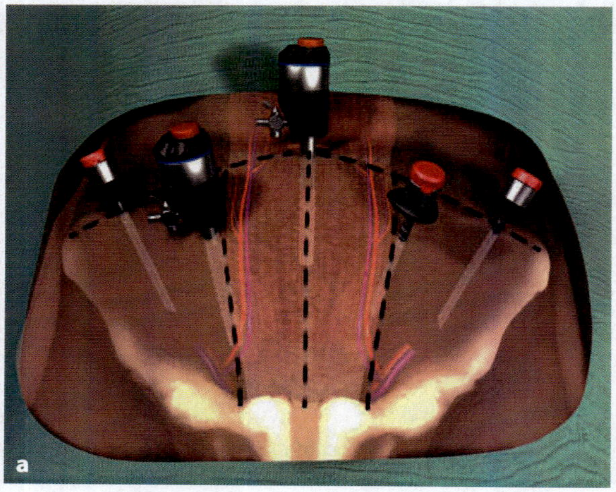

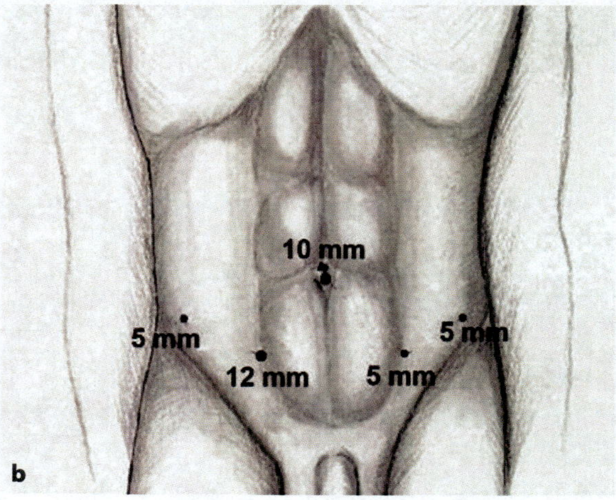

A five-port extraperitoneal or transperitoneal approach is used with the patient under general anaesthesia, in a modified Trendelenburg position (Step 1). The camera trocar is placed through the rectus muscle sheath on the right side just under the umbilicus. The left trocars are placed on the line between the umbilicus and anterior left iliac crest. The medial trocar is inserted 2–3 cm from the umbilicus and the lateral 2–3 cm from the iliac crest. The right trocars are placed as mirror images to the left ones. The insertion of the camera trocar for the transperitoneal approach is performed with either a Veress needle or the open Hasson technique. Alternatively, balloon dilation of the extraperitoneal space is performed.

Step 2: Entrance to the Retzius space and initiation of cystotomy

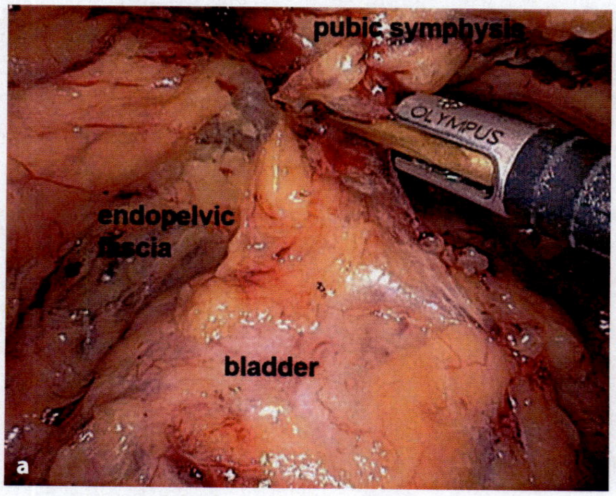

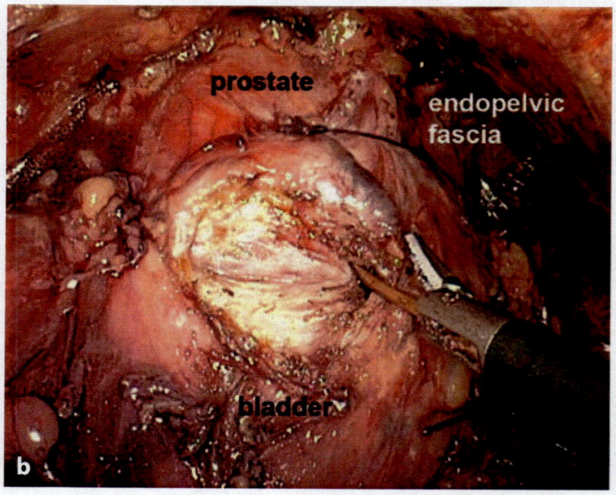

After mobilising the bladder (for the transperitoneal approach), the Retzius space is entered and the anterior surface of the prostate capsule is cleared of overlying fatty tissue (Step 2a). The extraperitoneal approach does not require bladder mobilisation as the Retzius space is accessed directly during the balloon dilation. A haemostatic back bleeding stitch is placed near the prostate base, which also allows the anterior traction of the prostate. A transverse cystotomy incision is made 1–2 cm proximal to the junction of the bladder and the prostate (Step 2b). An ultrasonic scalpel or J-hook electrocautery instrument is used because they provide accurate incisions and haemostasis.

Step 3: Cystotomy

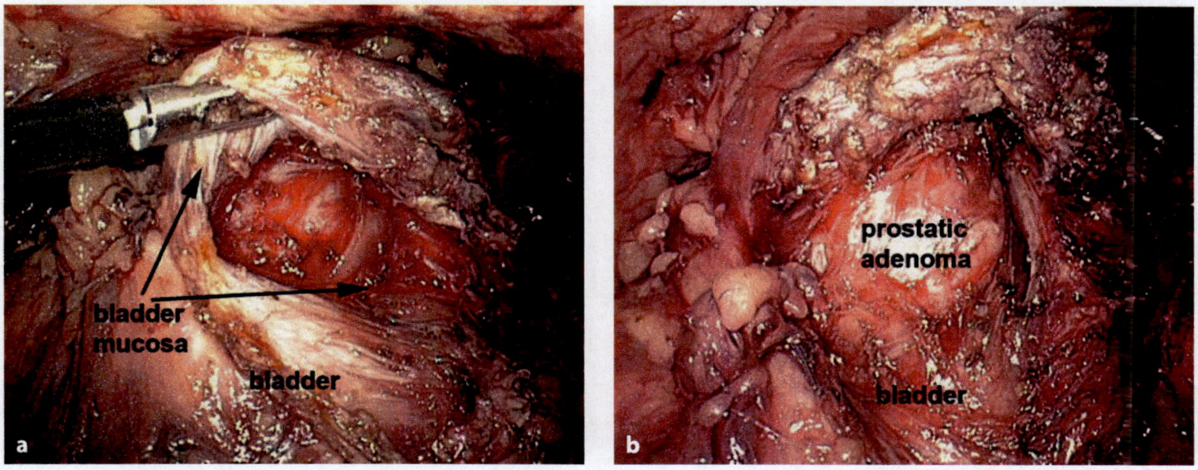

The anterior bladder neck is incised and the bladder lumen is entered (Step 3a). Alternatively, the incision could be made over the junction of the bladder and prostate as per the surgeon's preference. The prostate and bladder mucosa are visualised and should be carefully inspected. The ureteral orifices should be identified. The latter structures are usually close to the large medial lobes and may interfere with the adenoma excision, resulting in injury. In difficult cases, the bilateral insertion of double-J stent is advisable. The latter manoeuvre provides constant visualisation of the orifices and it is easier to avoid injuries. Step 3b shows a bulging large median lobe of the prostate with the bladder mucosa overlying the prostate.

Step 4: Traction of the medial lobe

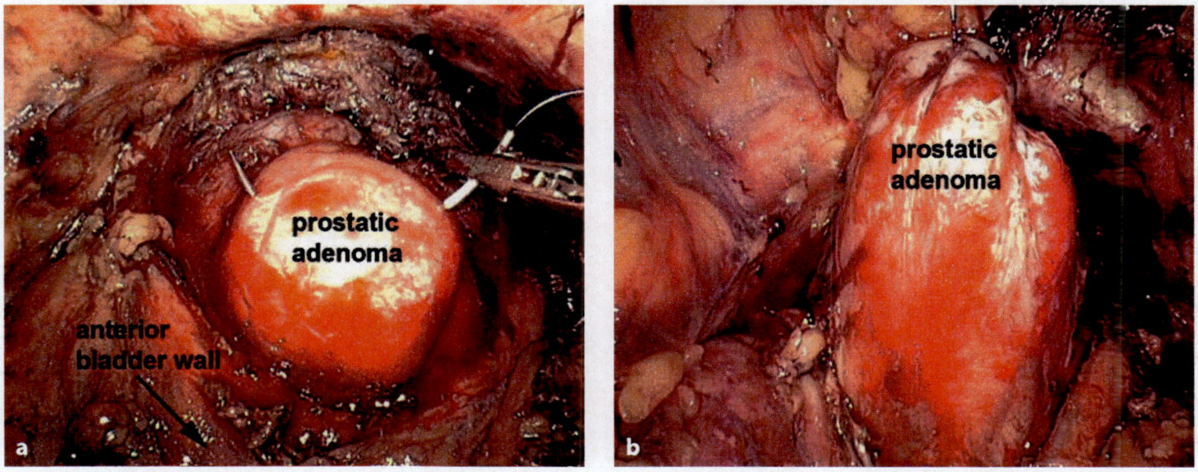

A large, bulging medial lobe can be retracted anteriorly in an efficacious manner with a figure-eight stay stitch. The suture is placed using a standard laparoscopic method or using a Keith needle or Carter-Thomason port closure needle device. Step 4a demonstrates the placement of retraction suture using a needle holder. The two ends of the stay stitch are retrieved and anchored outside of the anterior abdominal wall. Thus, continuous traction of the prostate adenoma towards the abdominal wall is applied and the dissection of the adenoma from the surrounding prostatic tissue is facilitated (Step 4b). Continuous retraction of the adenoma by the assistant using a grasper is not advisable.

Step 5: Bladder mucosal incision and subcapsular dissection plane

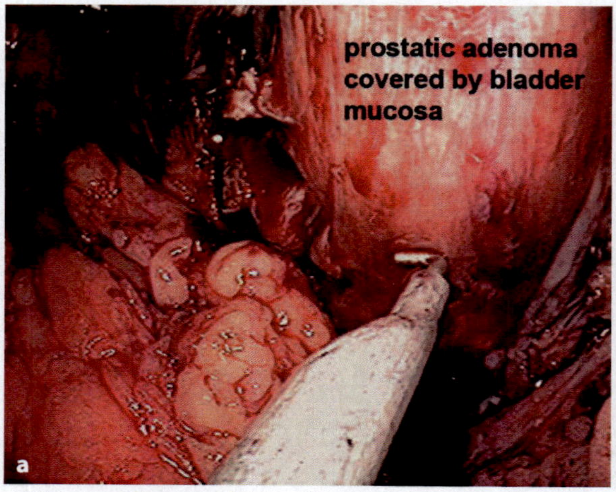

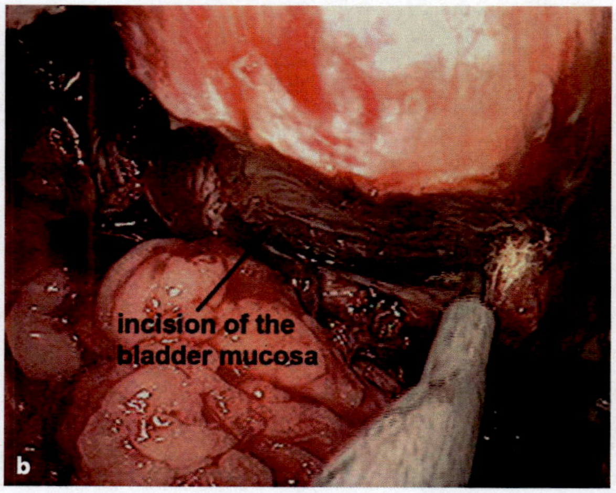

The excision of the prostatic adenoma is initiated by a horizontal posterior incision on the bladder mucosa overlying the prostate lobes at the site of the bladder neck (Step 5a). This semicircular mucosal incision is located between the 8 o'clock and 6 o'clock positions of the bladder neck and is extended up to the 4 o'clock position. The dissection plane is gradually deepened until the prostatic adenoma is identified by its characteristic white texture. Careful blunt and electrocautery dissection is performed to reach the proper subcapsular plane outside the prostate adenoma and inside the prostatic capsule (Step 5b). A Monocryl suture on a CT-1 needle is placed through the one of the lobes of the adenoma for retraction purposes. The retracted lobe is the first to be further dissected.

Step 6: Mucosal incision and initiation of adenoma enucleation

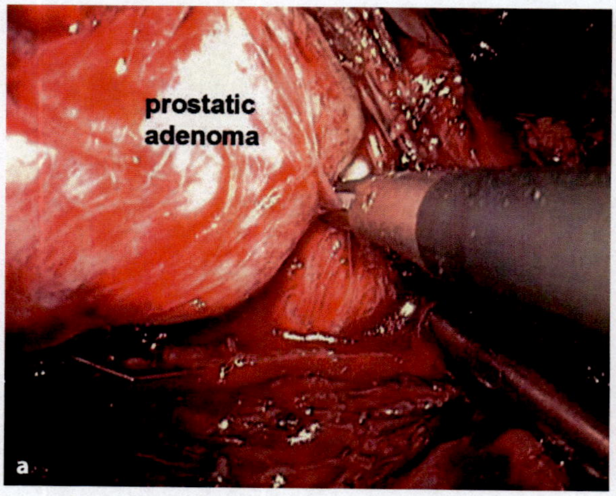

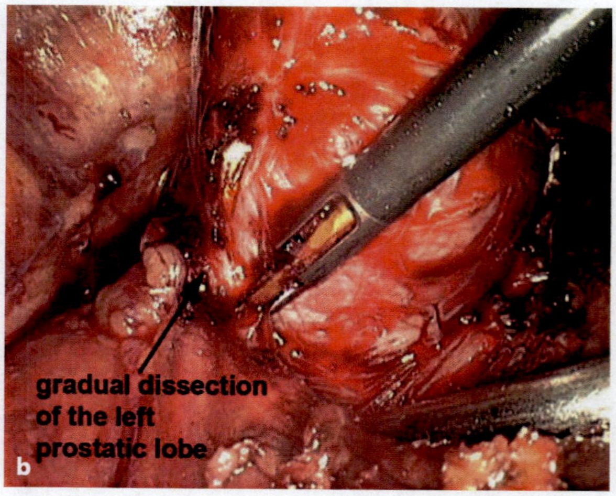

Semicircular movements, using J-hook electrocautery, ultrasonic scissors and/or a suction-irrigation cannula, progressively free the adenoma from the inside of the prostate capsule. The left lateral lobe is dissected first. Step 6a presents the dissection of adherences at the proximal side of the subcapsular plane between the left lobe and the prostatic capsule. The initial mucosal incision is completed circumferentially to provide adequate exposure to the underlying prostate (Step 6b). The assistant uses the suction cannula to provide tension to the opposite side and to facilitate the dissection. In fact, the cleavage plane between the prostatic adenoma and capsule is better identified by the latter manoeuvre.

Step 7: Adenoma enucleation

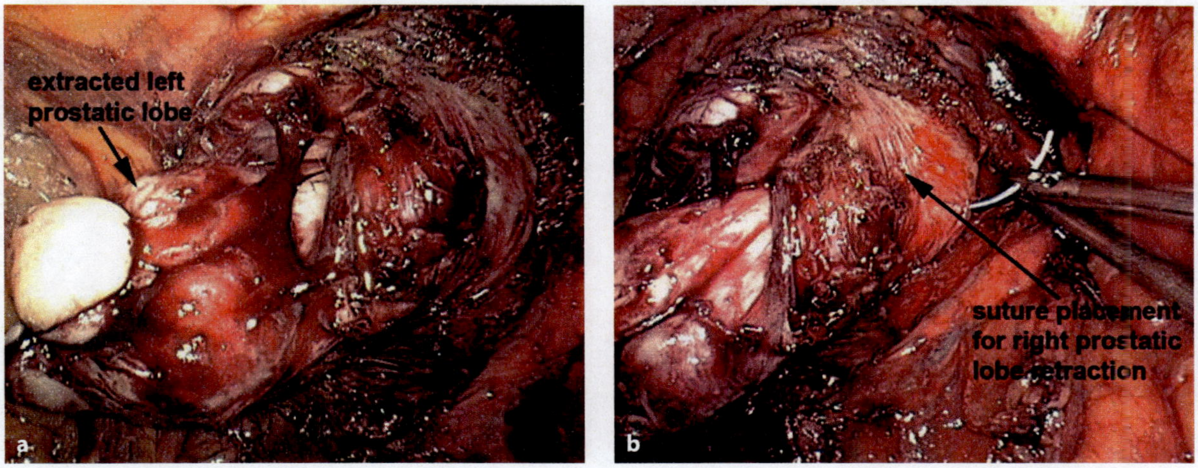

The dissection is extended distally through a largely avascular subcapsular plane towards the apex of the prostate. At the same time, the assistant provides suction and retraction as previously described. Haemostasis of bleeding blood vessels is ensured with electrocautery or the ultrasonic scalpel. Step 7a shows the left prostatic lobe mobilised completely from the capsule. The left lobe is mobilised first and the right lobe follows. Step 7b shows the placement of the retraction suture on the right prostatic lobe. The enucleation of the right lobe is identical to the described technique. Specific care should be taken at the apex of the prostate. The transection of the urethra includes a significant risk for injury to the external sphincter and avulsion.

Step 8: Enucleation with Sotelo prostatotomy

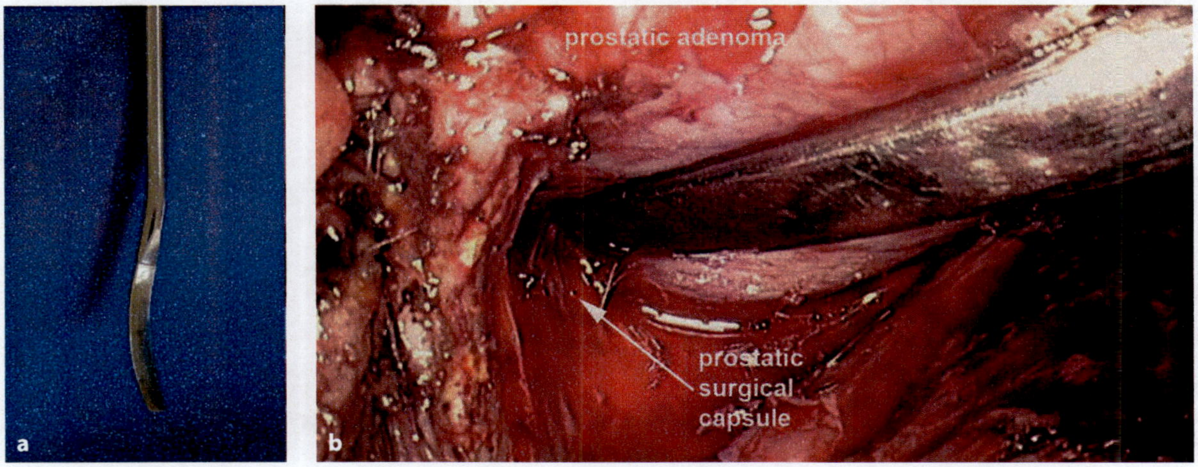

The adenoma is enucleated using a Sotelo prostatotome (Step 8), a metallic device similar to a curette or an osteotome. The instrument facilitates the dissection of the adherences between the adenoma and the capsula in the precise subcapsular plane (Step 8b). The instrument is used with a gently circumferential movement at the subcapsular plane and provides blunt division of the adenoma from the capsule. The curved shape of the instrument imitates the shape of the adenoma. The assistant provides tension by retracting the prostate on the side opposite the adenoma. It is important to avoid sharp dissection with the instrument with direction towards the apex of the prostate because this may cause injury to the sphincter. The dissection is facilitated using the Sotelo prostatotome.

Step 9: Transection of the urethra

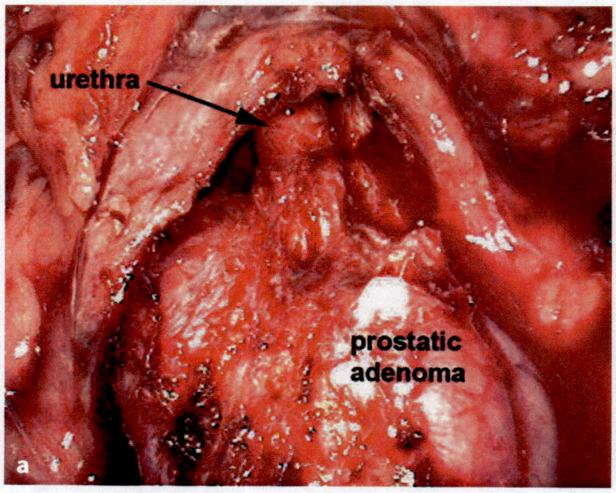

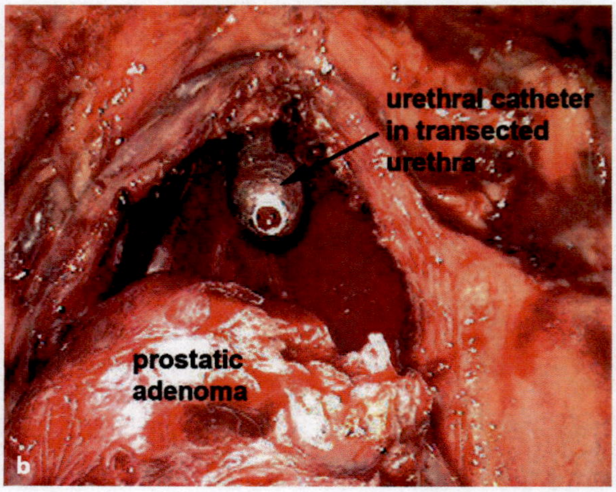

Step 9a demonstrates a mobilised urethra from the prostatic capsule adenoma. Both lobes are free and the only adherence of the adenoma is the urethra. Intracapsular urethral transection follows and the prostatic adenoma is removed (Step 9b). Specific care is taken at this point of the procedure. Injury to the external sphincter and avulsion should be avoided. Therefore, the transection should never be performed using the ultrasonic scalpel and only cold scissors are indicated. Coagulation should be avoided over or near the sphincter. During the dissection of the lobes near the apex, gentle traction should be applied to the adenoma because the risk of avulsion in such a delicate structure is high. A urethral catheter is inserted to facilitate the visualisation of the urethra.

Step 10: Haemostasis

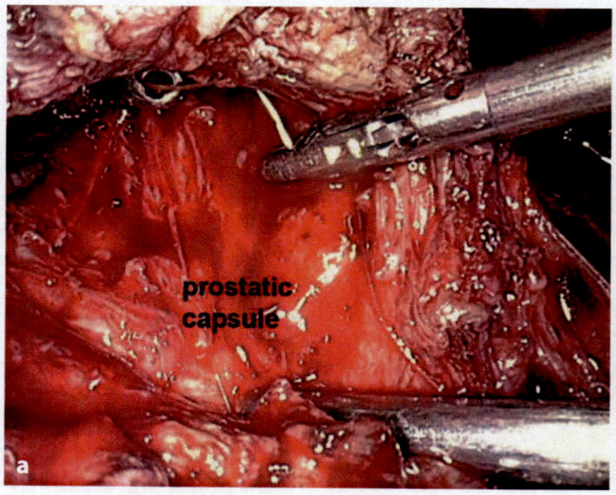

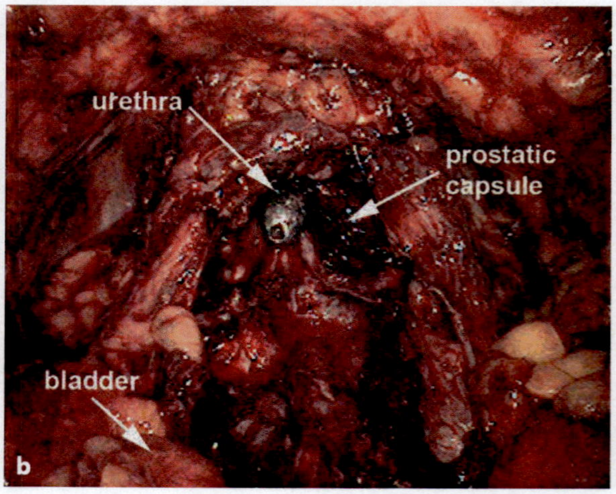

Every attempt is made to maintain good haemostasis during this dissection, so that enucleation proceeds under clear visualisation. If necessary, an ultrasonic scalpel or haemostatic figure-eight suture can be placed at the 4–5 and 7–8 o'clock positions at the proximal prostatic capsule. The latter sites are associated with the prostatic pedicles and the neurovascular bundles on the external lateroposterior side of the prostate. Significant bleeding is not uncommon at this site, and efficient insertion of these sutures is imperative. Step 10a presents the placement of the sutures at the above sites. Step 10b demonstrates the empty prostate capsule and the anatomical landmarks identified after the removal of the adenoma.

Step 11: Trigonisation

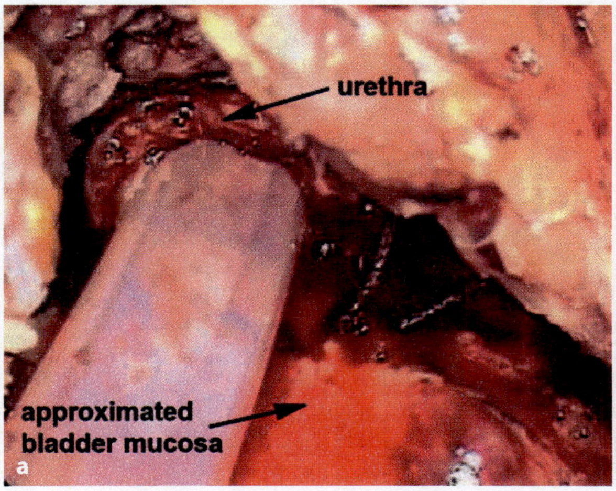

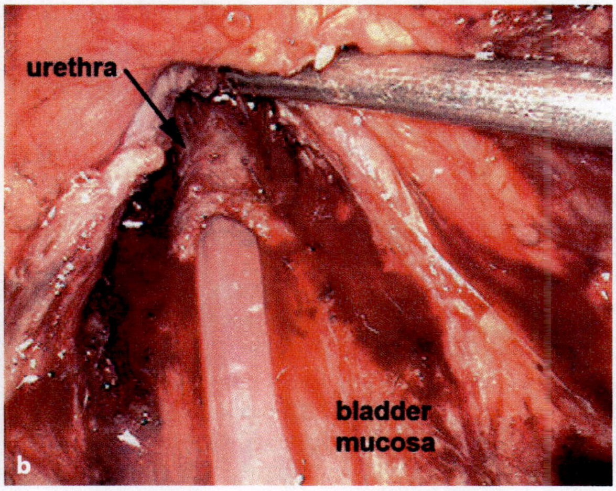

In case of a redundant or hypermobile incised edge of the bladder neck mucosa, the bladder neck stump is suture-approximated to the floor of the prostatic fossa or to the posterior wall of the urethra in an attempt to trigonise the fossa. Step 11a provides a close-up of the retracted and sutured posterior bladder neck mucosa to the level of the urethral stump. The sutures could be placed on the posterior wall of the prostatic fossa or the posterior urethral wall depending on the tension between the two structures. Step 11b shows a wider view of the trigonisation manoeuvre. The bladder neck mucosa has been sutured to the posterior urethra. Redundant bladder neck mucosa could function as a valve and interfere with urination postoperatively. The trigonisation attempts to stabilise the above tissue and prevent further unwelcome events.

Step 12: Closure of the bladder

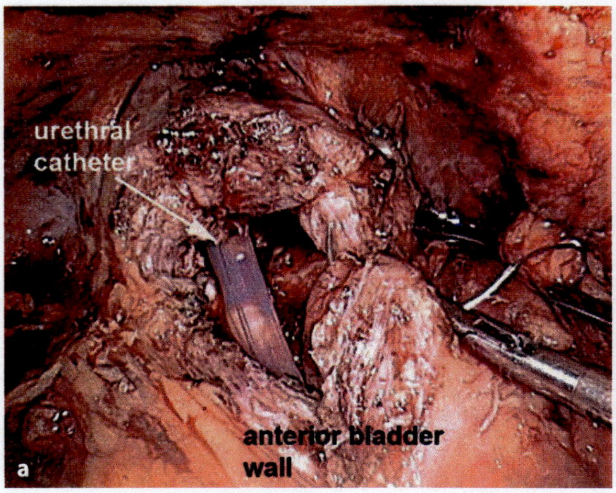

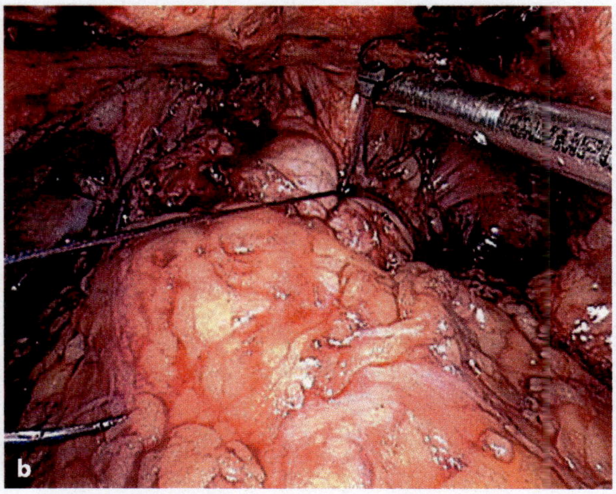

Once the surgeon is satisfied that there is adequate haemostasis, a three-channel Foley catheter (22 or 24 F) is inserted. The balloon is inflated with 25–30 cc of saline. Step 12a shows the initiation of closure of the transverse incision of the bladder. The transverse cystotomy is closed with a running Vicryl suture on a CT-1 needle in a watertight two-layer manner. Step 12b shows completed cystotomy closure. The irrigation is connected to the catheter and the watertightness of the closure is evaluated. A nonsuction drain is inserted. The prostatic adenoma is removed using an endobag via the incision of the lateral left trocar. Careful inspection of the operative field and extraction of the trocars follows. All incisions are closed.

Postoperative Management

- The continuous irrigation is usually removed after 12 h once the absence of bleeding has been confirmed
- The Foley urethral catheter is removed in 5–7 days

References

1. Mariano MB, Graziottin TM, Tefelli MV (2002) Laparoscopic prostatectomy with vascular control for benign prostatic hyperplasia. J Urol 167:2528–2529
2. Van Velthoven R, Peltier A, Laguna MP et al (2004) Laparoscopic extraperitoneal adenomectomy (Millin): pilot study on feasibility. Eur Urol 45:103–109
3. Sotelo R, Spaliviero M, Garcia-Segui A, Novoa J, Desai MM, Kaouk JH, Gill IS (2005) Laparoscopic retropubic simple prostatectomy. J Urol 173:757–760
4. Sotelo R, Clavijo R, Carmona O, Garcia A, Banda E, Miranda M, Fagin R (2008) Robotic simple prostatectomy. J Urol 179:513–515
5. Njinou Ngninkeu B, de Fourmestreaux N, Lufuma E (2007) Digitally-assisted laparoscopic prostatic adenomectomy: a preliminary report of 75 cases [abstract]. J Urol 177:578–579

3.10.2 LESS Adenomectomy

René Sotelo, Camilo Giedelman, Mihir Desai

Introduction

Surgical treatment of symptomatic benign prostatic hyperplasia (BPH) depends on the gland volume and includes open surgical enucleation, transurethral resection, and energy-based ablation. In general, enucleation techniques (i.e. open, laparoscopic or transurethral holmium:yttrium-aluminum-garnet enucleation) are preferred for moderate- to large-volume adenomas. These techniques provide removal of large-volume adenomas and durable long-term outcomes in comparison to transurethral ablative and resection procedures. Encouraging results of laparoscopic and robotic simple prostatectomies have been reported, and these techniques have become alternatives to open simple prostatectomy in select patients with lower urinary tract symptoms due to large-volume prostatic adenomas. More recently, the introduction of novel single-port devices has enabled the performance of many laparoscopic ablative and reconstructive procedures in a virtually scarless fashion through a solitary umbilical incision [1–3].

Laparoendoscopic single-site (LESS) adenomectomy can be performed by placing a single port device by transperitoneal approach in the umbilicus. The transperitoneal approach is more challenging since the bladder must be pushed dorsally and the enucleation cannot be facilitated using the finger. Moreover, the cystotomy incision has to be closed laparoscopically in a watertight manner at the end of the procedure. With the new prebent instruments, the transperitoneal approach is simplified but remains difficult to carry out.

Nevertheless, the procedure can also be performed by placing the device under pneumovesicum in a suprapubic incision and inserting it directly into the bladder. Standard or articulating laparoscopic instrumentation can be used [4, 5]. In this section, we focus on the transvesical approach.

Indications

Preoperative evaluation includes a thorough medical history and physical examinations. Also, digital rectal examination and routine laboratory tests are necessary and include prostate-specific antigen, International Prostate Symptom Score (IPSS) and quality of life (QOL) questionnaires, uroflowmetry and transrectal ultrasound (TRUS) evaluation with prostate volume measurement.

- Selection criteria are a symptomatic BPH and a gland weight of 60 g or more, as estimated by TRUS

Contra-indications

- Prostate cancer
- Morbid obesity
- Anticoagulation, antiplatelet therapy
- Anaesthetic contraindications

Preoperative Preparation

- The patient should pause antiplatelet or any anticoagulant therapy at least 8 days before surgery

Step 1: Operative setup and instrumentation

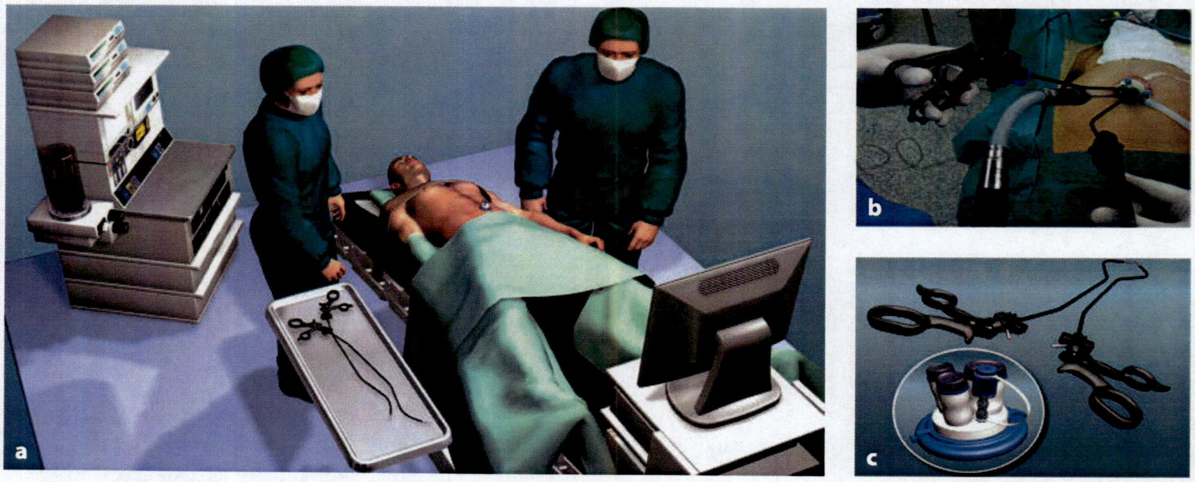

All procedures are performed under general anaesthesia with the patient in a modified low-lithotomy position (Step 1a). LESS adenomectomy can be performed by placing a single multilumen port via the transperitoneal approach in the umbilicus. Multilumen ports allow the insertion of several instruments simultaneously through the same incision. Specialised prebent instruments have been introduced to facilitate the performance of complex procedures through these ports. The combination of the above instruments and conventional laparoscopic instruments is also possible and frequently advisable. Endoscopic cameras of small diameter and special design should also be used. Step 1b and Step 1c show an ideal configuration for LESS surgery using prebent instruments and a camera with a bent shaft.

Step 2: Multilumen port insertion (transvesical approach)

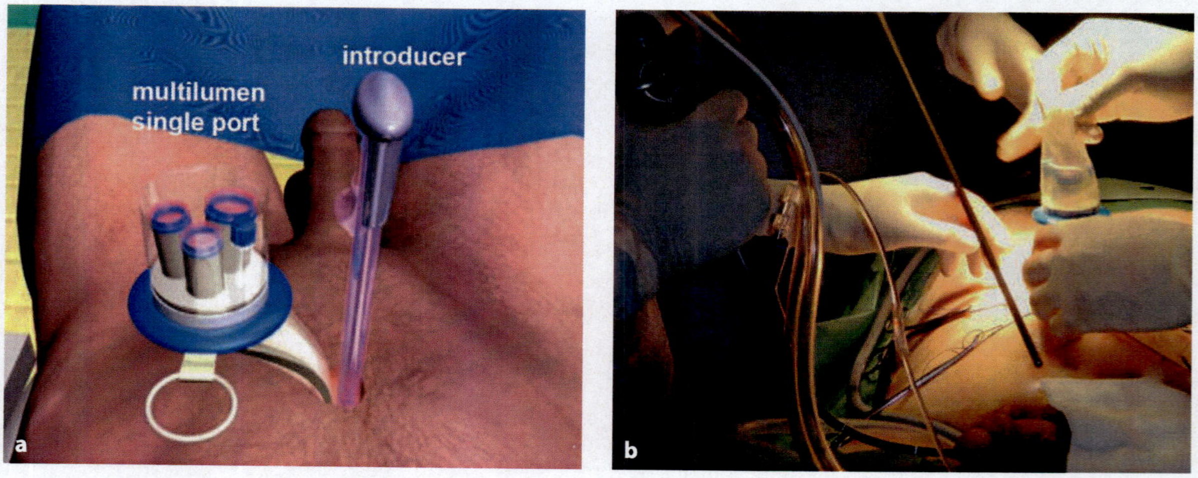

Initially, cystoscopy is performed for the evaluation of the prostate and the bladder is filled with normal saline. An approximately 2.5-cm-long skin incision is made down to the rectus fascia. The incision is located just above the pubis. The bladder wall is identified and cleared of any prevesical fat. Two 2/0 Vicryl stay sutures are placed. The bladder wall is entered sharply between the stay sutures and the inner ring of the Triport is inserted by an introducer into the bladder (Step 2a). The inner and outer rings are approximated by removing the slack on the plastic sleeve, thus clinching the abdominal and bladder walls between the rings of the Triport in an airtight seal (Step 2b).

Step 3: Multilumen port placement

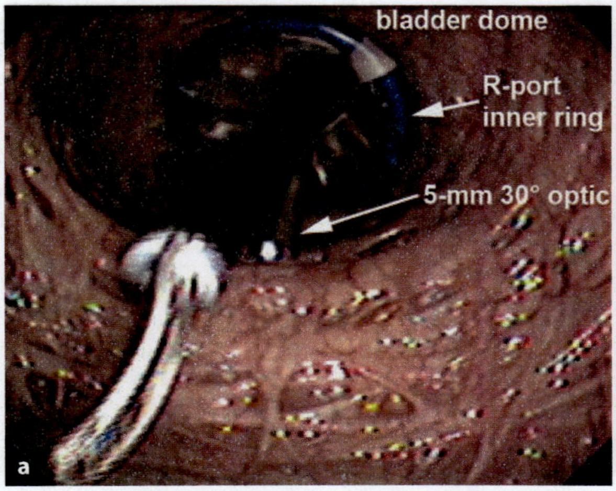

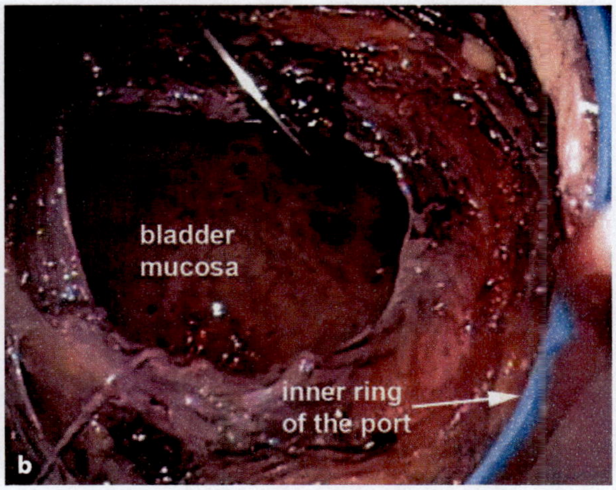

The valve of the Triport is inserted and the bladder is insufflated with carbon dioxide to create the pneumovesicum. The insertion and deployment of the Triport is monitored cystoscopically (Step 3a). Absorbable sutures are passed through the entire thickness of the vesical wall and are placed opposite each other. The sutures provide traction, facilitate the introduction of the trocar and are used for closure of the vesical defect at the end of the procedure. The incision of the fascia and the bladder should be less than 2.5 cm long since the inner ring of the Triport would be easily retracted outside the bladder. Step 3b shows the inner ring of the Triport to be outside of the bladder.

Step 4: Incision of bladder mucosa

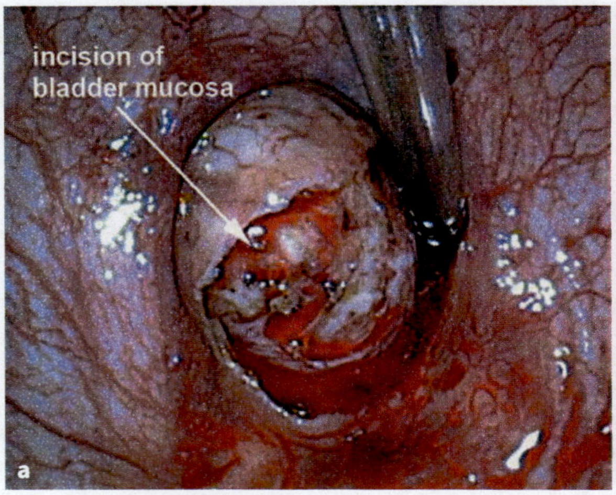

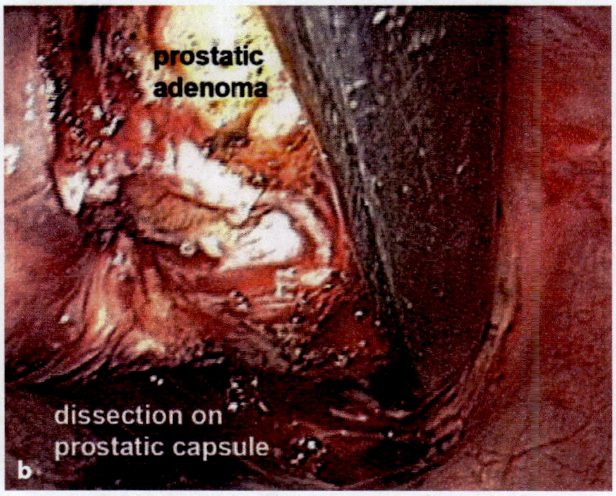

A U-shaped incision is made on the bladder mucosa, immediately over the adenoma extending between the 3 o'clock and 9 o'clock position (Step 4a). A reddish zone of mucosa is present immediately lateral to the internal meatus and serves as a reliable guide for creating the mucosal incision. The horizontal limb of the U-incision is made by using a hook electrode and dissecting to reach the whitish prostatic adenoma. The plane between the surgical capsule and the adenoma is created using the electrocautery hook and suction cannula. The circumferential mucosal incision follows. Separate excisions of each mobilised lobe of the adenoma provide superior visualisation of the adenoma (Step 4b).

Step 5: Enucleation of the adenoma (Sotelo prostatotomy)

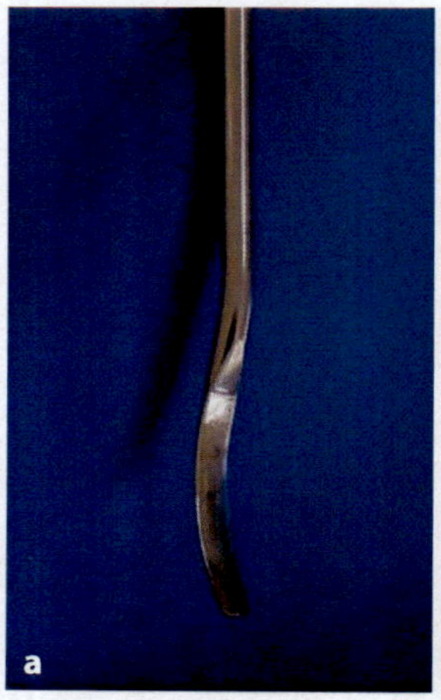

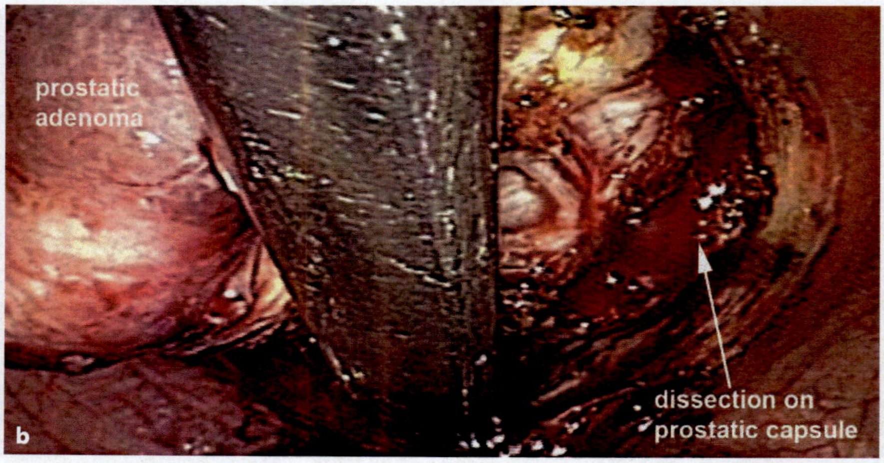

Several manoeuvres are used to facilitate the enucleation of the adenoma: the Sotelo prostatotome (Step 5a), a device similar to a curette or an osteotome, facilitates enucleation of the adenoma during laparoscopic simple prostatectomy. Its metallic, curvilinear tip, with a sharp cold knife on the distal side of the forceps, is used to dissect the margin between the adenoma and its capsule during the circumferential dissection of the adenoma (Step 5b). The instrument provides efficient and precise dissection of the adenoma.

Step 6: Finger enucleation of the adenoma and transurethral apical incision

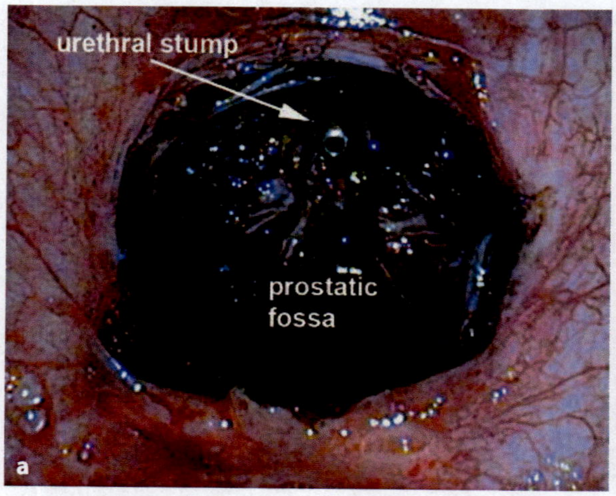

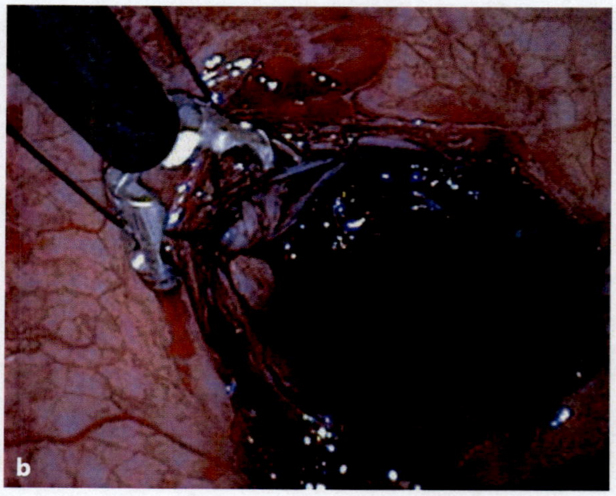

Another method for adenoma enucleation is the insertion of the right index finger through the port after the Triport valve is removed. The latter manoeuvre expedites the distal part of the enucleation. The left index finger is placed in the rectum to elevate the prostate. Once the finger dissection has been completed, the Triport valve is reattached. The pneumovesicum is re-established for the dissection of the urethra at the prostatic apex and the termination of the procedure. The latter method can be facilitated by the incision of the urethra with a bipolar resectoscope, immediately after the placement of the port (Step 6a) and before any dissection from cephalad direction (Step 6b).

Step 7: Haemostasis

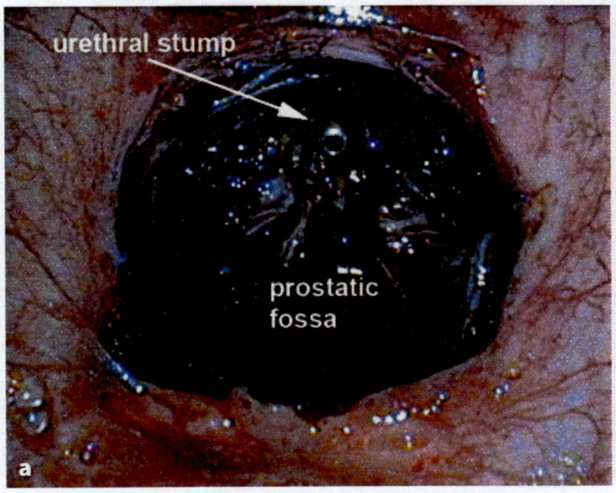

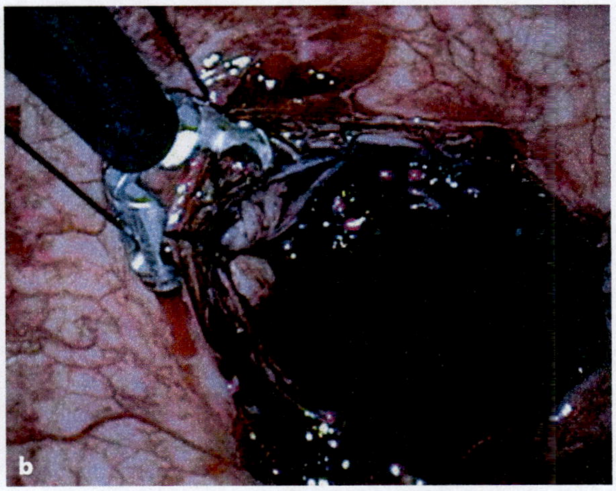

After removing the adenoma (Step 7a), haemostatic figure-eight sutures are made using an extracorporal knot pusher (Step 7b). The sutures are placed at the 4 and 8 o'clock positions of the prostatic capsule in order to control the main prostatic vessels. The lateral prostatic pedicles should be thoroughly checked and the pneumopressure should be reduced to ensure that there is no active bleeding. Any minor bleeding can be controlled with a monopolar or bipolar cautery. If there is still doubt, absorbable sutures could be placed.

Step 8: Trigonisation and closure of the bladder

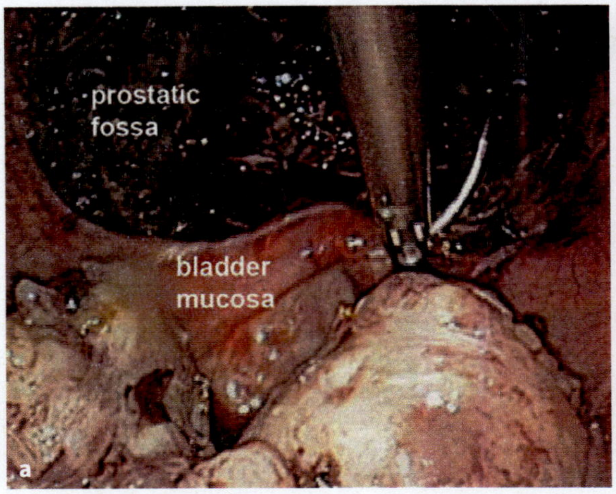

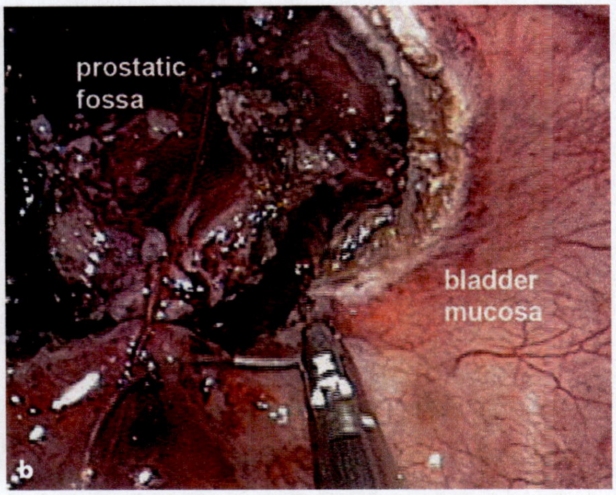

The prostatic adenoma is extracted through the Triport ring after dividing it into multiple pieces during extraction with Allis forceps. After adenoma removal, trigonisation of the prostatic fossa can be performed by suturing the posterior segment of the bladder neck stump (Step 8a) distally towards the apex of the prostatic fossa (Step 8b). The extracorporal knot pusher is useful for this task. The bladder neck opening is sutured using 3/0 Vicryl. The rectus fascia and skin are closed in a standard fashion.

Step 9: Suprapubic and urethral catheter insertion

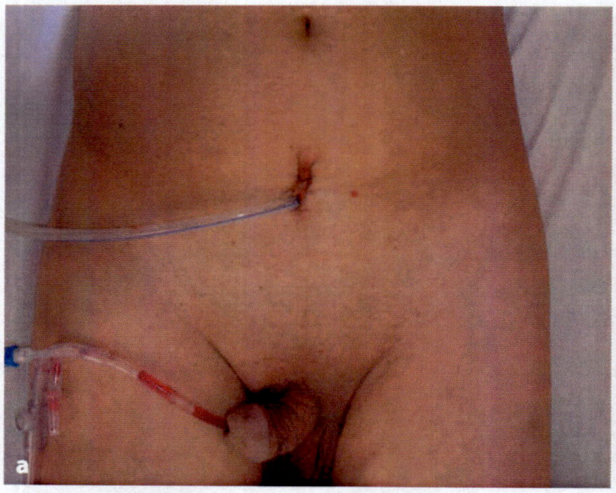
a

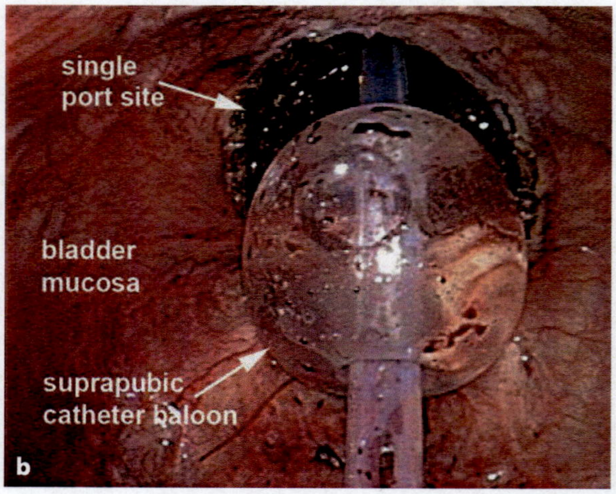

b

A suprapubic catheter can be inserted through the inner ring of the Triport depending on the amount of bleeding. The balloon is inflated and the Triport can be removed. Step 9a shows the suprapubic and the urethral catheter, which are left for the postoperative management of the patient. The diameter of the Triport ring is large enough for insertion of the suprapubic catheter balloon (Step 9b). Thus, correct placement of the catheter inside the bladder can be ensured. The stay sutures on the bladder wall can be tied along with any additional sutures, providing a watertight closure of the bladder incision.

Postoperative Management

- A suprapubic catheter remains in place for 2–3 days
- The Foley catheter is removed on the 6th postoperative day

References

1. Sotelo R, Spaliviero M, Garcia-Segui A, Novoa J, Desai MM, Kaouk JH, Gill IS (2005) Laparoscopic retropubic simple prostatectomy. J Urol 173:757–760
2. Sotelo R, Clavijo R, Carmona O et al (2008) Robotic simple prostatectomy. J Urol 179:513–515
3. Rane A, Rao P, Rao P (2008) Clinical evaluation of a novel laparoscopic port (R-Port) in urology and evolution of the single laparoscopic port procedures (SLIPP) and one port umbilical surgery (OPUS). Eur Urol Suppl 7:193
4. Sotelo R, Astigueta J, Desai M, Canes D et al (2009) Laparoendoscopic single-site surgery simple prostatectomy: initial report. Urology 74:626–630
5. Desai M, Aron M, Canes D, Fareed K, et al. (2008) Single-port transvesical simple prostatectomy: initial clinical report. Urology 72: 960–965

3.11 Transperitoneal Radical Prostatectomy

3.11.1 Transperitoneal Laparoscopic Radical Prostatectomy (Wide Excision and Nerve Sparing)

Bertrand Guillonneau, Heidi Rayala

Introduction

Since the first laparoscopic radical prostatectomy by Schuessler et al. in 1992 [1], the procedure has undergone rapid transformation, integrating the surgical principles of prostate cancer surgery as defined by Walsh with the minimally invasive approach of laparoscopy. Numerous groups have demonstrated consistently reproducible advantages to the laparoscopic approach, including reduced blood loss, shortened hospital stay and decreased postoperative analgesic requirements [2–4]. For these reasons, the laparoscopic approach has become increasingly favored by patients and surgeons alike. Yet, the laparoscopic approach to prostatectomy remains a divisive subject in the field of urology, with concerns of cost regarding the robotic assistance and learning curves often overshadowing oncologic and functional outcomes. As the field continues to mature and as laparoscopy (with or without robotic assistance) becomes a standard skill set of the incoming generation of urologic surgeons, it is presumed that the laparoscopic approach to prostatectomy will become the standard of surgical care.

Laparoscopic radical prostatectomy can be performed by either a trans- or extraperitoneal approach. We favour the transperitoneal approach because (1) we can perform a more extended lymph node dissection, (2) it allows a large working space, making the surgery more straightforward for those early in their learning curve, (3) it may be easier in the setting of prior mesh hernia repairs and (4) in our hands, it appears to exert less tension on the final bladder–urethra anastomosis. However, the extraperitoneal approach may provide protection from serious but uncommon surgical complications including bowel injury, intraperitoneal haemorrhage, and intraperitoneal urine leak. However, we believe such complications can be avoided in the transperitoneal approach with careful attention to the surgical steps by the well-trained surgeon.

Indications

- Biopsy-proven localised prostate cancer, patient life expectancy greater than 10 years and a patient who is not considered a candidate for active surveillance
- Salvage prostatectomy in the appropriate clinical framework

Absolute Contra-indications

- Pelvic lipomatosis
- Intracranial pathology (tumours, arteriovenous malformation or cerebral aneurysm), which may result in increased intracranial pressure with prolonged Trendelenburg position

Preoperative Preparation

- No specific dietary modifications or bowel preparation is necessary
- Low-molecular-weight heparin to prevent thrombotic complications in at-risk patients
- Preoperative cephalosporin 30 min prior to incision

Step 1: Patient position and trocar placement

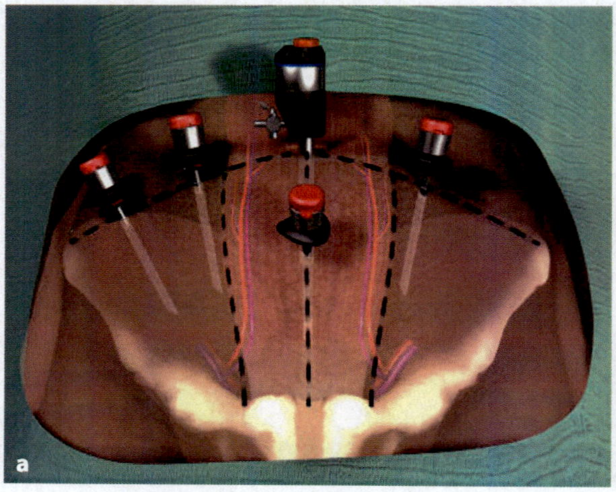

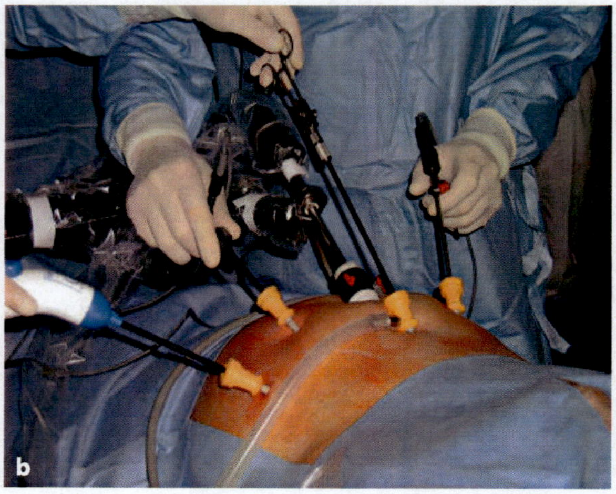

Transperitoneal access is obtained using a Veress needle approach as described in Sect. 1.2. Our preferred port placement includes a 10-mm periumbilical trocar for the 0° endoscope, two 5-mm working ports on both mid-clavicular lines slightly inferior to the umbilicus and lateral to the epigastric arteries, one 5-mm assistant port lateral to the right-sided working port, and a final 5-mm assistant port in the midline centred between the umbilicus and the symphysis pubis. We prefer to have a wide working angle between ports for the main surgeon. Pelvic lymph node dissection (PLND) is performed prior to prostatectomy. The patient is maintained in the Trendelenburg position for the majority of the procedure.

Step 2: Posterior approach and dissection of the seminal vesicles

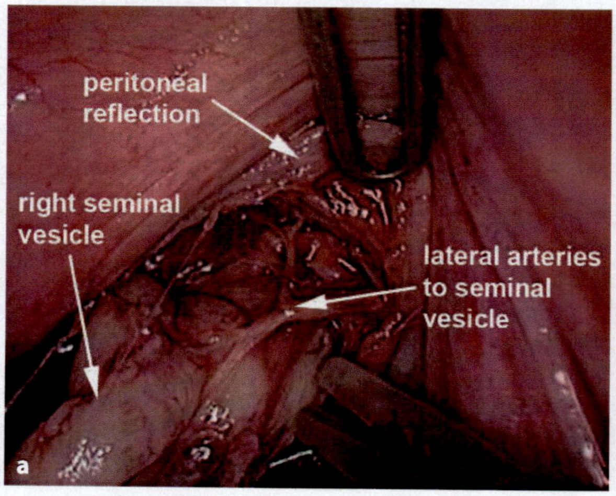

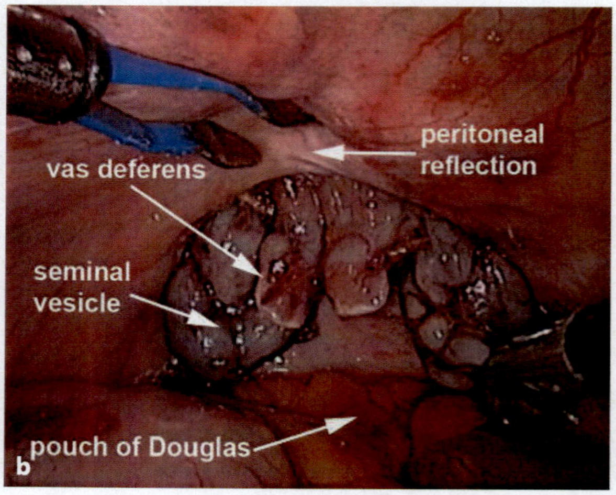

The line of Toldt is opened bilaterally at PLND. The colon is retracted out of the pelvis by the assistant, revealing the pouch of Douglas (if previous surgery, narrow pelvis, obesity or a deep cul-de-sac makes this difficult, the seminal vesicles are approached anteriorly after bladder neck transection). Open the peritoneum horizontally. The dissection continues until the seminal vesicles covered by Denonvilliers fascia are identified. This is incised horizontally and the vasa ampullae are found medially and followed laterally where they are clipped and transected. Three main vesicle arteries must be controlled: (1) the vesiculodeferential artery posterolateral to the vas, (2) a hypogastric branch to the vesicle tips (clip as it is close to inferior hypogastric plexus) and (3) posterior vessels from prostatic pedicles.

Step 3: Further posterior dissection and anterior bladder release

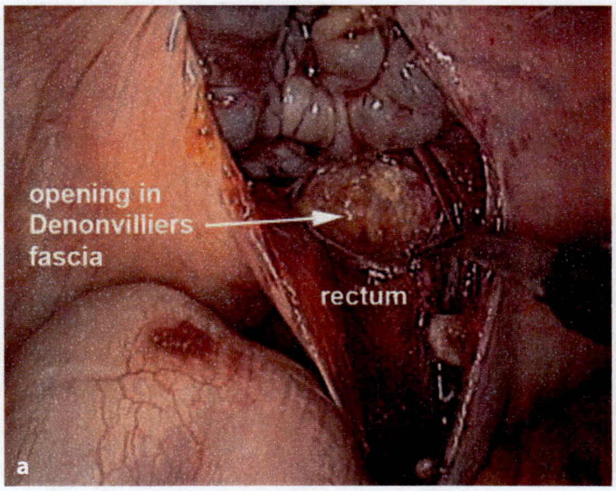

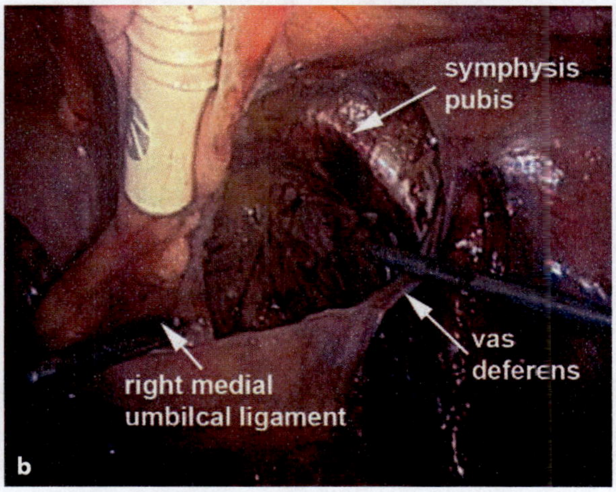

The seminal vesicles are freed and retracted superiorly by the assistant, allowing visualisation of Denonvilliers fascia. This is then incised horizontally on the posterior prostate to access the rectoprostatic plane. This incision should stay medial. Dissection continues along this plane as far as visualisation allows (Step 3a). Now the bladder is released off the anterior abdominal wall. The right medial ligament is retracted downwards and medially. The anterior peritoneum is entered anterior and lateral to the point where the vas deferens crosses the medial umbilical ligament. Starting on the right side, the peritoneum is incised lateral to the medial umbilical ligament, revealing an avascular plane anterior to the bladder that leads to the Retzius space. The bladder is kept attached anteriorly by its medial and median umbilical ligaments (Step 3b).

Step 4: Superficial dorsal vein and endopelvic fascia dissection

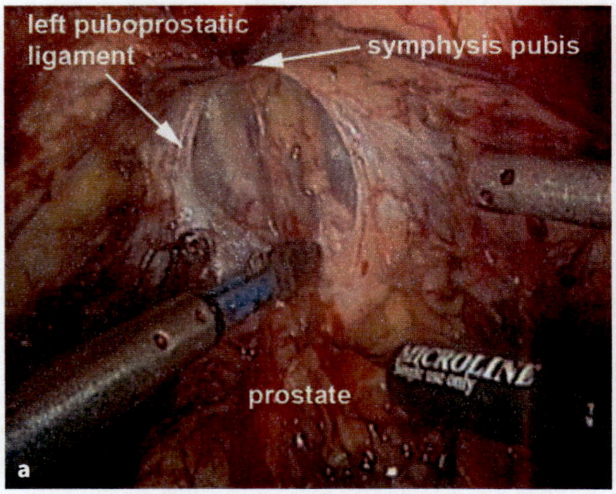

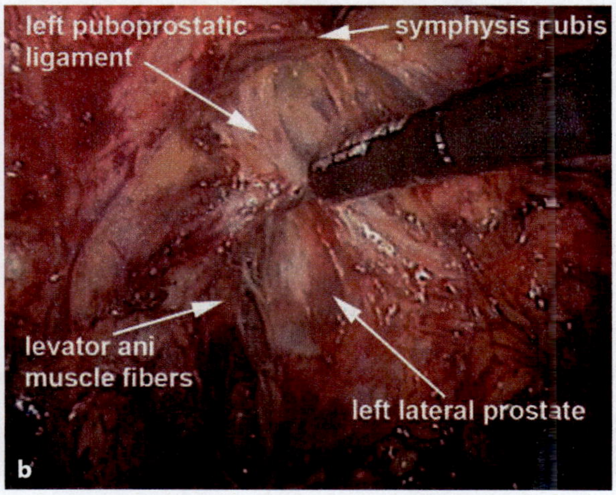

Clear the fatty tissue on both sides of the prostate to reveal the endopelvic fascia, puboprostatic ligaments and superficial dorsal vein running between the ligaments. The superficial dorsal vein is coagulated (Step 4a). The endopelvic fascia is incised at the base of the prostate and the plane between the levator ani fascia and the prostatic fascia is developed. The incision is continued anteriorly, sweeping the levator ani and investing fascia laterally from the prostate. When nerve sparing, this plane is not developed further posteriorly, as the neurovascular bundles may be injured. The puboprostatic ligaments are transected (Step 4b). We do not transect the dorsal vascular complex yet, as it sometimes causes bleeding and reduces visualisation.

Step 5: Transection of anterior and posterior bladder neck

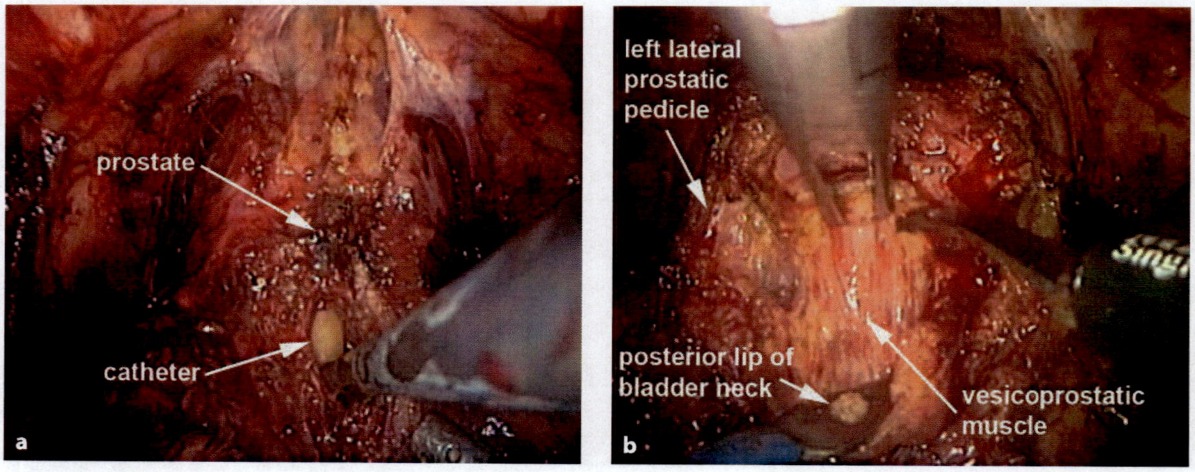

The bladder neck is incised horizontally because we do not aim to preserve the bladder neck. The bladder neck is recognised by a change of the detrusor fibres (from plexiform to longitudinal). The catheter is visualised and the tip brought up to the symphysis pubis (Step 5a). The scrub nurse provides countertraction on the external portion of the catheter to elevate the prostate. This allows the posterior bladder neck and ureteric orifices to be visualised. With downward traction on the posterior lip of the bladder neck, dissection continues at an angle that parallels the posterior bladder wall. The vesicoprostatic muscle is exposed and incised to reveal the seminal vesicles. The catheter is released, the posterior lip of the prostate grasped (Step 5b) and the seminal vesicles elevated superiorly by the assistant.

Step 6: Transection of lateral pedicles and extrafascial nerve sparing

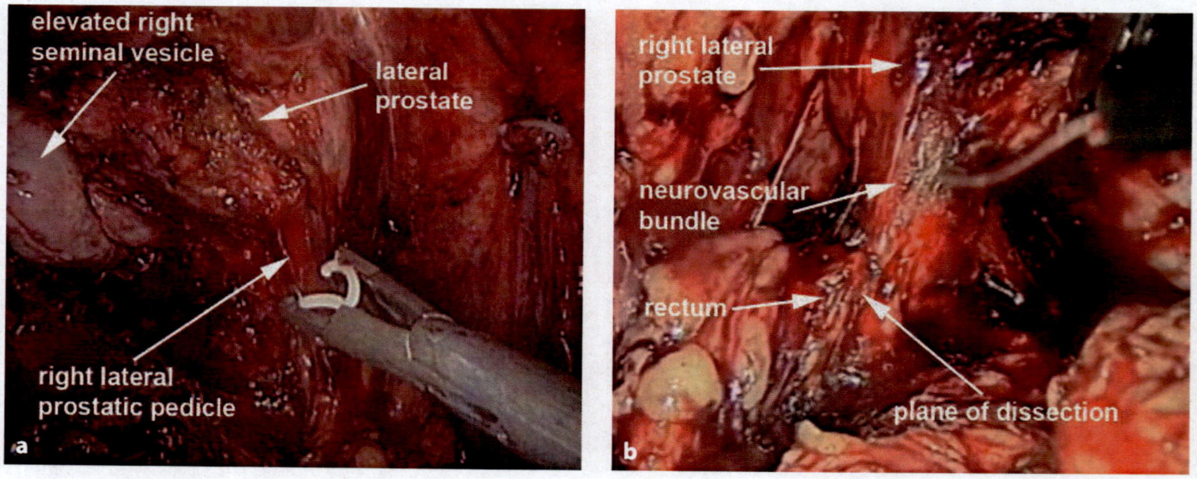

There are three approaches: an intrafascial dissection (between the prostatic capsule and the prostatic fascia), an interfascial dissection (lateral to the prostatic fascia and medial to the neurovascular bundle) and an extrafascial dissection (lateral to the levator ani fascia). It is important that the assistant retracts the seminal vesicles and vas away from the side of dissection to allow visualisation of the prostatic base and a clear line of transection. For the extrafascial technique, dissection begins lateral to Denonvilliers fascia at the lateral aspect of the prostatic pedicle. The dissection margin is wide to the seminal vesicles, prostate and laterally to the nerve bundles. Electrocautery can be used for haemostasis. Identifying the rectum during the posterior dissection is essential. Leave dissection of the distal prostate until the dorsal vascular complex (DVC) is transected.

Step 7: Interfascial and intrafascial nerve sparing

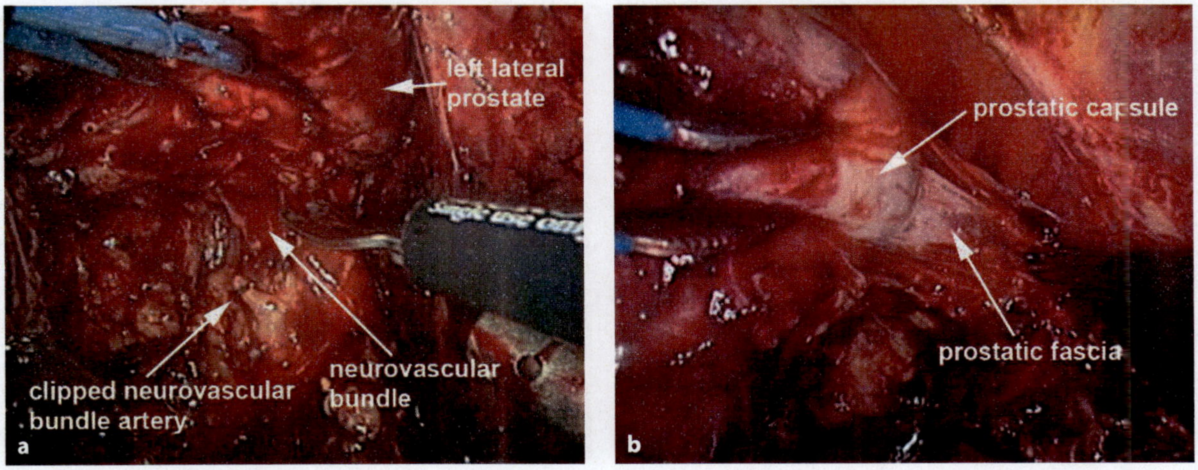

The interfascial technique partially preserves the neurovascular bundle. The prostatic fascia is resected and nerves lying closest to the prostate are ultimately sacrificed. The value of this approach is that the extent of nerve sparing can be adjusted along the length of the prostate according to preoperative tumour characteristics and imaging topography. The intrafascial dissection is functionally efficient, but it does pose a higher risk of positive surgical margin. The aim is to completely preserve the neurovascular bundle including the prostatic fascia. Following the contour of the prostate and beginning posteriorly along the incised Denonvilliers fascia, the neurovascular bundle along with the prostatic fascia is completely peeled off the capsule using blunt dissection (Step 7b).

Step 8: Transection and ligation of the dorsal vascular complex

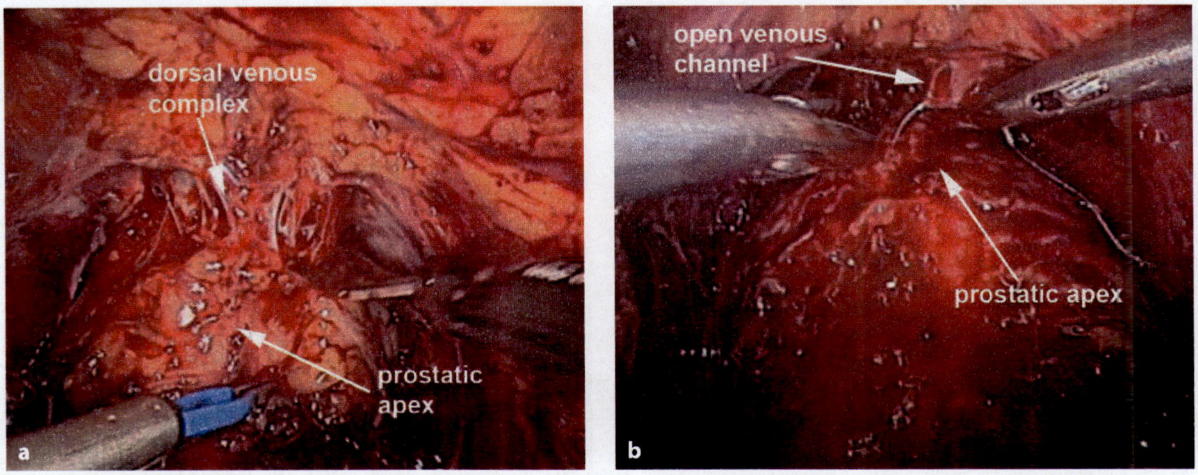

As the dissection continues towards the apex on either side, the DVC is better visualised. Intra-abdominal pressure can be increased up to 20 mmHg if excessive venous bleeding is noted. The DVC is incised sharply. The direction of incision is initially perpendicular to the vascular complex before coursing posteriorly towards the prostatic apical groove along the surface of the prostate. Retraction of the prostate to either side will allow a lateral view of the apex relative to the urethra and aid the angle of incision (Step 8a). Once the DVC is transected, the intra-abdominal pressure is decreased to 12 mmHg, and a 3/0 Vicryl on an RB1 needle, with a figure eight suture, closes the open venous channels. It may require two throws to bunch up the DVC (Step 8b).

Step 9: Dissection of the neurovascular bundle from the prostatic apex

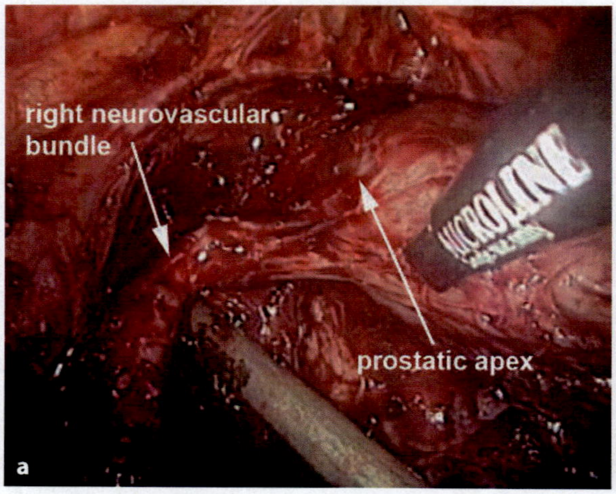

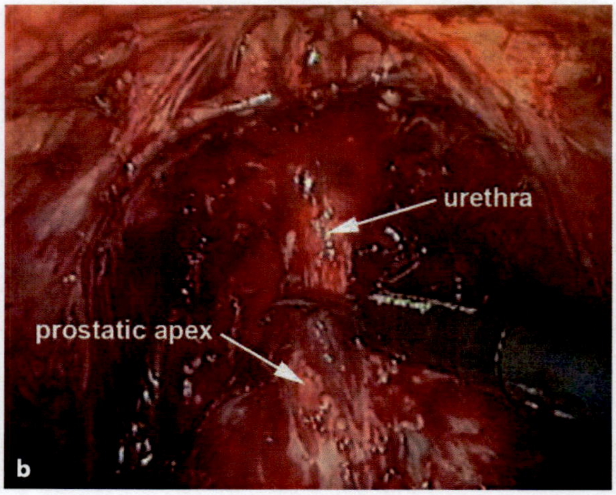

It is at this point in the dissection that the distal third of the prostate is best visualised because the prostate becomes more mobile and the remaining apex is dissected; if needed, a Béniqué sound can be used to help delineate the junction between the prostatic apex and urethra. The prostatic apex should be totally free from surrounding tissue. Lateral retraction of the entire prostate will allow visualisation of the urethra with respect to the posterior distal attachment of Denonvilliers fascia to the rectourethralis muscle, and any remaining attachments between the prostatic apex and underlying rectum can be incised. The urethra can then be transected perpendicular to its course, preserving its length and ensuring that the posterior lip of the prostate apex is not resected.

Step 10: Bagging the specimen and urethrovesical anastomosis

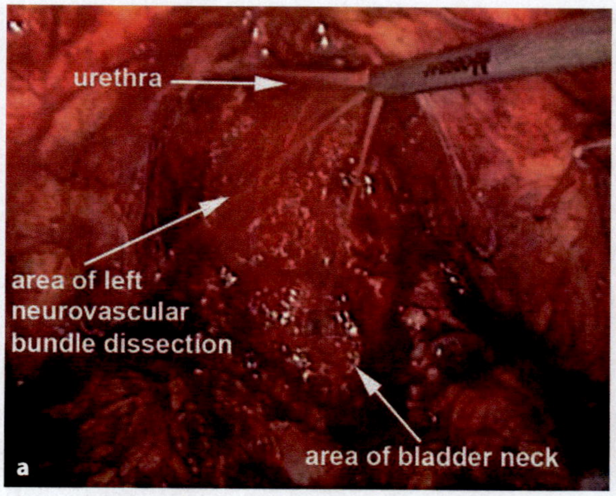

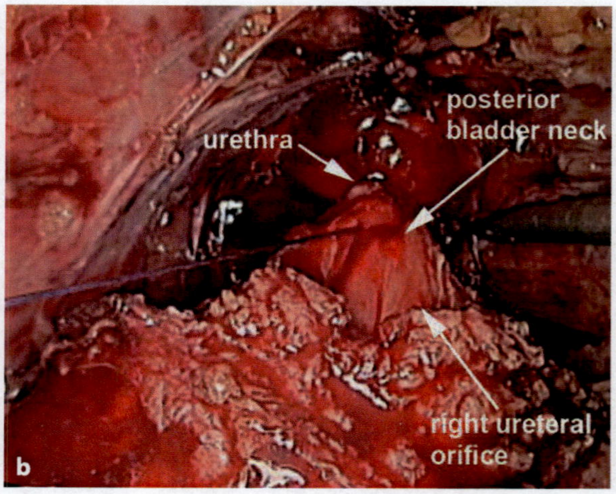

We place a 10-F bag through the camera port with a 5-F camera through the right lateral port. The specimen is then placed cephalad outside of the working field. If the tumour margins are suspicious, the prostate is extracted via the umbilical port site for frozen section before the anastomosis. The neurovascular bundle is assessed after copious irrigation (Step 10a). Small arteries need surgical clips or coagulation. Interrupted sutures are used for the anastomosis (theoretically less ischaemia and better approximation if urethra and bladder neck tension). Four interrupted 3/0 Vicryl sutures are used along the posterior anastomosis in an in-out (urethra-bladder) fashion with the knots inside (Step 10b). A Béniqué sound advances the needle into the urethra and prevents backwalling.

Step 11: Lateral and anterior urethrovesical anastomotic suturing

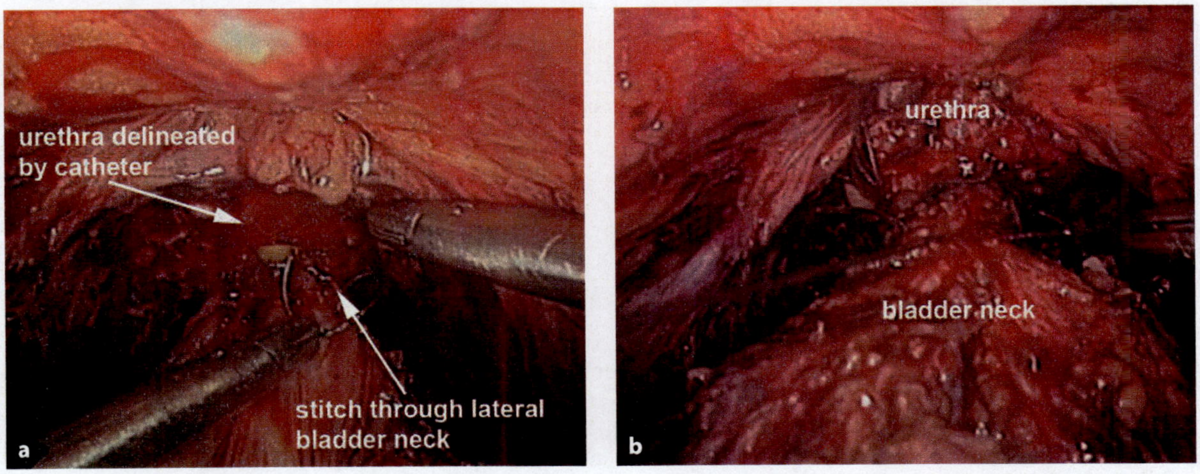

Two lateral Vicryl sutures are generally needed on either side. These are placed in an out-to-in fashion on the lateral bladder neck, followed by the in-to-out fashion on the urethra, such that the knot lies on the outside of the anastomosis (Step 11a). A final U-stitch encompasses the anterior bladder neck (out-to-in), anterior urethra (in-to-out), the free portion of the puboprostatic ligament and across to the contralateral puboprostatic ligament; the contralateral anterior urethra (out-to-in) and contralateral anterior bladder neck (in-to-out) will complete the urethral anastomosis and also provide suspension to the urethra (Step 11b).

Step 12: Closure of redundant bladder neck and final inspection

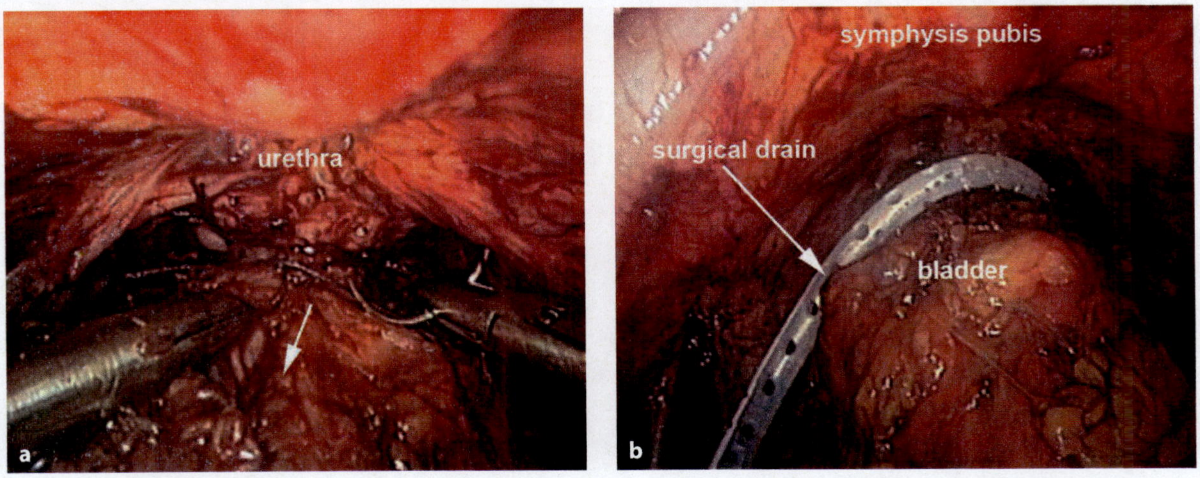

Using a running 3/0 Vicryl suture, redundant anterior bladder neck tissue is closed in a tennis-racket fashion (Step 12a). An 18-F Foley catheter is advanced into the bladder and the balloon is inflated with 10 ml of saline. The bladder is irrigated free of clots and after installation of 180 cc of fluid, any leaks are identified in the anastomosis. Any leaks visualised will require an additional suture. A surgical drain is brought through one lateral 5-mm port site and laid over the urethral anastomosis. The abdominal pressure is then decreased, the 5-mm trocars extracted and a final inspection of the surgical field is made. The umbilical camera port incision is lengthened to allow removal of the bagged specimen.

Postoperative Management

- Ketoralac and Vicodin for pain control
- Clear diet on the day of surgery, regular diet on postoperative day 1
- Low-molecular-weight heparin on 1st postoperative day and daily until discharge
- Remove surgical drain on day 1 if drain creatinine is equal to that of serum creatinine
- The pathway allows for discharge home on postoperative day 1
- Remove catheter day 5–8 without cystography unless anastomotic leak suspected

References

1. Schuessler WW, Kavoussi LR, Clayman RV, Vancaillie TG (1992) Laparoscopic radical prostatectomy: initial case report. J Urol 147:A246
2. Rassweiler J, Seemann O, Schulze M, Teber D, Hatzinger M, Frede T (2003) Laparoscopic versus open radical prostatectomy: a comparative study at a single institution. J Urol 169:1689–1693
3. Bhayani SB, Pavlovich CP, Hsu TS, Sullivan W, Su LM (2003) Prospective comparison of short-term convalescence: laparoscopic radical prostatectomy versus open radical retropubic prostatectomy. Urology 61:612–616
4. Guillonneau B (2008) The case for laparoscopic radical prostatectomy. J Endourol 22:2045–2046

3.11.2 Robot-Assisted Transperitoneal Radical Prostatectomy

Alexander Mottrie, Nazareno Suardi, Jamil Rehman, Mattia Sangalli

Introduction

The goal and outcome measure of robotic prostatectomy are those of open radical prostatectomy [1, 2]: complete removal of all prostatic tissue with minimal morbidity or deterioration of quality of life. As surgical cure rates for localised prostate cancer improve considerably, the functional sequelae of treatment (urinary continence and potency) have moved to the forefront in urologic oncology.

The introduction of robotic technology (da Vinci surgical robot) has enhanced the surgeon's ability to perform minimally invasive surgery with precision and perfection. The robot and its refinements in surgical techniques based on improved anatomical understanding have improved the quality of surgery, including oncological and functional outcome, with a steep decrease in morbidity. Robotic radical prostatectomy provides exposure and visualisation of the male pelvis not previously appreciated. Surgeons with extensive experience with the open approach to radical prostatectomy find that familiarity with anatomy and technique facilitates the acquisition of skills for robotic prostatectomy. The Aalst robotic prostatectomy technique, which has evolved over time, simultaneously addresses the competing goals of cancer control, preservation of surrounding normal tissues [3–5] and enhanced functional outcomes [6].

Indications

- Clinically localised prostate cancer
- Patients with life expectancy greater than 10 years

Contra-indications

- Advanced or metastatic disease
- Anaesthesia-related (cardiac, pulmonary and general medical status)

Preoperative Preparation

- Informed consent
- Mechanical bowel preparation: magnesium citrate, two bottles the evening before surgery
- Coagulation status (anticoagulants, including over the counter medications, stopped)
- Deep vein thrombosis prophylaxis: half dose of low-molecular-weight heparin is given before surgery and a full dose administered next day and treatment is continued for 4 weeks following surgery
- Antibiotic prophylaxis: a second-generation cephalosporin is administered. A bolus injection is given before inducing anaesthesia

Step 1: Patient position

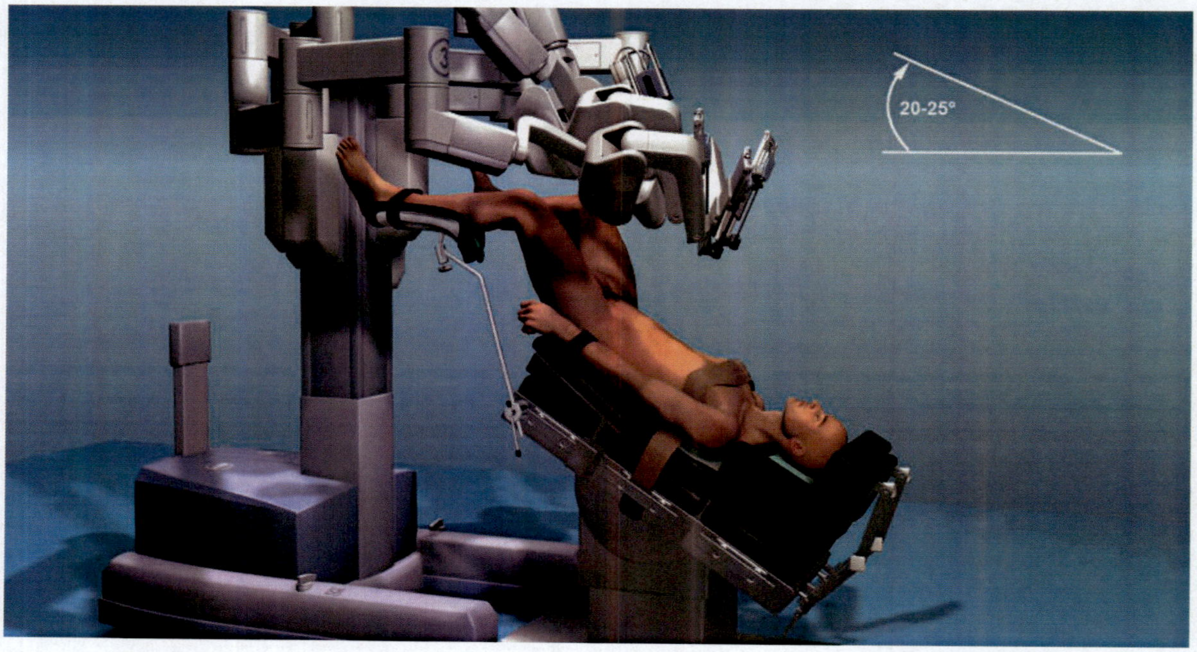

After general anaesthesia induction and orogastric tube placement, the legs are placed in a semi-lithotomy position to define the value of Trendelenburg position accordingly, with compression stockings and a sequential compression device for deep vein thrombosis prophylaxis, using well-padded Allen stirrups. Legs apart to allow free access to the perineal space and to facilitate the positioning of the robotic unit between the legs. The patient is then prepped and draped. An 18-F silicone Foley catheter is inserted, and the balloon is inflated to 15 ml.

Step 2: Trocar placement

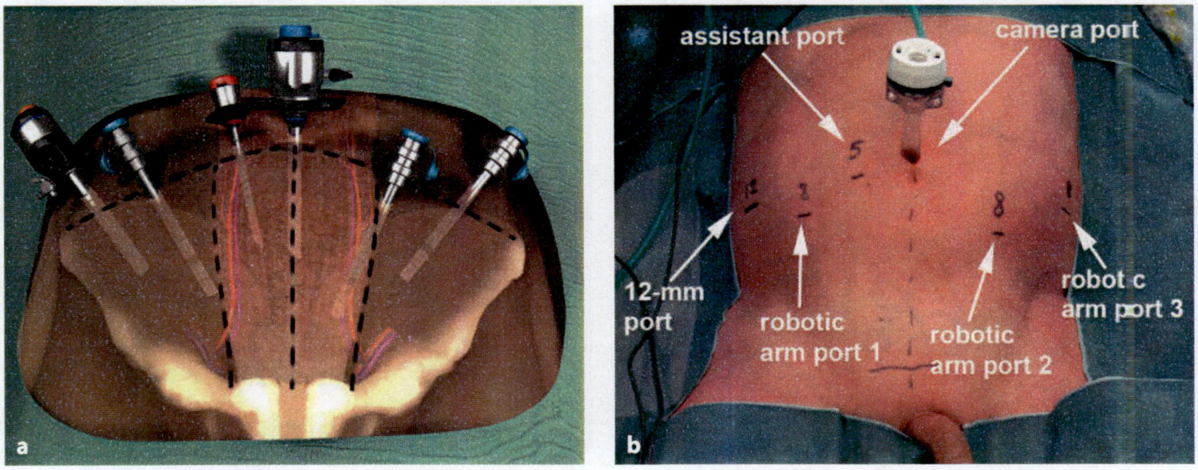

A 12-mm supraumbilical incision is made. A Veress needle is used to insufflate the abdomen (15 mmHg) supraumbilically followed by trocar placement (12-mm trocar). Two 8-mm instrument trocars are placed approximately 7–10 cm (one handbreadth) lateral of the umbilicus in the direction of the anterior superior iliac spine (approximately 2.5 cm lateral to the rectus muscle and 2 cm below the umbilicus). A 5-mm port is placed lateral to the camera port and superior to the right robotic port. A second 12-mm assistant port is placed 7–10 cm directly lateral to the right robotic port (approximately 5 cm above the anterior superior iliac spine in the anterior axillary line). A third 8-mm robotic port (for the fourth arm) is placed 7–10 cm lateral to the left robotic port 2 cm above and anteriorly to the anterior superior iliac spine.

Step 3: Mobilisation of the bladder

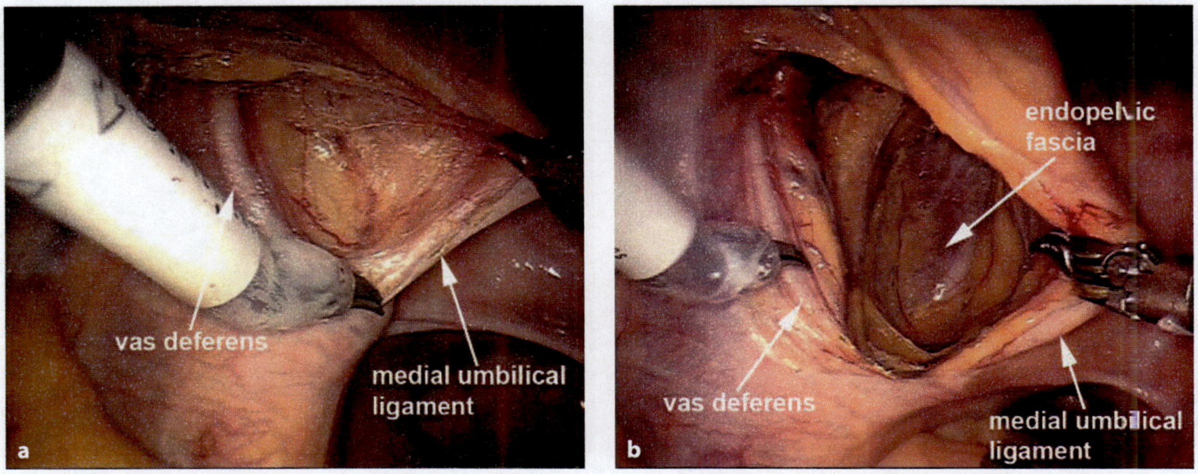

The opening of the peritoneum is made in a triangular space, which is defined by the umbilical ligament, the vas deferens and the abdominal wall (Step 3a). Each medial umbilical ligament is sequentially grasped and pulled downwards (caudally and medially) with countertraction provided by the fourth arm; the hot shears are used to incise the peritoneum lateral to the grasped ligament to access to retropubic space. This peritoneal incision is made in the described triangle and carried down to the vas deferens. An area of foamy bloodless fat tissue is seen. The space is opened using simple divergent traction of the graspers. It is continued to the lateral pelvic wall, until the endopelvic fascia is seen at the bottom bilaterally (Step 3b).

Step 4: Gaining access to the extraperitoneal Retzius space

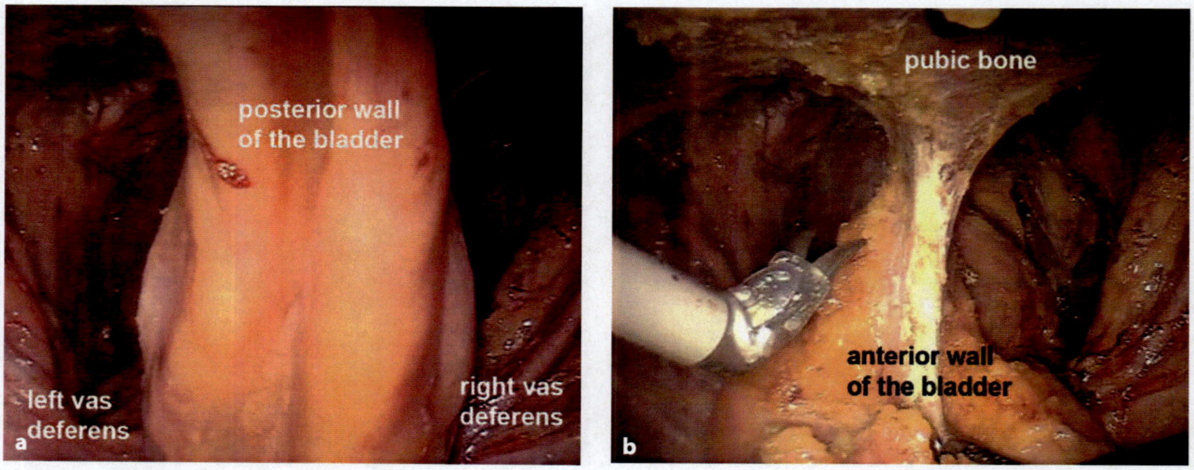

This dissection is continued medially to cut the urachus. The same technique is used on the contra-lateral side, and the bladder remains attached to the pubic bone by the prevesical fat tissue (Step 4a). Finally, the prevesical space behind the pubis is opened (Step 4b), until the bladder is completely detached.

Step 5: Opening the endopelvic fascia

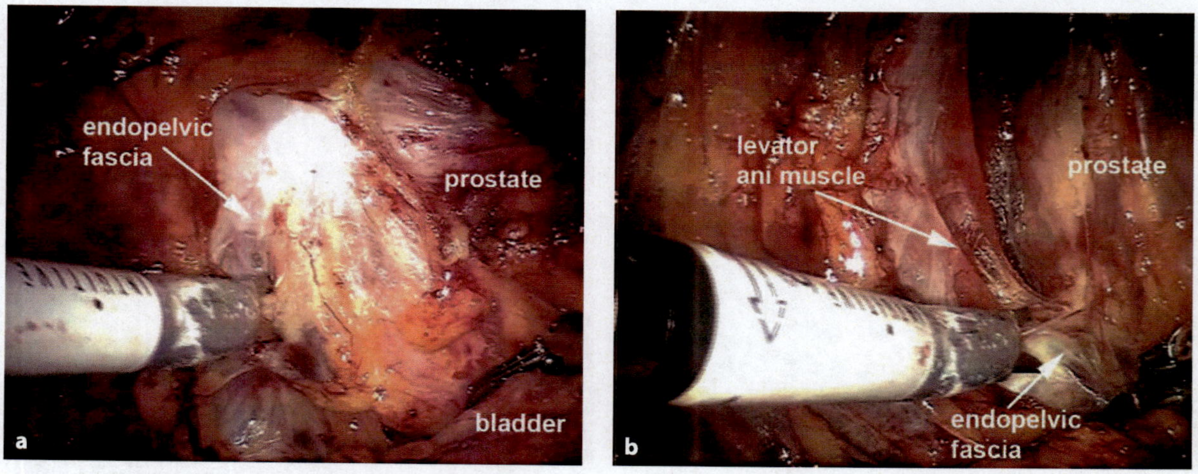

After complete mobilisation of the bladder, the periprostatic fat is removed from the endopelvic fascia and from the prostate. The puboprostatic ligaments, prostate, and prostatovesical junction and bladder are now clearly defined. The pelvic cavity, formed by the endopelvic fascia that covers the superior surface of the prostate, is incised on its line of reflexion to gain access to the lateral surface of the prostate gland in close contact with the fibres of the levator ani muscles (Step 5b).

Step 6: Identification of bladder neck

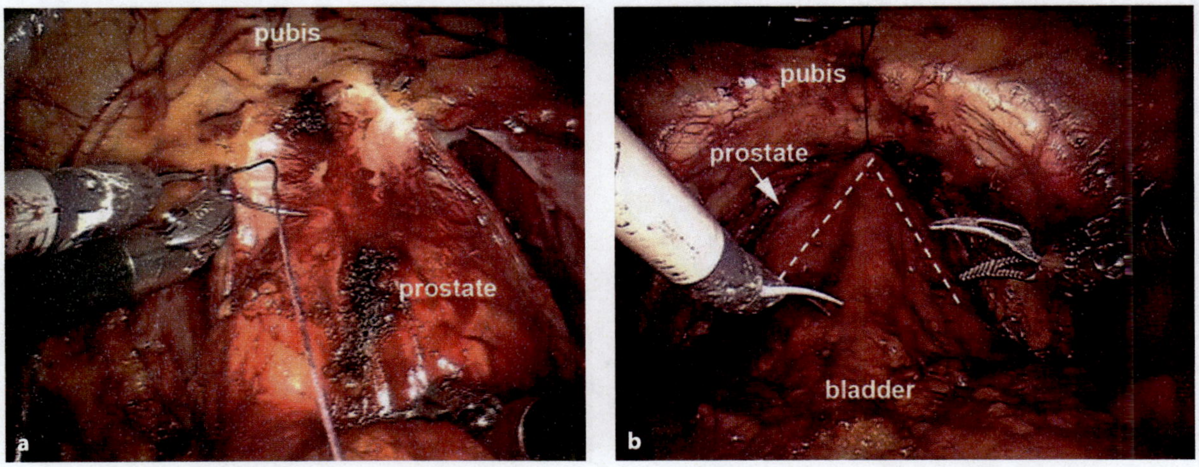

A holding stitch (Vicryl 2/0) is placed in the mid-prostate (Step 6a) and the prostate is lifted up. The bladder neck becomes visible as an inverted V on the prostate (Step 6b). Using the bipolar forceps, the bladder is bluntly pulled medially just beyond the junction with the prostate. The combination of gentle superior retraction of the bladder with traction on the catheter demonstrates a clear outline of the prostatovesical junction.

Step 7: Lateral bladder neck detachment and dissection

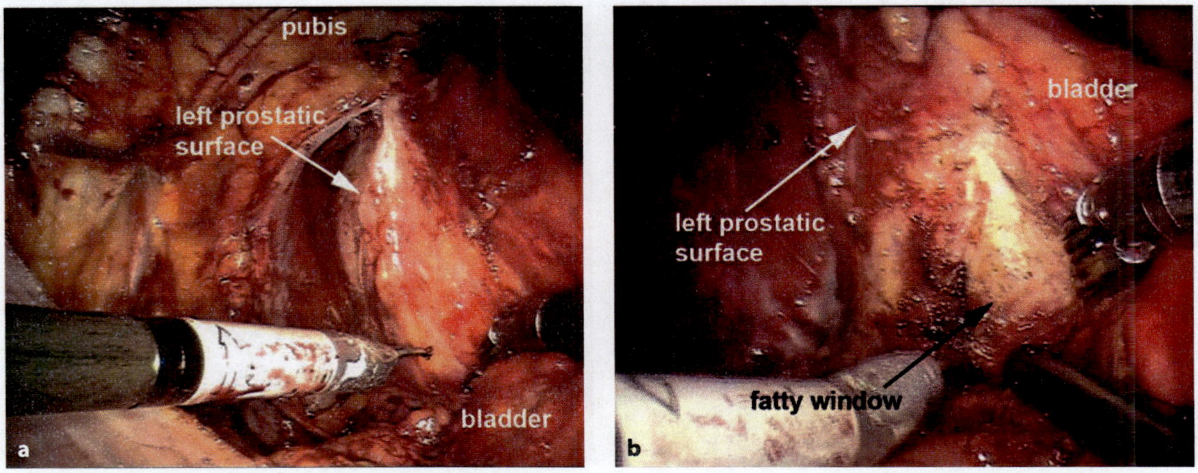

After deflation of the catheter balloon, the bladder neck is dissected using the Hot Shears with a lateral approach (Step 7a). The plane between the bladder neck and the prostate is identified laterally, on both sides of bladder neck, by following the curved contours of the prostatic base. The bladder and prostate are retracted and the prostatovesical junction is identified, and the dissection is completed until the posterolateral fatty window to the preseminal vesicles area is reached. The space between the base of the prostate and the bladder neck becomes more and more evident.

Step 8: Anterior bladder neck dissection

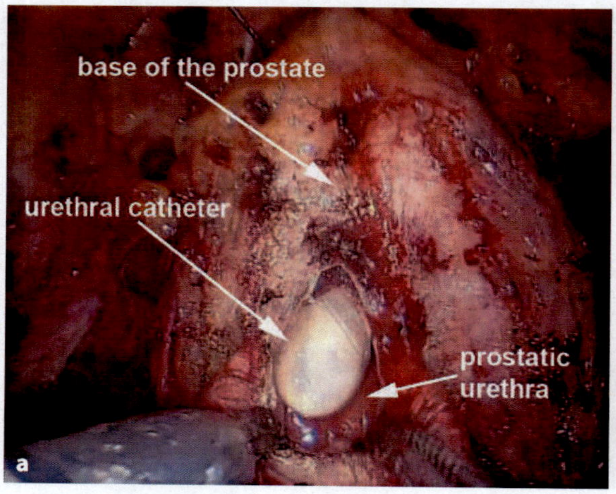

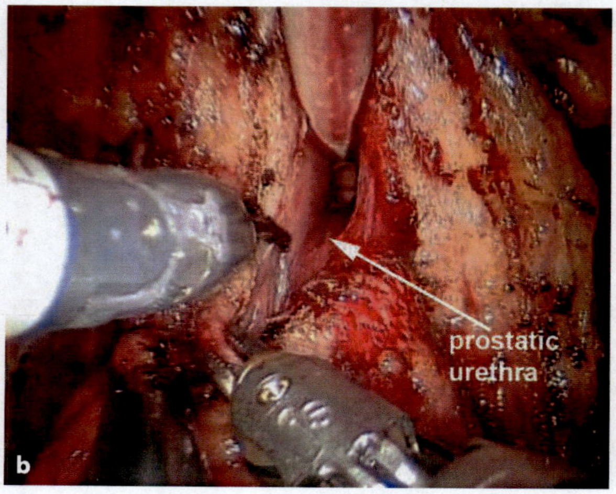

Anteriorly, the bladder neck incision is made in the midline and deepened, the Foley catheter is encountered and the bladder is entered (Step 8a). This allows visualisation of the posterior bladder neck immediately upon entering the bladder. As soon as the catheter is visible, it is grasped by the robotic fourth arm using ProGrasp forceps through the eye of the catheter. The robotic arm then pulls the catheter cephalad and anteriorly to prepare the posterior dissection (Step 8b).

Step 9: Posterior bladder neck dissection

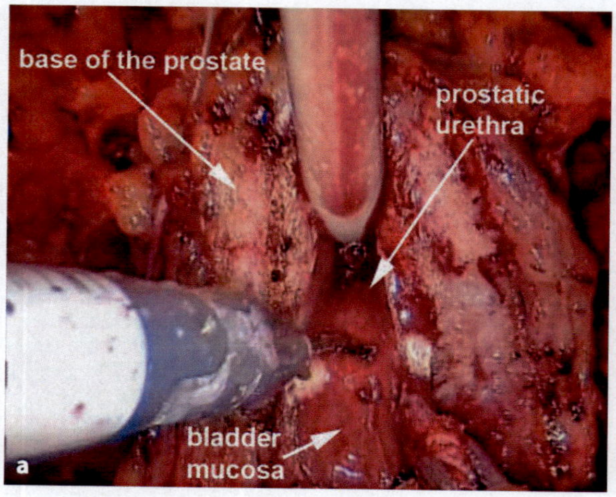

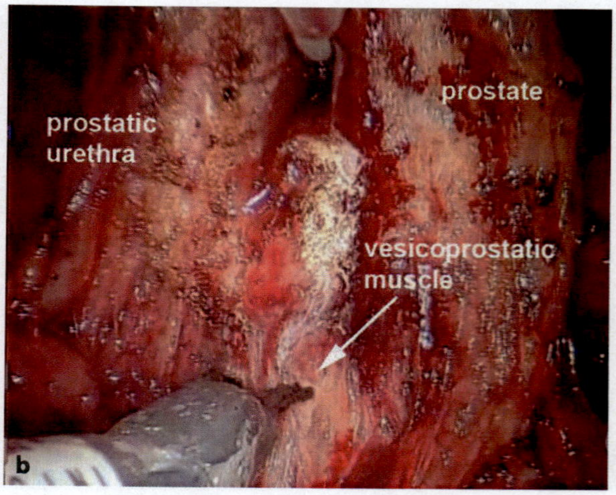

By dissecting the lateral sides first, the medial portion is better delineated. Starting laterally, use the bipolar forceps to grasp one side of the bladder opening and place on gentle traction, while using the shears to carefully dissect the lateral portion of the bladder neck from the prostate, following the fusion planes (Step 9a). With meticulous dissection, the posterior bladder neck is incised under direct vision. After the incision of the bladder neck, the anterior muscular layer of the Denonvilliers fascia (vesicoprostatic muscle) is encountered (Step 9b).

Step 10: Dissection of seminal vesicles and vas deferens

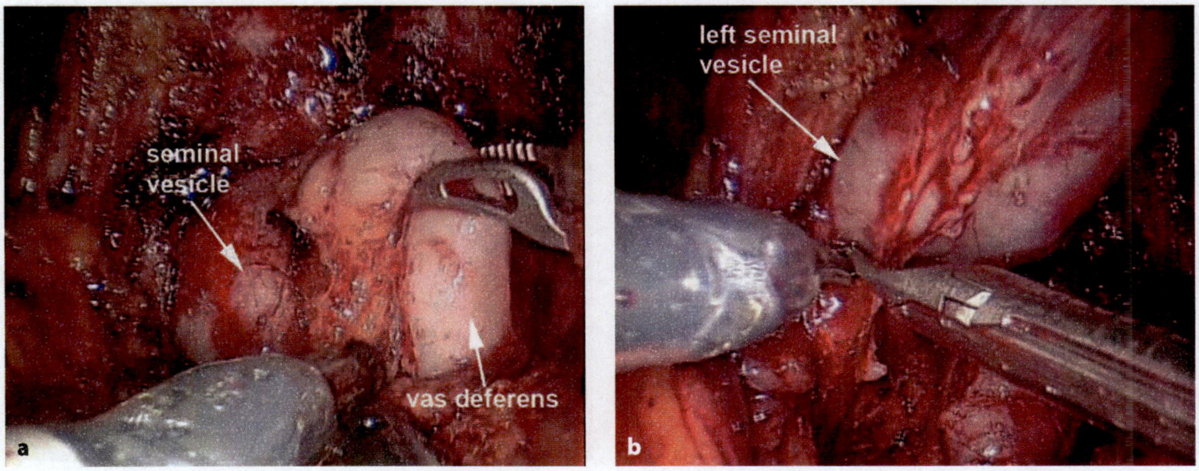

A transverse incision is made on anterior Denonvilliers fascia close to the prostate. There should be minimal use of cautery in the area of the seminal vesicles, in order to avoid injury to cavernous nerves. After isolation of the vas deferens (Step 10a), it is divided and the cut end is grasped to provide upward and cranial traction in order to dissect the vesicles. The tip of seminal vesicles is mobilised by clipping its arterial blood supply, then the seminal vesicles are dissected laterally. The remaining arterial branches supplying the seminal vesicles should be clipped and divided (Step 10b).

Step 11: Retroprostatic dissection I

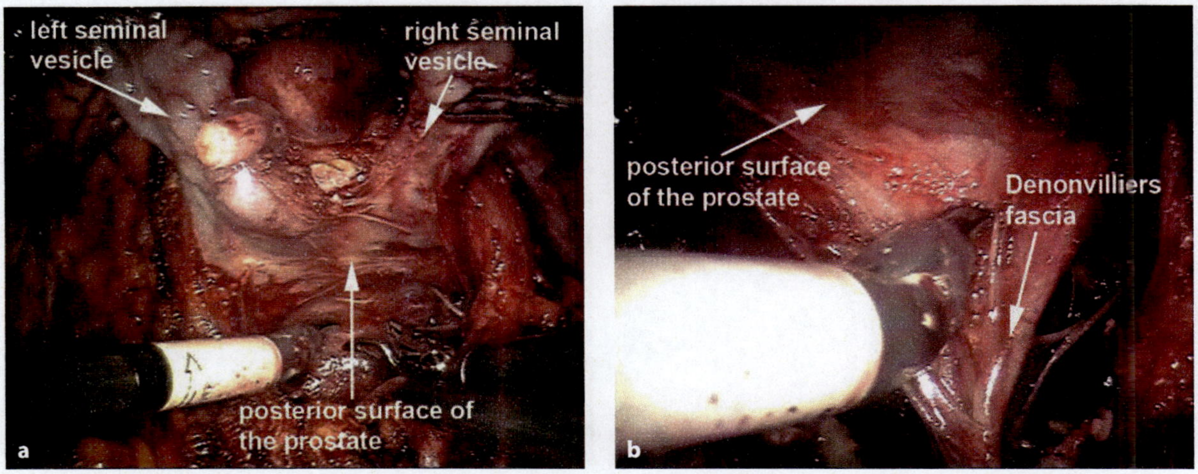

Meticulous sharp dissection at this step is essential: in low-risk patients in whom nerve preservation is feasible, the posterior layer of Denonvilliers fascia (which contains communicating nerve fibres) is left on the rectum, whereas in high-risk patients it is included with the specimen. The fourth arm is used to elevate the prostate superiorly and cranially by grasping the left seminal vesicle, while the assistant grasps the right seminal vesicle (Step 11a). An incision in the Denonvilliers fascia is made a few millimetres below the base of the prostate. The posterior Denonvilliers fascia has a characteristic pearly white appearance.

Step 12: Retroprostatic dissection II

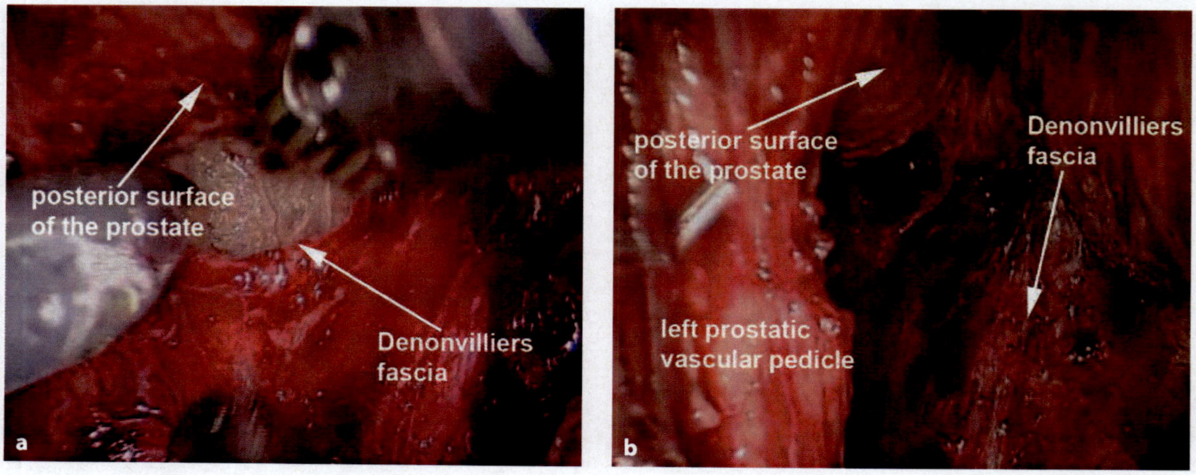

Once incised, the perirectal fat is visible covering the fascia propria of rectum and the incision is continued on the Denonvilliers fascia laterally along the entire width of the prostate (Step 12a). The rectum can be separated from the prostate using scissors, under direct vision. The plane between the rectum and prostate is defined by blunt and sharp dissection, continuing distally. The fascial space is dissected all the way down to the apex and laterally over the neurovascular bundles. In high-risk patients, the dissection between the prostate and rectum is performed along the anterior surface of the rectum, in contact with the fat, releasing the entire posterior surface of the prostate covered with Denonvilliers fascia down to the apex.

Step 13: Antegrade release of the neurovascular bundles

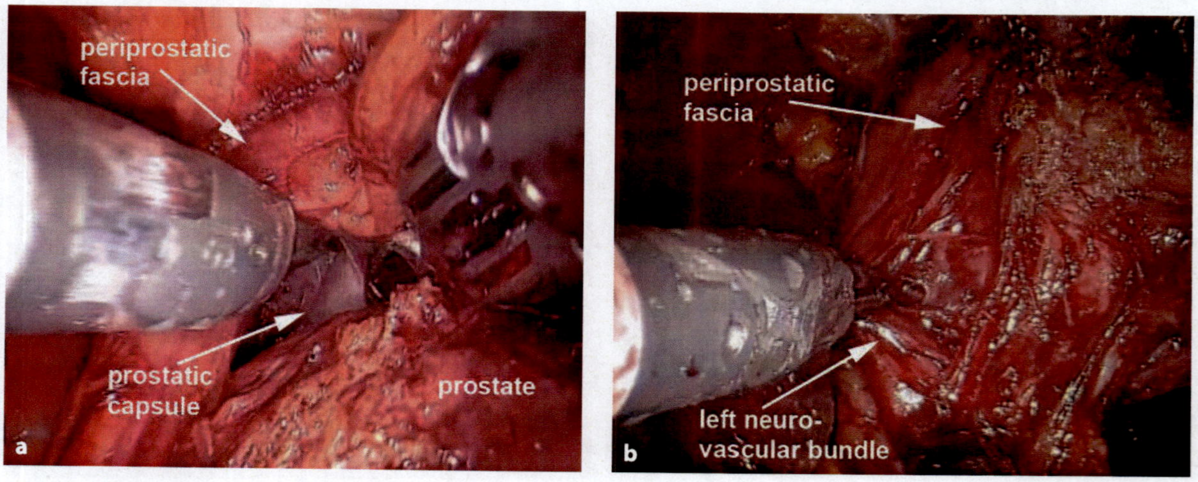

The neurovascular bundle should be released at least partially before division of the pedicles is begun. The dissection is accomplished between the prostate capsule and endopelvic fascial covering. The plane between the prostatic capsule and the prostatic fascia is accomplished (Step 13a). The visceral leaflet of the endopelvic fascia covering the prostate (periprostatic fascia or lateral prostatic fascia) is incised towards the puboprostatic ligaments or prostate apex. By doing so, a subtle groove appears on the posterolateral edge of the prostate, which helps to direct the dissection of the bundle toward the urethra. This manoeuvre releases the bundle laterally and the neurovascular bundle stands out and is progressively separated from the prostate (Step 13b).

Step 14: Selective control of prostate vascular pedicles

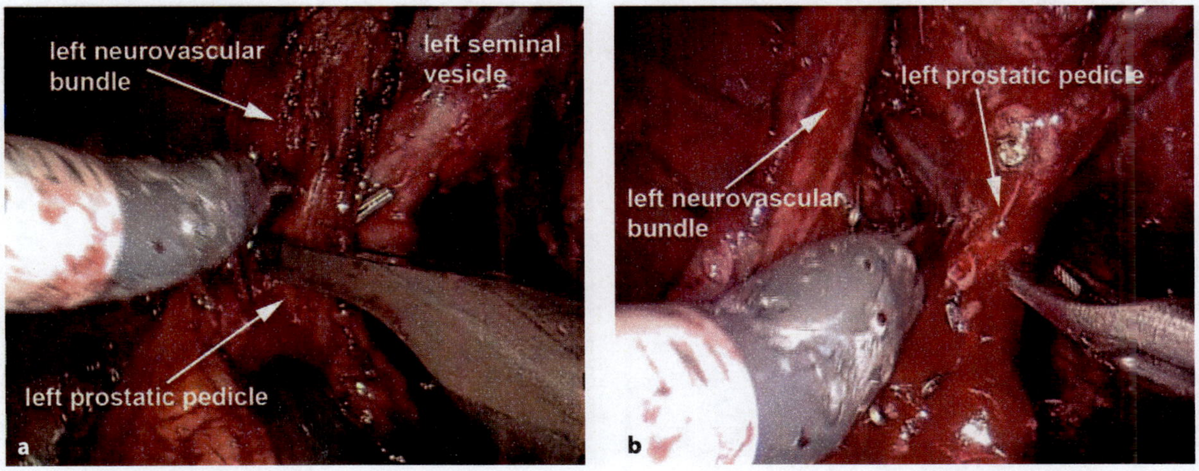

The prostatic vascular pedicles are separated by a thin fat plane from the posterolateral neurovascular bundles. Upwards, cranial and contralateral traction on the vas deferens and seminal vesicle exposes the lateral prostate pedicles (Step 14a). The pedicles are then dissected so that large Hem-o-lok clips can be placed to secure them (Step 14b). In high-risk patients, after ligation and division of prostatic pedicles, the prostatectomy is continued anteriorly with an extrafascial technique with resection of the prostatic fascia and of the neurovascular bundles up to the apex.

Step 15: Preservation of neurovascular bundles

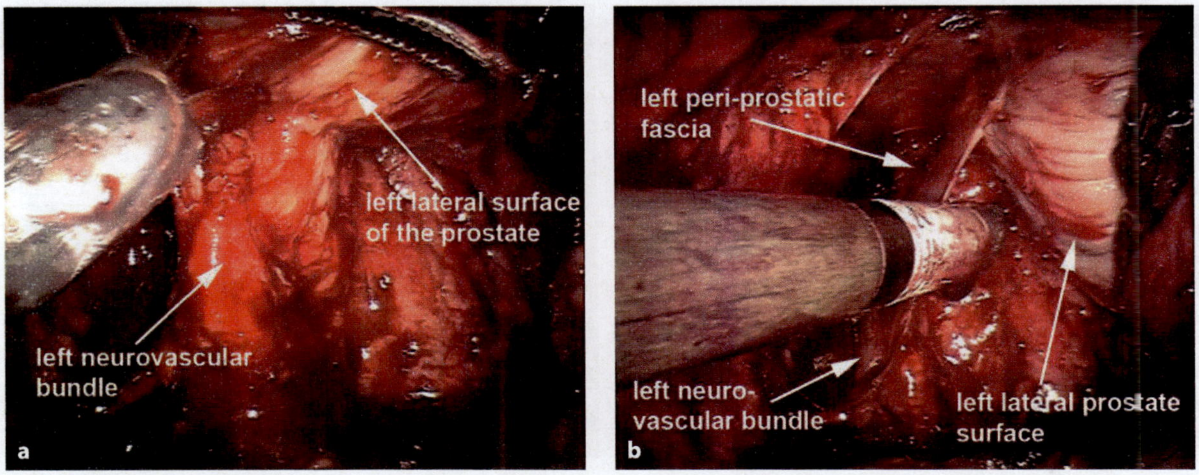

The dissection is carried along the lateral aspect of the prostate towards the apex under the endopelvic fascia, retracting the prostate medially (Step 15a). Small arterial and venous branches originating in the bundles and running towards the prostate (perforating branches) are secured with 2-mm clips. Both sharp and blunt dissection is performed and the bundles are swept laterally (Step 15b). The dissection is continued on both sides, until the prostatic apex is reached, ensuring the complete release of neurovascular bundles. The specimen is now attached only by the urethra and dorsal vein complex.

Step 16: Tangential division of dorsal venous complex

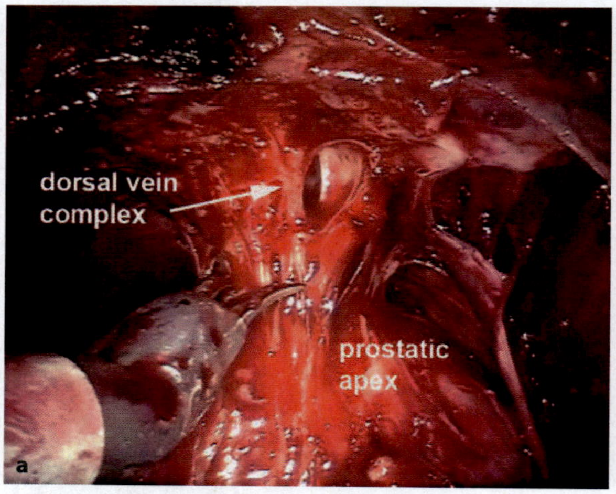

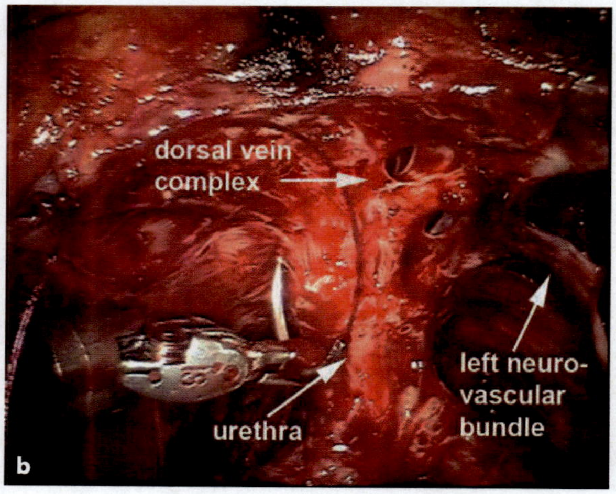

The prostate is pulled cephalad (holding the prostate traction suture with the fourth arm) and the intra-abdominal pressure is raised to 20 mmHg. The puboprostatic ligaments and the dorsal vein complex are divided tangentially close to the prostate until the avascular plane separating the urethra from the venous complex is reached (Step 16a). After completion of the dissection, the dorsal venous complex is ligated in a running fashion with a 3/0 Monocryl suture on a UR-6 needle, passing the needle under the dorsal vein complex in a cephalad direction (Step 16b).

Step 17: Apical and urethral dissection

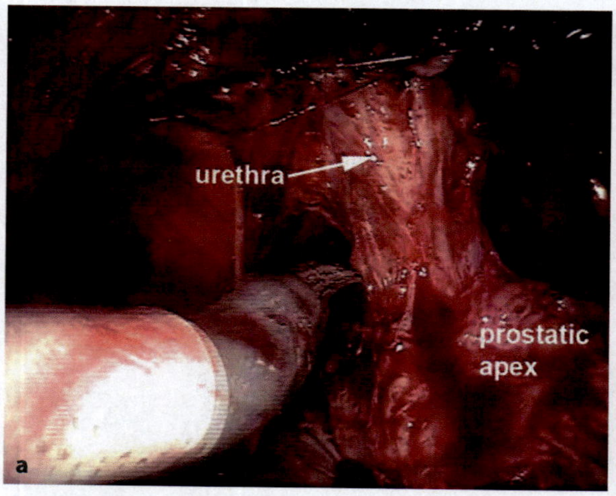

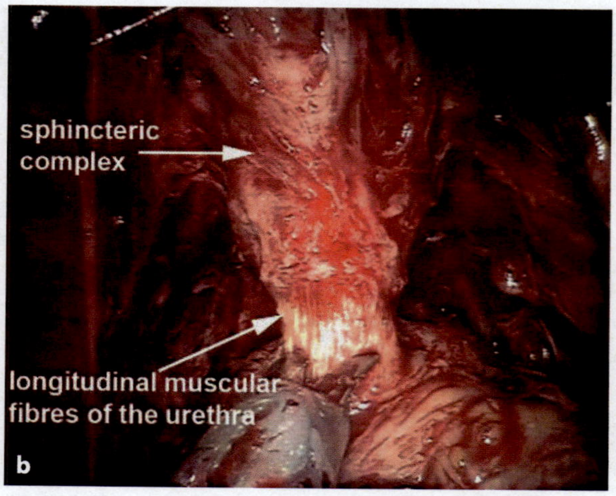

The best way to visualise the urethra is to dissect along the contour of the prostate around the apex very closely. Division on both sides of the apical pillars (Walsh pillars) and pushing fascia to delineate the urethra allows the urethra to stand out quite distinctly. The dissection is extended distally. The lateral dissection separates any residual attachment between the bundles and lateral surface of the prostate. The anterior urethral wall is opened just below the apical limit, exposing the Foley catheter. The posterior wall and the underlying rectourethralis muscle are then divided close to the prostate with a cold knife while retracting the prostate cephalad. The division of the rectourethralis muscle completely frees the specimen, which is placed in an endoscopic bag.

Step 18: Posterior musculofascial plate reconstruction (Rocco stitch)

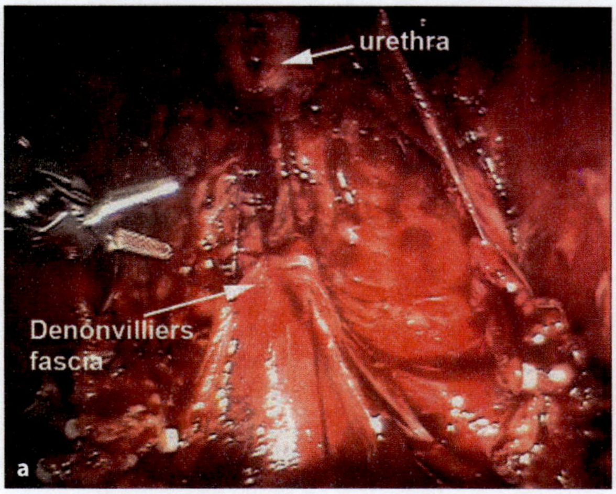

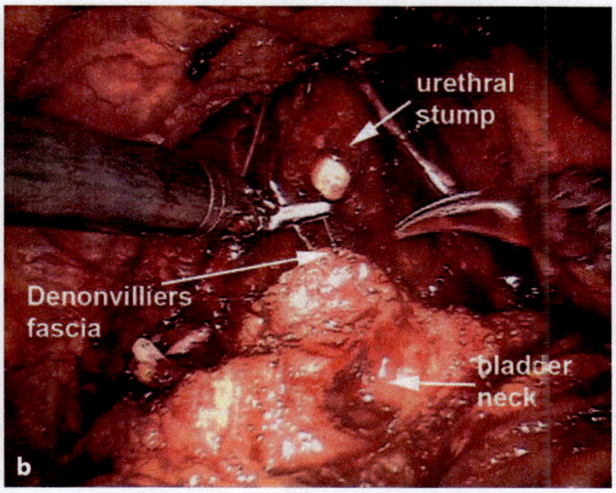

The posterior layer of Denonvilliers fascia (fibrous layer) is sutured to the posterior sphincteric complex by a running suture (3/0 Monocryl on a UR-6 needle) from left to right (Step 18a). This suture is then continued back to left in a second layer incorporating the anterior layer of Denonvilliers fascia (muscular) into the urethrovesical anastomosis. This restores the posterior anatomy connecting the fascia to the urogenital diaphragm (Step 18b).

Step 19: Urethrovesical anastomosis

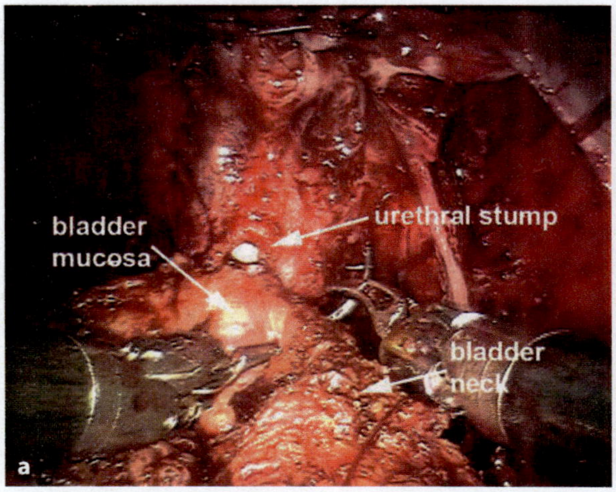

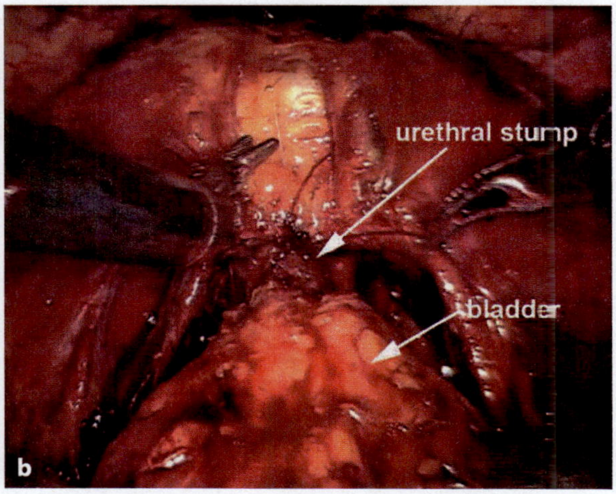

The urethrovesical anastomosis is performed with the single knot technique described by Van Velthoven (using two 20-cm 2/0 sutures on a 5/8 needle, whose tails are centrally knotted together). The running stitch is initiated by placing both needles outside-in through the bladder neck and inside-out on the urethra starting at 5 o'clock (Step 19a) and runs first left (clockwise) and then right (anti-clockwise). The bladder neck is advanced to approximately the urethra by gently applying progressive traction on the sutures. An 18-Charrière catheter is placed in the bladder and the balloon is filled with 10 cc of saline.

Postoperative Management

- Early mobilisation
- Oral intake on day of surgery
- Full diet on postoperative day 2
- Drain is removed on postoperative day 1
- The Foley catheter is removed on postoperative day 5
- Patient is discharged home after catheter removal

References

1. Walsh PC (1998) Anatomic radical prostatectomy: evolution of the surgical technique. J Urol 160:2418
2. Myers R (1994) Radical prostatectomy: pertinent surgical anatomy. Atlas Urol Clin North Am 2
3. Tewari A, Takenaka A, Mtui E, Horninger W, Peschel R, Bartsch G, Vaughan ED (2006) The proximal neurovascular plate and the tri-zonal neural architecture around the prostate gland: importance in the athermal robotic technique of nerve-sparing prostatectomy. BJU Int 98:314–323
4. Takenaka A, Leung RA, Fujisawa M, Tewari AK (2006) Anatomy of autonomic nerve component in the male pelvis: the new concept from a perspective for robotic nerve sparing radical prostatectomy. World J Urol 24:136–143
5. Costello AJ, Brooks M, Cole OJ (2004) Anatomical studies of the neurovascular bundle and cavernosal nerves. BJU Int 94:1071–1076
6. Mottrie A, Van Migem P, De Naeyer G, Schatteman P, Carpentier P, Fontayne E (2007) Robotic-assisted laparoscopic radical prostatectomy: oncologic and functional results of 184 cases. Eur Urol 52:746–750

3.12 Endoscopic Extraperitoneal Radical Prostatectomy (EERPE)

3.12.1 EERPE – Conventional Endoscopic Technique

3.12.1.1 Wide-Excision Endoscopic Extraperitoneal Radical Prostatectomy

Jens-Uwe Stolzenburg, Minh Do, Anja Dietel, Alan Mc Neil, Rowan Casey, Mathias Winkler, Christopher Anderson, Michael Truss, Kevin Turner, Ian Dunn, Evangelos N. Liatsikos

Introduction

In 2003, we described our own initial experience with 70 endoscopic extraperitoneal radical prostatectomies (EERPEs) by an entirely extraperitoneal retropubic approach for radical prostatectomy [1]. Our initial results demonstrated that the combination of the advantages of minimally invasive surgery and the retropubic open approach not only provided functional and oncological results similar to those of transperitoneal laparoscopic radical prostatectomy, but also complete avoidance of intraperitoneal complications. In the course of time, we have performed more than 3,000 cases with a continuously improving technique, which has been standardised as a first-line therapy for localised prostate cancer [2, 3].

There are no specific selection criteria or special contra-indications for EERPE in comparison to radical retropubic prostatectomy. Previous abdominal surgery does not have a negative impact on the overall operative times or the complication rates [4]. EERPE in patients with previous mesh placement from totally extraperitoneal hernioplasty (TEP) or transabdominal preperitoneal hernioplasty (TAPP) is technically demanding but remains feasible and safe. Nevertheless, port placement and technique should be adapted to individual patient characteristics [5]. Inexperienced laparoscopists should also avoid salvage prostatectomy after brachytherapy, external beam radiotherapy or after high-intensity focused ultrasound (HIFU) [6].

Based on the preoperative staging, there are two different techniques: wide-excision EERPE and intrafascial nerve-sparing (ns)EERPE. Both wide-excision and intrafascial nerve-sparing procedures will be presented step by step in the next two sections.

Indications

- The indications for EERPE are the same as for open radical retropubic prostatectomy
  - Clinically localised prostate cancer (T1 and T2) is the major indication. The life expectancy of the patients should be at least 10 years
  - According to the European Association of Urology Guidelines, surgery can be considered as a therapeutic alternative in clinical T3a prostate cancer
  - However, pelvic lymphadenectomy may not be possible in previous laparoscopic or endoscopic extraperitoneal hernia mesh placement due to adhesions

Contra-indications

- Serious cardiac conditions or insufficiency
- High intracranial and intraocular pressure (risk of haemorrhage)
- Uncorrected coagulopathy

Relative contra-indications (depending on the experience of the surgeon)	• Obesity • Prior major abdominal surgery (including the lower abdomen) • Prior inguinal hernia repair with mesh placement • Prior transurethral resection of the prostate • Very large prostate • Presence of large middle lobe • Asymmetric prostate • Extensive pelvic fibrosis (gun shot injury, orthopaedic trauma surgery) • Salvage prostatectomy after brachytherapy, external-beam radiation and HIFU • Clinical T3 cancer
Preoperative Preparation	• An enema on the evening before surgery • Broad-spectrum antibiotics are administered perioperatively

Step 1: Patient position and trocar placement

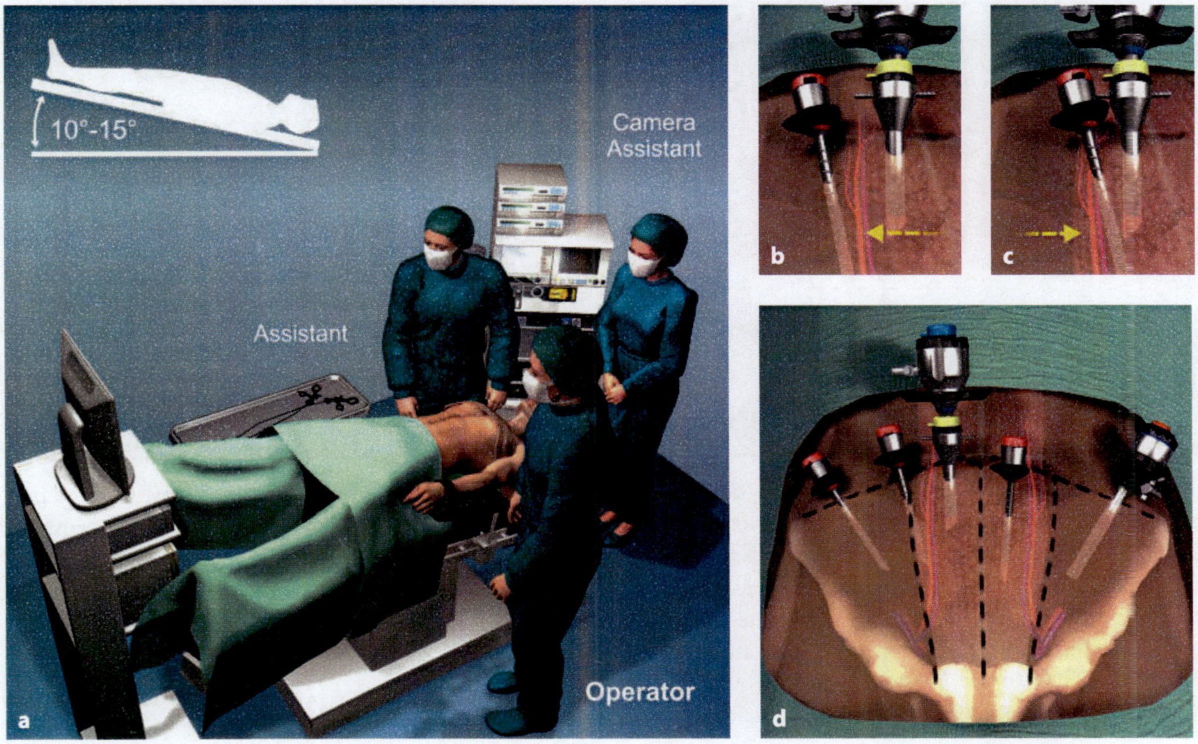

The patient is placed in a dorsal supine position with legs slightly apart, as described in Sect. 3.2. The surgeon stands to the left of the patient with an assistant opposite. The camera-holder stands behind the head of the patient (Step 1a). A Foley catheter is inserted under sterile conditions. Once the preperitoneal space has been created, one Hasson type optical trocar, one 12-mm trocar and three 5-mm trocars are placed as described in Sect. 3.4 (Step 1c). A 0° optical laparoscope is used during the whole procedure. In extremely obese or very tall patients, all trocars should be placed 2–3 cm caudally for optimal access to the retropubic space. The right paramedian port placement may be moved medially or laterally depending on the position of the epigastric vessels (Step 1b).

Step 2: Incision of endopelvic fascia

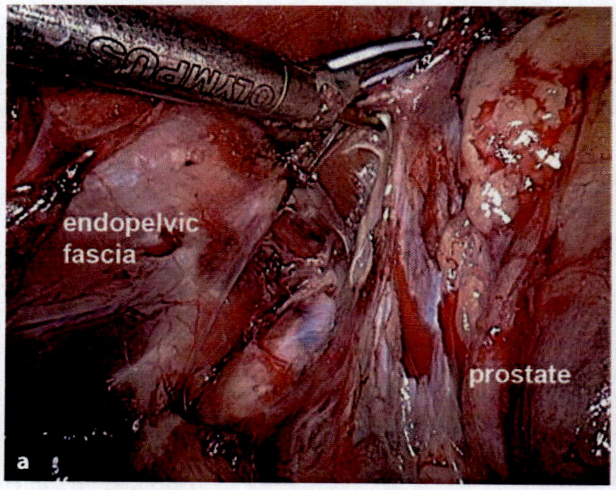

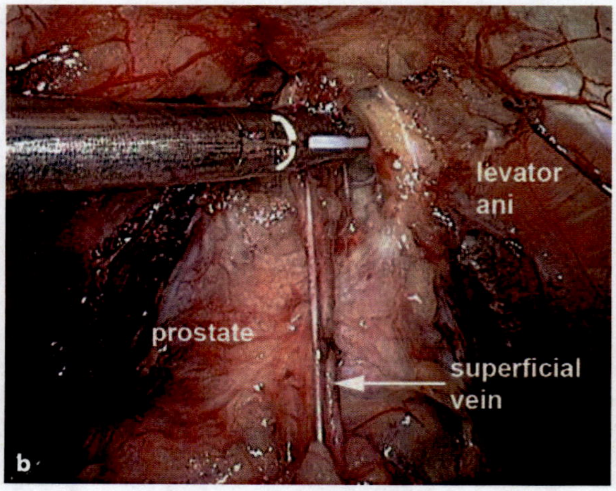

The endopelvic fascia is incised on both sides. Blunt dissection is performed proximally towards the apex. Sharp dissection might be necessary towards the apex in case of adhesions (use the SonoSurg device to avoid bleeding) (Step 2a). The prostate is retracted medially by the assistant to free any fibres of the levator ani that remain attached to the prostate. The fatty and areolar tissue is swept gently from the anterior surface of the bladder neck, from the anterior surface of the prostate and the endopelvic fascia. The use of the bipolar forceps is advised. The superficial branch of the dorsal vein has to be exposed (Step 2b), coagulated and cut using the SonoSurg device.

Step 3: Cutting the puboprostatic ligaments and ligation of the Santorini plexus

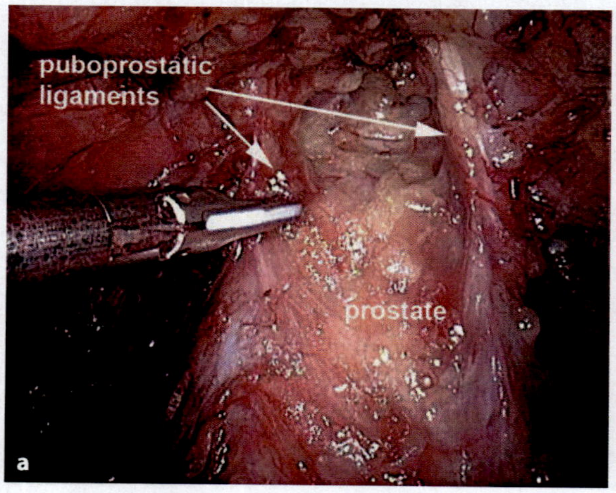

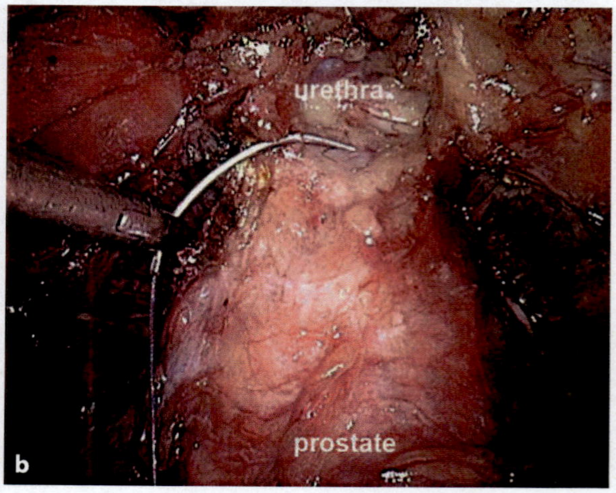

Both puboprostatic ligaments are fully dissected with cold scissors or the SonoSurg device. The Santorini venous plexus is situated directly under the ligaments (Step 3a). Be careful not to cut too deeply. The next step is the ligation of Santorini plexus, which is clearly visible from the lateral side. A 2/0 Polysorb GS-22 needle (slightly straightened; Step 3b) is then used and guided from left to right in the plane below the dorsal venous complex, and the plexus is then ligated. During this step, the assistant pushes the prostate dorsocranially to elongate the urethra. If the initial ligation is not sufficient pass a second suture with the same needle. The urethral catheter should be manipulated to ensure that it has not been entrapped by the suture.

Step 4: Ventral and lateral bladder neck dissection

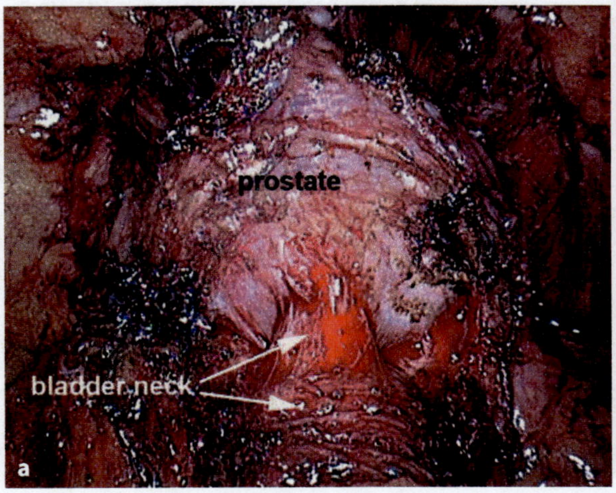

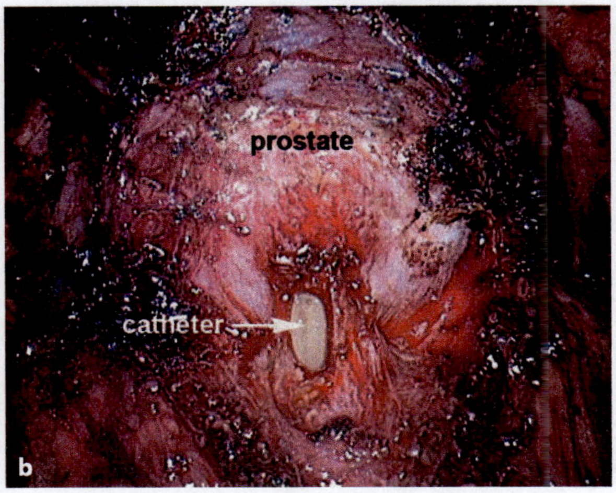

The bladder neck is dissected with blunt and sharp dissection gradually, aiming to define the longitudinal musculature of the bladder neck (Step 4a). A transverse incision is made in this muscle with the SonoSurg device. This superficial incision is enlarged and deepened from 9 to 3 o'clock to identify the longitudinal musculature of the bladder neck. The assistant and the operator now push the bladder dorsally and the bladder neck is cut and the catheter becomes visible (Step 4b). When the correct plane between the prostate and bladder is not clearly seen, bladder neck dissection should be performed more proximally. It is better to have a wider bladder neck than to risk a positive margin here.

Step 5: Posterior bladder neck dissection

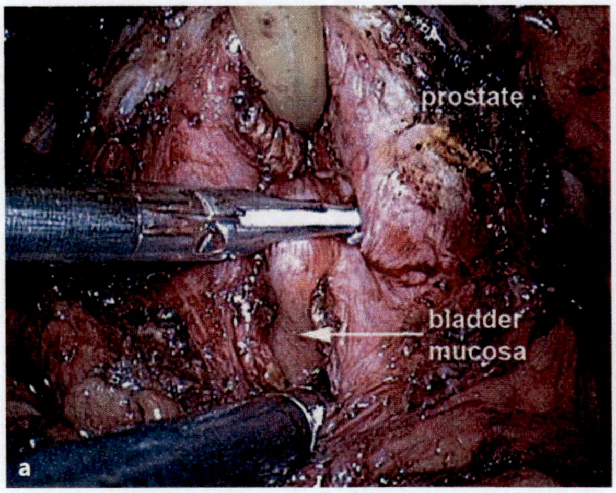

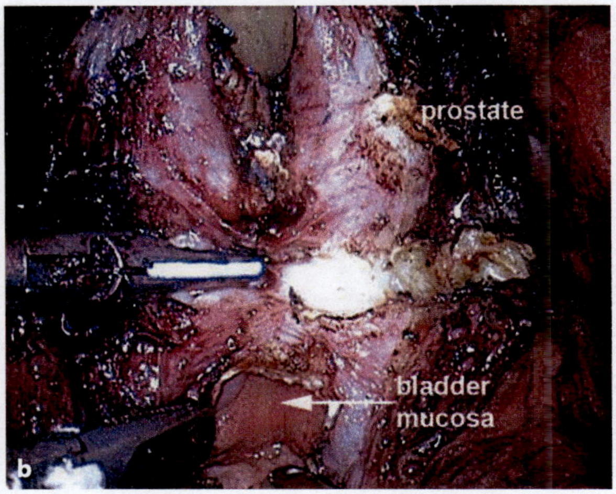

The catheter is then pulled up into the retropubic space under continuous traction by the assistant. The posterior bladder neck is transected using the SonoSurg device following a perpendicular plane to access the vas and seminal vesicles. In case of lost orientation during dissection, go back to the midline, identify bladder neck mucosa and recommence. The bladder neck is first completely divided between the 5 and 7 o'clock position, as in Step 5b. Then the surgeon bluntly enlarges this space. The most common mistake is to dissect too oblique and end up within the prostate. The end point of the posterior bladder neck dissection is the identification of the anatomical landmarks of the ampulla of the vas deferens.

Step 6: Lateral bladder neck dissection and dissection of the vas

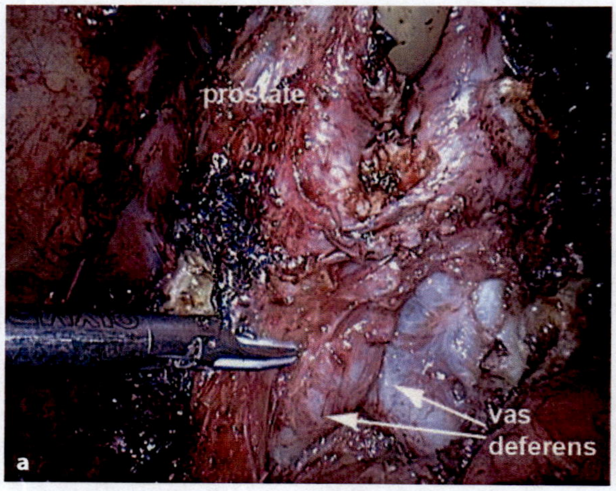

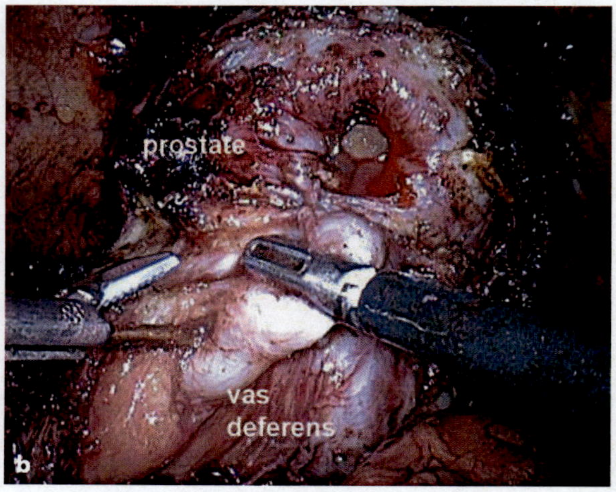

When both vas are identified, the posterior bladder neck dissection is extended laterally in both directions. The dissection of the whole posterior bladder neck including the lateral fascias provides easier access to the vas and seminal vesicles (Step 6a). Both vas should now be freed and divided close to the level of the seminal vesicle tips (dissection too close to the prostate makes the seminal vesicle dissection more difficult). Once the left vas is divided, the assistant grasps and pulls it contra-laterally towards the pubic bone to aid seminal vesicle dissection (Step 6b). The assistant must push the bladder down with the suction to allow better access to the vas, seminal vesicles and their vessels. The same manoeuvre is performed on the other side.

Step 7: Seminal vesicle dissection and Denonvilliers fascia incision

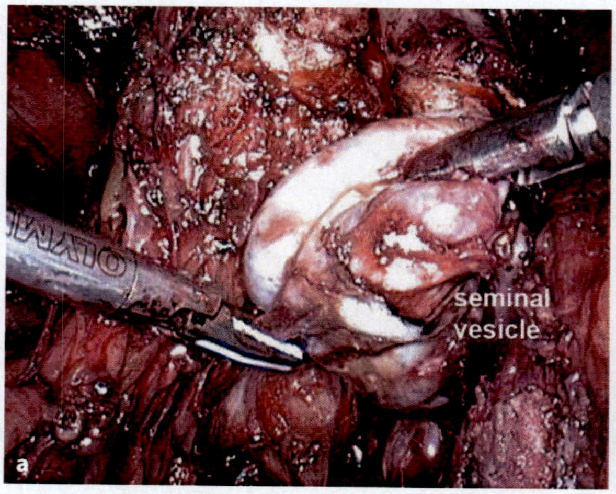

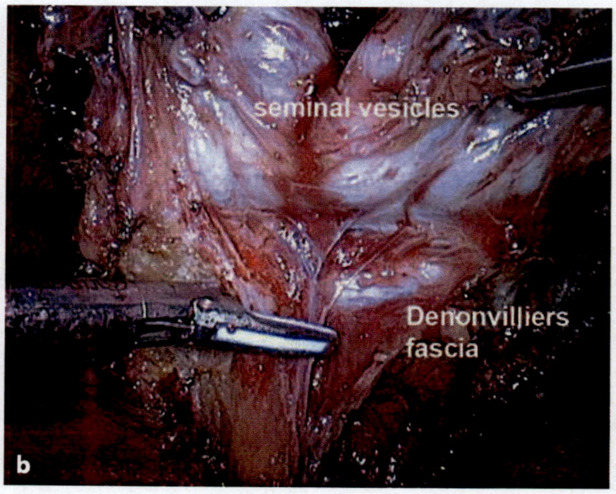

The seminal vesicles are identified slightly laterally to the vas. The assistant retracts the seminal vesicle medially and cranially with the forceps in the right hand, and with the suction in the left hand, the bladder is pushed down (Step 7a). The small arteries of the seminal vesicle have to be dissected using the SonoSurg device to prevent bleeding. Both the surgeon and the assistant now retract the seminal vesicles in a craniolateral direction, exposing the posterior layer of the Denonvilliers fascia. A horizontal incision is made on this layer (Step 7b) and the yellow prerectal fatty tissue is visualised. The dissection is continued as far as possible towards the apex of the prostate in the midline.

Step 8: Prostatic pedicle and neurovascular bundle dissection

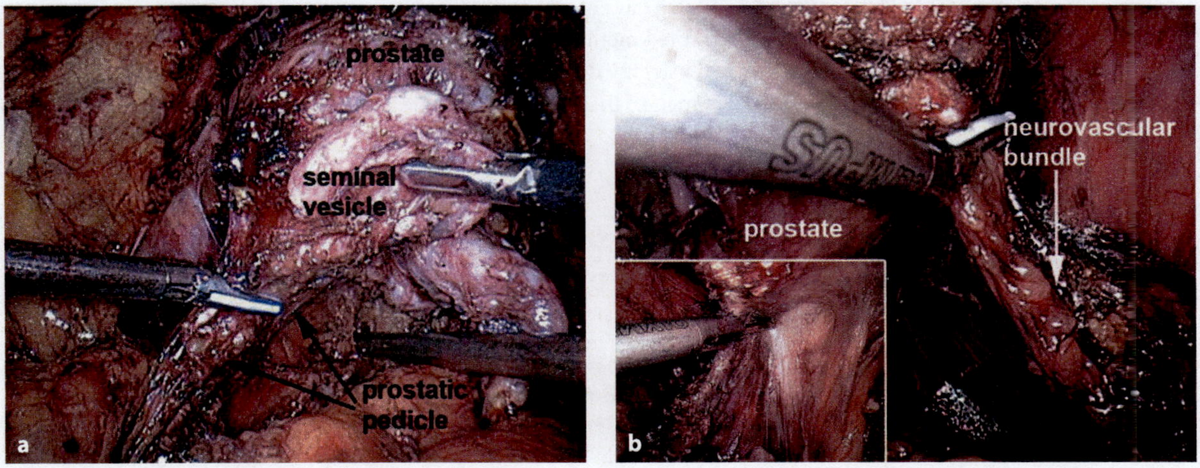

The next manoeuvre is designed to place the prostatic pedicles on tension. To accomplish this, the assistant again elevates the left seminal vesicle in a contra-lateral cranial direction out of the pelvis. In that way, the left prostate pedicle can easily be identified as a cord structure (Step 8a). The pedicle and the neurovascular bundle are then dissected using the SonoSurg device. Step 8b demonstrated the dissection of the neurovascular bundle on the right side. This dissection is performed to a point just cephalad to the prostate apex and the urethra (inset). When the assistant continues to maintain the traction on the base of the seminal vesicle, the prostate is pulled increasingly out of the pelvis and this aids dissection.

Step 9: Apical dissection and urethrovesical anastomosis

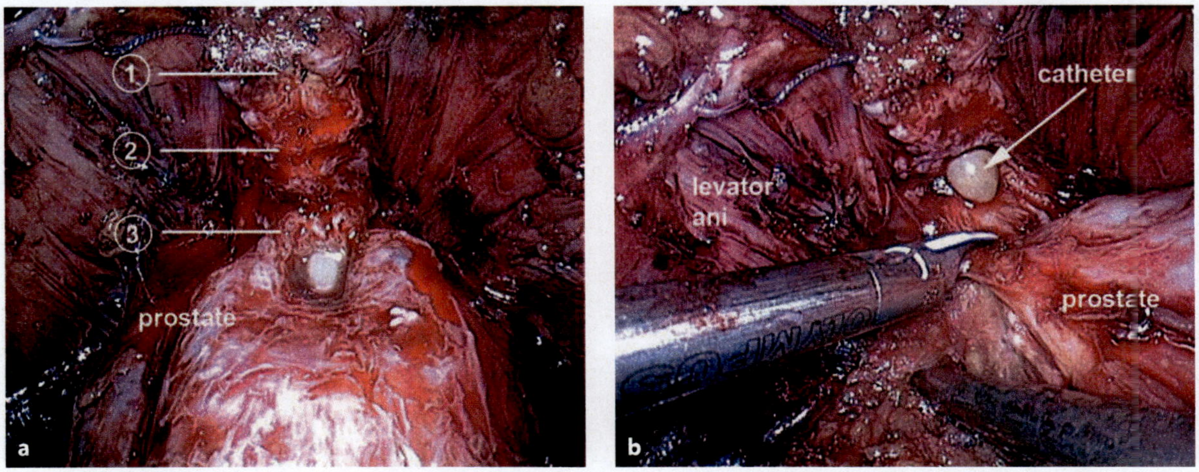

Apical dissection is a five-step procedure (Step 9a): dorsal venous plexus division (1), anterior urethral wall division (junction between external striated sphincter and apex of the prostate) (2), identification, preservation and opening of the longitudinal urethral smooth muscle layer anteriorly (3), urethral mucosa division caudal to the verumontanum (4, not shown), final posterior urethral detachment (5; Step 9b). The final detachment (5) is performed dorsolaterally to avoid rectal injury. The assistant retracts the prostate contralaterally out of the pelvis and pushes the rectum down. When the prostate is completely freed from its surrounding structures, it is placed in an endoscopic retrieval bag, removed, and sent for frozen section. The trocar is inserted again to perform the urethrovesical anastomosis (see Sect. 3.12.1.2).

Postoperative Management

- Drain is removed on day 1
- Catheter removed on day 5 or 6 if no leak at retrograde cystography
  - Minor leak requiring 3–7 extra days of catheterisation
- There is no unanimously accepted method of categorisation of anastomotic leakage in the literature. Even though there are no strictly defined criteria, we have attempted a categorisation facilitating postoperative management of these patients in Stolzenburg et al. [7]

References

1. Stolzenburg JU, Do M, Rabenalt R, Pfeiffer H, Horn L, Truss,MC, Jonas U, Dorschner W (2003) Endoscopic extraperitoneal radical prostatectomy (EERPE) – initial experience after 70 procedures. J Urol 169:2066–2071
2. Stolzenburg JU, Rabenalt R, DO M, Ho K, Dorschner W, Waldkirch E, Jonas U, Schütz A, Horn L, Truss MC (2005) Endoscopic extraperitoneal radical prostatectomy: oncological and functional results after 700 procedures. J Urol 174:1271–1275
3. Stolzenburg JU, Kallidonis P, Minh D, Dietel A, Häfner T, Dimitriou D, Al-Aown A, Kyriazis I, Liatsikos EN (2009) Endoscopic extraperitoneal radical prostatectomy: evolution of the technique and experience with 2400 cases. J Endourol 23:1467–1472
4. Stolzenburg J-U, Ho KM, Do M, Rabenalt R, Dorschner W, Truss MC (2005) Impact of previous surgery on endoscopic extraperitoneal radical prostatectomy. Urology 65:325–231
5. Stolzenburg J-U, Anderson C, Rabenalt R, Do M, Ho K, Truss M (2005) Endoscopic extraperitoneal radical prostatectomy (EERPE) in patients with prostate cancer and previous laparoscopic inguinal mesh placement for hernia repair. World J Urol 27:1–5
6. Stolzenburg JU, Bynens B, Do M, Rabenalt R, Katsakiori PF, Liatsikos E (2007) Salvage laparoscopic extraperitoneal radical prostatectomy after failed high-intensity focused ultrasound and radiotherapy for localized prostate cancer. Urology 70: 956–960
7. Stolzenburg JU, Gettman MT, Liatsikos EN (eds) (2007) Endoscopic Extraperitoneal Radical Prostatectomy: Laparoscopic and Robot-Assisted Surgery. Springer, Berlin Heidelberg, New York

3.12.1.2 Nerve-Sparing Endoscopic Extraperitoneal Radical Prostatectomy

Jens-Uwe Stolzenburg, Minh Do, Thilo Schwalenberg, Anja Dietel, Alan Mc Neil, Rowan Casey, Christopher Anderson, Panagiotis Kallidonis, Evangelos N. Liatsikos

Introduction

Despite the different approaches for radical prostatectomy, the key to better results is the understanding of the anatomy of the bladder neck, urethra and the neurovascular bundles [1, 2]. Based on our recently published anatomical studies, nerve and puboprostatic ligament-preserving techniques supplemented the original EERPE technique, leading to the development of the nerve-sparing (ns)EERPE and improving potency and early continence. However, the most recent and promising refinement of the EERPE procedure is the intrafascial nerve-sparing EERPE [3, 4]. In intrafascial nerve-sparing radical prostatectomy, the pelvic plexus, the neurovascular bundle and the prostatic plexus – a distribution of nerve fibres on the lateral surface of the prostate – are preserved in order to maintain neurovascular integrity [5]. The preservation of additional neural tissue located in the periprostatic fascia as performed in intrafascial nsEERPE is associated with significantly better functional outcome with a limited effect on the radical nature of the surgery. It is therefore an effective cancer procedure which provides further decreases in procedure-related morbidity [6].

Indications

- Clinically organ-confined prostate cancer
- No palpable induration at the apex or posterolateral margins of the prostate. In selected cases, intraoperative frozen section may be helpful to decide whether a nerve-sparing technique is possible
- Patients with PSA less than 10 ng/ml and Gleason sum under 7 traditionally are regarded as candidates for a nerve-sparing procedure
  a. Patients with a less favourable profile may be considered on an individual basis. In patients with a palpable lesion or Gleason score of 7, intraoperative frozen section may be helpful in this setting
  b. Newer normograms taking into account the percentage of tumour infiltration per biopsy, the total number of biopsies and the number of positive biopsies may aid decision making in the future.
- Preoperative erectile function sufficient for intercourse. This is a relative indication since the return to complete continence is also better in patients who had a nerve-sparing procedure. Therefore, a nerve-sparing procedure may also be indicated in patients with impaired sexual function

Contra-indications

- Gleason score 8–10 prostate cancer.
  - If unilateral Gleason 8 disease, a nerve-sparing procedure may be performed contralaterally by an experienced surgeon
- Fixation of the neurovascular bundle to the prostatic capsule (intraoperative decision)
- Tumour invasion within the neurovascular bundle (intraoperative frozen section)
- Induration at the apex or posterolateral borders of the prostate

Preoperative Preparation

- An enema on the evening before surgery
- Broad-spectrum antibiotics are administered perioperatively

Step 1: Mobilisation of periprostatic fascia and puboprostatic ligaments

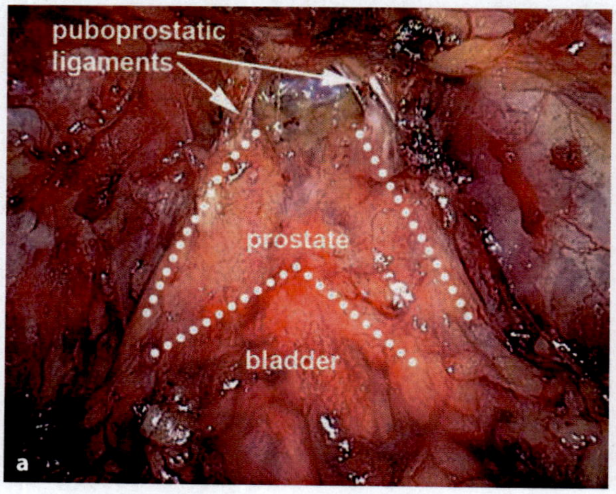

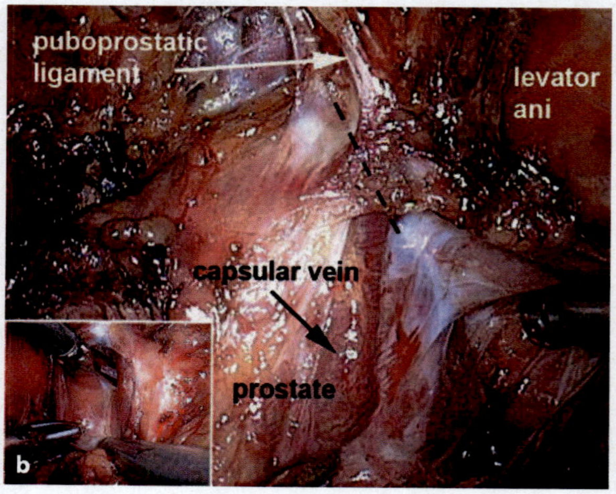

The bladder neck, the prostate and the endopelvic fascia are completely exposed. The superficial branch of the deep dorsal vein complex is fulgurated with bipolar forceps and divided. A plane is developed between the prostate and its thin overlying fascia (periprostatic fascia), as seen in Step 1a. This can be performed in most cases bluntly. A sharp incision is made only toward the apex medially to the puboprostatic ligaments (dashed line Step 1b). This manoeuvre preserves the puboprostatic ligaments on both sides. When the right plane has been developed, a shiny fascia covering the levator ani is apparent.

Step 2: Ventral bladder neck dissection

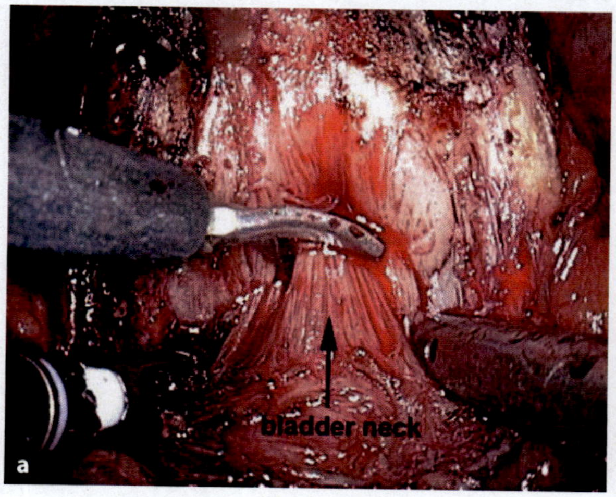

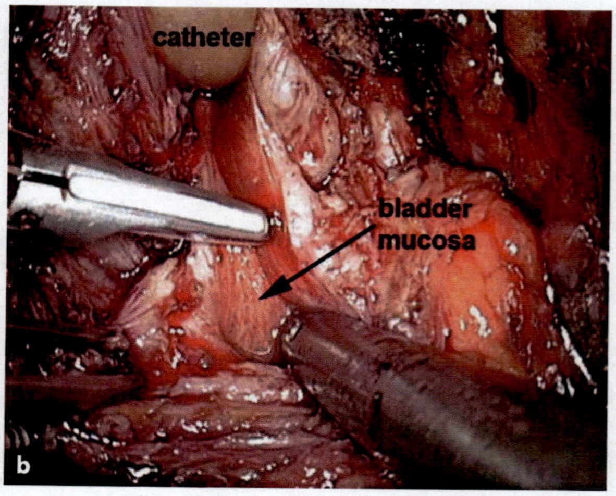

The next step is the bladder neck dissection. It is performed gradually, aiming to define the longitudinal musculature of the bladder neck (Step 2a). This longitudinal musculature is only evident surrounding the urethra at the bladder neck. When cutting the bladder neck, the assistant (using suction) and the operator (using the forceps in the left hand) have to push the bladder dorsally. Thus, the bladder neck becomes clearly visible. It is completely incised and the catheter becomes visible. The catheter is then pulled up into the retropubic space by the assistant under continuous tension. The bladder neck dissection is now continued in the lateral and posterior direction (Step 2b).

Step 3: Dissection of the vas and mobilisation of seminal vesicles

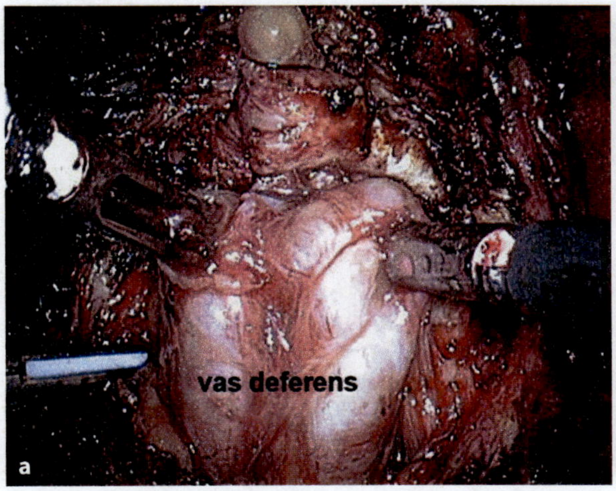

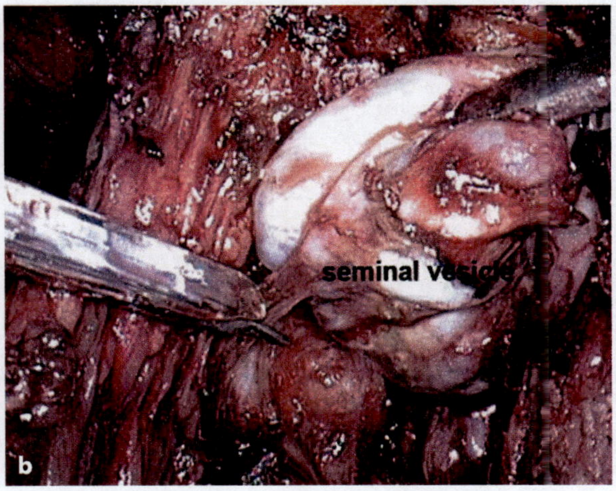

The posterior bladder neck is completely dissected. The main difference to wide excision is the restricted window behind the bladder due to the lateral attachments, which must be preserved (fascias, nerves and vessels). The anatomical landmarks of the ampullary segments of the vas are then visualised (Step 3a) and dissected with the SonoSurg device. After the division of the vas the seminal vesicles are freed. Blunt and sharp dissection avoiding the use of electrocautery is recommended, especially during dissection of the seminal vesicle tips. The seminal vesicles are completely freed and care must be given to the vessels, which should be clipped (Step 3b), especially at the tip of the seminal vesicles.

Step 4: Stripping Denonvilliers fascia

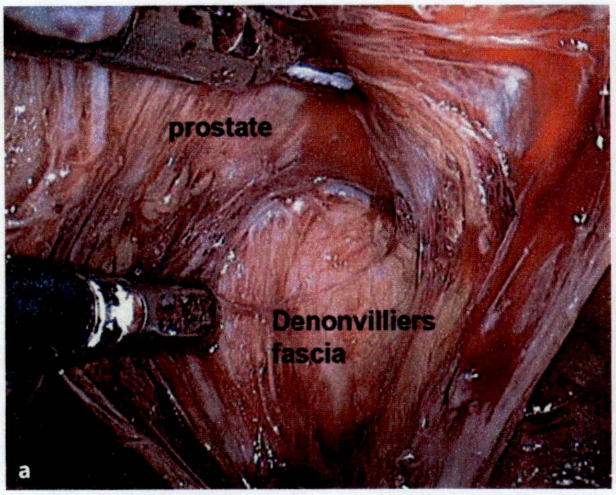

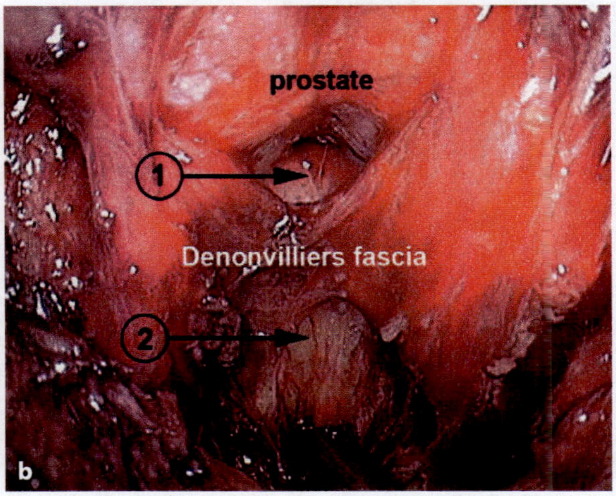

After complete mobilisation of both seminal vesicles, the surgeon and the assistant retract the seminal vesicles in a craniolateral direction, exposing the posterior layer of Denonvilliers fascia. Denonvilliers fascia is now stripped down from the prostatic capsule, as seen in Step 4a (intrafascial plane). Step 4b shows the intrafascial plane (1) as well as the conventional (interfascial) plane (2), where the Denonvilliers fascia is incised and the prerectal fatty tissue becomes visible. The blunt dissection is continued as far as possible towards the apex of the prostate, strictly in the midline in order to avoid injury to the neurovascular bundles.

Step 5: Prostatic pedicle dissection

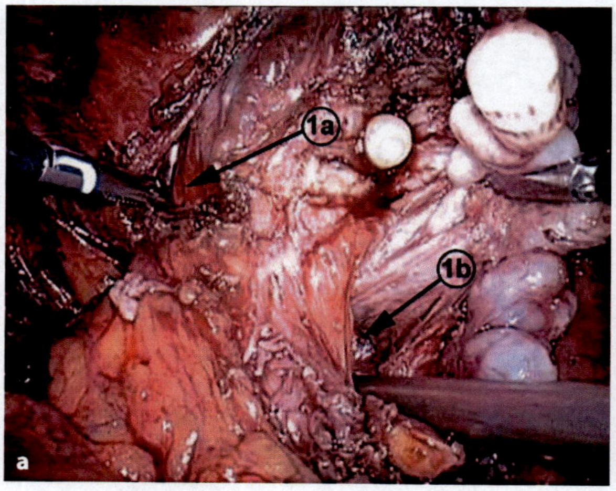

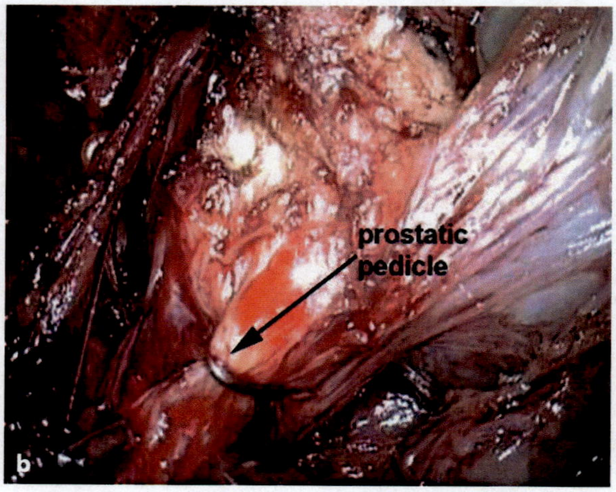

At this point of the procedure, two planes have been developed: laterally (1a) as well as medially (1b). The shiny surface of the prostatic capsule is clearly seen. The prostatic pedicle (between these two planes) is now clipped close to the prostate and cut step by step (Step 5b). It is advisable to proceed with the clipping and cutting in small steps. Care has to be taken to avoid inadvertent injury to the neurovascular bundle. Therefore, the pedicles are cut with cold scissors. No energy (SonoSurg, the UltraCision device or electrocautery) should be used at this point of the procedure.

Step 6: Mobilisation of the neurovascular bundle and the periprostatic fascia

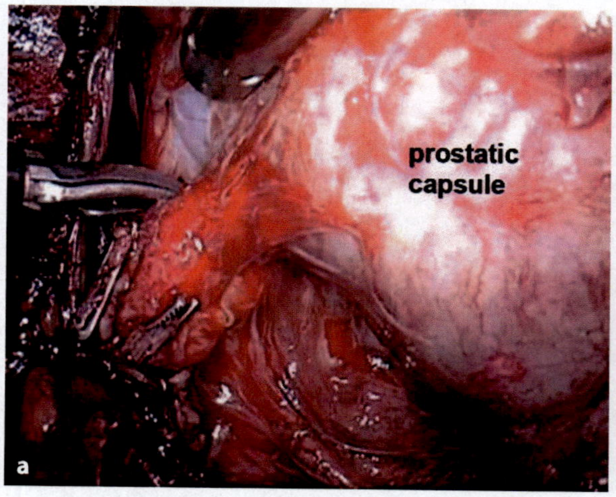

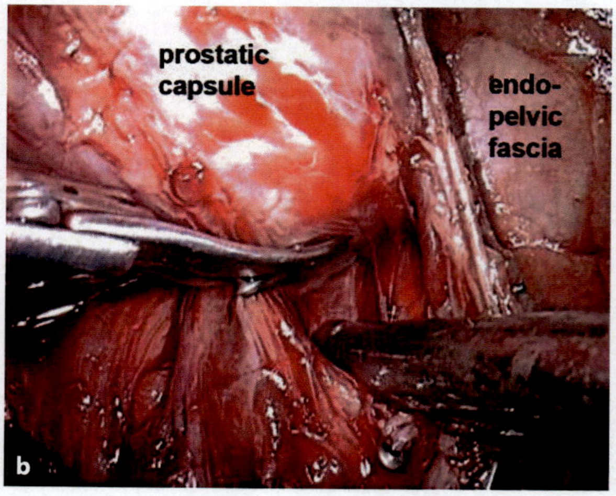

When the main prostatic pedicle has been fully dissected, the remaining neurovascular bundle including the periprostatic fascia can be detached from the prostatic capsule, in most cases bluntly, using atraumatic graspers. Small capsular vessels can be clipped by small clips and divided. To facilitate the dissection on the left side (Step 6a), the assistant retracts the left seminal vesicle with his right forceps and pushes the lateral side of the prostate with his left instrument. The blunt dissection can be completed on both sides to free the entire posterior and posterolateral surface of the prostate. The same process is repeated on the right side (Step 6b). During the whole dissection, the white shiny surface of the prostate capsule can be seen.

Step 7: Apical mobilisation and ligation of the Santorini plexus

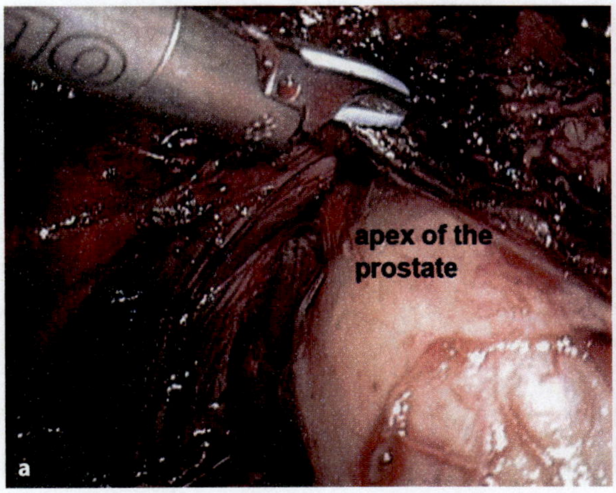

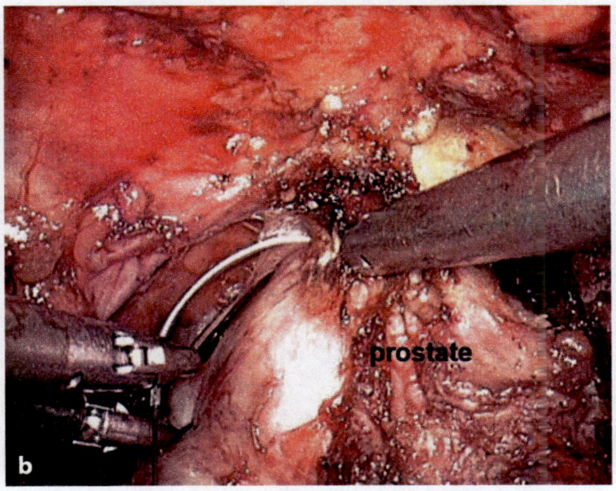

The prostate is now pushed into the pelvis contralaterally to provide good access to the apex and the urethra. The mobilised puboprostatic ligaments and the remaining puboprostatic fascia on the lateral surface of the prostate are now completely detached from the urethra and the apex. Only the ventral tissue on the prostate can be dissected with the SonoSurg (Step 7a). The rest of the dissection must be done bluntly. After full mobilisation, the Santorini plexus is clearly visible from the lateral side. A 2/0 Polysorb GS-22 needle (slightly straightened) is then used and guided from left to right in the plane below the dorsal venous complex, and the plexus is thus ligated (Step 7b). A second ligation with the same suture provides optimal haemostasis. The catheter is manipulated to ensure it has not been included.

Step 8: Apical dissection

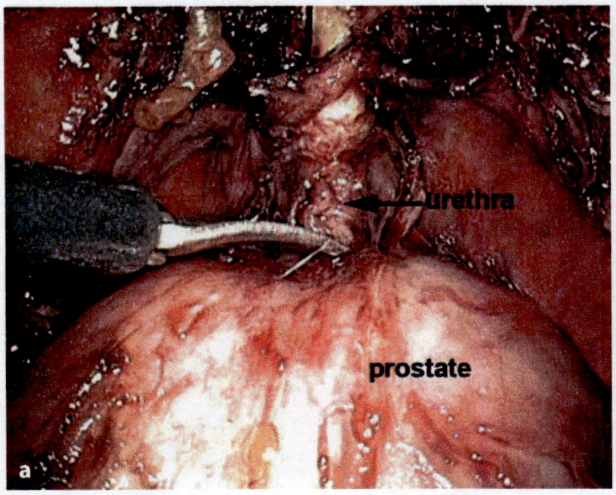

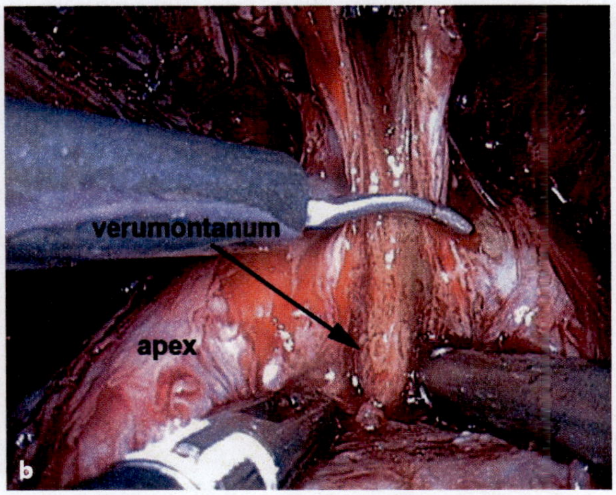

The apical dissection is a five-step procedure, as has been described in Sect. 3.12.1.1. It starts with the dissection of the Santorini plexus (1). This is performed laterally to medially. For the entire apical dissection, make sure that the catheter is inserted within the urethra and visible at the proximal end. The next step is the ventral dissection of the border between the prostate and the urethra (external sphincter) (2). The smooth muscular inner layer of the urethra (Step 8a) should be completely exposed and cut (3). The assistant retracts the catheter towards the symphysis with the forceps on the right hand, and pushes the prostate down with the suction in the left hand (Step 8b). The dissection of the urethra is continued posteriorly and distally to the verumontanum (4).

Step 9: Apical dissection and haemostasis

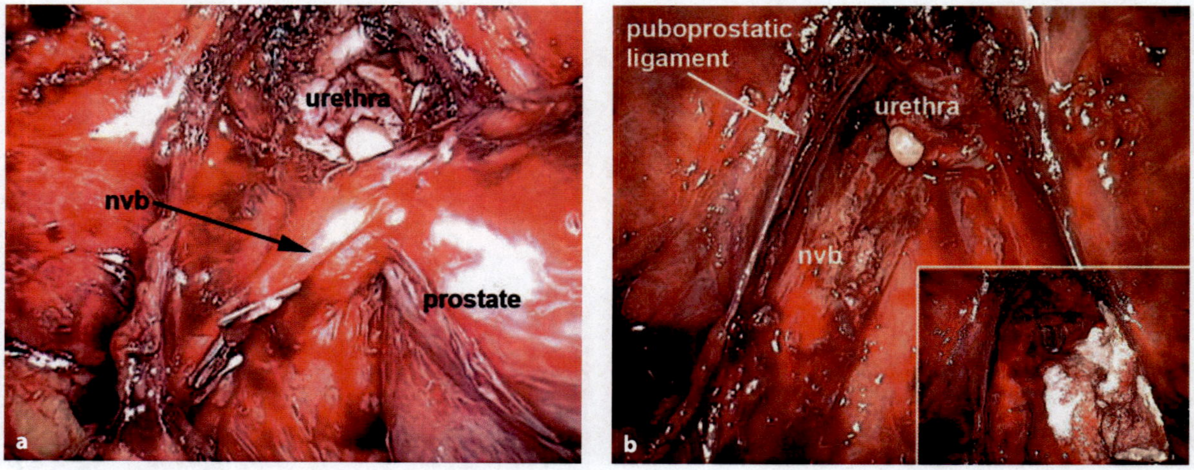

The final detachment of the posterior urethra is performed dorsolaterally (5) to avoid any injury to the neurovascular bundles and the rectum (Step 9a). The assistant retracts the seminal vesicle contra-laterally out of the pelvis and also pushes the prostate laterally.

Step 9b shows the intraoperative field after complete detachment of the prostate in a bilateral nerve-sparing prostatectomy. The preserved neurovascular bundles (nvb) are seen bilaterally. Haemostasis is now checked and where there is minor bleeding from the neurovascular bundle (surface haemorrhage and slow venous oozing), TachoSil (NYCOMED Austria GmbH, Vienna, Austria) (inlay Step 9b) or FloSeal (Baxter, Deefield, IL, USA) can be used. Arterial bleeding must be either clipped or sutured (4/0 Vicryl) depending on the location to the neurovascular bundles.

Step 10: Urethrovesical anastomosis

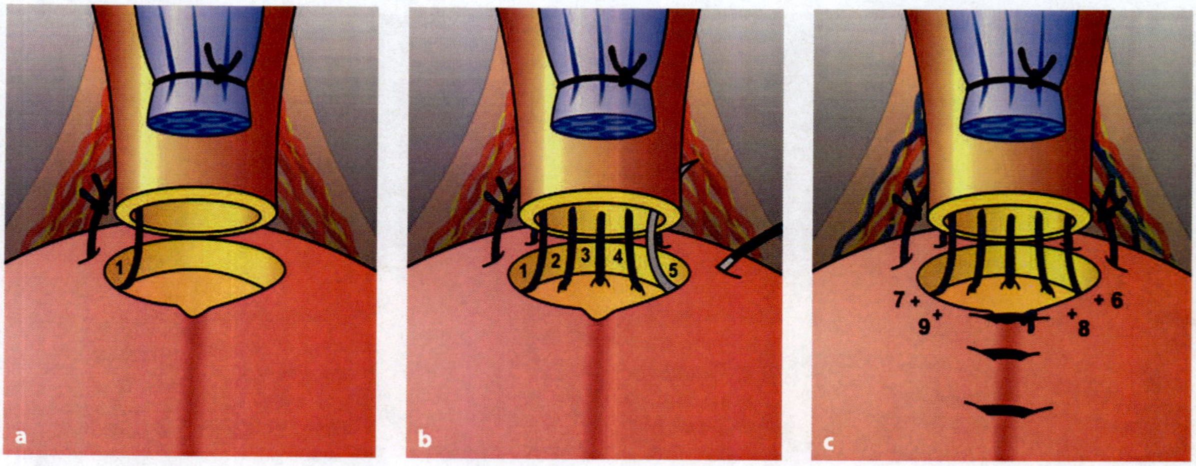

In principle, the anastomosis can be performed with an interrupted or a running suture. We prefer the interrupted suture technique. Depending on the size of the bladder neck, eight to nine sutures are necessary for watertight anastomosis. In case of a widely open bladder neck, bladder neck closure (ventrally) should also be performed prior to the final stitches. The sequence and method of suture placement is clearly shown in this figure. When there is tension (very seldom) to the urethra, do not attempt to approximate the bladder to the urethra with the first stitch. Secure the knot of the first suture before full approximation. Make sure that the bladder is empty. The final approximation can be reached with the next stitch.

Postoperative Management

- See Sect. 3.12.1.1 on wide-excision EERPE

References

1. Stolzenburg JU, Schwalenberg T, Horn LC, Neuhaus J, Constantinides C, Liatsikos EN (2007) Anatomical landmarks of radical prostatectomy. Eur Urol 51:629–639
2. Schwalenberg T, Neuhaus J, Liatsikos E, Winkler M, Löffler S, Stolzenburg JU (2009) Neuroanatomy of the male pelvis in respect to radical prostatectomy including three-dimensional visualization. BJU Int 105:21–27
3. Stolzenburg JU, Rabenalt R, Tannapfel A, Liatsikos EN (2006) Intrafascial nerve-sparing endoscopic extraperitoneal radical prostatectomy. Urology 67:17–21
4. Stolzenburg JU, Rabenalt R, Do M, Schwalenberg T et al (2008) Intrafascial nerve-sparing endoscopic extraperitoneal radical prostatectomy. Eur Urol 53:931–940
5. Stolzenburg JU, Gettman MT, Liatsikos E (2007) Endoscopic Extraperitoneal radical Prostatectomy: Laparoscopic and Robot-Assisted Surgery. Springer, Berlin
6. Stolzenburg J-U, Kallidonis P, Do M et al (2010) A comparison of outcomes for interfascial and interfascial nerve-sparing radical prostatectomy. Urology 76:743–751

3

3.12.2 Robot-Assisted Extraperitoneal Radical Prostatectomy

Ingolf A. Tuerk, Evangelos Liatsikos, Panagiotis Kallidonis, Christopher Anderson, Jens-Uwe Stolzenburg

Introduction

Robot-assisted extraperitoneal laparoscopic radical prostatectomy (eRALP) provides access to the prostate without interfering with the peritoneal cavity [1]. Thus, bowel-related complications are minimised [2,3]. Nevertheless, the decision between a transperitoneal or extraperitoneal approach to robot-assisted prostatectomy remains the surgeon's [1].

Indications, Contra-indications, Preoperative Preparation

See Sect. 3.12.1.

Step 1: Patient position and development of extraperitoneal space

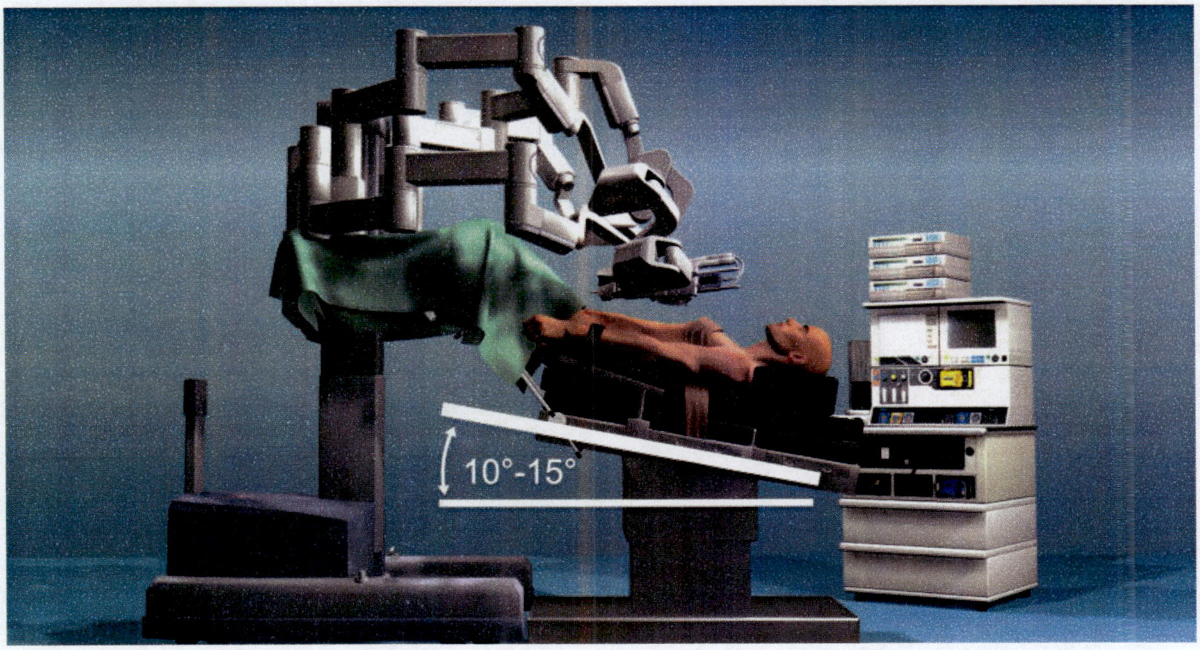

The patient is in the supine position with the legs slightly abducted so that the robotic system can be positioned between them. An infraumbilical incision laterally to the midline is continued down to the posterior rectus sheath and a balloon trocar is inserted to prepare the extraperitoneal space of Retzius (see Sect. 3.4).

Step 2: Trocar placement

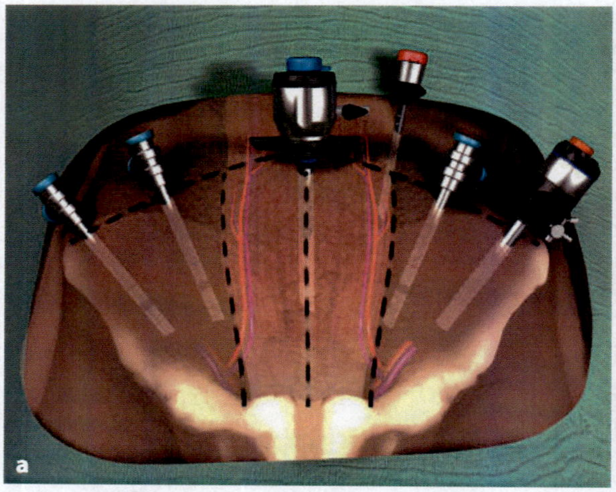

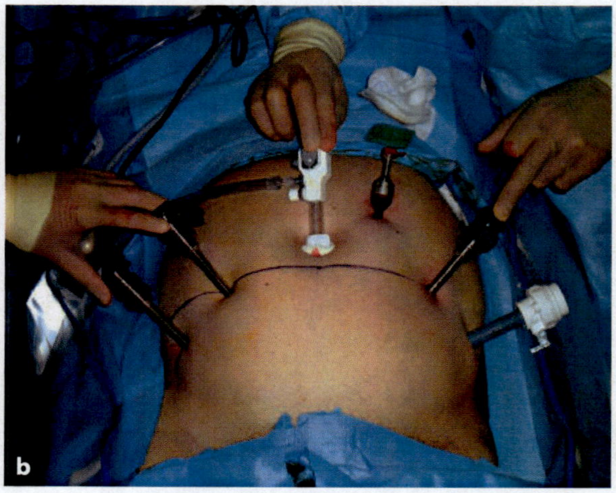

The camera trocar (12 mm) is placed at the site of the initial incision. The arrangement of the trocars for the extraperitoneal approach is different from the transperitoneal approach. Despite the use of the six-port technique for radical prostatectomy, the two working robotic trocars inserted on both lateral edges of the rectus muscle are placed in a 2-cm caudal position in comparison to the one used for the transperitoneal approach. The assistant working trocars are placed on the same sites. On the assistant's lateral right trocar, a fourth robotic arm could be docked if a four-arm robotic system is available.

Step 3: Development of the extraperitoneal space and insertion of the remaining trocars

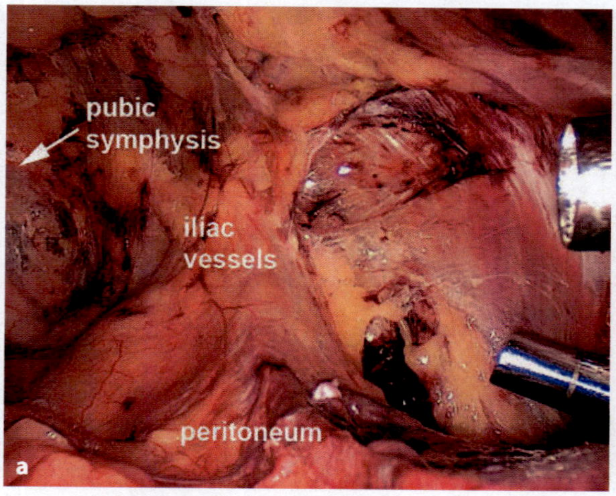

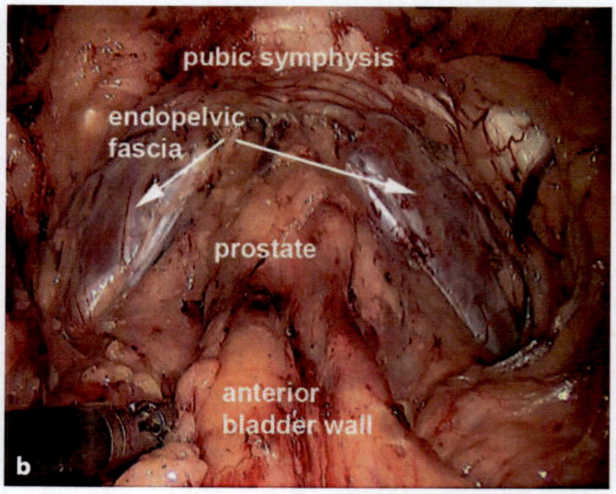

Conventional laparoscopic instruments are used for the gradual extension of the extraperitoneal space to both sides in an attempt to create more space for the insertion of the lateral right and left trocars. Alternatively, the camera could be used with careful sweeping moves to develop these spaces and the trocars are inserted afterwards. Step 3a shows the extended extraperitoneal space to the right. Docking of the robotic arms follows, and the retropubic space is developed along with the endopelvic fascia using gentle sweeping movements (Step 3b).

Step 4: Pelvic lymph node dissection

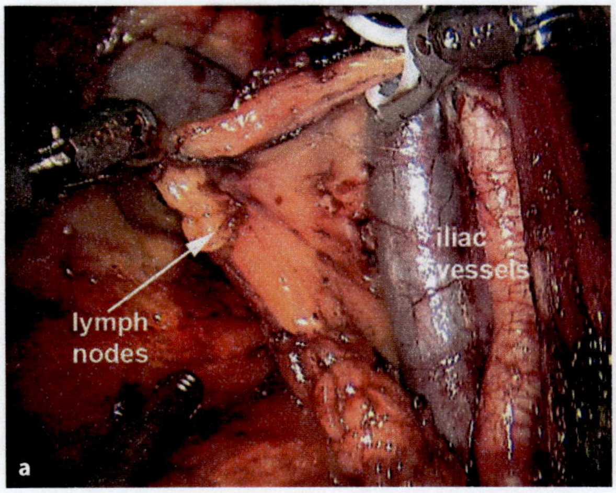

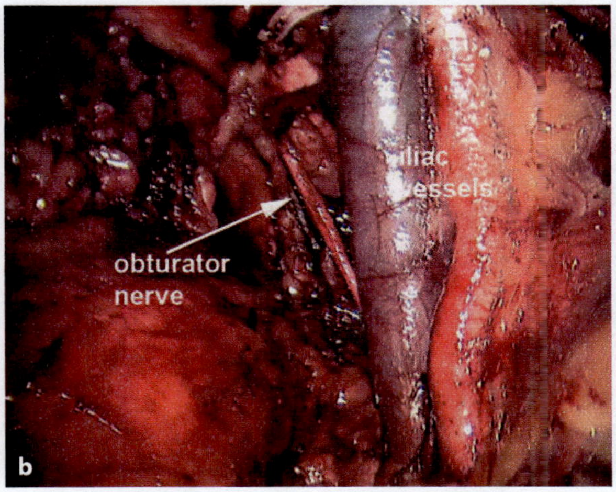

Pelvic lymph nodes are dissected when indicated. The procedure usually precedes the prostatectomy but can be done afterwards. The fatty tissue overlying the iliac vessels and located in the obturator fossa is carefully excised. A combination of the clips and coagulation is used for the ligation of lymph vessels (Step 4a). Lymph node dissection leaves iliac vessels and obturator fossa free of fatty tissue (Step 4b). The iliac, obturator and epigastric vessels as well as the obturator nerve interfere with the operative field. Thus, the one robotic arm gently retracts the aforementioned structures while the other dissects the fatty tissue. The use of the four-arm system for retraction should be considered.

Step 5: Preparation of dorsal venous complex

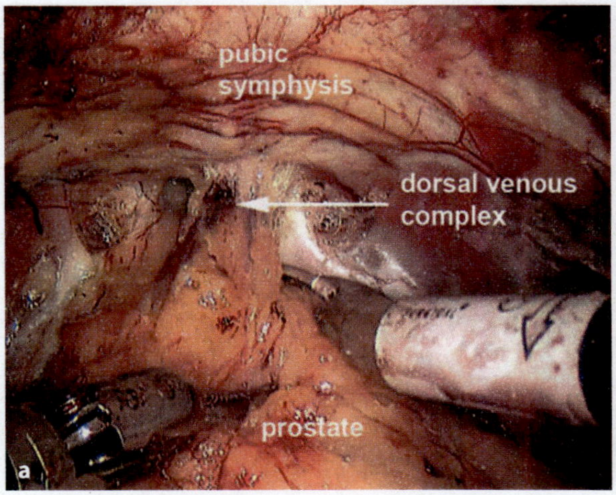

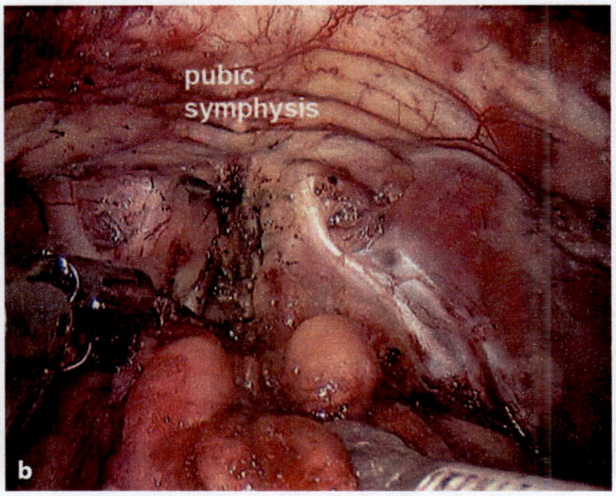

Step 5a presents the dissection of the fatty tissue overlying the dorsal venous complex. Superficial branches of the dorsal venous complex are ligated using coagulation (Step 5b). At this point, the fourth arm is used for the retraction of the bladder in the dorsal direction. Otherwise, the bladder could be retracted by the assistant in the same direction using laparoscopic graspers. The dissection should remain on a superficial plane as the underlying dorsal venous complex is a site of significant bleeding during radical prostatectomy.

Step 6: Incision of the endopelvic fascia

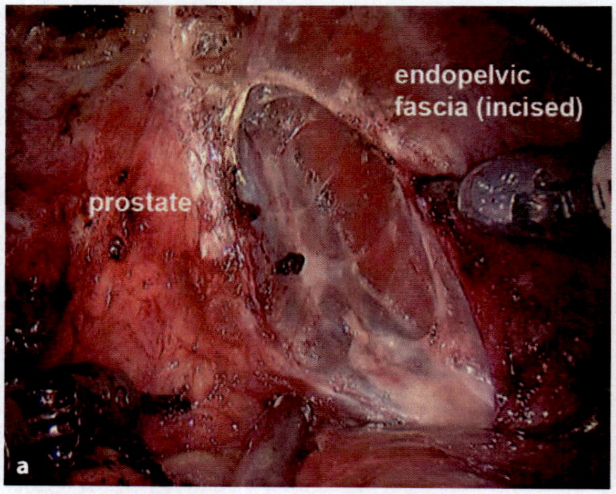

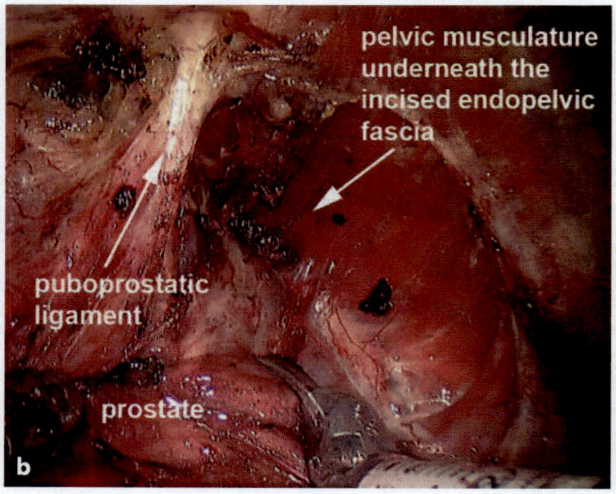

The endopelvic fascia is incised to reveal the lateral aspect of the prostate and the underlying pelvic floor musculature (Step 6a). The incision of the endopelvic fascia is a point distinguishing the interfascial from the intrafascial technique for nerve preservation during radical prostatectomy. The endopelvic fascia is not incised during the intrafascial approach and the latter fascia is preserved along with the remaining fascias surrounding the prostate as well as the neurovascular bundles. Step 6b demonstrates the incision of the endopelvic fascia to be carried anteriorly towards the dorsal venous complex.

Step 7: Dissection of the puboprostatic ligaments

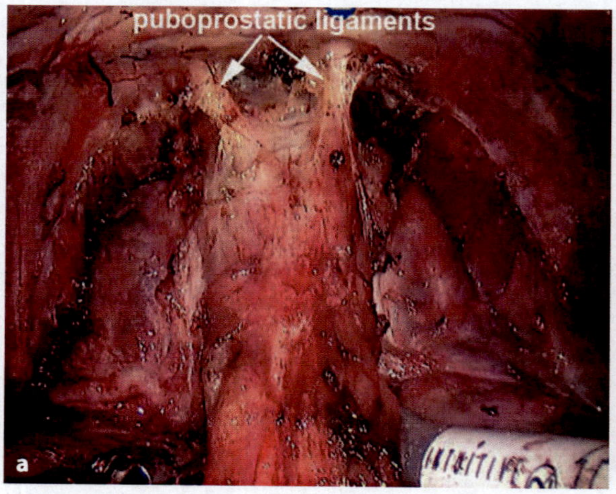

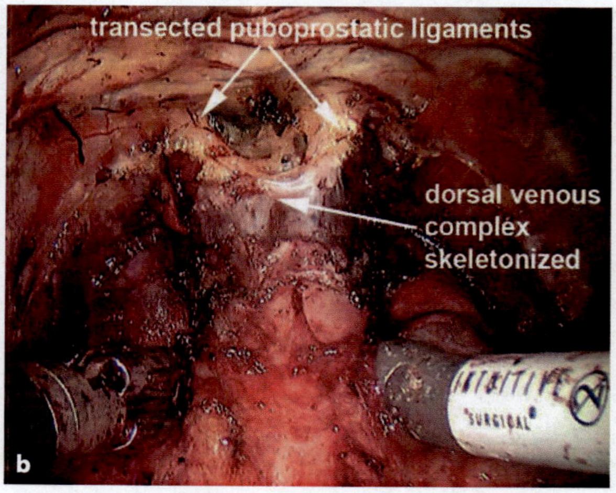

The endopelvic fascia has been dissected to the dorsal venous complex in Step 7a. The puboprostatic ligaments can be preserved in an attempt to improve early postoperative continence. Nevertheless, the effect of puboprostatic ligament preservation in continence remains a controversial issue in the literature. The intrafascial nerve-sparing technique also preserves the puboprostatic ligaments. The authors favour preserving the ligaments since their experience shows that early continence is improved. Step 7b shows the puboprostatic ligaments to be transected and the dorsal venous complex prepared for ligation.

Step 8: Ligation of the dorsal venous plexus (Santorini plexus)

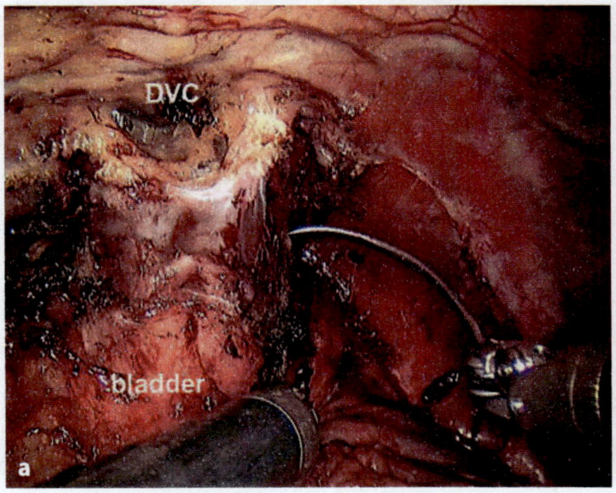

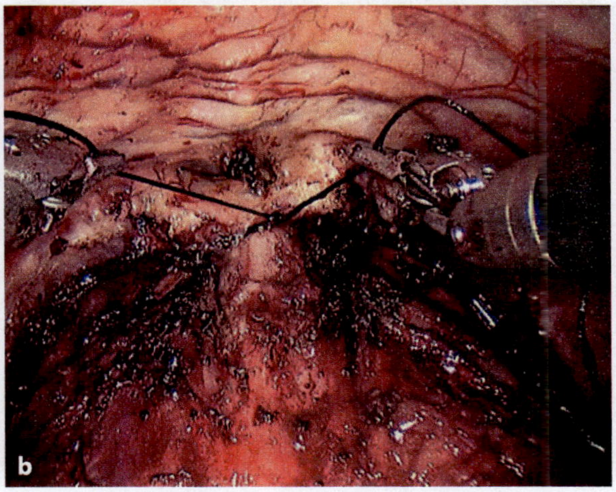

A 0 Vicryl suture on a CT-1 needle is guided from right to left between the dorsal venous complex and the anterior urethral wall (Step 8a). An intracorporal knot is tied and the ligation of the Santorini plexus is achieved (Step 8b). The efficient preparation of the Santorini plexus prior to its ligation is important for the adequate ligation of the plexus and the prevention of urethral injury. A second suture can be placed if deemed necessary. The fourth arm should retract the prostate in the dorsal and cephalad direction during the ligation of the plexus.

Step 9: Bladder neck dissection

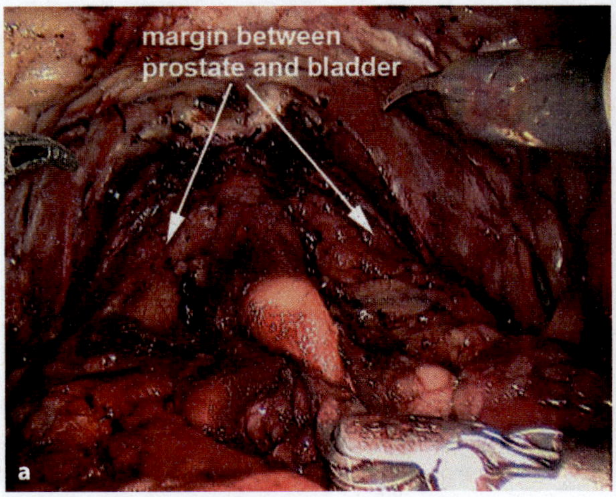

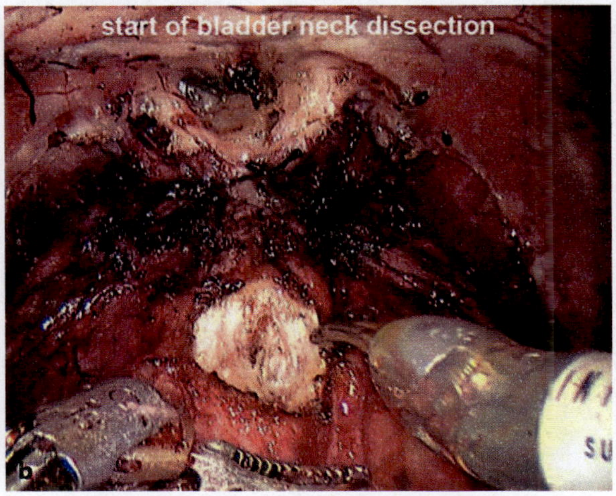

The fourth arm of the robotic system facilitates the visualisation of the margin between the prostate and the bladder by grasping of the bladder and providing tension (Step 9a). If the margin is not clear, an inflated urethral catheter balloon could be moved in the bladder lumen by the assistant. The latter manoeuvre facilitates the identification of the margin. The dissection of the bladder neck starts at the 12 o'clock position and progresses along the margin between the prostate and the bladder in an effort to depict the longitudinal musculature of the bladder neck (Step 9b).

Step 10: Incision of bladder neck

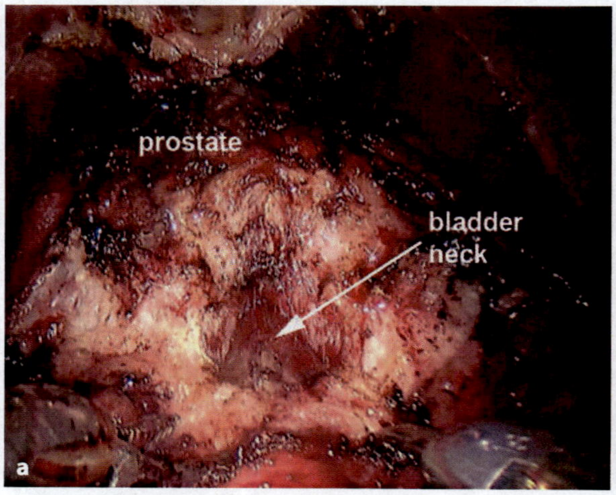

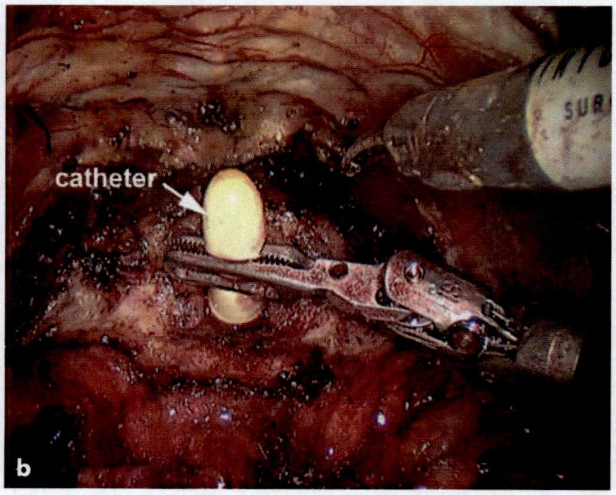

Step 10a shows the elongation of the incision of the bladder neck from 10 o'clock to the 2 o'clock position. The dissection is guided by the longitudinal musculature of the bladder. When the anterior portion of the bladder neck is dissected, the urethral catheter is revealed, allowing the fourth arm to grasp the catheter (Step 10b) and retract it ventrally. The urethral catheter represents a landmark for the dissection of the posterior bladder neck and the spermatic vesicles. The preservation of the bladder neck is possible by gradual dissection in small steps alternatively on both sides.

Step 11: Preparation for the dissection of the posterior bladder neck

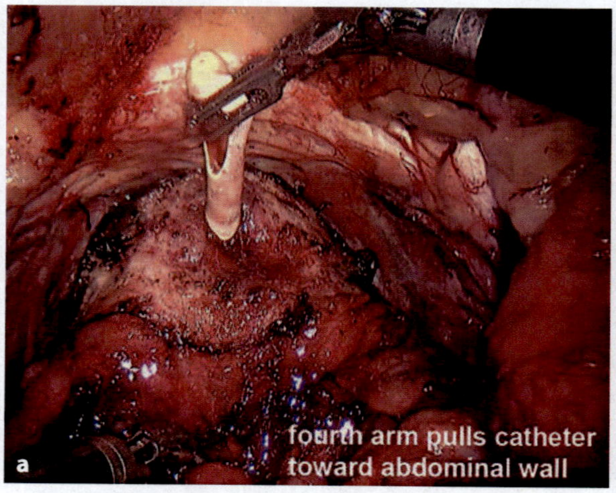

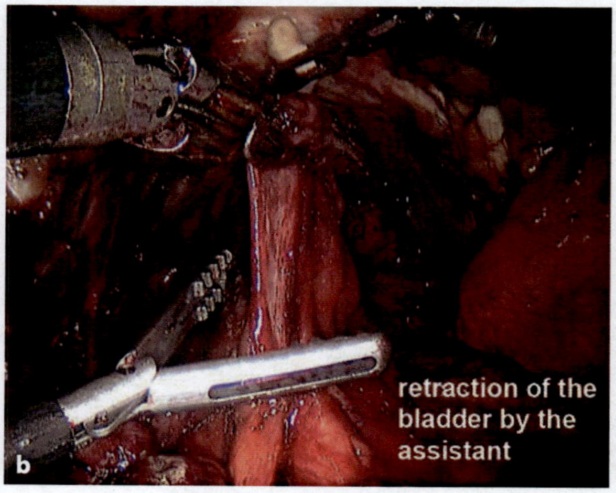

Step 11a shows the ventral retraction of the urethral catheter, which puts the prostate and the surrounding structures under tension. The catheter is pulled ventrally and at the same time the catheter is stabilised on its external side on the operating table draping. Thus, greater tension can be applied on the catheter and its surrounding structures. A conventional laparoscopic grasper is used by the assistant to provide traction to the bladder, facilitating the dissection of the posterior segment of the bladder neck (Step 11b).

Step 12: Dissection of the posterior bladder neck

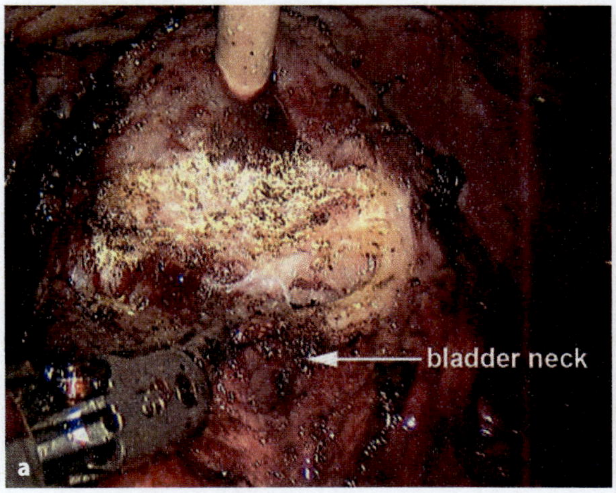

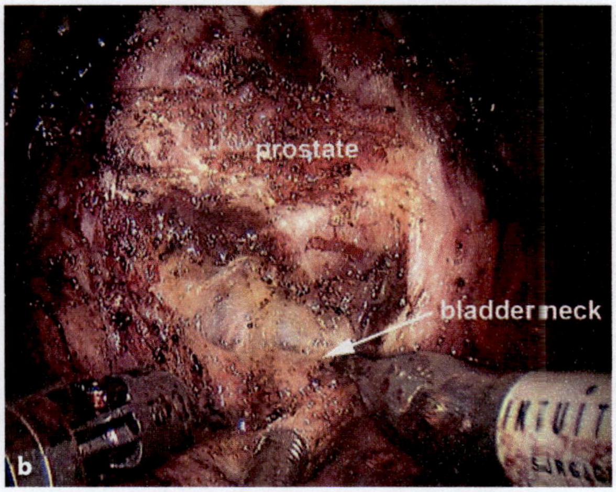

The dissection of the posterior bladder neck follows. It is important for the dissection to be performed through the correct plane because it is easy to dissect the posterior of the prostate or the posterior bladder wall. Step 12a demonstrates the semicircular dissection of the posterior bladder neck, which should be done in a stepwise fashion. The dissection is continued towards the posterior of the prostate and bladder neck aiming to expose the seminal vesicles (Step 12b). The identification of the seminal vesicles designates the complete dissection of the posterior bladder neck.

Step 13: Preparation of the seminal vesicles

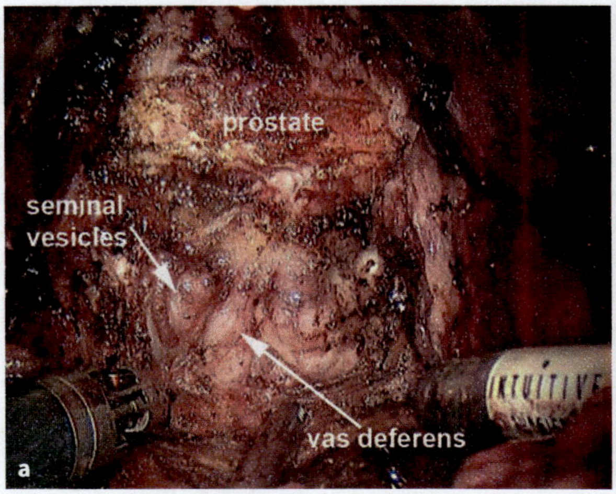

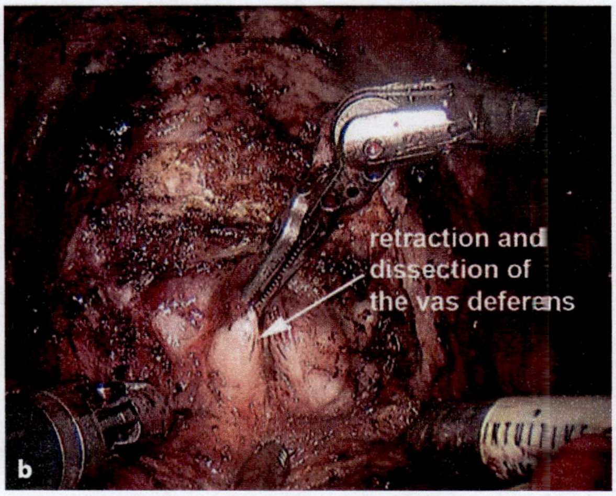

The ampullae and seminal vesicles are mobilised with sharp and blunt dissection. In Step 13a, the seminal vesicles and the vas deferens are identified. The fourth arm is used for the retraction of the vas deferens (Step 13b). The latter manoeuvre provides exposure of the ipsilateral vesicle, which is prepared using blunt and sharp dissection. The vas deferens is also transected. Care is taken to avoid any injury to the pelvic plexus and the neurovascular bundle, which run in close proximity to the tips of the seminal vesicles. Thus, the preservation of the tips of the seminal vesicles should be considered for nerve-sparing prostatectomy.

Step 14: Mobilisation of the seminal vesicles

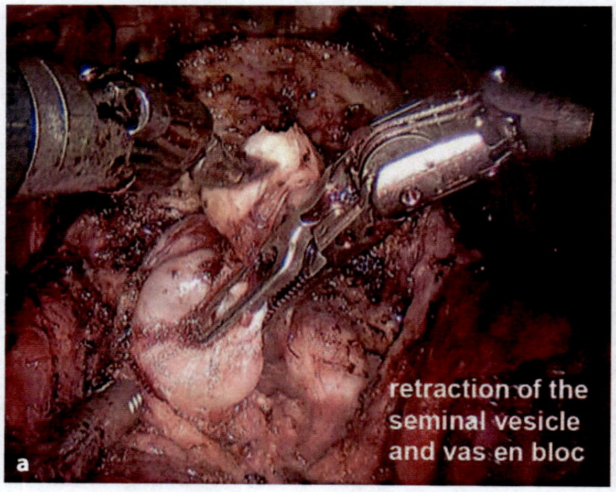

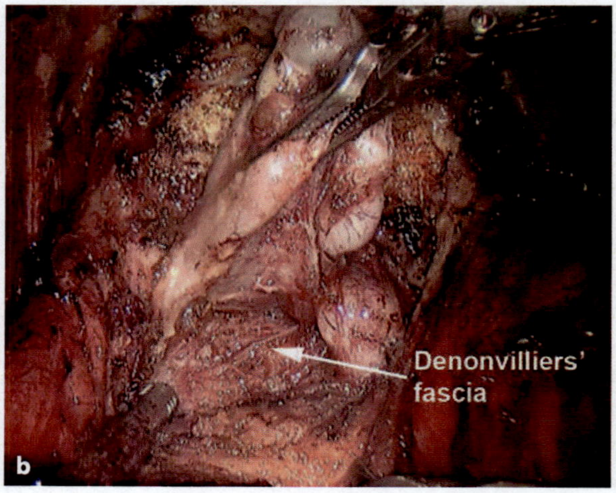

As the seminal vesicles are released from their attachments, the fourth arm is useful to provide traction by grasping the seminal vesicles and retracting them in a ventral direction. Step 14a shows the use of the fourth robotic arm for the latter manoeuvre, The mobilisation and retraction of the one seminal vesicle is followed by the mobilisation of the contralateral vesicle. The ventral retraction of both vesicles reveals the Denonvilliers fascia (Step 14b). The fourth arm is used for the retraction. The Denonvilliers fascia is a natural barrier for extending the dissection towards the prostatic apex.

Step 15: Stripping down the Denonvilliers fascia

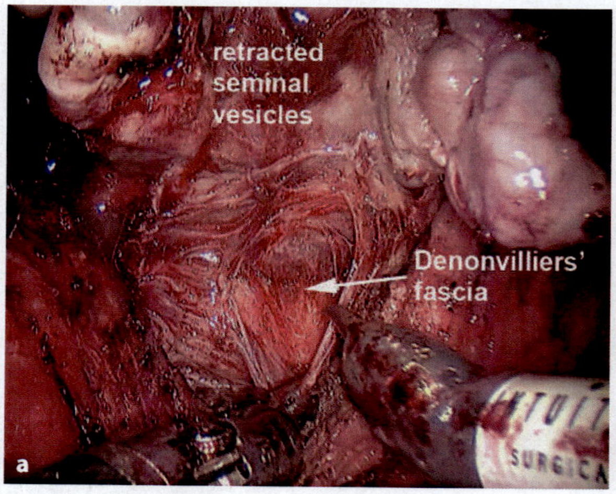

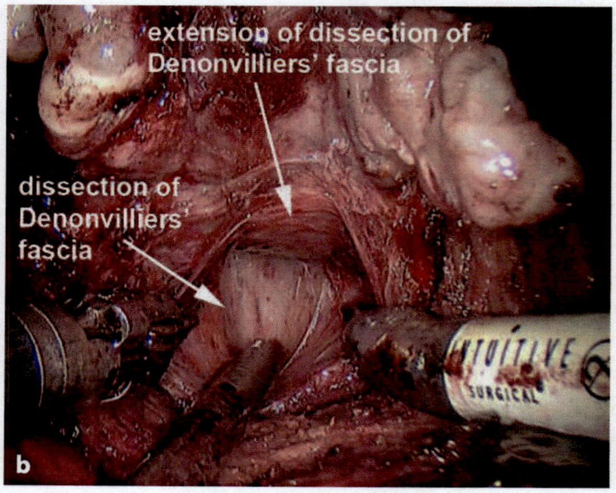

The Denonvilliers fascia is accessible after the mobilisation of the seminal vesicles (Step 15a). Blunt dissection and stripping down of the fascia from the prostate takes place (intrafascial plane). The dissection remains strictly in the midline in order to avoid injury to the neurovascular bundles while the plane is directed towards the apex of the prostate (Step 15b). The rectum should be mobilised away from the prostate as extensively as possible since the latter step is important for the preservation of the neurovascular bundles later.

Step 16: Dissection of the prostatic pedicles

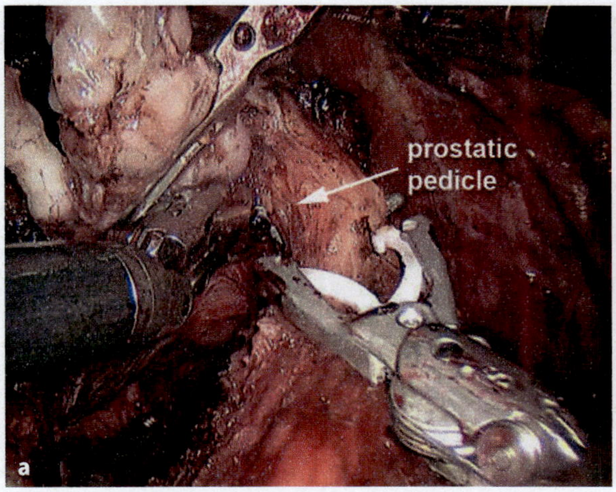

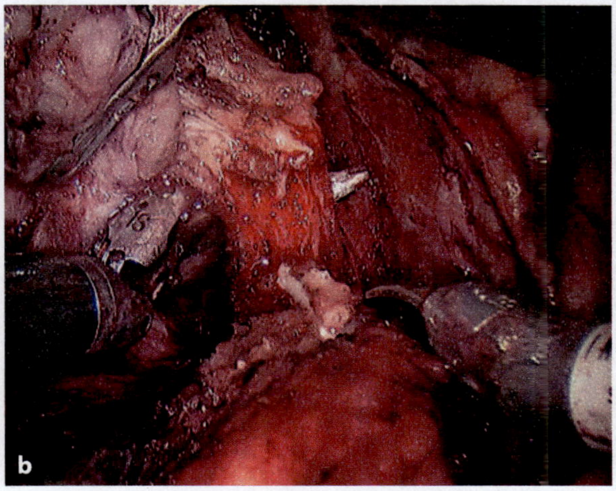

The prostate is still attached by the pedicles and the apex. The incision of the endopelvic fascia and the blunt dissection of Denonvilliers fascia created two planes to facilitate prostatic pedicle dissection. The shiny surface of the prostatic capsule is clearly seen medially and laterally. The fourth arm is used to retract the seminal vesicles ventrally, allowing clear exposure of the prostatic pedicle.

The prostatic pedicles are then clipped and cut in stepwise fashion (Step 16a). The pedicles should be divided between clips and the cutting should be performed in small steps directly on the surface of the prostatic capsule in an attempt to prevent inadvertent injury to the ipsilateral neurovascular bundle (Step 16b).

Step 17: Development of the neurovascular bundles

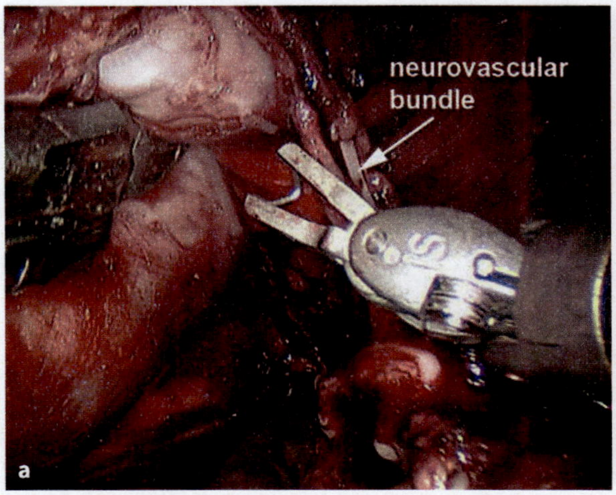

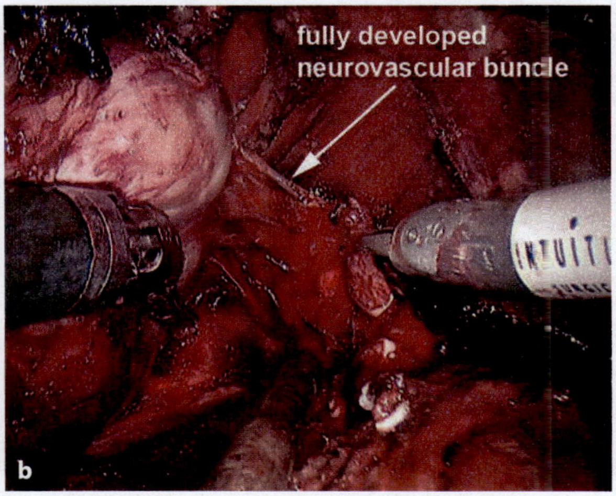

When the dissection of the opposite prostatic pedicles is completed, the prostate is mobilised from the neurovascular bundle towards the apex. Retracting the prostate to the opposite side facilitates dissection. The use of energy-free dissecting instruments is advisable. Step 17a shows the application of metal clips (5 mm) on the neurovascular bundle (NVB) in an attempt to provide haemostasis. The cutting of the bundle follows. The gradual development of the NVB using clips prior to cutting provides adequate haemostasis. Coagulation, which could result in damage to the NVB, is prevented. Step 17b shows a fully developed NVB up to the level of the prostatic apex.

Step 18: Dissection of the dorsal venous plexus

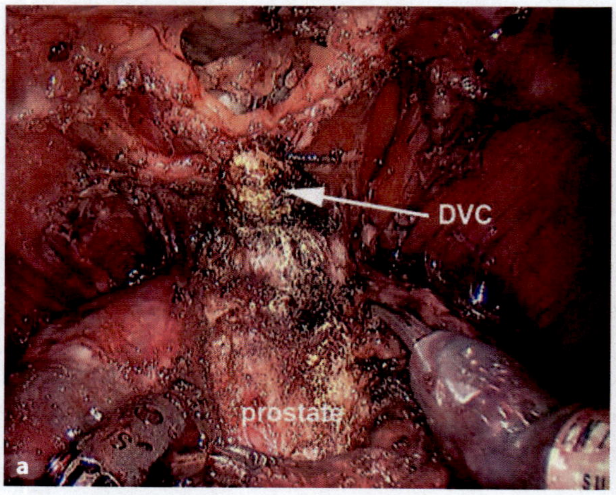

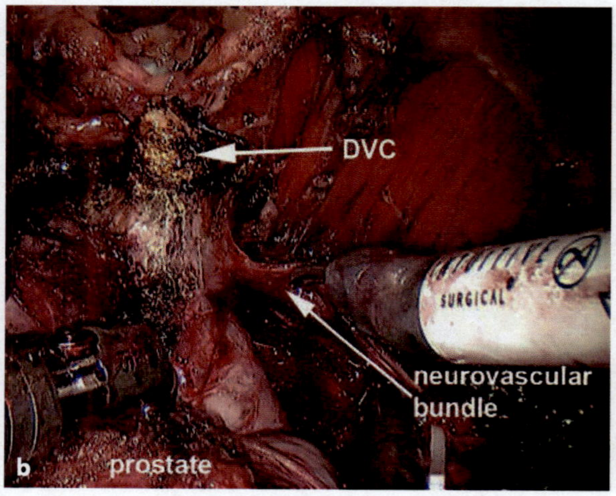

The prostate from the urethra is sharply dissected at the apex when the prostate is released from its surrounding fascias, the bladder, prostatic pedicles and the neurovascular bundles. The apical dissection starts with the division of the dorsal venous plexus with monopolar scissors (Step 18a). The previously ligated dorsal venous complex is unlikely to bleed. Nevertheless, an additional suture could be used to manage any bleeding. The NVB is carefully released from the apex of the prostate (Step 18b). After the Santorini plexus is divided, the border between the apex of the prostate and the urethra is exposed.

Step 19: Dissection of the urethra

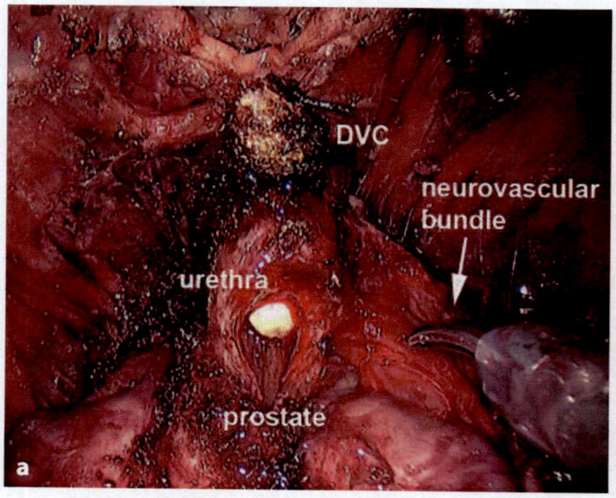

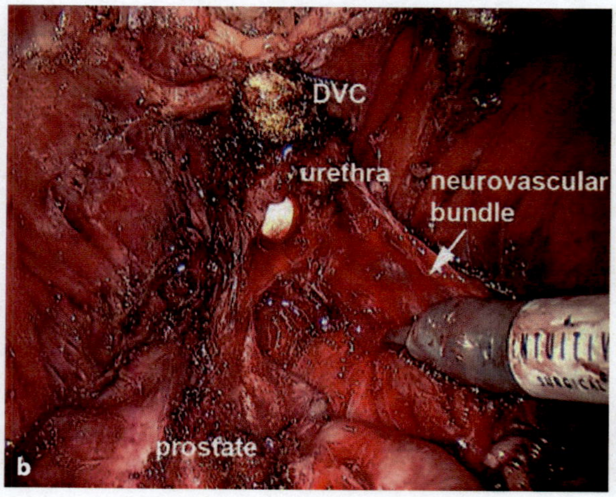

The division of the urethra starts by sharp dissection of the junction between the striated part of the urethral sphincter and the apex of the prostate. The urethra with the external sphincter is dissected from the apex in small carefully performed steps, extending the dissection plane laterally to both sides. The inner smooth layer of urethra becomes visible, is then dissected and the urethral catheter becomes visible. The inner layer should be dissected as close to the prostate as possible in order to preserve urethral length (Step 19b). The posterior urethra is dissected with scissors, while the fourth robotic arm gently retracts the prostate in a cephalad direction.

Step 20: Inspection and haemostasis of the operative field

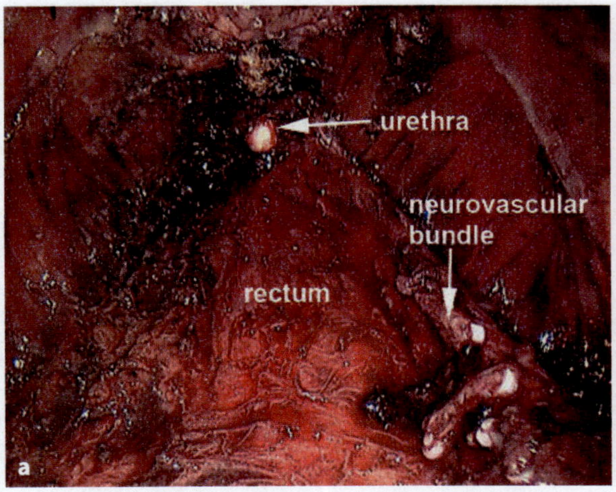

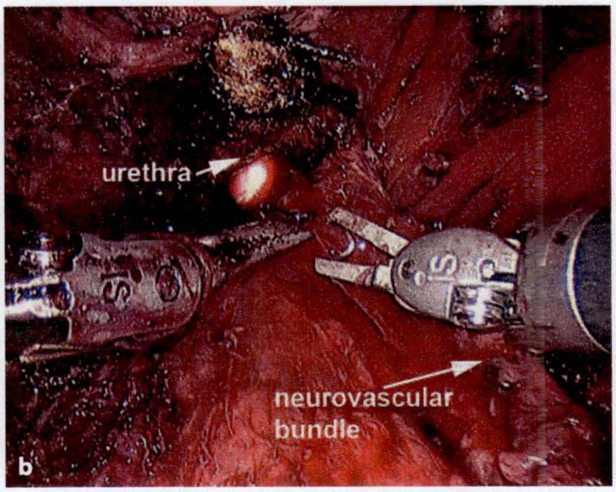

After the complete removal of the prostate, the operative site for the detection of bleeding should be inspected. Step 20a presents a case of unilateral NVB preservation. Note that the right NVB is visible while the left NVB has been excised. Bleeding is evident on the NVB and should be controlled. Clips should be used instead of coagulation in case of bleeding from the NVBs. In addition, haemostatic material (i.e. Tachosil, FloSeal) could be placed on the NVB to prevent bleeding due to venous oozing. Selective suturing of the NVB is also indicated as a haemostatic method.

Step 21: Initial sutures of the vesicourethral anastomosis

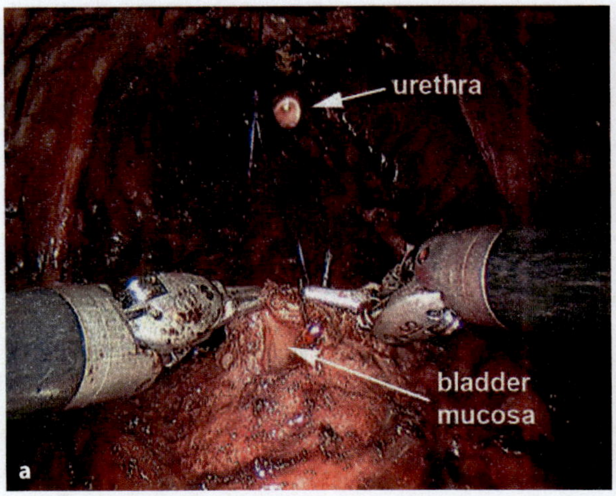

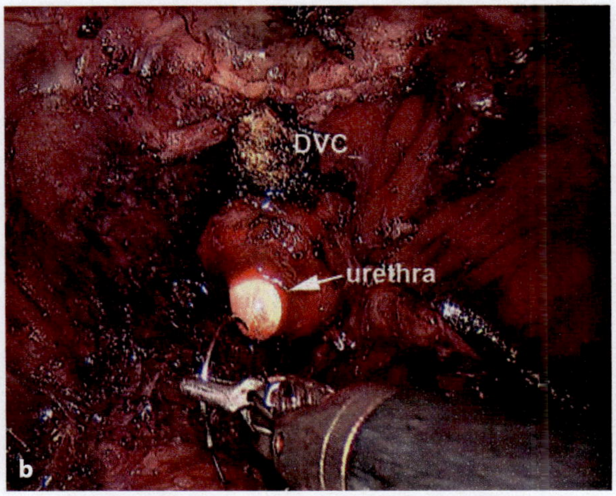

The vesicourethral anastomosis is carried out with continuous suturing. For this purpose, two 3/0 Monocryl sutures with an RB-1 needle have been knotted together with a Lapra-Ty clip at their end. The first stitch is passed through the detrusor muscle of the bladder and the second through the bladder neck (Step 21a). Then the first suture to the urethra is stitched (Step 21b). All stitches are directed from outside to inside at the bladder and from inside to outside at the urethra. Careful manipulation of the needle during suturing is important as the urethra and bladder are delicate structures. The urethral catheter is a landmark for suturing the urethra.

Step 22: Accomplishment of vesicourethral anastomosis

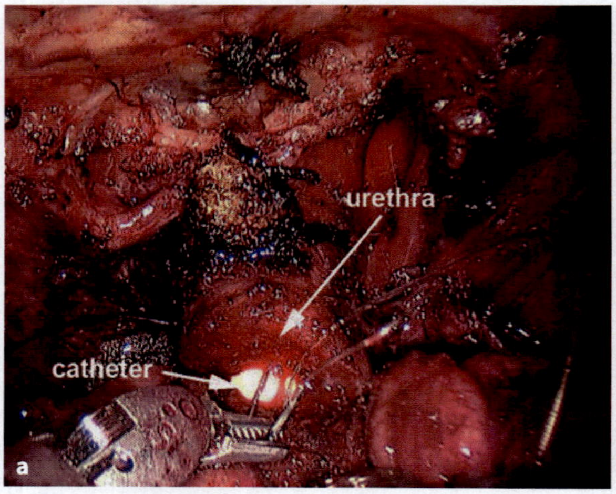

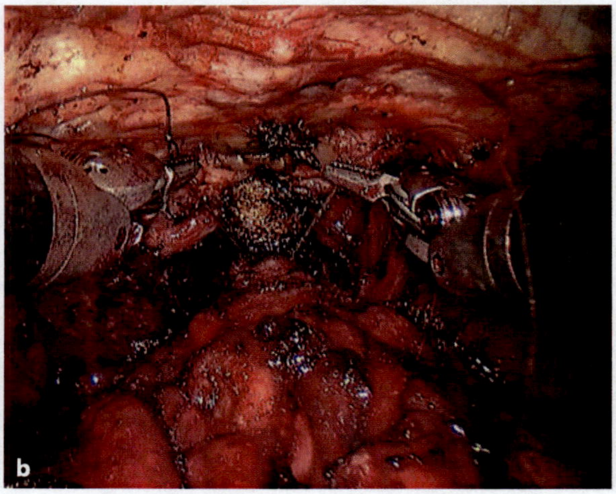

When the first three passes between the bladder and urethra have been performed, the bladder is retracted to the urethra. Each end of the suture is used to complete one side of the anastomosis. The dorsal aspect of the anastomosis is completed and a new silicon urethral catheter is inserted to serve as a guide for the rest of the sutures (Step 22a). Complete suturing of the anastomotic circumference is followed by tying a knot between the two sides of the suture (Step 22b). Saline (approximately 200 cc) is injected through the urethral catheter to check that the anastomosis is watertight.

Step 23: Bladder neck suspension

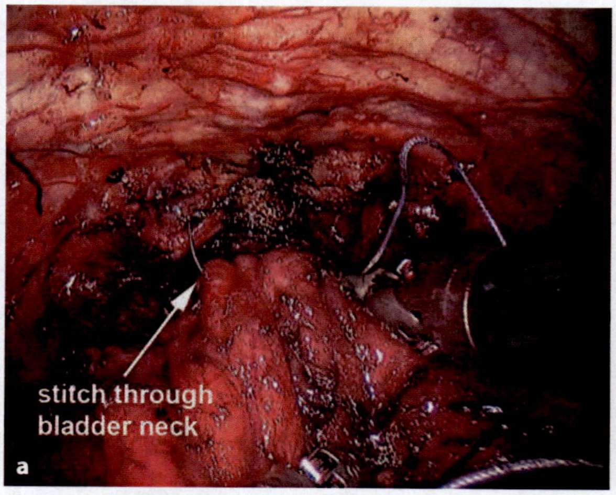

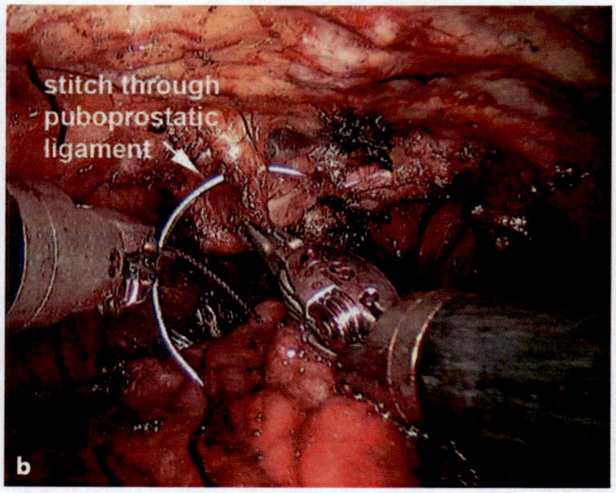

Bladder neck suspension (BNS) has been proposed to improve early postoperative continence after RALP [4]. Although the exact mechanism contributing to continence is unclear, the performance of BNS should be considered. A 2/0 Vicryl suture (SH needle) is passed at the bladder neck (Step 23a) to the puboprostatic ligament (Step 23b) and an intracorporal knot is tied. A 16-F non-suction drain is placed through a 5-mm port. An endoscopic bag containing the specimen is removed through a 12-mm trocar port site. Before the removal of the trocars, the operative field and trocars should always be meticulously inspected for bleeding sites.

Postoperative Management

- Oral or intramuscular analgesia is sufficient
- Drain removal on day 1 postoperatively in case of minimal output
- Fluid diet on the evening of the procedure
- Normal diet and mobilisation of the patient from day 1
- Urinary catheter removed on day 5 after cystography
- Discharge home day 3
- Pelvic floor exercises are advisable
- Initiation of phosphodiesterase 5 inhibitors could be considered

References

1. Atug F, Castle EP, Woods M, Srivastav SK, Thomas R, Davis R (2006) Transperitoneal versus extraperitoneal robotic-assisted radical prostatectomy: is one better than the other? Urology 68:1077–1081
2. Atug F, Thomas R (2007) Transperitoneal versus extraperitoneal robotic-assisted radical prostatectomy: which one? Minerva Urol Nefrol 59:143–147
3. Madi R, Daignault S, Wood DP (2007) Extraperitoneal vs intraperitoneal robotic prostatectomy: analysis of operative outcomes. J Endourol 21:1553–1557
4. Patel VR, Coehlo RF, Palmer KJ, Rocco B (2009) Periurethral suspension stitch during robotic-assisted laparoscopic radical prostatectomy: description of the technique and continence outcomes. Eur Urol 56:472–478

Chapter 4

Paediatric Urology

CONTENTS

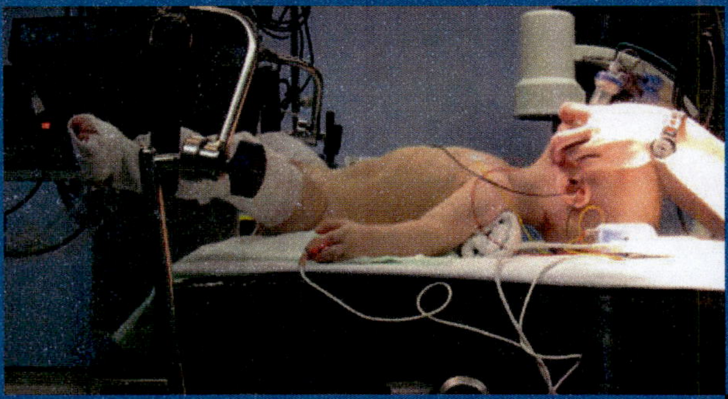

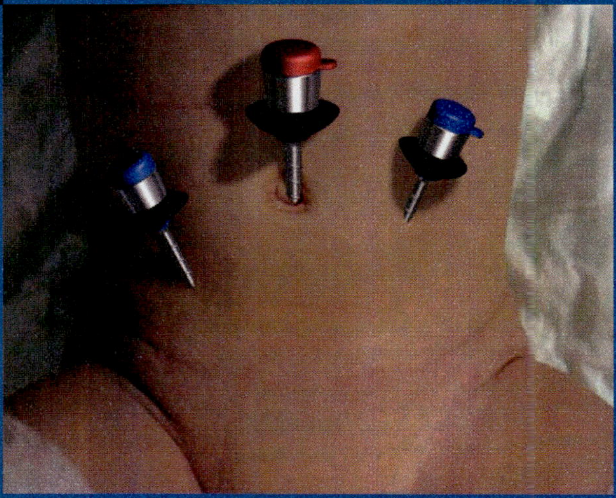

J.-U. Stolzenburg, I. Türk, E. Liatsikos: *Laparoscopic and Robot-Assisted Surgery in Urology*
DOI: 10.1007/978-3-642-00891-7_4, © Springer-Verlag Berlin Heidelberg 2011

4.1 Pyeloplasty

Holger Till, Jens-Uwe Stolzenburg

Introduction

Laparoscopic dismembered pyeloplasty was first described in 1993 and has gained increasing popularity since then [1, 2]. Today pediatric urologists all over the world consider this procedure feasible and safe even in children younger than 1 year of age. However, not only small instruments (2–3 mm) are required, but also the surgical expertise in suturing in very limited spaces. Whether a pyeloplasty should be approached laparo- or retroperitoneoscopically continues to be the subject of lively debate [1, 3, 4]. Some authors argue that transgression of the peritoneal cavity entails distinct disadvantages. They indeed are performing a minimal invasive pyeloplasty in the retroperitoneum with great success [5]. However, range of motion is limited, especially in smaller children, due to the small space between the 12th rib and the iliac crest. The following description will focus on the laparoscopic transperitoneal approach.

Indications

- International standards for pelvic–ureteric junction obstruction (PUJO)

Contra-indications

- Cardiac defects
- Multiple abdominal operations

Preoperative Preparation

- Empty urinary bladder (bladder catheterisation)
- Single-shot antibiotics

4

Step 1: Patient position and trocar placement

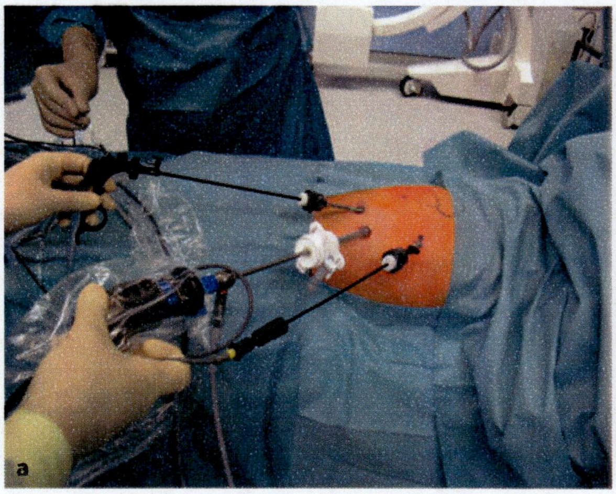

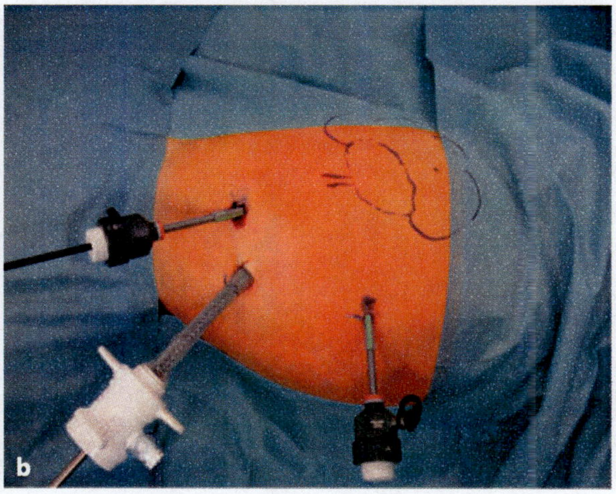

The patient is positioned in a semilateral position (Step 1a) and secured to the table with straps so that additional tilting is possible. The surgeon and the assistant stand on the contra-lateral side. Through a periumbilical incision, a 5-mm port and a 30° laparoscope are inserted. Pneumoperitoneum is maintained at 10–12 mmHg. Two additional 3-mm ports are inserted in the midline between the umbilicus and xiphoid, as well as in the ipsilateral lower quadrant (Step 1b). In a right-sided PUJO, a fourth port may be necessary to elevate the liver. Most surgeons would place this in the left upper quadrant.

Step 2: Mobilisation of the renal pelvis and resection of the PUJO

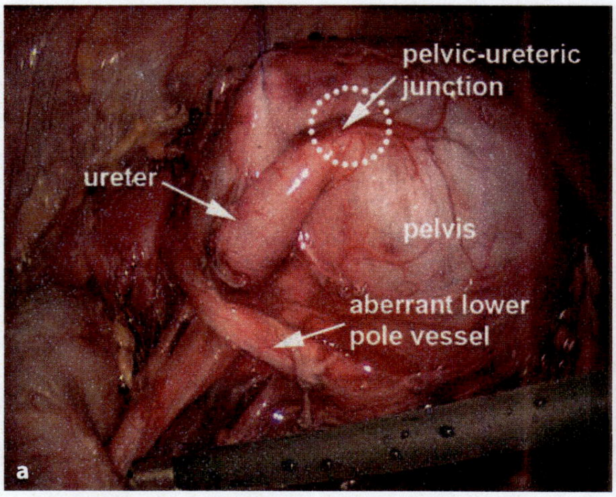

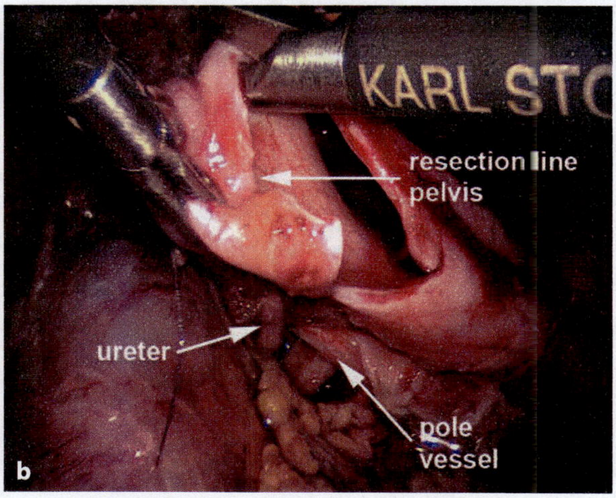

The colonic flexure is mobilised, the Gerota fascia is opened and the pelvic–ureteric junction (PUJ) is identified. At this point, a hitch stitch may be advisable, which elevates and stabilises the renal pelvis (Step 2a): A 4/0 monofilament suture over a straight needle is introduced percutaneously, passed through the lower pole of the renal pelvis and returned outside. If an aberrant lower pole vessel is suspected, this should be clarified at this point. A loop around these vessels may be helpful. Furthermore, a 6/0 Vicryl stitch to the medial border of the ureter below the PUJO may be advisable to facilitate orientation and minimal tissue trauma during later dissection. The renal pelvis is opened above the obstruction (Step 2b). The redundant renal pelvis is excised.

Step 3: Ureteric mobilisation, vessel transposition and ureteric spatulation

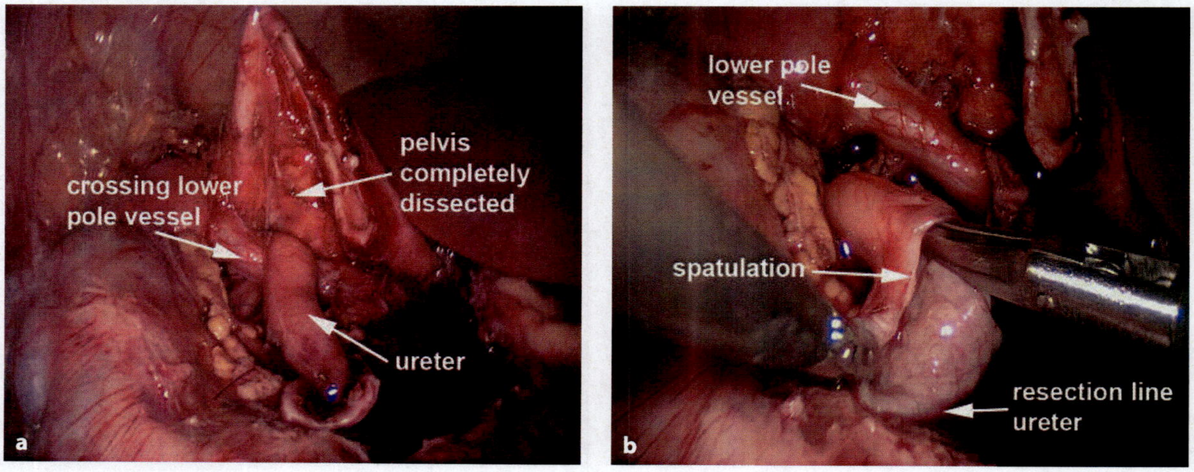

In cases of an aberrant lower pole vessel, which crosses the ureter (Step 3a), the ureter must now be transposed to the front. After the PUJO is resected, the ureter is transposed, spatulated and anastomosed (Step 3b). Alternatively, some authors leave the PUJO attached at this point of the operation and spatulate it as well, before resecting it later during the pyeloplasty. Atraumatic manipulation of the ureter is very important and may be achieved by handling it with the marking stitch or atraumatic forceps.

Step 4: Performing the pyeloplasty

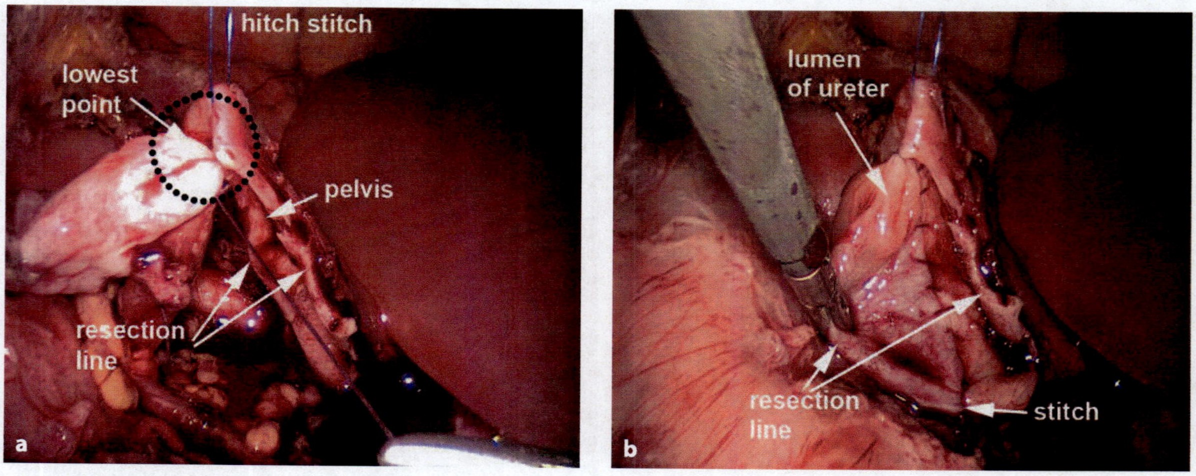

For the pyeloplasty, we prefer a running suture of the posterior wall. Therefore, a 5/0 or 6/0 suture on a 3/8 needle (passing through a 3.5-mm trocar) is introduced (length, 12–15 cm). The anastomosis between the reduced pelvis and the spatulated ureter is started at the lowest (most distal) point, taking an outside-in/inside-out stitch, as depicted in Step 4a. After passing the needle from behind the knot to the front, the reconstruction is continued with an outside-in-outside stitch on the posterior wall and then continued in a running fashion until the final knot is placed on the outside (Step 4b).

Step 5: Ureteric stent insertion

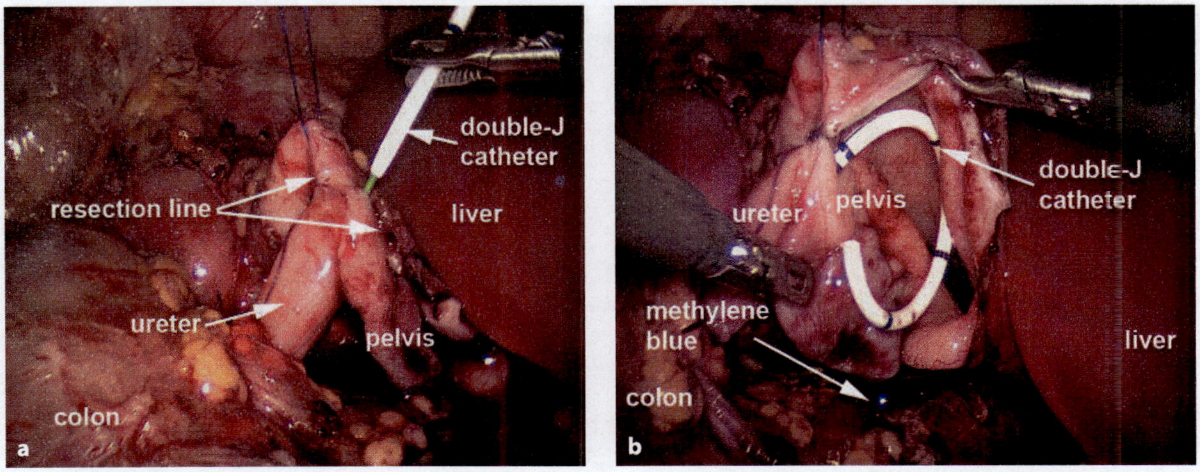

The decision "to stent or not to stent" should not depend on the laparoscopic approach, but on the surgeon's preference in general. The authors prefer a transanastomotic, internal double-J stent, which is employed after completion of the posterior wall. To achieve this, a flexible guidewire is inserted transabdominally into the proximal ureter and advanced into the bladder. A 4-F or 5-F double-J stent (depending on the child's size) is passed over the guidewire into the bladder (Step 5a). The proximal end of the double-J stent is placed in the renal pelvis (Step 5B). An intravesical position is confirmed by fluoroscopy or filling the bladder with methylene blue and watching for blue-coloured urine dripping out of the stent.

Step 6: Completion of pyeloplasty

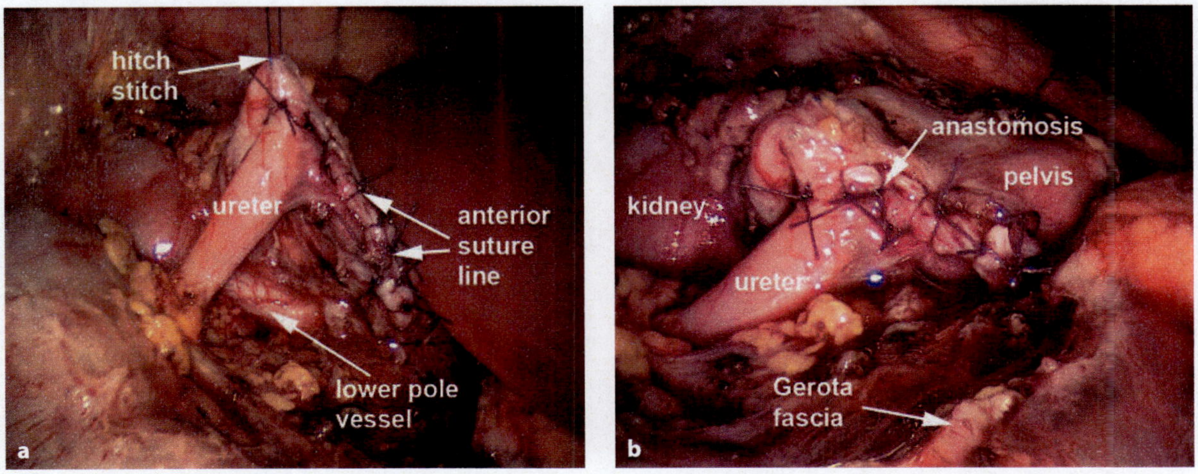

The anterior portion of the pyeloplasty is completed with a continuous or interrupted suture (Step 6a; note the posterior position of the lower pole vessels). The hitch stitch is released and the pyeloplasty is inspected to ensure that there is no anastomotic tension or kinking (Step 6b). If the anastomosis appears to be watertight, a retroperitoneal drain can be placed but is not necessary. Instead, the Gerota fascia can be used to cover the pyeloplasty.

Postoperative Management

- Mobilisation and feeding on the day of surgery
- Analgesia until discharge
- Antibiotic prophylaxis until the double pigtail stent is removed 3–4 weeks after surgery
- MAG3 diuretic renal renography 3 months after removal of the stent

References

1. Eden CG (2007) Minimally invasive treatment of ureteropelvic junction obstruction: a critical analysis of results. Eur Urol 52:983–989
2. Janetschek G, Peschel R, Frauscher F (2000) Laparoscopic pyeloplasty. Urol Clin North Am 27:695–704
3. Tan HL (1999) Laparoscopic Anderson-Hynes dismembered pyeloplasty in children. J Urol 162:1045–1047
4. Jarrett TW, Chan DY, Charambura TC, Fugita O, Kavoussi LR (2002) Laparoscopic pyeloplasty: the first 100 cases. J Urol 167:1253–1256
5. Yeung CK, Tam YH, Sihoe JD, Lee KH, Liu KW (2001) Retroperitoneoscopic dismembered pyeloplasty for pelvic–ureteric junction obstruction in infants and children. BJU Int 87:509–513

4.2 Laparoscopic Treatment of Impalpable Undescended Testis

Holger Till, Ulrike Waldschmidt

Introduction

Impalpable testis represents a major malformation amongst the spectrum of undescended testis (UDT). This term suggests that the testis may be found intra-abdominally. Consequently, a diagnostic laparoscopy is indicated in order to detect the testis and define its anatomical position [1, 2]. In children with bilateral impalpable testis, the possibility of an intersex should be considered. In unilateral cases, basically three different testicular pathologies can be encountered [3–5]:

a) A blind-ending vas deferens or cordal-like structure with no testicular remnant (also called vanishing testis)
b) A well-developed testis close to the internal inguinal ring (also called peeping testis)
c) A high intra-abdominal testis with short spermatic vessels

Indications

- Any boy with impalpable UDT should undergo laparoscopic exploration, once the clinical examination and an inguinal ultrasound have remained negative. The timing of surgery depends on multiple factors and international guidelines differ considerably. However, it has been widely accepted that the status of the testis should be assessed within the first 12 months of life

Contra-indications

- Multiple abdominal operations are considered as a relative contra-indication (note though that the child in Step 1a, undergoing diagnostic laparoscopy for UDT, had previously had a transverse upper abdominal incision)

Preoperative Preparation

- Usually no elaborate preoperative work-up or patient preparations are necessary. Again, only bilateral cases of impalpable UDT deserve a specific workup for intersex. Most cases can be scheduled as an outpatient procedure. Immediately before starting the laparoscopy, one should empty the urinary bladder

Step 1: Patient position and trocar placement

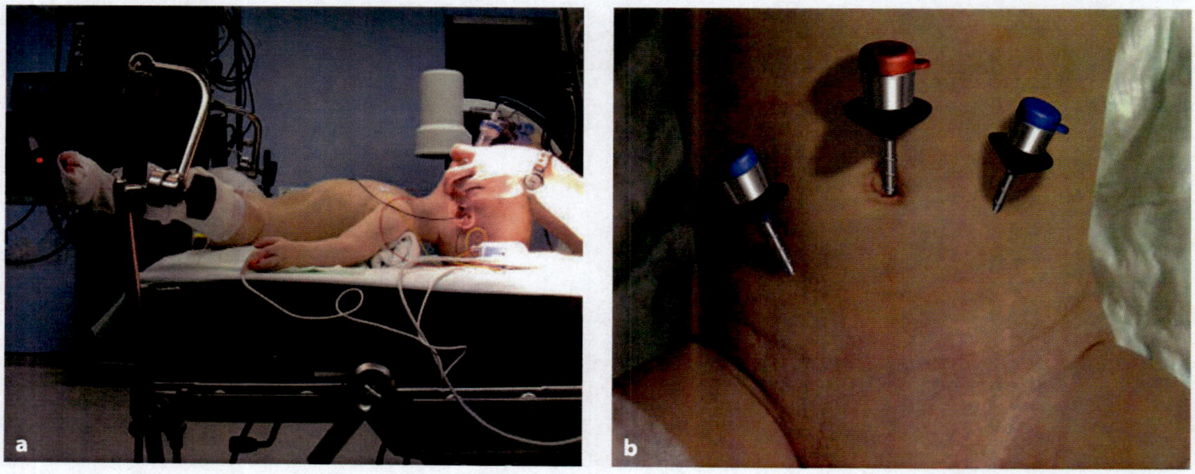

The patient is placed supine. If a Fowler-Stephens orchidopexy (FSO) is planned, it may be advisable to spread the legs in order to gain sterile access to the scrotum. The monitor should be positioned at the patient's feet. Both surgeons stand on the contra-lateral side, close to the child's head. A 3- to 5-mm port and a 30° scope are inserted through a periumbilical incision with pneumoperitoneum at 6–8 mmHg pressure. If the diagnostic inspection reveals a pathology, which requires further manipulation, two more working ports (3 mm) may be employed in the right and left abdomen (Step 1b). Alternatively, a 5-mm single-port device (see Sect. 4.3 on varicocelectomy) or TriPort can be used.

Step 2: Diagnostic laparoscopic findings: vanishing and peeping testis

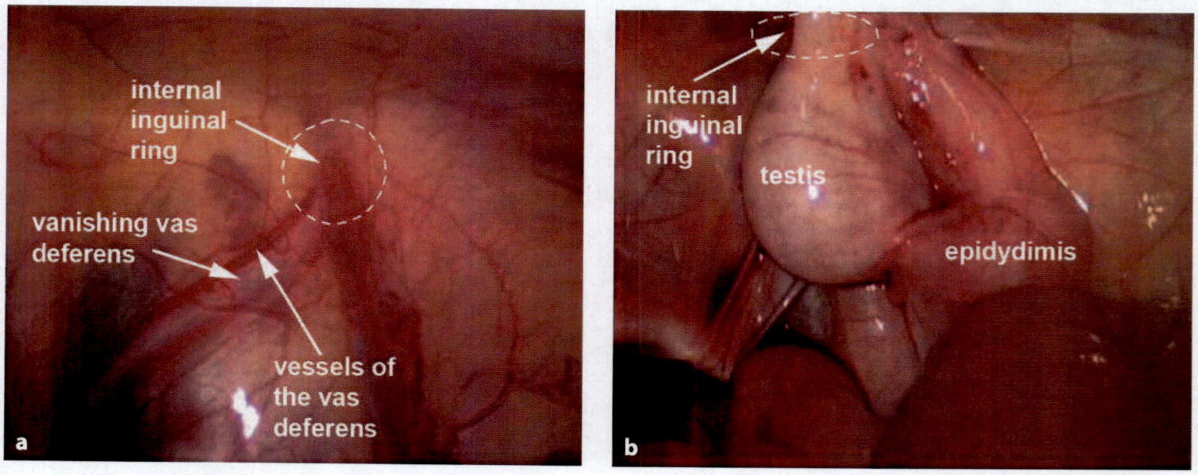

During diagnostic laparoscopy, the testis is identified and its position is assessed. If a vanishing testis is present (as in Step 2a), no further steps are necessary and the procedure can be terminated. If the surgeon has any doubt that the vas deferens does not end blindly but may lead into a testicular remnant within the inguinal canal, he may manipulate the peritoneum close to the vas deferens to visualise the testis. Finally, simultaneous inguinal exploration could be considered. In cases of a so-called peeping testis, which is close to the internal inguinal ring, as seen in Step 2b, simultaneous conventional orchidopexy is recommended.

Step 3: Further variant: high intra-abdominal testis

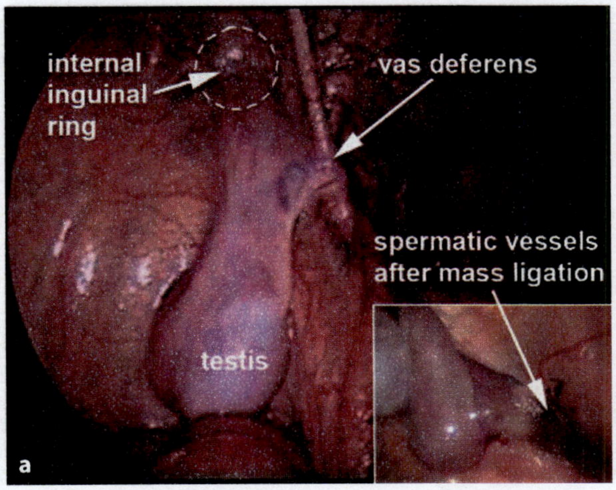

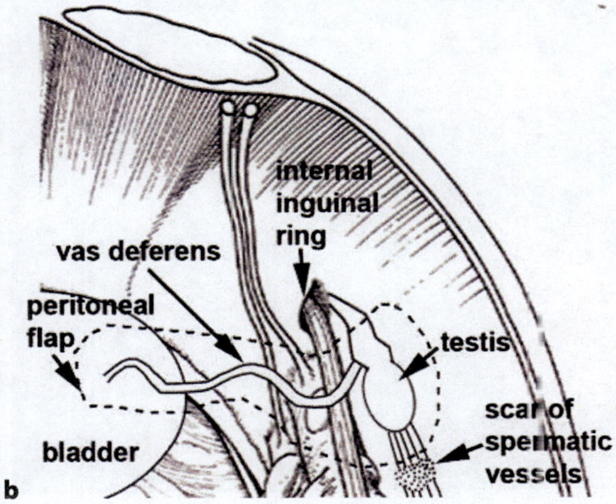

A high intra-abdominal testis with very short spermatic vessels is seen in Step 3a. It must be decided now whether this pedicle will allow the testis to reach the scrotum. Some authors estimate the adequate length by trying to swing this testicle to the contra-lateral internal inguinal ring. If there is not adequate length one should continue with an FSO. The testis is supplied by several arteries (the spermatic, vassal, gubernacular arteries). In FSO part 1, the spermatic vessels are divided using an electrocautery hook or a harmonic scalpel (Step 3a, inset). This generates collateral arteries. In FSO part 2 (most authors wait for 3–6 months), a large peritoneal pedicle including the testis and vas with its vessels is dissected (Step 3b, dotted lines). The testis will be brought down on this pedicle into the scrotum.

Step 4: Fowler-Stephens orchidopexy (part 2)

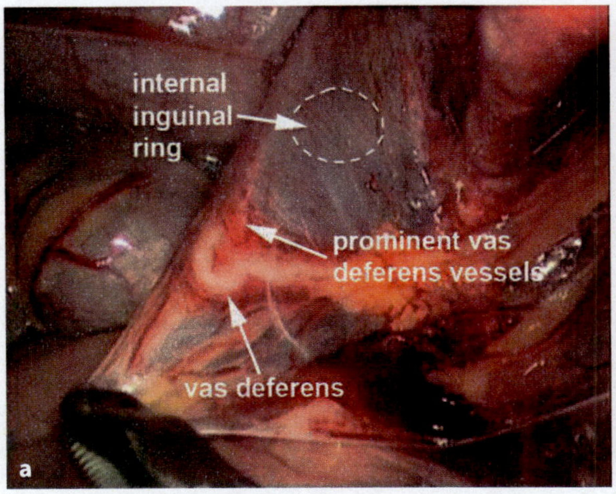

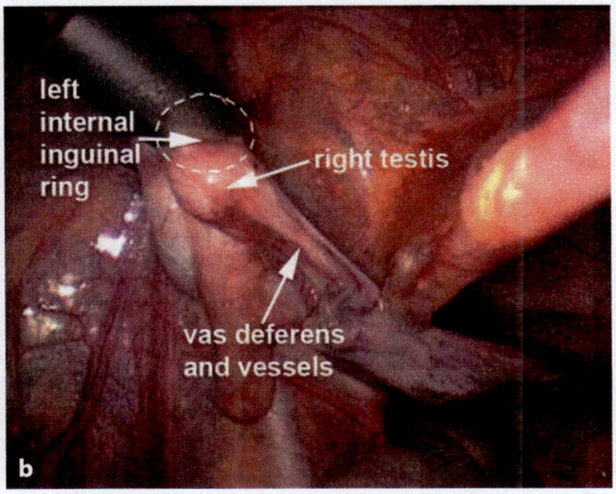

Three to six months after FSO part 1, the testis is examined for volume and consistency and excised only if severe atrophy has taken place. Step 4a demonstrates the peritoneal pedicle hosting the vas deferens and some prominent vessels, which have developed after mass ligation. If the testis looks rather normal, a wide peritoneal flap is excised around the testis and the vas deferens. This incision and dissection should extend over the external iliac vessels down towards the bladder in order to provide sufficient length to bring the testis into the scrotum. Adequate length of the peritoneal pedicle has been achieved once the testis reaches the contra-lateral internal inguinal ring with its peritoneal pedicle. Step 4b shows that the right-sided testis reaches to the left internal inguinal ring.

Step 5: Orchidopexy

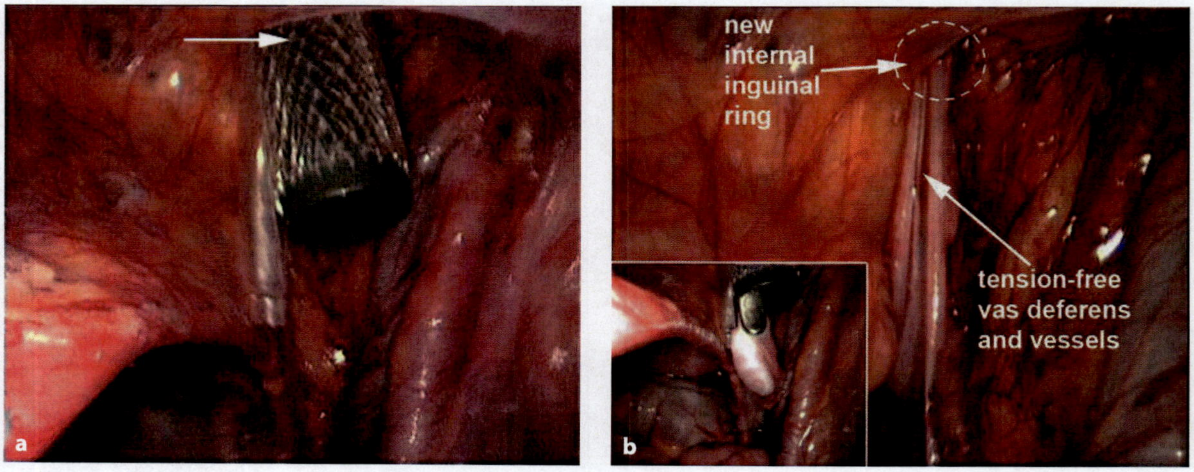

There are two options for bringing the testis into the scrotum: if the inguinal canal is patent (which is usually not the case in impalpable UDT), a straight grasper can be passed through the inguinal canal to catch the testis. Bringing it down through the inguinal canal is a longer route. The shorter route would be through a new defect close to the inferior epigastric vessels. To create this, a subdartos pouch is fashioned. A dissector is passed bluntly under laparoscopic guidance medial to the inferior epigastric vessels into the abdomen. This tract is dilated using a Veress needle and a 10-mm STEP (expandable) trocar (Step 5a). The testis is pulled (Step 5b, inset) through the trocar into the scrotum and sutured to the dartos fascia. A tension-free pedicle (Step 5b) must be ensured.

Postoperative Management

- Discharge on the same day if possible
- Long-term follow-up for atrophy and infertility of the testis [4, 5]

References

1. Bruijnen CJ, Vogels HD, Beasley SW (2008) Review of the extent to which orchidopexy is performed at the optimal age: implications for health services. ANZ J Surg 78:1006–1009
2. Mathers MJ, Sperling H, Rübben H, Roth S (2009) The undescended testis: diagnosis, treatment and long-term consequences. Dtsch Arztebl Int 106:527–532
3. Virtanen HE, Bjerknes R, Cortes D, Jørgensen N, Rajpert-De Meyts E, Thorsson AV, Thorup J, Main KM (2007) Cryptorchidism: classification, prevalence and long-term consequences. Acta Paediatr 96:611–616
4. Thorup J, Cortes D (2009) Surgical treatment and follow up on undescended testis. Pediatr Endocrinol Rev 7:38–43
5. Murphy F, Paran TS, Puri P (2007) Orchidopexy and its impact on fertility. Pediatr Surg Int 23:625–632

4.3 Varicocoelectomy

Holger Till, Jens-Uwe Stolzenburg

Introduction

Varicocoele is defined as an abnormal dilatation of the pampiniform plexus. It usually occurs on the patient's left side, probably due to an impaired drainage of the left spermatic veins into the renal vein. However, it is important to rule out Wilms tumour, which may compromise the renal venous flow [1]. Generally, varicocoele is classified into three grades: grade 1, only palpable during Valsalva manoeuvre; grade 2, palpable but not visible in a standing patient; grade 3, visible ("bag of worms"). Clinically most patients with varicocoeles are asymptomatic, although scrotal discomfort and even acute pain (possibly due to microthrombosis) have been reported [1]. Pathophysiologically, whether the increased venous blood stagnation causes testicular atrophy and infertility continue to be debated [2, 3]. Nevertheless, the surgical options are either selective ligation of enlarged veins (Bernardi) [4] or mass ligation of the spermatic vessels (Palomo) [5]

Indications

- Varicocoele grade 2–3
- Clinical symptoms
- Testicular atrophy
- Impaired fertility

Contra-indications

- Cardiac defects
- Multiple abdominal operations

Preoperative Preparation

- Empty urinary bladder via catheterisation

Step 1: Patient position and trocar placement

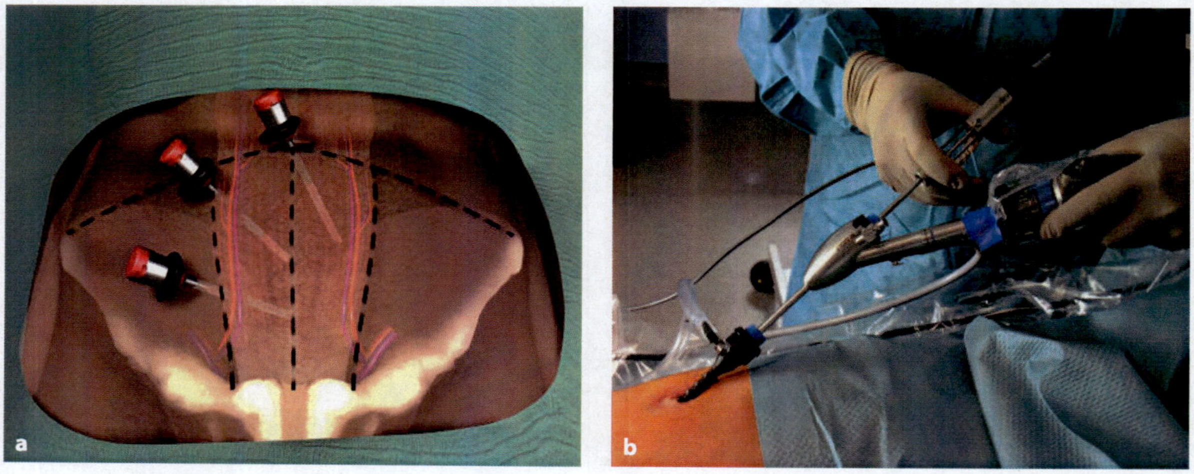

Varicocoelectomy in children can be performed either as a three-port technique (Step 1a) or as a single-port operation (Step 1b). Most surgeons prefer three ports, 3–5 mm each. The patient is placed supine with the surgeon and assistant both on the contra-lateral side. The first trocar is inserted at the umbilicus followed by pneumoperitoneum of 10–12 mmHg. Two 3- to 5-mm ports are placed in the contralateral abdomen (Step 1a) using a 5-mm scope, 30°. From an ergonomic point of view, it seems preferable to change the scope to the middle port and manipulate through the lateral ports. Recently, a 5-mm single-port scope has become available hosting a 5-mm working channel. This instrument makes a single-port varicocoelectomy feasible (Step 1b; note the 3.5-mm bipolar coagulator inserted into the working channel).

Step 2: Identification of landmarks

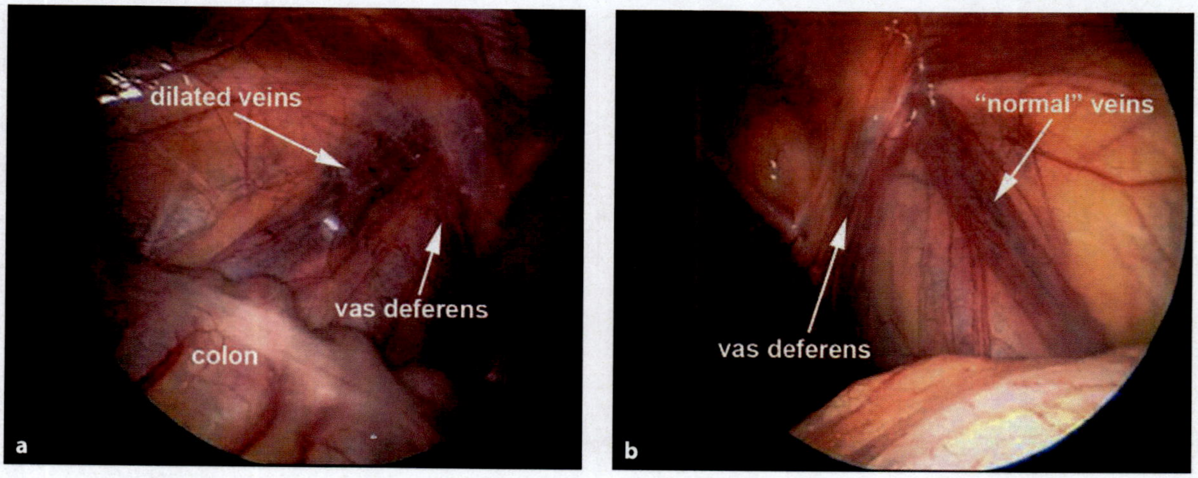

The surgical landmarks of this operation include the vas deferens after it crosses over the iliac artery and vein, the spermatic vessels and internal inguinal ring (Step 2a). The spermatic vessels are easily visualised in the retroperitoneum. Even with a pneumoperitoneum with 10–12 mmHg of pressure, the dilatation of the left spermatic veins (as seen in Step 2a) becomes obvious in comparison to the same patient's normal right side (as seen in Step 2b).

Step 3: Peritoneal incision

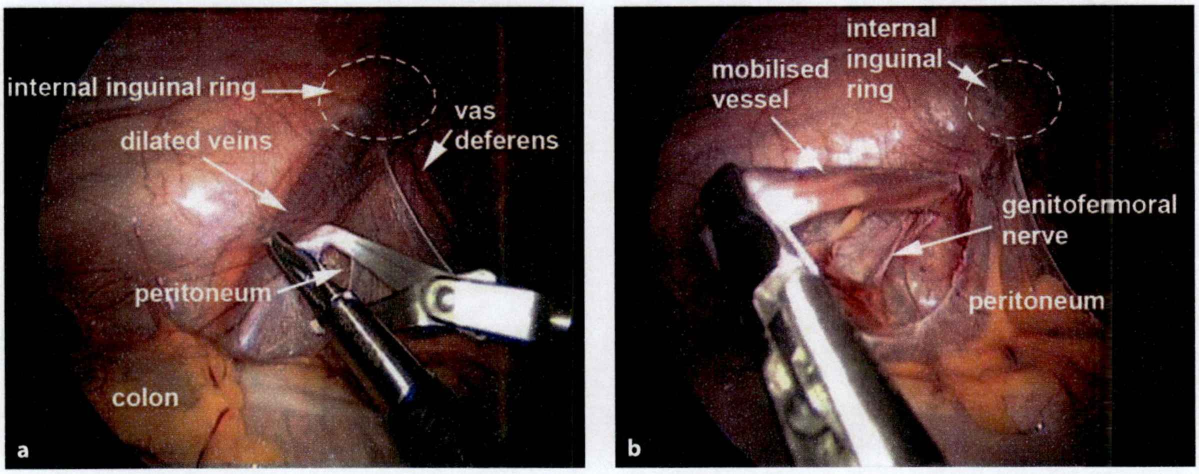

Paying close attention to the course of the vas deferens, the peritoneum is incised about 2 cm proximally to the internal inguinal ring, just above the spermatic vessels, as seen in Step 3a. Standard scissors, an electrocautery hook or a harmonic scalpel can be used to perform this step. Thereafter, the spermatic vessels are mobilised completely and lifted off the posterior pelvic wall (Step 3b). The genitofemoral nerve, which is usually located posteriorly, must be clearly identified and carefully preserved.

Step 4: Division of the varicose vessels

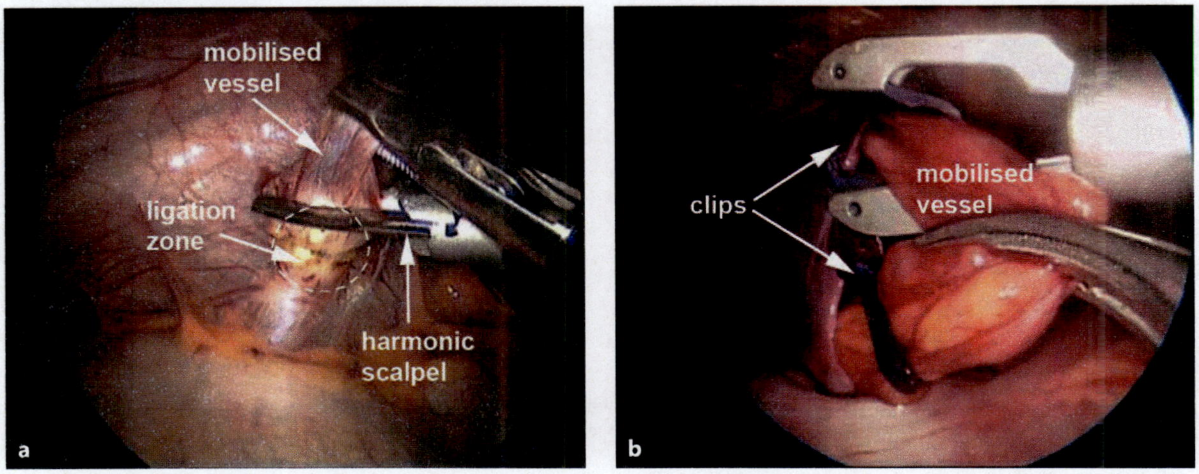

If possible, the testicular artery should be identified visually or with a laparoscopic ultrasound probe. In case of doubt, a mass ligation of the spermatic vessels, including the artery, is recommended in order to avoid recurrence of the varicocoele, since the testis should survive on the remaining two arteries from the gubernaculum and the vas deferens. Thus the ligation of the varicose veins is carried out with either the harmonic scalpel, as demonstrated in Step 4a, or laparoscopic clips (Step 4b) or electrocautery.

Step 5: Lymphatic preservation and peritoneal closure

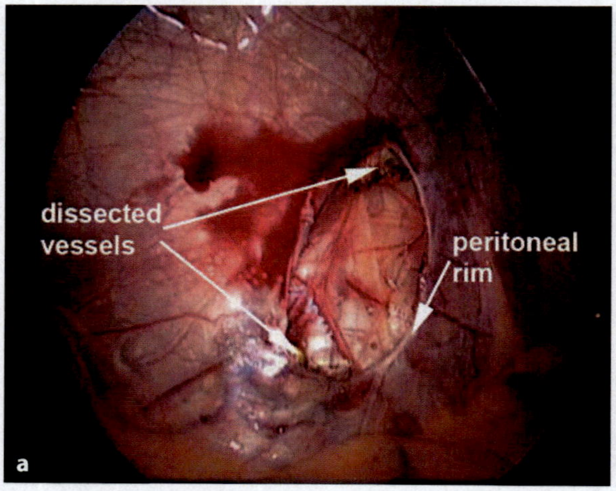

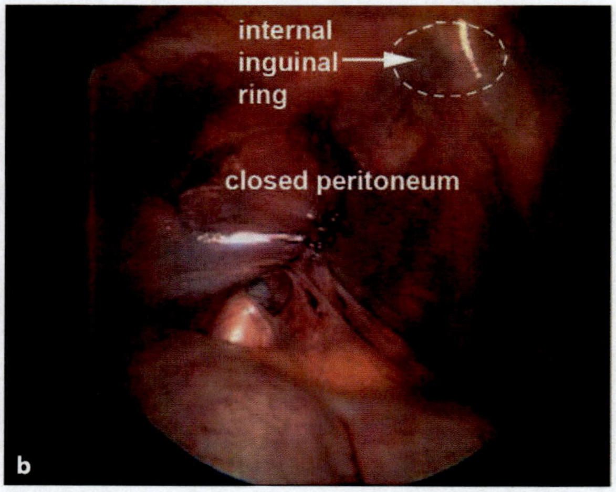

Injection of isosulfan blue into the subdartos pouch helps to identify and preserve the lymphatic vessels. Preservation of lymphatic channels helps to prevent postoperative complications such as the development of a hydrocoele in the scrotum. The most important aspect of the procedure is the complete dissection of the vessels to prevent recurrence of the varicose veins (Step 5a). The peritoneal window may be closed using an absorbable interrupted or running suture, as in Step 5b. Again, care must be taken to avoid inadvertent suturing of the genitofemoral nerve during this step.

Postoperative Management

- Discharge on the same day if possible
- Long-term follow-up necessary to check for testicular atrophy or hydrocoele/lymphocoele formation

References

1. El-Saeity NS, Sidhu PS (2006) Scrotal varicocele, exclude a renal tumour. Is this evidence based? Clin Radiol 61:593–599
2. Smith R, Kaune H, Parodi D, Madariaga M, Rios R, Morales I, Castro A (2006) Increased sperm DNA damage in patients with varicocele: relationship with seminal oxidative stress. Hum Reprod 21:986–993
3. Agarwal A, Deepinder F, Cocuzza M, Agarwal R, Short RA, Sabanegh E, Marmar JL (2007) Efficacy of varicocelectomy in improving semen parameters: new meta-analytical approach. Urology 70:532–538
4. Salem HK, Mostafa T (2009) Preserved testicular artery at varicocele repair. Andrologia 41:241–245
5. Méndez-Gallart R, Bautista-Casasnovas A, Estevez-Martínez E, Varela-Cives R (2009) Laparoscopic Palomo varicocele surgery: lessons learned after 10 years' follow-up of 156 consecutive pediatric patients. J Pediatr Urol 5:126–131

Chapter 5

Miscellaneous

CONTENTS

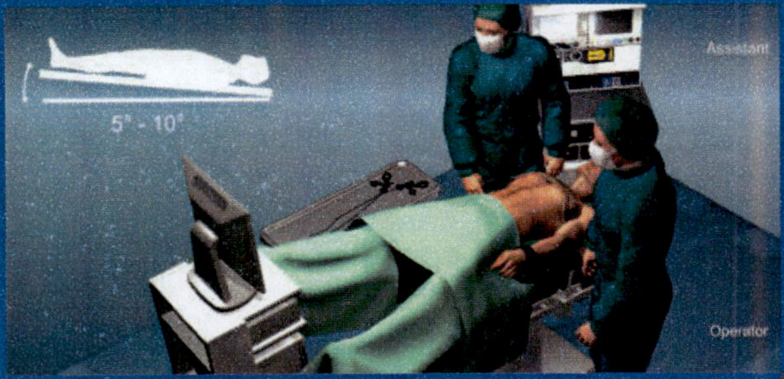

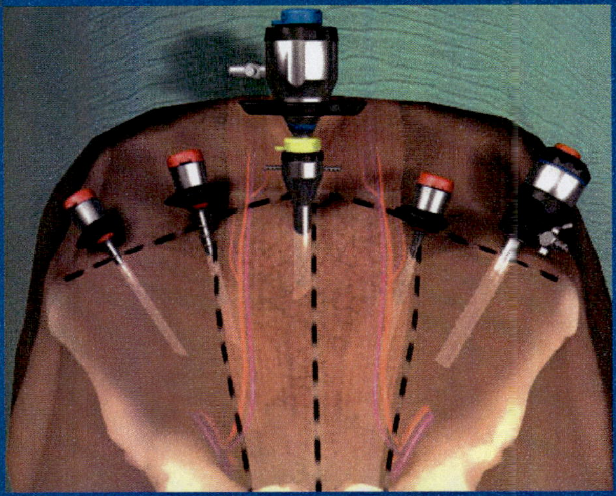

J.-U. Stolzenburg, I. Türk, E. Liatsikos: *Laparoscopic and Robot-Assisted Surgery in Urology*
DOI: 10.1007/978-3-642-00891-7_5, © Springer-Verlag Berlin Heidelberg 2011

5.1 Extraperitoneal Hernia Repair with Mesh Placement

Jens-Uwe Stolzenburg, Evangelos N. Liatsikos, Thilo Schwalenberg, Tim Häfner, Minh Do

Introduction

There are two main surgical access techniques to reach the preperitoneal space and place the synthetic mesh for inguinal hernia repair. The transabdominal (transabdominal preperitoneal technique, TAPP) or the extraperitoneal route (totally extraperitoneal technique, TEP). Both of these laparoscopic techniques use the principle of tension-free hernia repair, covering the hernial defect and potential sites for recurrence.

We favour the preperitoneal mesh technique (TEP) for the repair of inguinal hernias because of its direct access to the posterior inguinal anatomy and the clear visibility of all possible hernial defects. It is technically easier and quicker to perform than the transperitoneal technique. The trend in laparoscopic/endoscopic surgery towards the TEP repair has shown it to be equally effective but with fewer complications [1, 2]. The technique completely avoids intraperitoneal entry and therefore its complications. Staples or stitches are not necessary for fixation of the mesh.

The extraperitoneal endoscopic hernia repair can also be safely performed concurrently with endoscopic extraperitoneal radical prostatectomy [3, 4].

Indications

- All inguinal hernias including recurrent hernias

Contra-indication

- Incarcerated hernias
- Children

Preoperative Preparation

- Empty urinary bladder (if necessary bladder catheterisation)
- Single-shot broad-spectrum antibiotics

Step 1: Operative setup and dissection of the preperitoneal space

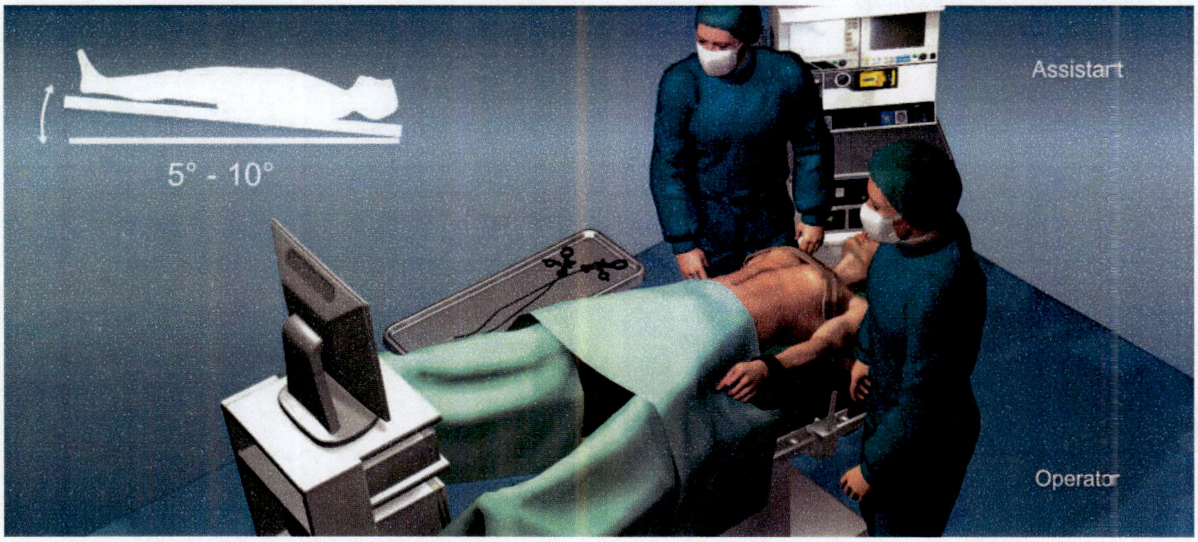

The patient is placed in a dorsal supine, 5–10° Trendelenburg position. The first surgeon stands on the contralateral side to the hernia. A 15-mm paraumbilical incision is made (left side, left inguinal hernia; right side, right inguinal hernia). The balloon trocar dissection of the preperitoneal space, the placement of optical trocar (Hasson type), and CO_2 insufflation (pressure, 12 mmHg) are performed as described in Sect. 3.4.

Step 2: Trocar placement

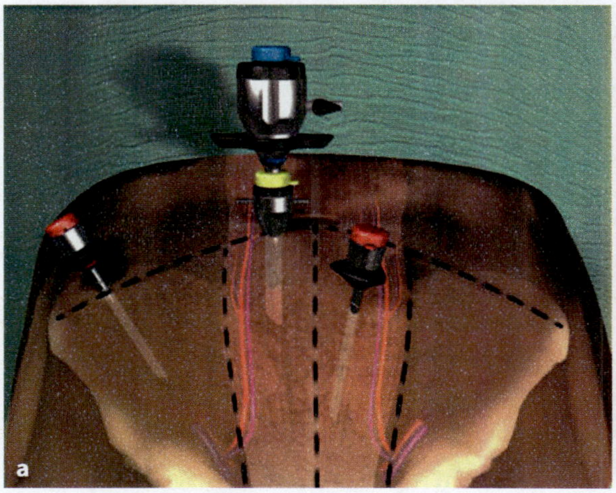

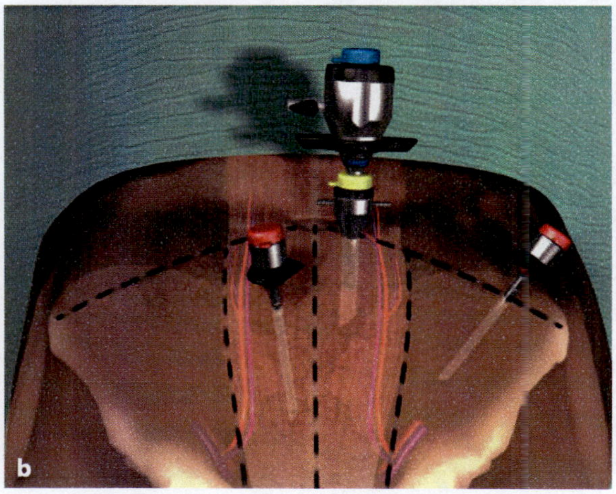

A 5-mm trocar is placed in a left paramedian position (in cases of right inguinal hernia) and as cranially as possible under direct visual control. The creation of the preperitoneal space is continued with blunt dissection. A second 5-mm trocar is placed as laterally as possible cranial to the anterior superior iliac spine (Step 2a). Step 2b shows the trocar placement for left inguinal hernia. In the case of bilateral hernia repair, place the first 5-mm trocar as cranially and laterally as possible (on the side of the paraumbilical incision). Free the preperitoneal space along the pubic arch across to the other side. In some cases, a third 5-mm trocar placed suprapubically in the midline is necessary (suturing, difficult dissection).

5

Step 3: Dissection of hernial sac (medial hernia)

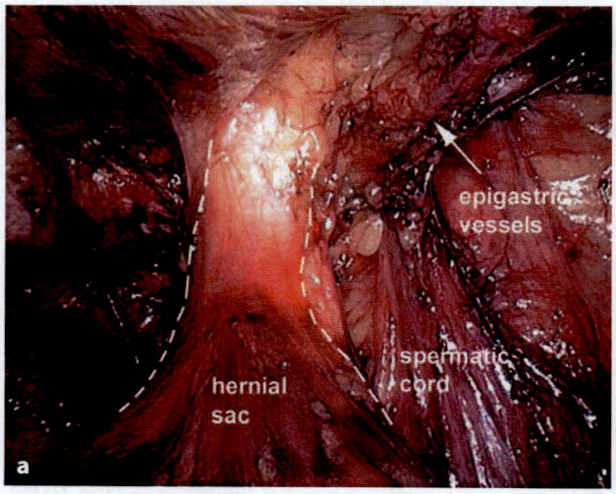

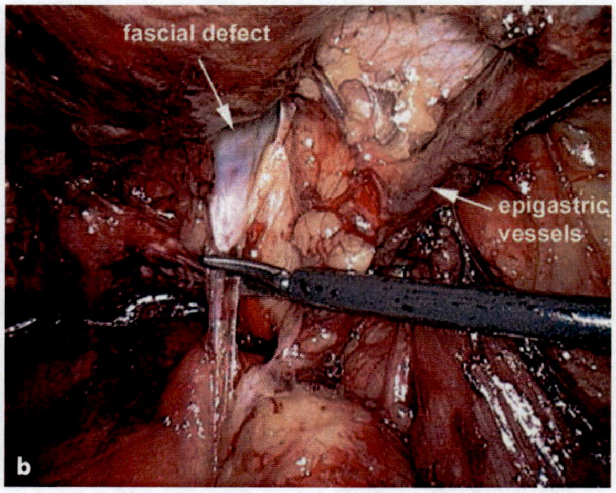

In direct (medial) hernias, the hernial sac (peritoneum) is found medial to the epigastric vessels. During the creation of the preperitoneal space, the medial fascial defect becomes clearly visible after balloon dissection. Traction and counter-traction manoeuvres are used to reduce the hernial sac. In many patients, the dissection of the medial hernial sac is nearly completely done by the balloon during initial dissection of the preperitoneal space.

Be aware that in cases with a large direct hernial defect one must cut and place the final mesh in an asymmetrical fashion underneath the cord, making sure that the medial aspect of the mesh is larger.

Step 4: Dissection of hernial sac (lateral hernia)

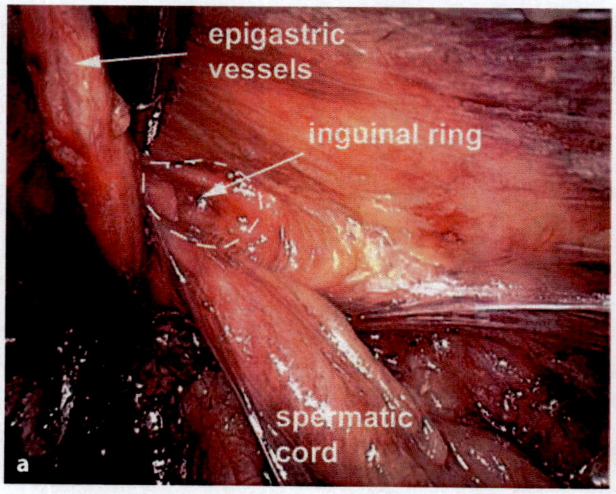

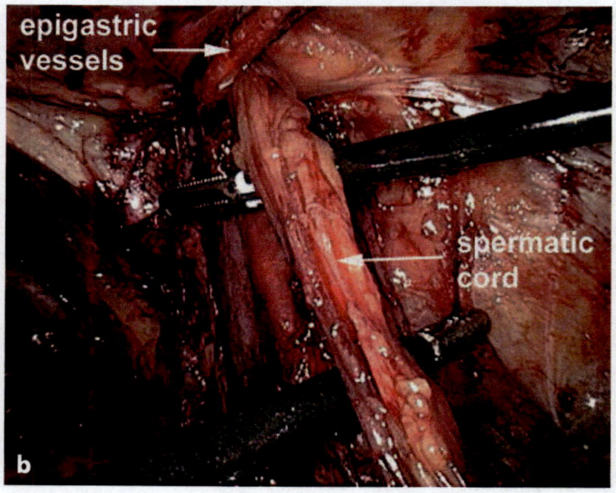

In indirect (lateral) hernias, the peritoneal sac will travel on the anteromedial aspect of the spermatic cord as it enters the internal ring. The hernial sac is carefully dissected free from the cord. If the hernia sac cannot be completely and sufficiently retracted (i.e. large indirect inguinal–scrotal hernia), the hernial sac can be divided at the level of the internal inguinal ring. Care should be taken during the incision not to injure the bowel within the hernial sac. Closure (suturing) of any peritoneal defect is essential. Contact between the bowel and the mesh could cause adhesions and probable ileus. The entire spermatic cord is elevated and an opening is created posteriorly for the insertion of the mesh. This space should not be too small to avoid folding the mesh once in place.

Step 5: Preparation of the synthetic mesh

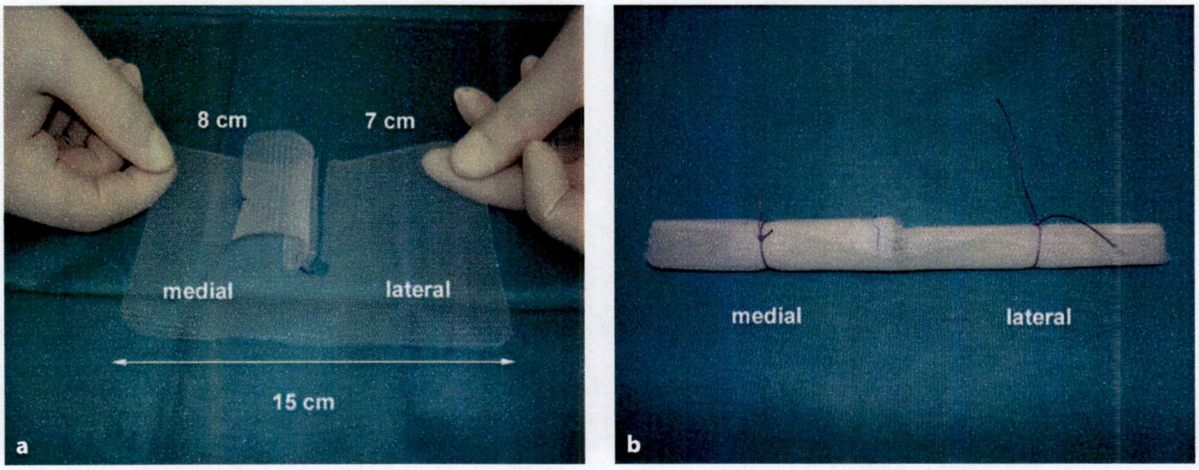

The synthetic mesh (e.g. Prolene 10 × 15 cm) is prepared extracorporally. A 6-cm incision is made in the middle of the mesh, and a 0.5-cm hole is cut out for the spermatic cord. When a large medial hernia is to be repaired, the medial aspect of the mesh should be larger. The incision in the mesh is covered by a further 4×6-cm Prolene mesh. This additional patch is secured with 2/0 Prolene running suture. The next steps are needed to insert and place the mesh around the spermatic cord. The flap is temporarily fixed at the medial aspect of the main mesh by a stay suture (Step 5). The mesh is rolled up and fixed by two loose ties, leaving the suture long on the lateral aspect and short on the medial aspect. This enables easy recognition and placement in-situ.

Step 6: Mesh placement

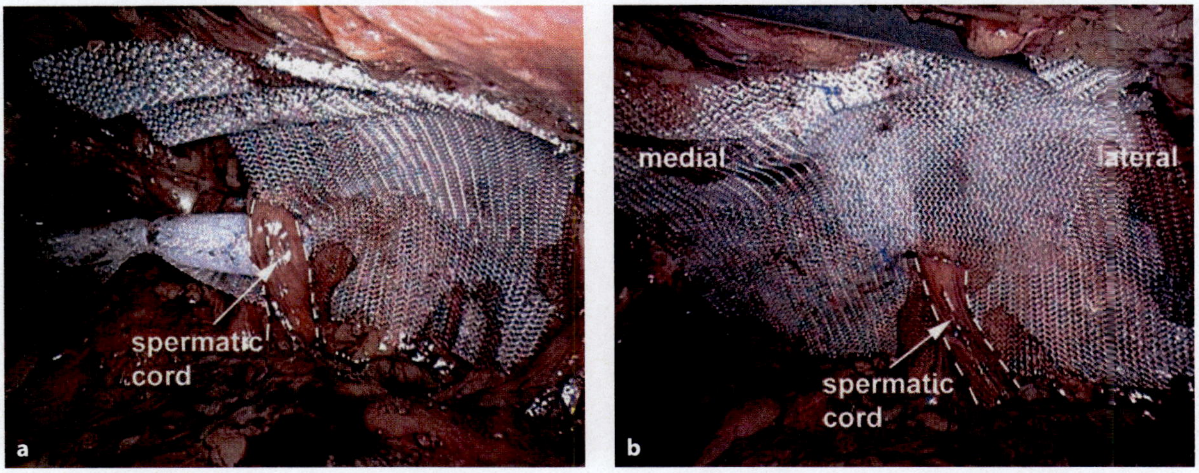

The mesh roll is inserted through the 12-mm optical trocar and placed under the spermatic cord. The stay sutures are cut in sequence (first lateral, second medial and third the flap stay suture) and the mesh is subsequently unfolded around the spermatic cord. Thus, the mesh covers the hernial orifices and the entire space from the symphysis pubis in the midline to the anterior superior iliac spine laterally. If hernias are bilateral, two pieces of mesh (the same size) should be used and overlapped medially. After releasing the carbon dioxide at the end of the procedure, the mesh is anchored to the abdominal wall by intra-abdominal pressure alone. Placing the mesh around the spermatic cord prevents any possibility of its dislocating or migrating. Staples or stitches are not used for fixation of the mesh.

5

Postoperative Management

- Remove drain on the first postoperative day (if present)
- Resumption of normal activities in 7 days

References

1. Ramshaw BJ, Tucker JG, Duncan TD, Heithold D, Garcha I, Mason EM, Wilson JP, Lucas GW (1996) Technical considerations of the different approaches to laparoscopic herniorrhaphy: analysis of 500 cases. Am Surg 62:69–72
2. Kraehenbuehl L, Schaefer M, Feodorovici MA, Buechler MW (1998) Laparoscopic hernia surgery: a overview. Dig Surg 15:158–166
3. Stolzenburg JU, Pfeiffer H, Nehaus JM, Sommerfeld M, Dorschner W (2001) Repair of inguinal hernias using the mesh technique during extraperitoneal pelvic lymph node dissection. Urol Int 67:19–23
4. Stolzenburg JU, Rabenalt R, Dietel A, Do M, Pfeiffer H, Doschner W (2003) Hernia repair during endoscopic (laparoscopic) radical prostatectomy. J Laparoendosc Adv Surg Tech 13:27–31

5.2 Extraperitoneal Colposuspension

Stefan Orth, Florian Wissing, Orietta Dalpiaz, Christoph Guball, Michael C Truss

Introduction

For more than 30 years, modified open colposuspension was the gold standard in the treatment of female stress urinary incontinence [1–3]. Minimally invasive sling procedures are currently the standard of care in most female patients with genuine stress urinary incontinence (SUI) without pelvic organ prolapse (POP). A complete preoperative evaluation, including videourodynamics is required to diagnose anatomical abnormalities and characterise bladder dysfunction. In some cases of SUI with a combined lateral defect or a moderate combined vertical descent, reconstruction of the anatomical defect is warranted to prevent early failure [4]. In such cases, an endoscopic colposuspension is a valid option. Minimally invasive colposuspension can be performed by either a trans- or extraperitoneal approach [3, 5]. We prefer the extraperitoneal approach. This limits the space created to what is necessary eliminating intraperitoneal complications. Our extraperitoneal approach is identical to the endoscopic radical prostatectomy setup (see chapter 3.4 and 3.12)

Indications

- SUI with a combined lateral defect or a moderate combined vertical descent

Contra-indications

- Morbid obesity
- Multiple prior procedures resulting in likely extensive adhesions
- Prior mesh hernia repairs on both sides

Preoperative Preparation

- Transurethral bladder catheterisation and drainage
- Disinfection including the vagina
- Broad-spectrum antibiotic prophylaxis

Step 1: Patient position, extraperitoneal approach and trocar placement

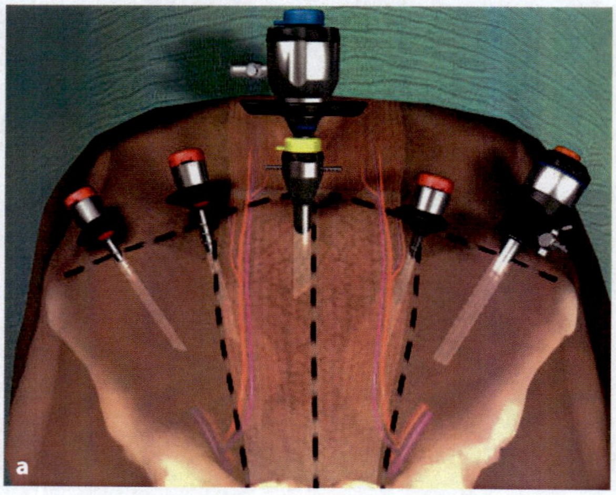

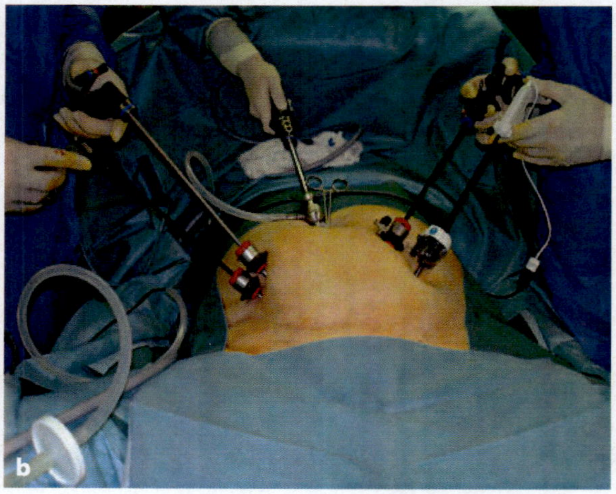

The patient is placed in a flat, or low, lithotomy position, with arms by the side. A moderate Trendelenburg position of up to 10° and slight break in the middle of the table can be helpful. An infraumbilical skin incision is made. The anterior rectus sheath is incised, through which the balloon dilatator is passed, superficial to the posterior fascia. Balloon inflation opens the retropubic space. The anatomical landmarks of the symphysis pubis and Cooper ligaments should be identified at this point. The (0°) camera port is established using a (10-mm) Hasson trocar. Other ports to be placed include two 5-mm working ports inferior to the umbilicus (one lateral to the epigastric arteries with the other more distal and lateral) and two 5-mm assistant ports on the right side identical to the left-sided working ports, as shown in Step 1a and Step 1b.

Step 2: Preparation of the vaginal fascia

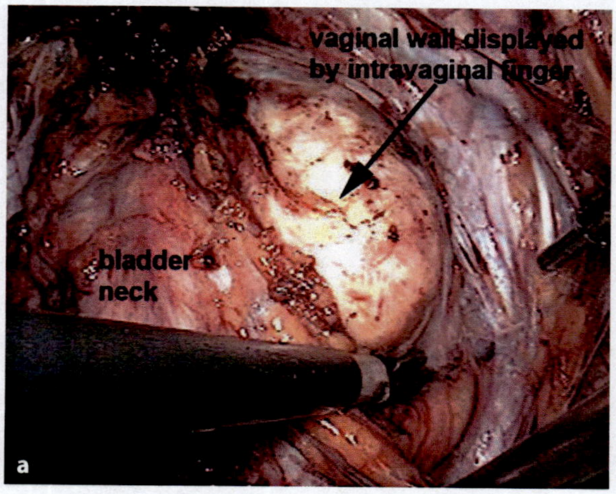

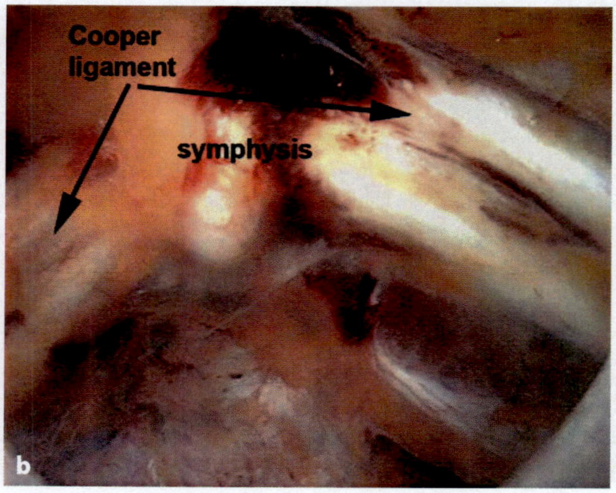

Fatty tissue is removed from the vaginal fascia with bipolar forceps until a clear view is obtained. The assistant then applies traction to the urinary catheter to delineate the exact position of the bladder neck (Step 2a). With the operator's finger placed intravaginally, the optimal position of the first stitch on the vaginal wall is easily identified. The assistant retracts the bladder neck with the suction device (Step 2b).

Step 3: Positioning the first stitch

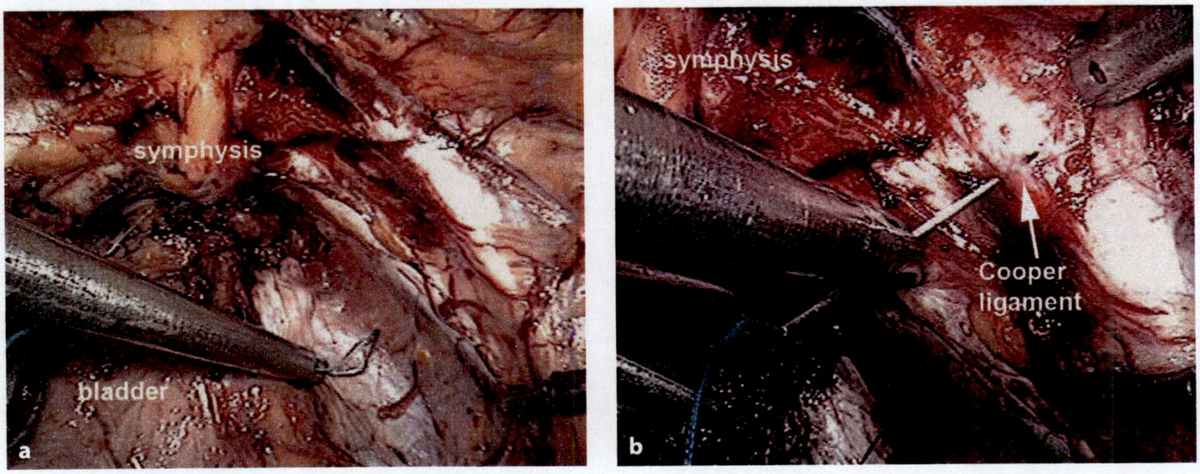

With the suction device, the assistant helps in the positioning of the first stitch on the vaginal tissue, as the operator's left index finger remains in the vagina (Step 3a). Moving the urinary catheter provides confirmation of urethral position. We use a 2/0 (nonabsorbable) Ethibond suture on an SH needle. The needle is passed through the vaginal wall (excluding mucosa) and then through the Cooper ligament (Step 3b). As the suture is tensioned, the knot is secured by the assistant's forceps when optimal elevation of the anterior vaginal wall is achieved, before tying.

Step 4: Positioning the second and third stitches

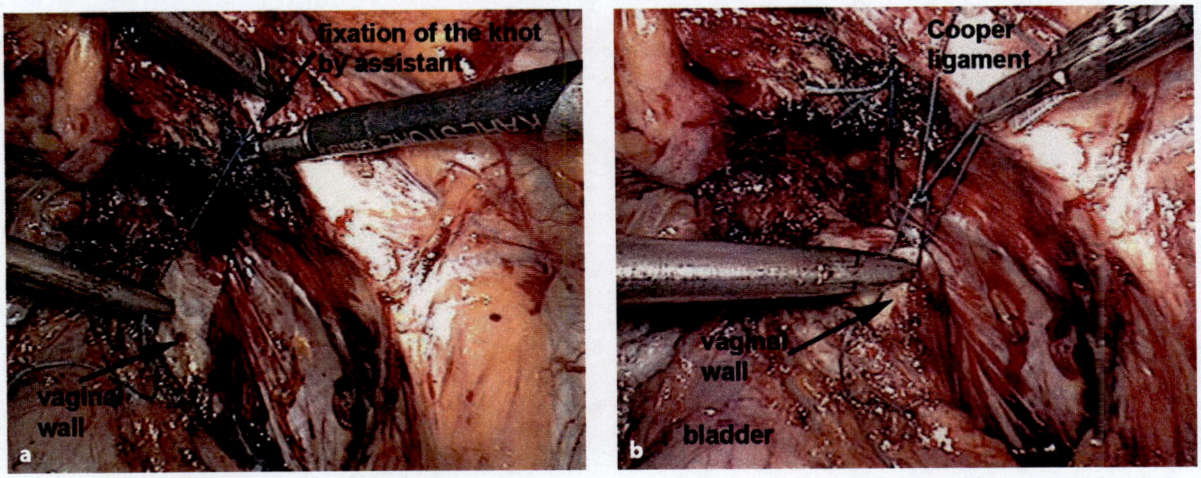

The second stitch is made craniolaterally to the first, with an at least 1.5-cm separation from the very sensitive bladder neck region (Step 4a). A third stitch can be placed if space permits. Care must be taken to avoid bladder or ureteric injury (Step 4b). Check for any bleeding and coagulate as necessary with bipolar forceps.

Step 5: Positioning stitches on the other side

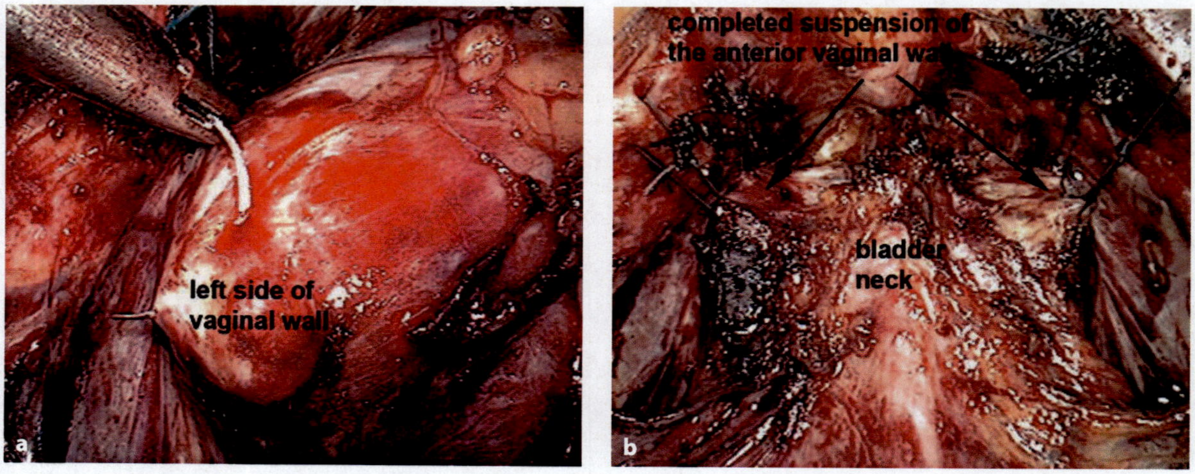

The same procedure is performed on the other side (Step 5a). Adequate and stable elevation of the anterior vaginal wall is essential for success.

Bladder integrity is confirmed through cystoscopy. A surgical drain is not routinely required. Any inadvertent peritoneal breach can be left unclosed. Make a final inspection for hemostesis and remove the trocars under vision (Step 5a, Step 5b).

Postoperative Management

- Removal of the urethral catheter after 24 h
- Voiding protocol and ultrasonographic measurement of post-void residual volume
- Light activities with no heavy lifting or straining for 6 weeks

References

1. Cowan W, Morgan HR (1979) A simplified retropubic urethropexy in the treatment of primary and recurrent urinary stress incontinence in the female. Am J Obstet Gynecol 133:295–298
2. Petri E (1989) Die Kolposuspension zur Behandlung der weiblichen Harninkontinenz. Akt Urol 20:138–142
3. Goepel M, Bross S (2009) Stress incontinence in women. Is there still an indication to perform the Burch colposuspension and the fascial sling. Der Urologe Ausg A 48:487–490
4. Richardson DA (1991) The evaluation of different surgical procedures. In Ostergard, DR, Bent AE (eds) Urogynecology and Urodynamics, 3rd edn. Williams & Wilkins, Baltimore pp 413–421
5. Wallwiener D, Grischke EM, Rimbach S, Maleika A, Kaufmann M, Bastert G (1995) Endoscopic colposuspension (Retziusscopy versus laparoscopy). An effective extension of the surgical spectrum of stress incontinence? Geburtshilfe und Frauenheilkunde 55:235–239

5.3 Fistula Repair

5.3.1 Rectourinary Fistula Repair

René Sotelo Noguera, Juan Carlos Astigueta, Eudo Herrera Morillo

Introduction

Rectourinary fistulae (RUF) are uncommon communications between the lower urinary system and the rectum. Although they may develop in patients with inflammatory bowel disease and perirectal abscesses, they most frequently appear as an iatrogenic complication of extirpative or ablative prostate procedures. A review of complications after radical prostatectomy in the Medicare population revealed a 1% incidence of RUF. Other ablative treatments to the prostate are related to an RUF incidence of 0.4–8.8% after brachytherapy, 0–6% after external beam radiotherapy and 0.4% after cryotherapy [1].

Conservative management is initially attempted, consisting of urinary diversion, broad-spectrum antibiotics, and parenteral nutrition. Nevertheless, the latter approach typically fails. If the fistula has not closed within 3–6 months, it is unlikely to do so. The surgical management of RUF includes transanal, transanorectal, transsphincteric, transabdominal, perineal, and combined techniques. There are no data clearly favouring any one of the approaches [2]. We will focus on the laparoscopic approach [3–5].

Indications

- Rectourethral fistulae
- Rectovesical fistulae

Contra-indications

- The same contra-indications as for any laparoscopic procedure

Preoperative Preparation

- Full mechanical bowel preparation the day before surgery. Enemas are useful to clear mucous in the distal 25 cm of rectosigmoid stump
- Antibiotics covering enteric flora are given perioperatively
- The patient is induced to general anaesthesia

Step 1: Identification of the fistula: rectourethral fistulae

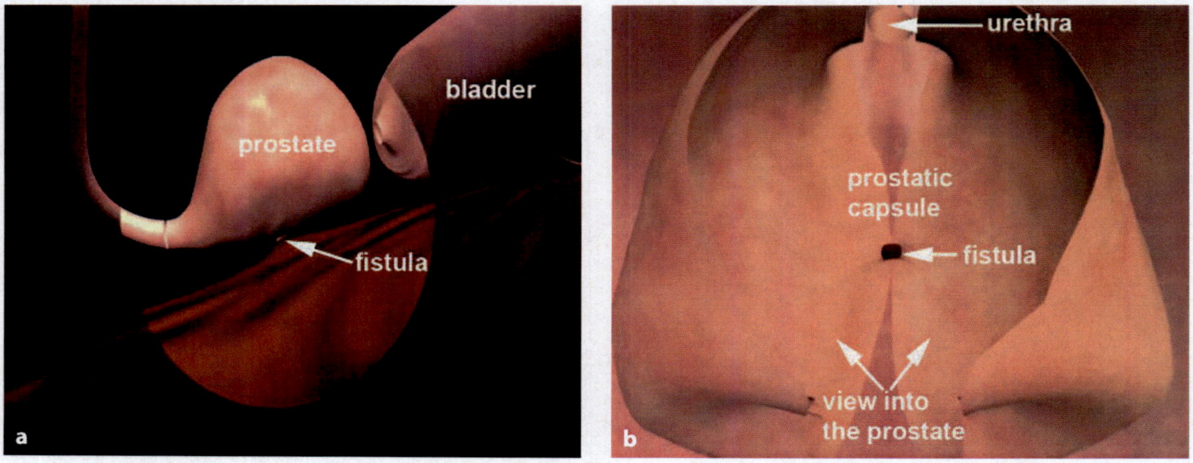

Fistulae between the prostatic urethra and the rectum usually develop after ablative therapies or surgery for benign prostatic hyperplasia. Management of recto-urethral fistulae includes the following surgical steps: (1) excision of the remaining prostate capsule, (2) closure of the rectum and (3) tissue interposition. During the transperitoneal approach, the omentum is used, while the neurovascular bundles and periprostatic fascia are brought together in the midline when an extraperitoneal approach is employed, and (4) urethrovesical anastomosis is then performed in the standard fashion.

Step 2: Identification of the fistula: rectovesical fistula

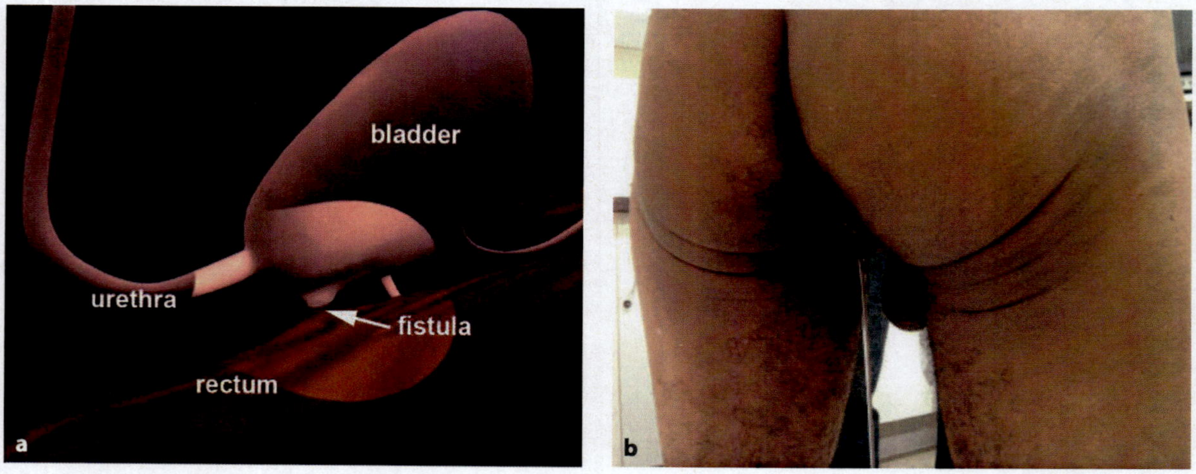

The development of rectourinary fistula after radical prostatectomy usually occurs along the vesicourethral anastomotic line. Intensive inflammation, haematoma or persistent urine leakage at the site of anastomosis may be responsible for the formation of the rectovesical fistula postoperatively. Step 2a is a schematic presentation of the rectovesical fistula. A fistula between bladder neck (anastomotic line) and the rectum results in loss of urine through the rectum or the passage of faeces and/or gas to the bladder. Step 2b shows the characteristic clinical presentation of the rectourinary fistula with loss of urine through the rectum.

Step 3: Cystographic confirmation of the rectovesical fistula

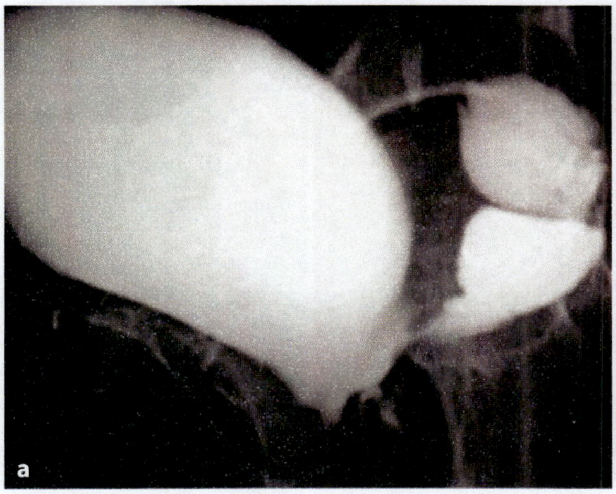
a

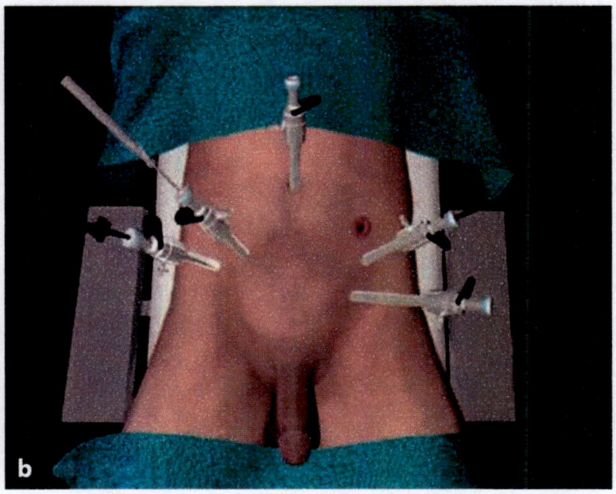
b

Step 3a presents the cystographic confirmation of a rectourinary fistula at the site of vesicourethral anastomosis after radical prostatectomy. The administration of the contrast through a urethral catheter results in leakage of the contrast to the rectum. The presence of gas in the bladder can also be expected. A voiding cystography, barium enema or sigmoidoscopic examination may demonstrate the communication between the rectum and the bladder. Cystoscopic examination is the most useful diagnostic procedure and reveals severe localised inflammatory reaction from which bowel contents may exude. Catheterisation of the fistula tract is possible.

Step 4: Cystoscopy, catheterisation of the ureters and fistula

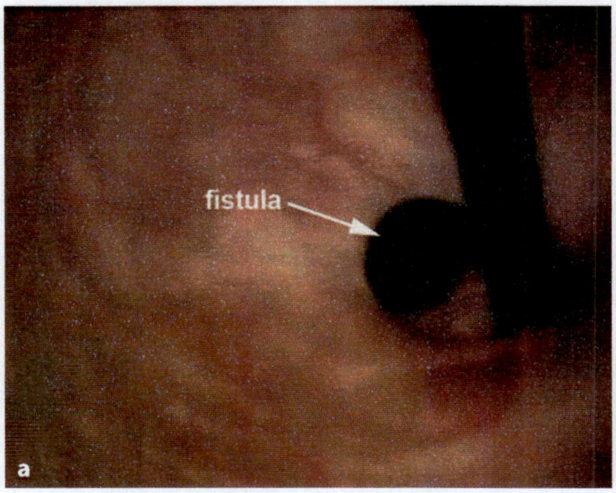

a

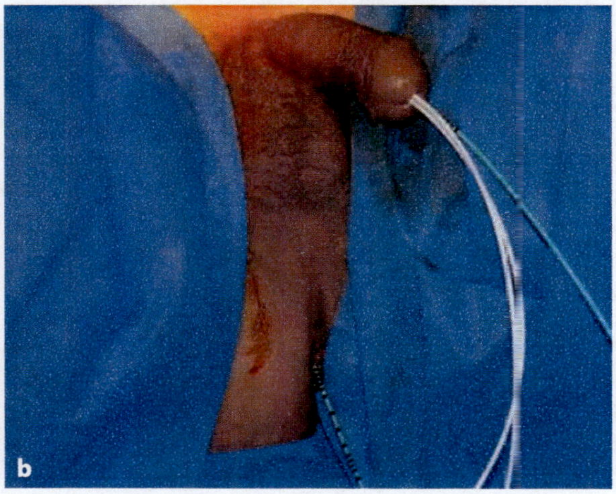
b

The patient is placed in a low lithotomy and steep Trendelenburg position. Sequential compression stockings are used to the lower extremities. Initially, cystoscopy is performed and bilateral ureteral catheterisation takes place. The latter manoeuvre facilitates ureteral identification and prevents ureteral injury during excision and closure of the fistula. The orifice of the fistula is identified and a ureteral catheter with a different colour from those used for the ureters is inserted. The catheter is passed through the fistulous tract into the rectum and retrieved through the anus. The latter manoeuvre facilitates the identification of the fistulous tract during the excision. Step 4b demonstrates a patient with all the necessary stents in place ready for the initiation of the laparoscopic reconstruction.

Step 5: Cystotomy

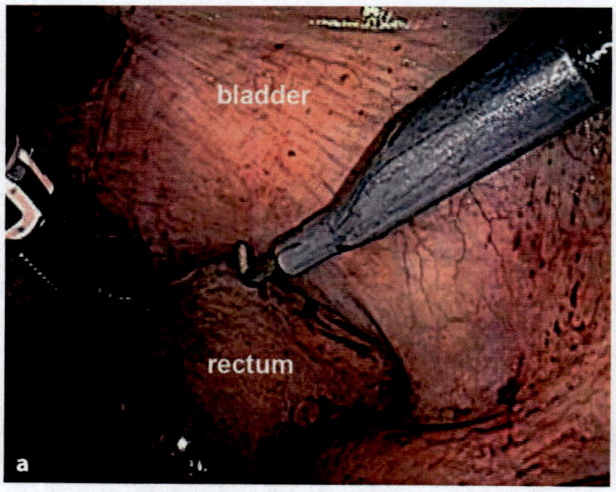

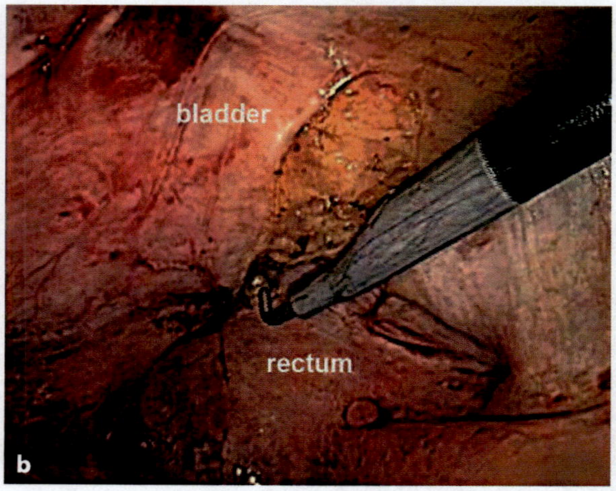

A five-port transperitoneal approach is used, as shown in Step 3b. The arrangement of the trocars is similar to laparoscopic radical prostatectomy. The port configuration could be oriented to the left or right in an attempt to avoid interfering with the usually existing colostomy. After the establishment of pneumoperitoneum and trocar placement, adhesiolysis is carefully performed. An omental flap is retrieved from the site of the right gastroepiploic artery. A vertical midline posterior cystotomy is created with ultrasonic shears (Step 5a) and carried distally to the posterior aspect of the fistulous tract (Step 5b).

Step 6: Cystotomy and dissection of the fistulous tract

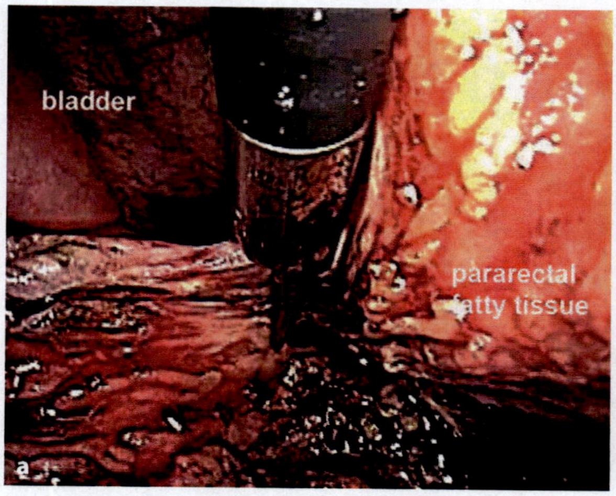

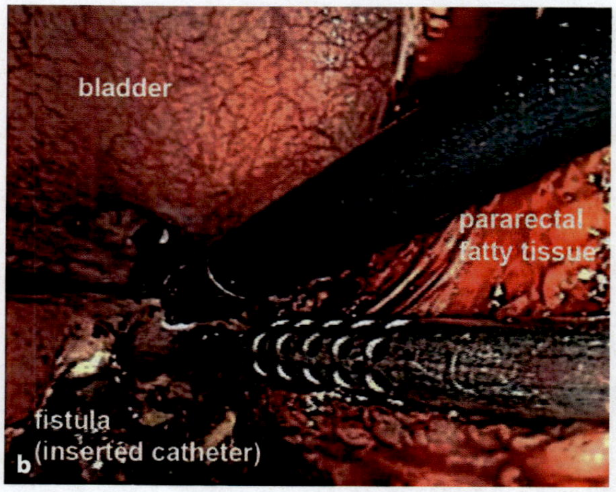

The incision on the posterior wall of the bladder is continued in the direction of the catheter that defines the fistula. The dissection is performed using ultrasonic shears and is guided in a plane between the bladder and the rectum by the prerectal fatty tissue (Step 6a). The incision of the posterior vesical wall results in the exposure of the posterior aspect of the ureteral catheter inserted in the fistulous tract (Step 6b). The catheter is a landmark that will guide the dissection of the fistula throughout the procedure.

Step 7: Exposure of the fistulous tract

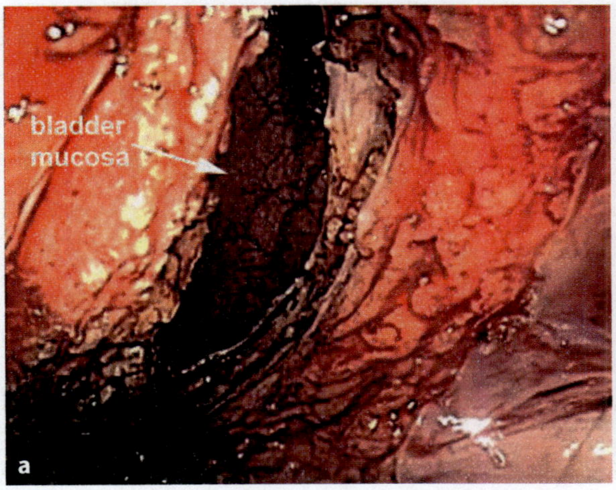

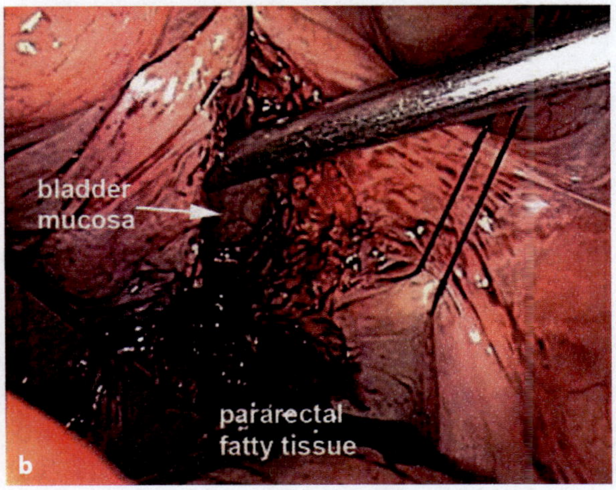

Step 7a demonstrates the cystotomy of the posterior wall. The edges of the incision to the bladder can be retracted laterally in an efficacious manner in an attempt to expose the fistulous tract adequately. A suture is placed at each side of the incision. These sutures can be placed using a Keith needle or a Carter-Thomason port closure needle device. The two ends of the stitch are retracted and anchored outside of the anterior abdominal wall, resulting in adequate exposure of the fistulous tract. Step 7b presents both sides of the bladder incision to be retracted by the aforementioned sutures.

5

Step 8: Identification of the fistulous tract and initiation of the excision

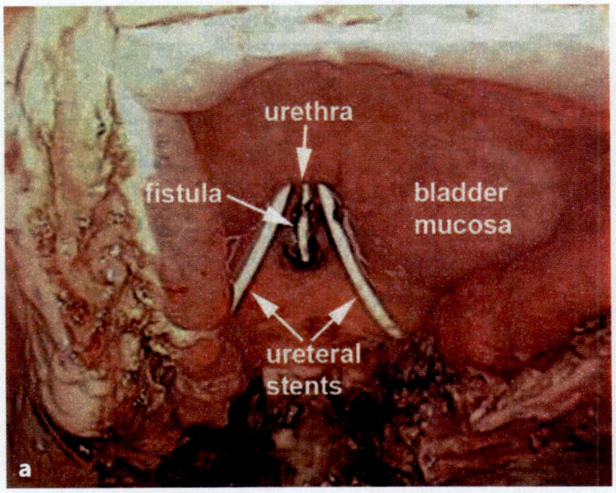

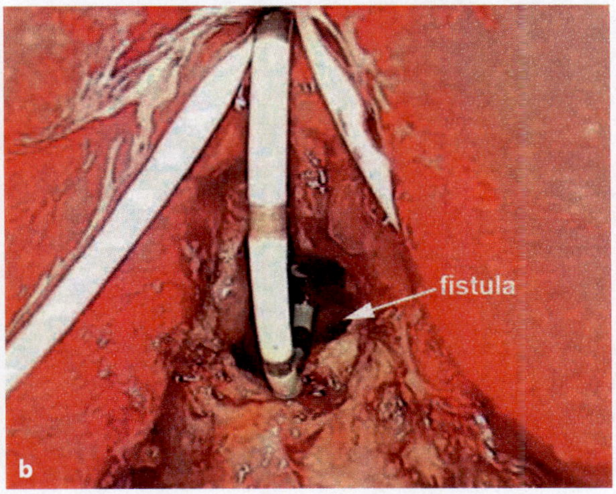

The communication of the bladder and the rectum is identified (Step 8a). The ureteral catheters designate the ureteral orifices, while the ureteral stent in the orifice of the fistula shows one side of the tract. Nonviable or necrotic tissue will be excised up to the point viable well-vascularised tissue is identified. The excision of the fistulous tract has started in Step 8b and the orifice of the fistula is wider as some of the surrounding tissue has been excised. The tract is close to the urethra and the care should be taken to avoid injury to the urethra and the sphincter.

Step 9: Excision of the fistulous tract

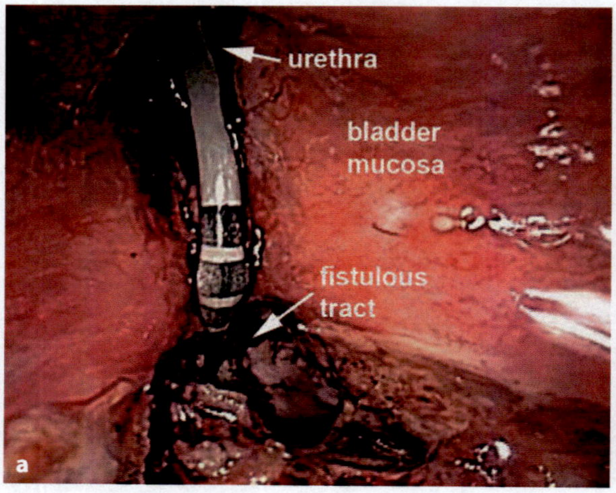

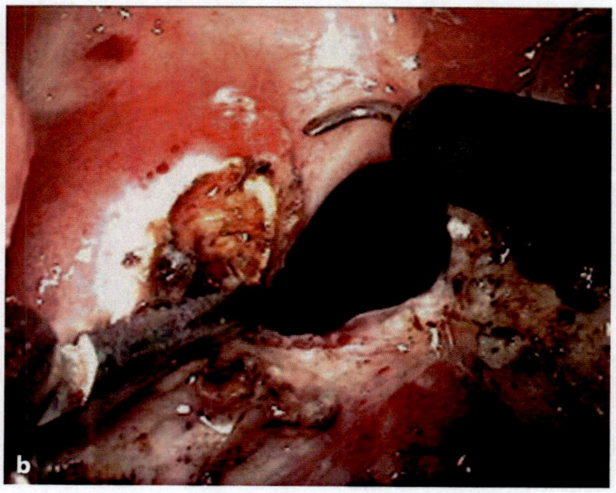

The excision of the fistulous tract is extended so that the communication between the bladder and the rectum become visible. The plane of excision should be directed away from the urethra and sphincter while performing meticulous wide dissection of the tract to separate the two organs. Note in Step 9a the direction of the excision which is carried away from the urethra. The dissection is performed using ultrasonic shears, J-hook electrocautery and laparoscopic scissors with or without coagulation in various combinations (Step 9b).

Step 10: Closure of the rectum

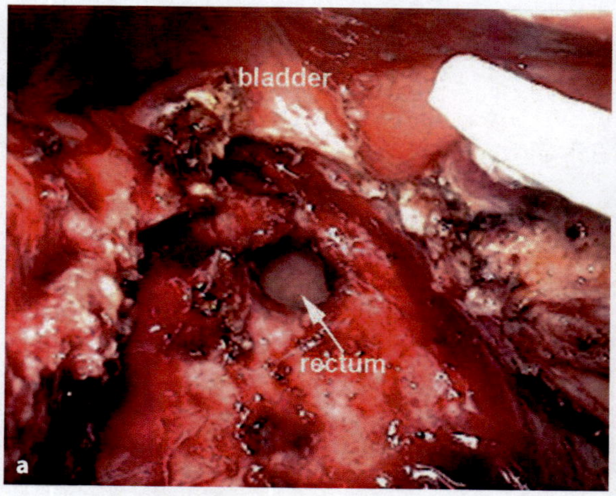

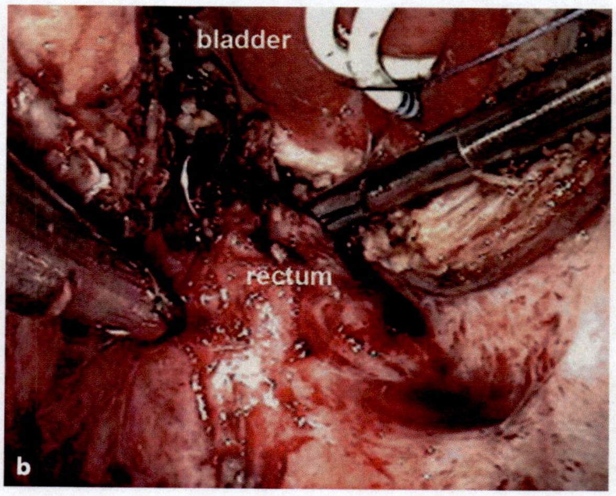

The resection of the fistulous tract is continued and eventually the communication between the bladder and the rectum is visible. In Step 10a, the fistulous tract has been resected and the rectum mucosa is visible through a defect left after the excision of the rectal orifice of the fistulous tract. At this point, the rectum should be closed. A 2/0 Monocryl suture on a UR-6 needle is used. The closure is performed in an interrupted one-layer fashion. The knots are tied on the outer surface of the rectum (Step 10b).

Step 11: Tissue interposition and closure of the bladder

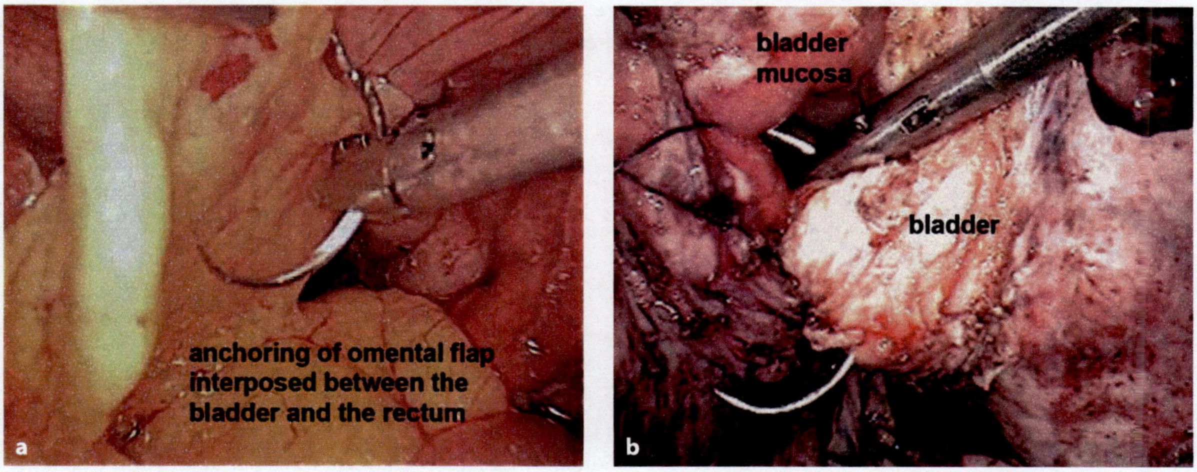

Intact omentum can be brought down to serve as a tissue interposition to bolster the repair. In case the omentum's length is inadequate, the ultrasonic shears can be used to make incisions and create an omentum pedicle flap. Careful planning is critical for the preservation of the omental vascular supply. The initial suture of the rectal closure is used to anchor the interpositioned tissue (Step 11a). Bladder closure is performed in one layer using a 2/0 Monocryl running suture. The suturing line runs in a superior direction (Step 11b). The closure is not completed until the suprapubic tube is placed.

Step 12: Drainage, colostomy, incision closure

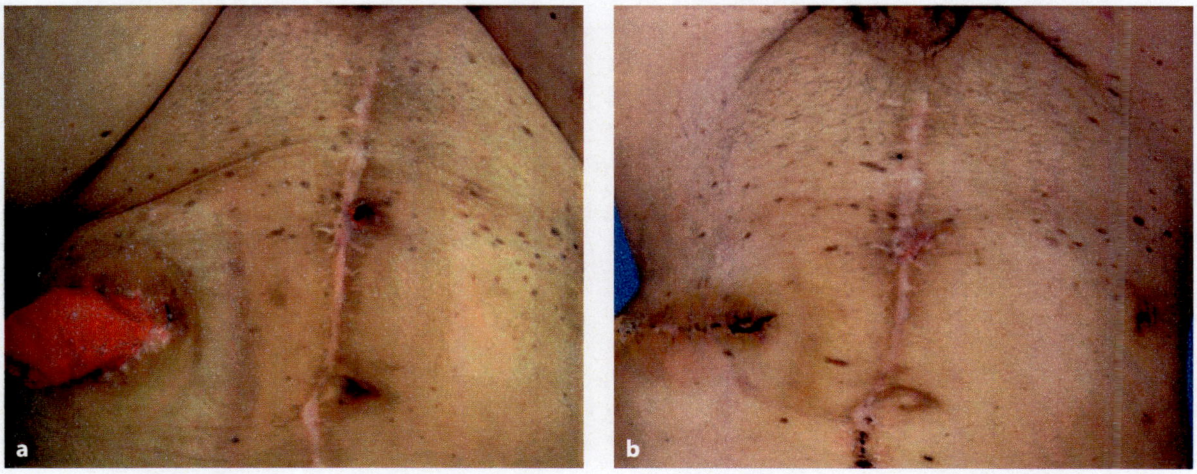

An extraperitoneal suprapubic tube is placed under laparoscopic guidance and the closure of the bladder is completed. The bladder is filled with saline to ascertain that watertight closure has been achieved. In addition, a urethral catheter and a Blake drain are placed. A colostomy can be created if deemed necessary (Step 12a). There is no need for repositioning the patient. Careful haemostasis and drain location confirmation takes place before removing the trocars; fascial closure of the trocar sites follows. Step 12b presents the postoperative appearance of the patients after the removing all drains and the restoration of the colostomy has been performed according to the postoperative schedule.

Postoperative Management

- It is important to maintain the patency of the urethral catheter and suprapubic tube by preventing clot obstruction and retention
- The catheters are irrigated only if there is suspicion of obstruction
- Prophylactic antibiotics are administered
- The urethral catheter and Blake drain are removed on the 3rd postoperative day
- The suprapubic tube is removed at 2 months after obtaining normal cystography
- At 4 months, bowel continuity is restored with laparoscopic assistance

References

1. Benoit RM, Naslund MJ, Cohen JK (2000) Complications after radical retropubic prostatectomy in the Medicare population. Urology 56:116–1120
2. Shin PR, Foley E, Steers WD (2000) Surgical management of rectourinary fistulae. J Am Coll Surg 191:547–553
3. Sotelo R, Garcia A, Yaime H, Rodríguez E, Dubois R, Andrade RD, Carmona O, Finelli A (2005) Laparoscopic rectovesical fistula repair. J Endourol 19:603–607
4. Sotelo R, Mirandolino M, Trujillo G, Garcia A, de Andrade R, Carmona O, Sánchez L, Rodriquez E, Finelli A (2007) Laparoscopic repair of rectourethral fistulas after prostate surgery. Urology 70: 515–518
5. Sotelo R, de Andrade R, Carmona O, Astigueta J, Velasquez A, Trujillo G, Canes D (2008) Robotic repair of rectovesical fistula resulting from open radical prostatectomy. Urology 72:1344–1346

5.3.2 Vesicovaginal Fistula Repair

René Sotelo Noguera, Roberto Garza Cortés

Introduction

Vesicovaginal fistulae (VVF) may be treated by different surgical techniques, either transvaginal or transabdominal (extra- or transvesical). The selection of the approach is based on the surgeon's preference. However, there is still controversy over the ideal approach and time of repair [1, 2]. In general, a vaginal approach is associated with lower morbidity, diminished blood loss and post-operative bladder irritability in comparison to the transabdominal approach. Furthermore, this technique may be performed in the outpatient setting. The results are often equal to those achieved with an abdominal approach [3]. The abdominal approach is indicated in case of another intra-abdominal condition requiring simultaneous surgical management. The abdominal method is also used when the fistula is lying high and/or on the vaginal vaults. Laparoscopy can be an alternative to the abdominal approach for managing VVF. Nezhat et al. initially reported laparoscopic VVF repair in 1994 [4]. Sotelo et al. reported the largest laparoscopic series. The latter group used a trans-vesical approach that led expeditiously to the fistulous tract without the need for additional vaginal incisions or further dissection of the vesicovaginal space [5]. Moreover, the laparoscopic approach enables a limited cystotomy, which is associated with less morbidity in comparison to the historical O'Connor procedure. During the latter procedure, the bladder is bivalved to the level of the fistula. In general, the advantages of laparoscopy include magnification of the operative field, efficient haemostasis, decreased hospital stay and shorter convalescence.

Indications

- Inadequate exposure related to a high or retracted fistula in a narrow vagina
- Close proximity of the fistulous tract to the ureter
- Associated pelvic pathology that requires surgery
- Multiple fistulae
- Morbid obesity
- Failure in a previous open surgical approach

Contra-indications

- Generalised peritonitis
- Uncorrected or uncorrectable coagulopathy
- Severe co-morbidities contra-indicating any surgical management

Preoperative Preparation

- It is necessary to clearly explain to the patient the type of procedure that will be performed. It is important to address the novelty of the technique and its recent development as a therapeutic option. Risks and complications should be discussed, as well as the possibility of open surgery, owing to anatomical variations or unforeseen complications that might require the open approach
- Most patients are surgically managed after 2 months of unsuccessful conservative management. In case of conservative management failure, a urethral catheter is avoided (if possible) until the day of surgery

Specific Patient Preparation

- Soft diet, at home
- The evening before the procedure, antegrade bowel preparation
- Fasting from 10:00 p.m. on the day before surgery
- Patient is admitted on the day of the procedure
- Preoperative administration of an intravenous broad-spectrum antibiotic (quinolone or cephalosporin)

Step 1: Cystoscopy and catheterisation of the ureters and fistula, port placement

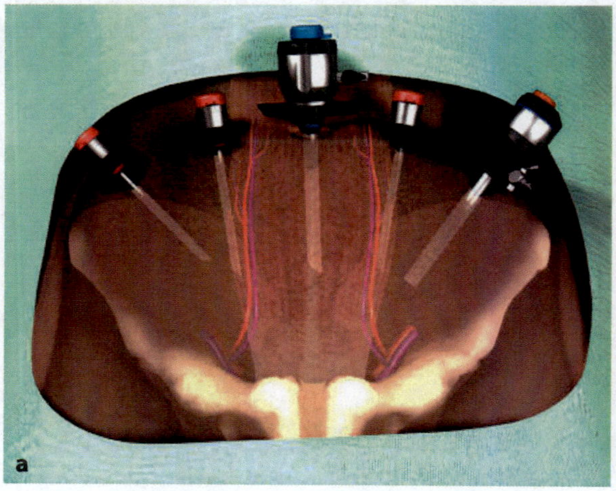
a

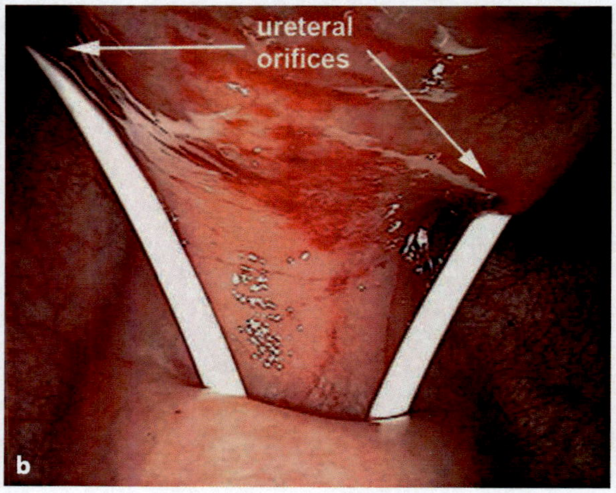

b

The patient is placed in dorsal lithotomy position. Cystoscopy is performed and both ureters are cannulated with 5-F ureteric catheters. The latter manoeuvre facilitates the identification of ureteral orifices and the course of the ureters. A ureteral catheter of a different colour is inserted through the bladder, advanced along the fistulous tract into the vagina and retrieved at the introitus. For large fistulae, a Foley catheter instead of a ureteral catheter can be used through the bladder. Port placement follows. A standard five-port transperitoneal approach, similar to that employed in laparoscopic prostatectomy, is used.

Step 2: Creation of omental flap, cystotomy

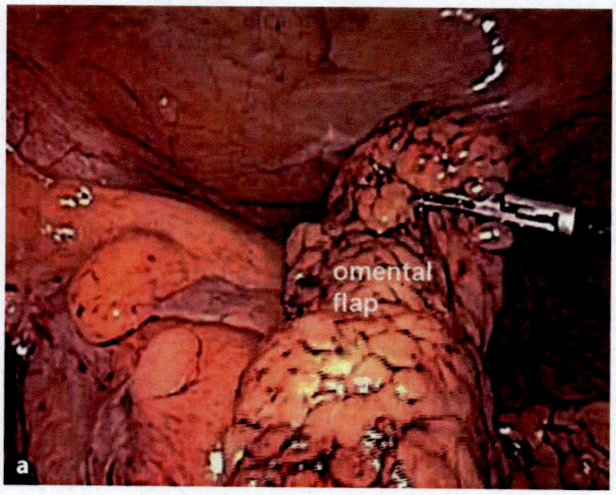

a

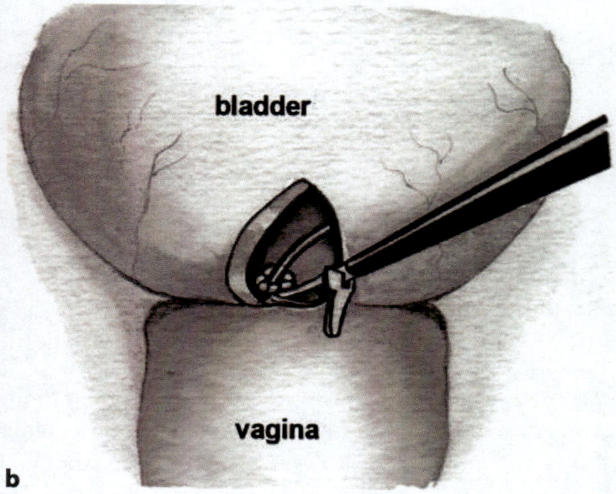

b

A sponge retractor is inserted into the vagina via the introitus to retract the vagina posteriorly. Once in the abdominal cavity, the first step is to dissect any adhesions. A omental flap is created from the site of the right gastroepiploic artery (Step 2a). The first step to repair the fistula is the dissection of the posterior bladder wall. A vertical bladder incision will be performed, creating a small cystotomy that dissects vertically towards the fistula. Step 2b is a schematic of the cystotomy. It is important to remember that the latter transvesical approach leads to the fistulous tract expeditiously.

Step 3: Identification of the bladder and initiation of cystotomy

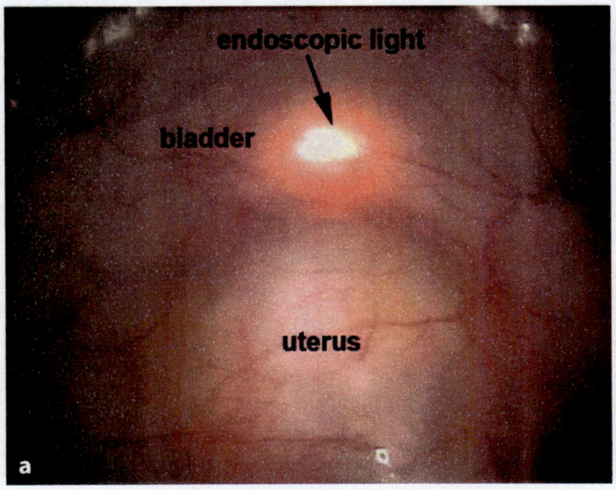

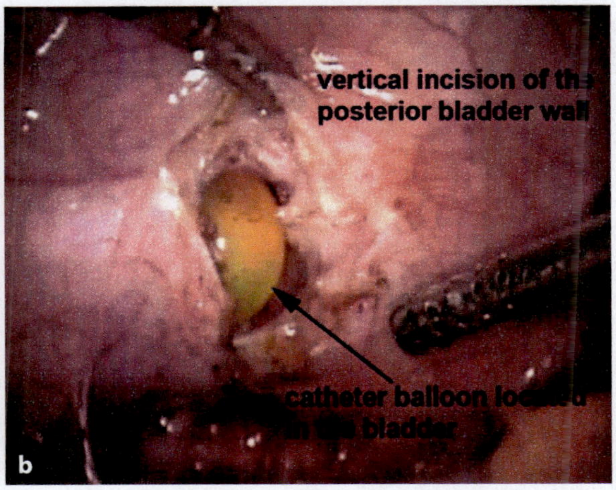

The identification of the site between the bladder and the vagina is facilitated by the insertion of a cystoscope, which is used to provide endoscopic light guidance to the bladder. Step 3a shows the endoscopic light designating the bladder and the bulging of the uterus to the peritoneal cavity, which could be used as landmarks for the identification of the site where the cystotomy should take place. An incision to the overlying peritoneum is made and the bladder is then opened by a vertical incision. The previously inserted urethral catheter is visible (Step 3b).

Step 4: Cystotomy

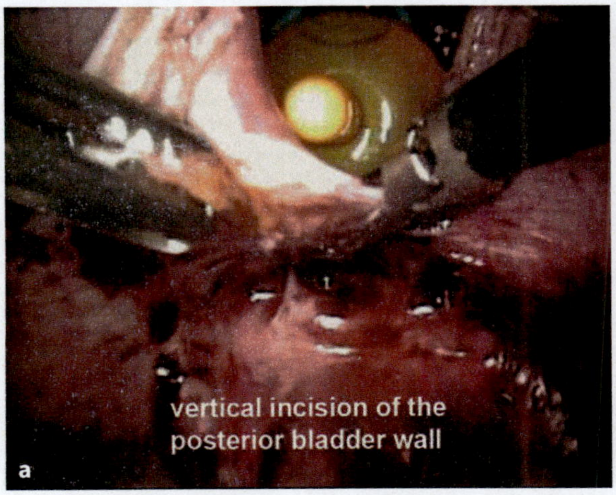

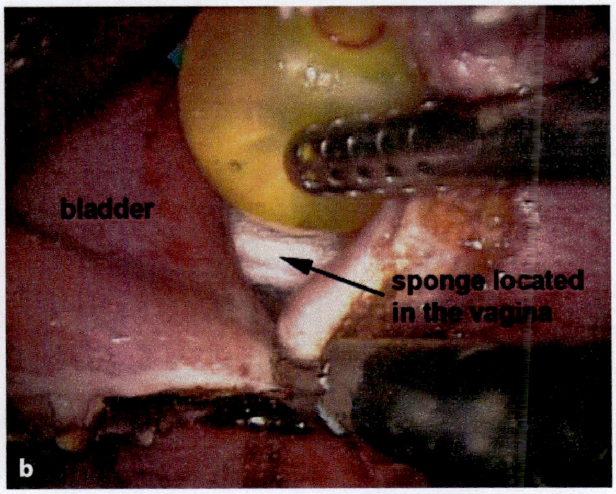

The incision directed vertically to the posterior bladder wall is extended (Step 4a). The incision is directed towards the bladder neck. The posterior aspect of the urethral catheter balloon and the sponge retractor inserted in the vagina are exposed and the fistulous tract is resected with direction to the vagina (Step 4b). For the performance of cystotomy, ultrasonic shears in combination with laparoscopic graspers are adequate. Nevertheless, the use of J-hook electrocautery or laparoscopic scissors is an alternative.

Step 5: Exposure of the vesicovaginal communication

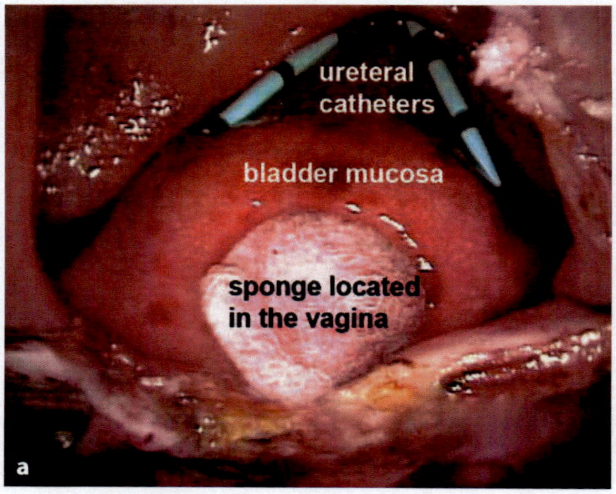

a

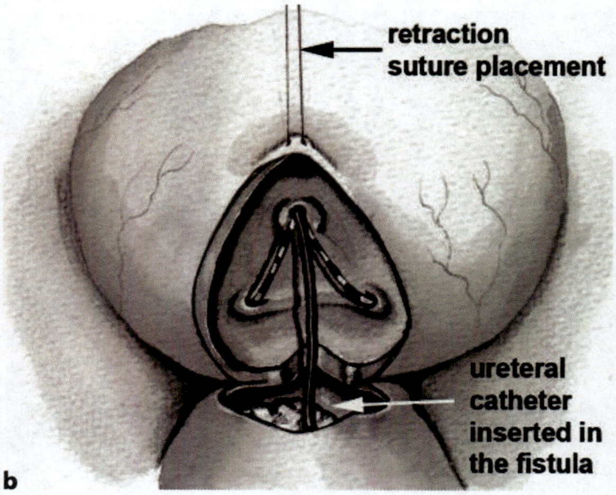

b

The resection of the fistulous tract is facilitated when the edges of the bladder incision are retracted laterally to expose the communication of the bladder to the vagina (Step 5a). A suture is placed at each side of the incision. Placement of these sutures can be performed using a Keith needle or a Carter-Thomason port-closure needle device. The two ends of the stitch are retracted and anchored outside of the anterior abdominal wall, resulting in adequate exposure of the fistulous tract. Alternatively, a single stay suture on the superior edge of the cystotomy could be used to retraction. A schematic of the latter method is presented in Step 5b.

Step 6: Excision of the fistulous tract

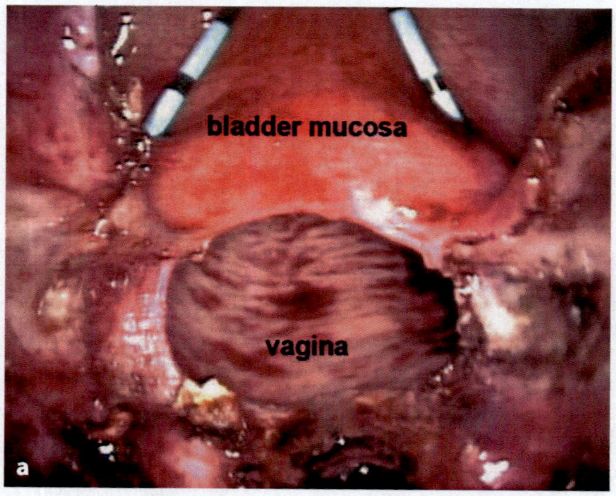

a

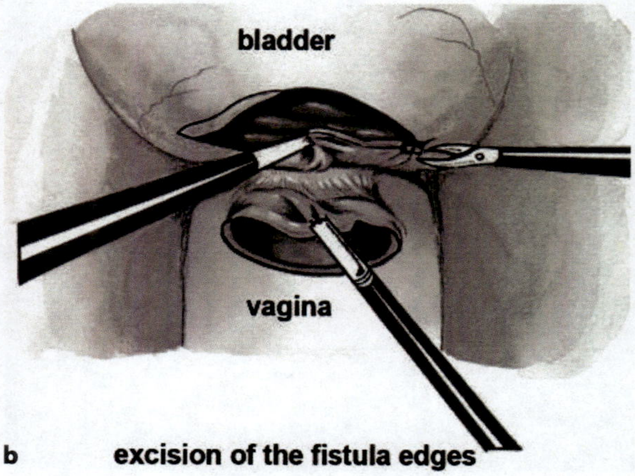

b excision of the fistula edges

When communication between the vagina and bladder is visualised, the sponge retractor is withdrawn (Step 6a) and a Foley catheter is placed in the vagina. The balloon is inflated with 70 cc of saline to prevent loss of pneumoperitoneum. Dissection is continued until the fistula is completely separated from the vagina. Step 6b shows the excision of the fibrous tissue edges of the fistula with laparoscopic scissors. All fibrotic and necrotic tissue should be excised. It is important to avoid injuring the ureteral orifices or the urethra during the wide excision of the fistulous tract.

Step 7: Closure of the vagina and bladder

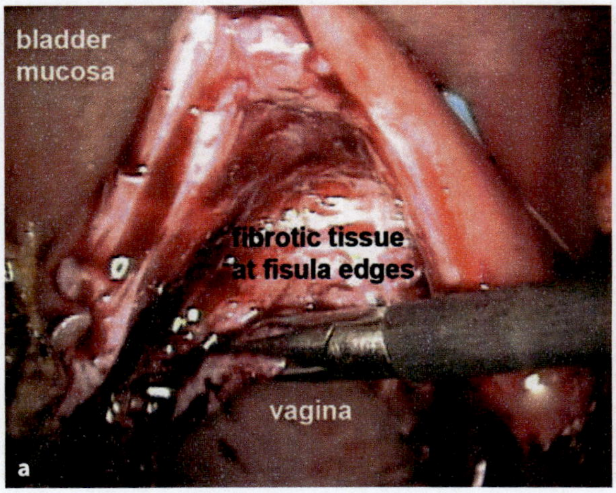

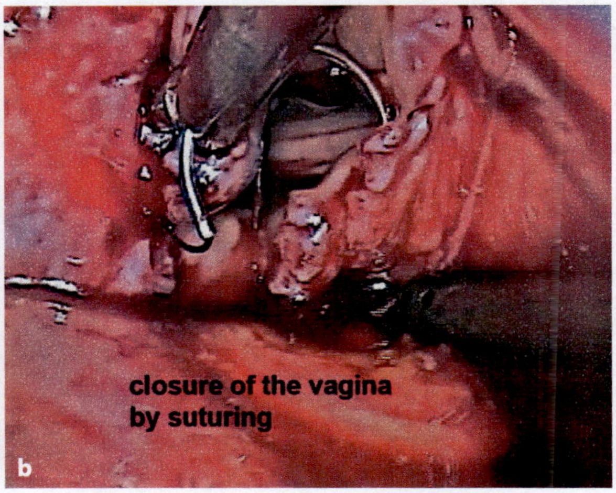

The creation of tissue flaps that are adequate for the tension-free closure of the vagina and the bladder requires further dissection of the tissue surrounding the fistulous tract. A combination of laparoscopic scissors and grasper are used for the task. Step 7a shows the site of a vesicovaginal fistula after the excision of the tract.

Excessive tissue at the vaginal wall could be used for the closure of the lesion. The latter is closed horizontally with a running 2/0 Monocryl suture on a CT-1 needle (Step 7b). The closure of the bladder defect and the cystotomy never presents a challenge.

Step 8: Tissue interposition

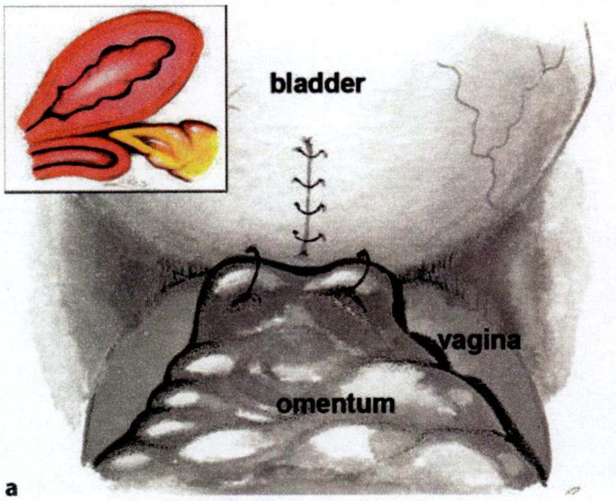

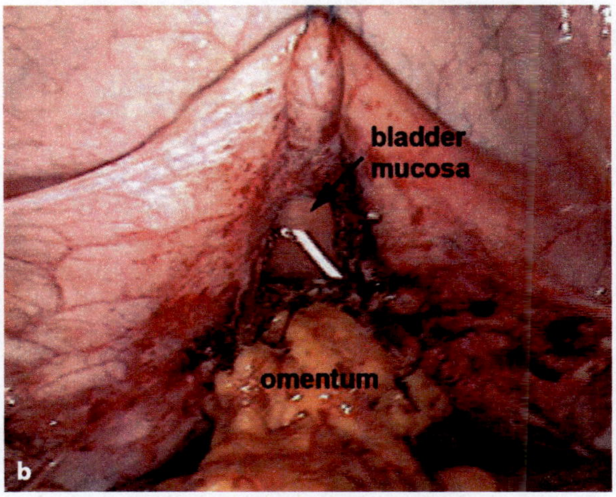

Step 8a is a schematic presenting the concept of bladder and vagina reconstruction as well as tissue interposition. Two sutures are placed in the anterior wall of the vagina, distal to the closure line. These sutures are used to anchor the tissue that has been previously prepared for interposition. Step 8b shows the omental flap anchored over the anterior wall of the vagina. The repaired vaginal lesion is fully covered by the omental flap. Recurrence of the fistula is prevented by the interposition of omental tissue. Alternatively, a peritoneal flap obtained superior and lateral to the bladder dome can be used.

Step 9: Closure of the bladder

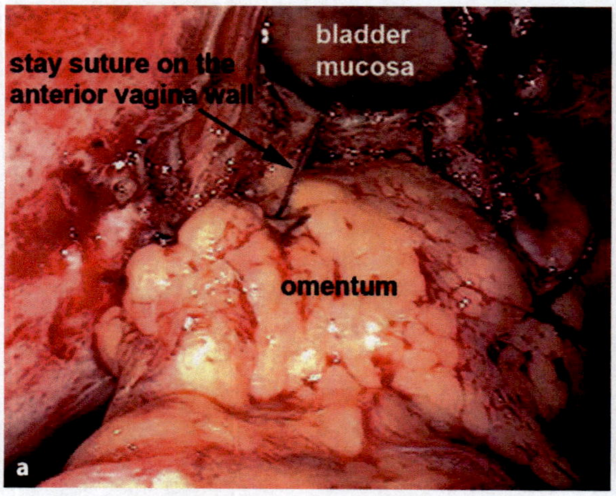

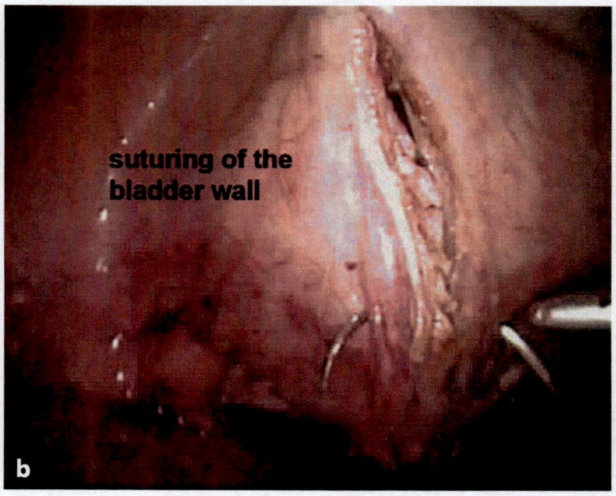

Step 9a shows the omental flap interposition to be completed. The vaginal defect is closed and covered by the flap and the bladder remains open. The posterior bladder wall is closed vertically with a running 2/0 Monocryl on a CT-1 needle suture. The suturing begins at the distal apex and continues proximally (Step 9b). Cystoscopic guidance can be used to facilitate the closure.

An additional running closure of the bladder serosa is performed with an absorbable suture. The ureteral catheters are removed. A 20-F urethral catheter is then inserted to maintain bladder drainage. The bladder is then filled with saline to confirm a watertight closure. A suprapubic cystostomy tube is not used. A drain is placed in the pelvis.

Postoperative Management

- Immediate care
- Two or three more doses of selected intravenous antibiotic
- Prevention of urethral catheter obstruction
- Irrigation of the bladder only if necessary
- Outpatient care
- Drain removal at 2 or 3 days
- Oral antibiotic of choice for 10 days
- Removal of urethral catheter at 10 days, after completion of cystography
- Sexual abstinence for 2 months
- Patients are advised not to use tampons

References

1. Raz S, Bregg K, Nitti V, Sussman E (1993) Transvaginal repair of vesicovaginal fistula using a peritoneal flap. J Urol 150:56–59
2. Blaivas JG, Heritz DM, Romanzi LJ (1995) Early versus late repair of vesicovaginal fistulas: vaginal and abdominal approaches. J Urol 153:1110–1112
3. Raz S (1995) Editorial comment on: Early versus late repair of vesicovaginal fistulas: vaginal and abdominal approaches. J Urol 153:1112–1113
4. Nezhat CH, Nezhat F, Nezhat C, Rottenberg H (1994) Laparoscopic repair of a vesicovaginal fistula: a case report, part 2. Obstet Gynecol 83:899–901
5. Sotelo R, Mariano MB, Garcia-Segui A, Dubois R, Spaliviero M, Keklikian W, Novoa J, Yaime H, Finelli A (2005) Laparoscopic repair of vesicovaginal fistula. J Urol 173:1615–1618